8th
EDITION

DORLAND'S DICTIONARY OF MEDICAL ACRONYMS & ABBREVIATIONS

ELSEVIER

Elsevier
1600 John F. Kennedy Blvd.
Ste 1600
Philadelphia, PA 19103-2899

Dorland's Dictionary Of Medical Acronyms & Abbreviations,   ISBN: 978-0-323-93260-8
Eighth Edition

Previous editions copyrighted 2016 by Elsevier, Inc., and 2009, 2005, 2001, 1997, 1992, 1987 by Saunders, an imprint of Elsevier, Inc.

Editor and Lexicographer: Sean Webb
Content Development Specialist: Rebecca Gruliow
Publishing Services Manager: Catherine Jackson
Senior Project Manager/Specialist: Carrie Stetz
Design Direction: Maggie Reid

Printed in the United States of America

Last digit is the print number: 9   8   7   6   5   4   3   2   1

Working together
to grow libraries in
developing countries

www.elsevier.com • www.bookaid.org

PREFACE

This eighth edition of *Dorland's Dictionary of Medical Acronyms & Abbreviations* is the third edition to be published since the original author, Stanley Jablonski, passed away. The book has been well received over the years, and the author's enthusiasm and love of medical vocabulary, even vexingly obscure abbreviations, are evident in its pages. The responsibility of maintaining this volume now resides with the developer of the *Dorland's* dictionaries, who is aware of the tradition of excellence associated with this dictionary.

The content remains the familiar, convenient resource that has served users for more than three decades. The print book retains its format of boldface abbreviations followed by run-in meanings, which enables it to include as many entries as larger, more cumbersome books while remaining a manageable size. As a bonus, you can obtain an eBook of this title by following the instructions on the inside front cover.

The abbreviations and acronyms are presented alphabetically. Several hundred new additions and changes have been made, including the addition of COVID-19-related entries presented in their own section as well as interspersed throughout the book. This edition retains the Abbreviations to Avoid because they may be misconstrued; explanations of the potential sources of confusion are included. The lists of commonly used symbols have been retained and updated. Listings for organizations have been updated—new ones added, name changes incorporated where appropriate, and outdated names removed.

The current editor of *Dorland's Dictionary of Medical Acronyms & Abbreviations* would like to express his appreciation for the work that has been handed down from the previous author and editors, and looks forward to maintaining the book's high standards. Because new acronyms and abbreviations are constantly being coined, this volume can never really be complete. If you do not find an acronym or abbreviation or a definition that you are searching for, we invite you to submit your suggestions for the next edition. You can do this at DorlandsOnline.com by clicking on "Suggest a Term." Just tell us that it is for *Dorland's Dictionary of Medical Acronyms & Abbreviations.* You can be sure your contributions will be much appreciated.

SEAN WEBB, MFA
Editor and Lexicographer

Acknowledgements

The publisher thanks Stanley Jablonski for his dedication in developing this book and updating the early editions. We also thank the previous lexicographers, Douglas Anderson and Michelle Elliott, whose contributions to recent editions extended the high standards that Mr. Jablonski set. We are indebted to them for the rich trove of content that provided the basis for this new edition.

CONTENTS

Symbols

The Greek Alphabet

Capital	Lower Case	Letter Name	Transcription
A	α	alpha	a
B	β	beta	b
Γ	γ	gamma	g
Δ	δ	delta	d
E	ε	epsilon	e
Z	ζ	zeta	z
H	η	eta	ē
Θ	θ	theta	th
I	ι	iota	i
K	κ	kappa	k
Λ	λ	lambda	l
M	μ	mu	m
N	ν	nu	n
Ξ	ξ	xi	x
O	ο	omicron	o
Π	π	pi	p
P	ρ	rho	r
Σ	σ,ς	sigma	s
T	τ	tau	t
Y	υ	upsilon	y (sometimes u)
Φ	φ	phi	ph
X	χ	chi	ch (sometimes kh)
Ψ	ψ	psi	ps
Ω	ω	omega	ō

Symbols Commonly Used in Pedigrees

□	male	(□)(○)	adopted
○	female		half sibling
◇	sex unspecified		
□—○	mating or marriage	○ ◇	stillbirth or abortion
□—○	consanguinity	□—○	no offspring
□⌐○	illegitimate offspring	■ ●	affected offspring
□—⫸○	divorce	■ ●	proband, propositus, or index case
□—○—□	multiple marriage	◧ ◑	heterozygotes for autosomal recessive
dizygotic twins		⊙	carrier of sex-linked recessive
monozygotic twins		⊘ ∅	death
4 ③	number of children of sex indicated		

Symbols Commonly Used in Physical Therapy Documentation

Ⓑ	bilateral	Ⓛ	left
Ⓒ	cue	Ⓡ	right
Ⓓ	dependent	Ⓢ	supervision
HH Ⓐ	hand held assist	std Ⓦ	standard walker
Ⓘ	independent	wh Ⓦ	wheeled walker

Mathematics and Statistics

α	probability of Type I error	e	base of natural logarithms
β	probability of Type II error	F	F statistic
$1-\beta$	power (of a statistical test)	f	frequency, function
χ^2	chi-square	H_0	null hypothesis
Cov_{AB}	covariance of A and B	H_1	alternative hypothesis
CV	coefficient of variation	H_a	alternative hypothesis
D	nonparametric statistic	ln	natural logarithm
d	parametric statistic	m	median
E	expectancy	μ	population mean

N	population size	$\times$	multiplied by, times
n	sample size	$\div$, /	divided by
ν	degrees of freedom	$=$	equals
P	probability	$\sim$	approximately
p	probability that event will occur	$\cong$	congruent to, approximately equal to
$P(A)$	probability that event A will occur	$\approx$	approximately equal to
$P(A\backslash B)$	probability that, given event A, event B will occur (conditional probability)	$\neq$	not equal to
		$>$	greater than *(on The Joint Commission "Do Not Use" List)*
q	probability that an alternative event will occur (equal to $1/p$)	$\geq$	greater than or equal to
r	sample correlation coefficient	$\ngtr$	not greater than
R	rate	$<$	less than *(on The Joint Commission "Do Not Use" List)*
ρ	population correlation coefficient		
r_s	Spearman's rank correlation coefficient	$\leq$	less than or equal to
		$\nless$	not less than
Σ	summation	$\equiv$	identical to
s	sample standard deviation	$\sqrt{}$	square root
s^2	sample variance	$\sqrt[3]{}$	cube root
σ	population standard deviation	$!$	factorial
σ^2	population variance	$\%$	percent
SD	standard deviation	∞	infinity
SE	standard error	$\binom{n}{k}$, $_nC_K$	binomial coefficient
t	(Student's) t-test variable	$*$	estimate (biased), used over a symbol
x	abscissa		
T	sample mean	$\wedge$	estimate (unbiased), used over symbol
$|x|$	absolute value of x	$\subset$	is a subset of
y	ordinate	$\supset$	contains as a subset
$+$	plus	$\cap$	("cap") intersection
$-$	minus	$\cup$	("cup") union
$\pm$	plus or minus		

Miscellaneous Symbols

Symbol	Meaning	Symbol	Meaning
Ⓐ	axilla (temperature)	+++	increased
ⓐx	axilla (temperature)		moderately active
Ⓗ	hypodermic		moderately severe
ⓗ	hypodermic	++++	large amount
Ⓜ	intramuscular		pronounced reaction
Ⓥ	intravenous		severe
Ⓛ	left	++/+	2 plus on the right, 1 plus on the left
Ⓜ	murmur	0/0	zero on either side
ⓜ	mouth	(+)	significant
	by mouth	−	absent
	murmur		alkaline
Ⓞ	by mouth		decreased
	oral		diminished
%DV	percent daily value		minus
Ⓡ	rectal		negative
	rectum	(−)	insignificant
	right	±	plus or minus
0	absent		positive or negative
	no response	(±)	possibly significant
+	acid	1×	once
	and	×2	twice
	increased	2×	twice
	plus	/	divided by
	positive		of
	present		per
	slight trace	°	degree
++	moderate		hour
	normally active	1°	first degree
	noticeable reaction		one hour
	trace		primary

2°	secondary	ΔA	change in absorbance
	second degree	ΔpH	change in pH
	two hours	Δt	time interval
3°	tertiary	↗	deviated
	third degree		displaced
	three hours		increase
24°	24 hours		increasing
̈∥	two	↑	elevated
′	foot		gas
	minute		increased
	univalent		increasing
″	inch	↑↑	extensor response, Babinski sign
	second		testes undescended
	bivalent		
:	is to	△	up
	ratio	↙	decrease
::	as (in ratios)		decreasing
∴	therefore	↓	decreased
#	fracture		decreasing
	gauge		deficiency
	has been done		deficit
	has been given		depressed
	number		diminished
	pounds		precipitate
@	at *(on the Joint Commission "Do Not Use" List)*	↓↓	bilaterally descended
			both down
∞	indefinitely more		plantar response, Babinski sign
	infinite		testes descended
	infinity	▽̣	down
Δ	change	↑V	increase due to in vivo effect
	difference	↓V	decrease due to in vivo effect
	Gibbs free energy	↑C	increase due to chemical interference during the assay
	prism diopter		

↓C	decrease due to chemical interference during the assay	√c̄	check with
		φ	none
→	causes	∨	systolic blood pressure
	distal	∧	diastolic blood pressure
	no change	∟	right lower quadrant right angle
	reaction proceeds to the right	⌐	right upper quadrant
	results in	⌐	left upper quadrant
	transfer to	⌐	left lower quadrant
	yields	∠	angle
←	caused by	∠E	angle of entry
	derived from	∠X	angle of exit
	is due to	∘∘	male
	reaction proceeds to the left	♂	male
⇌	reversible reaction	♀	female
?	doubtful	*	birth
	equivocal		not verified
	flicker		presumed
	possible	†	dead
	questionable		death
	unknown		died
‖	parallel	℞	recipe, take
	parallel bars	℥	ounce
⊖	normal	f℥	fluid ounce
c̄	with	℈	scruple
s̄	without	♏	minim
✔	check	ℨ	drachm, dram
	observe for	f℥	fluidrachm, fluidram
✔'d	checked		

ABBREVIATIONS TO AVOID

The following information has been adapted from The Joint Commission (2020) and the Institute for Safe Medication Practices (ISMP).*

The Joint Commission prohibits the use of these abbreviations in orders, handwritten documentation, or on preprinted forms. This applies to all orders and all medication-related documentation that is handwritten (including free-text computer entry) or on preprinted forms.

The Joint Commission list is part of the Information Management standards; it does not currently apply to preprogrammed health information technology systems such as electronic medical records or computerized provider order entries. When such systems are implemented or updated, effort should be made to eliminate the use of dangerous abbreviations, acronyms, symbols, and dose designations from the software.

U, u (unit)	"U" can be mistaken for a "0" (zero), the number "4" (four), or "cc" (cubic centimeters); write out "unit"
IU (International Unit)	"IU" can be mistaken for "IV" (intravenous) or the number "10" (ten); write out "International Unit"
Q.D., QD, q.d., qd (daily); Q.O.D., QOD, q.o.d., qod (every other day)	They can be mistaken for each other or other abbreviations; write out "daily" and "every other day"
Zeros after decimals and lack of zeros before decimals	The decimals might not be seen and therefore "1.0" can be mistaken for "10" or ".2" (0.2) can be mistaken for "2" (a trailing zero may be used when a value being reported needs to be precise)
Medication abbreviations "MS," "MSO₄," and "MgSO₄"	Abbreviations for "morphine sulfate" and "magnesium sulfate" can be confused for one another; write out "morphine sulfate" and "magnesium sulfate"

*Copyright ISMP 2021. Permission is granted to reproduce material with proper attribution for internal use within healthcare organizations. Other reproduction is prohibited without written permission from ISMP.

The Joint Commission suggests that these abbreviations, acronyms, and symbols not be used.

Less than (<) and greater than (>) symbols	Can be confused for the number "7" or letter "L"; spell out terms
Abbreviation of drug names	Many abbreviations cause confusion between drugs, particularly when the same abbreviation is used for multiple drugs
Apothecary units	Not all health care providers use these units and they can be confused with metric units; use metric units instead
@ ("at" symbol)	@ can be confused with the number 2; write out "at"
CC, cc	Can be confused with the abbreviation for "units"; use "ml" or "milliliters" instead
μg (micrograms)	"μg" can be misread as "mg" (milligrams); use "mcg" or write out "micrograms"

the ISMP suggests that these abbreviations not be used.

AD, AS, AU (right ear, left ear, both ears) OD, OS, OU (right eye, left eye, both eyes)	Abbreviations for eyes and ears can be mistaken for each other; write out the appropriate term
BT (bedtime)	Can be mistaken as BID (twice daily); write out "bedtime"
D/C (discharge or discontinue)	The intended meaning can be misconstrued causing unintended discontinuation of medication or unapproved discharge; write out "discharge" and "discontinue"
IJ (injection)	Can be mistaken for "IV" or intrajugular; write out "injection"
IN (intranasal)	Can be mistaken for "IM" or "IV"; write out "intranasal" or use the abbreviation "NAS"
HS (half strength) hs (at bedtime, hours of sleep)	They can be mistaken for each other; write out "half-strength" and "bedtime"
o.d. or OD (once daily)	Can be mistaken as "right eye" (OD, oculus dexter); write out "once daily"
OJ (orange juice)	Can be mistaken as OD or OS (right or left eye); write out "orange juice"
per os (by mouth, orally)	"os" can be mistaken as "left eye" (OS, oculus sinister); write out "by mouth" or "orally," or use "PO"
qhs (at bedtime)	Can be mistaken as "qhr" or every hour; write out "at bedtime"
qn (nightly)	Can be mistaken as "qh" (every hour); write out "nightly"
q1d (daily)	Can be mistaken as "q.i.d." (4 times daily); write out "daily"
SC, SQ, subq (subcutaneous)	SC be mistaken as SL (sublingual); SQ can be mistaken as "5 every"; the "q" in "sub q" can be mistaken as "every"; write out "subcut" or "subcutaneous"

ss (sliding scale [insulin] or $^1/_2$ [apothecary])	Can be mistaken as "55"; write out "sliding scale," or use "one-half" or "$^1/_2$"
SSRI (sliding scale regular insulin)	Can be mistaken as "selective-serotonin reuptake inhibitor"; write out "sliding scale (insulin)"
SSI (sliding scale insulin)	Can be mistaken as "strong solution of iodine" (Lugol's); write out "strong solution of iodine"
i/d (one daily)	Can be mistaken as "tid"; write out "1 daily"
TIW or tiw (3 times a week)	Can be mistaken as "3 times a day" or "twice in a week"; write out "3 times weekly"

COVID-19 Acronyms and Abbreviations

The acronyms and abbreviations presented here are commonly used in information pertaining to COVID-19. They are not intended to reflect or support any opinions or guidance regarding the care of patients who have contracted COVID-19.

2019-nCoV	2019 novel coronavirus (initial name for SARS-CoV-2)
AGP	aerosol-generating procedure
ACE2	angiotensin-converting enzyme 2
AIIR	airborne infection isolation room (formerly known as negative pressure isolation room)
APF	assigned protection factor
APR	air-purifying respiratory (particulate respirators, gas masks)
ARD	acute respiratory disease
ARDS	acute respiratory disease syndrome
ARI	acute respiratory infection
ASR	air-supplying respirator
B.1.1.529	Omicron variant of SARS-CoV-2 (includes BA.1, BA.1.1, BA.2, BA.3, BA.4, and BA.5 lineages)
B.1.1.7	Alpha variant of SARS-CoV-2 (also called United Kingdom variant)
B.1.351	Beta variant of SARS-CoV-2 (also called South Africa variant)
B.1.427/B.1.429	Epsilon variant of SARS-CoV-2
B.1.525	Eta variant of SARS-CoV-2
B.1.526	Iota variant of SARS-CoV-2
B.1.617.1	Kappa variant of SARS-CoV-2
B.1.617.2	Delta variant of SARS-CoV-2 (also called India variant)
B.1.621, B.1.621.1	Mu variant of SARS-CoV-2 (also called Colombia variant)
C.37	Lambda variant of SARS-CoV-2 (also called Peru variant)
3 C's	closed spaces, crowded places, close-contact settings
CAPR	controlled air purifying respirator
CDC	Centers for Disease Control and Prevention

COVID-19	coronavirus disease 2019 (caused by SARS-CoV-2)
CQ	chloroquine (phosphate)
CSG	*Coronaviridae* (or Coronavirus) Study Group
CT	community transmission
CTAP	Coronavirus Treatment Acceleration Program
ECMO	extracorporeal membrane oxygenation
EHFR	elastomeric half-facepiece respirator
Epi	epidemic (as in Epi-curve)
EUA	emergency use authorization
FFR	filtering facepiece respirator (includes N95 masks)
GCQ	general community quarantine
GISAID	Global Initiative on Sharing all Influenza Data
HCP	health care personnel
HCQ	hydroxychloroquine
HEPA	high-efficiency particulate air (filter respirator)
IPC	infection prevention and control (measures)
MAB, Mab, mAb	monoclonal antibody
MERS-CoV	Middle East respiratory syndrome coronavirus (emerged in 2012)
MEURI	Monitored Emergency Use of Unregistered Interventions Framework
MIS-C	multisystem inflammatory syndrome in children (associated with COVID-19)
N95	NIOSH-certified mask that filters at least 95% of airborne particles
NIOSH	National Institute for Occupational Safety and Health
NIV	noninvasive ventilation
P.1	Gamma variant of SARS-CoV-2 (also called Brazil variant)
P.2	Zeta variant of SARS-CoV-2
PAPR	powered air-purifying respirator
PCR	polymerase chain reaction (test)
PEM	postexertion malaise
PHSM	public health and social measures
PPE	personal protective equipment
PUI	patient under investigation
SARS-CoV	severe acute respiratory syndrome coronavirus (emerged in 2002)

SARS-CoV-2	severe acute respiratory syndrome coronavirus-2; the virus that causes COVID-19 (initially named 2019 novel coronavirus or 2019-nCoV)
SOFA	sequential (sepsis-related) organ failure assessment (scale)
VOC	variant of concern
VOI	variant of interest
VTM	viral transport media
WHO	World Health Organization

A

A abnormal; abortion; absolute temperature; absorbance; acceptor; accommodation; acetone; acetum; achondroplasia; acid; acidophil, acidophilic; acromion; actin; *Actinomyces*; activity; adenine; adenoma; adenosine; admittance; adrenalin; Adriamycin; adult; age; akinetic; alanine; albino; albumin; allergologist, allergy; alveolar gas; ambulation; ampere; amphetamine; ampicillin; amplitude; anaphylaxis; androsterone; anesthetic; angstrom, Ångström unit; anode; *Anopheles*; antagonism; anterior; antibody; antrectomy; apical; aqueous; area; argon; artery; assist; atomic weight; atrium; atropine; auricle; auscultation; axial; axilla, axillary; before [L. *ante*]; blood group A; ear [L. *auris*]; mass number; subspinale; total acidity; tumor limited to the bowel [Dukes classification]; tumor limited to the mucosa; uppercase Greek letter alpha; water [L. *aqua*]; year [L. *annum*]

Å Ångström unit

Ā antinuclear antibody; cumulated activity

A1 aortic first sound; prostatic tumor less than 5%

A₁ aortic first sound

A-1, 2, 3, 4, 5 anterior cerebral artery segments 1, 2, 3, 4, 5

AI, AII, AIII angiotensin I, II, III

A2 prostatic tumor more than 5%

A₂ aortic second sound

a absorptivity; acceleration; accommodation; acidity; activated; ampere; anode; anterior; area; arterial; arterial blood; artery; atto-; autopsy; before [L. *ante*]; thermodynamic activity; total acidity; water [L. *aqua*]

α lowercase Greek letter *alpha*; angular acceleration; first [chemical compounds]; optical rotation; probability of type I error; solubility coefficient

a- atto- [10^{-18}]

a sample y intercept of straight line

ā before [L. *ante*]

2AA 2-aminoanthracene

AA abampere; abdominal aorta; acetabular anteversion; acetic acid; achievement age; active alcoholic; active assistive [range of motion]; active avoidance; acupuncture analgesia; acute appendicitis; adenine arabinoside; adenylic acid; adjuvant arthritis; adrenal androgen; adrenocortical autoantibody; African American; aggregated albumin;

aggregative adherence; agranulocytic angina; alcohol abuse; Alcoholics Anonymous; allergic alveolitis; alopecia areata; alveolo-arterial; aminoacetone; amino acid; aminoacyl; amyloid A; anaplastic astrocytoma; antiarrhythmic agent; anticipatory avoidance; antigen aerosol; aortic amplitude; aortic aneurysm; aortic arch; aplastic anemia; arachidonic acid; ascending aorta; atlantoaxial; atomic absorption; Australia antigen; autoanalyzer; automobile accident; axonal arborization

A&A aid and attendance; awake and aware

A–a alveolar-arterial; alveolar-atrial

aA abampere

aa amino acid; arteries

AAA abdominal aortic aneurysm/aneurysmectomy; acne-associated arthritis; acquired aplastic anemia; acute anxiety attack; alacrima, achalasia, addisonianism [syndrome]; American Ambulance Association; American Association for Anatomy; androgenic anabolic agent; aneurysm of ascending aorta; angiography of abdominal aorta; apply to affected area; area agency on aging; aromatic amino acid; arrest after arrival

AAAA American Academy of Anesthesiologist Assistants

AAAAI American Academy of Allergy, Asthma & Immunology

AAAASF American Association for Accreditation of Ambulatory Surgical Facilities

AAACN American Academy of Ambulatory Care Nursing

AAAD aromatic amino acid decarboxylase

AA/AD alcohol abuse/alcohol dependence

AAAE amino acid activating enzyme

AAAHC Accreditation Association for Ambulatory Health Care

AAAHE American Association for the Advancement of Health Education

AAAI American Academy of Allergy and Immunology; Association for the Advancement of Artificial Intelligence

AAALAC Association for Assessment and Accreditation of Laboratory Animal Care [International]

AAAM Association for the Advancement of Automotive Medicine

AAANA American Academy of Ambulatory Nursing Administration

AAAP American Academy of Addiction Psychiatry

AAAS American Association for the Advancement of Science

AAASPS African-American Antiplatelet Stroke Prevention Study

AAAV avian adeno-associated virus

AAB American Association of Bioanalysts; aminoazobenzene

AABB American Association of Blood Banks; axis-aligned bounding boxes

AABCC alertness (consciousness), airway, breathing, circulation, cervical spine

AABH Association for Ambulatory Behavioral Healthcare

AABS automobile accident, broadside

AABV *Ascogaster argentifrons* bracovirus

AAC abnormal anterior coaptation; antibiotic-associated [pseudomembranous] colitis; antimicrobial agent−induced colitis; augmentative and alternative communication

AACA acylaminocephalosporanic acid; American Association of Clinical Anatomists

AACAP American Academy of Child and Adolescent Psychiatry

AACC American Association for Clinical Chemistry

AACD aging-associated cognitive decline; American Academy of Cosmetic Dentistry

AADA Abbreviated Antibiotic Drug Application

AACE acute acquired comitant esotropia; American Association of Clinical Endocrinologists

AACEM Association of Academic Chairs of Emergency Medicine

AACG acute angle closure glaucoma

AACH American Academy on Communication in Healthcare

AACHP American Association for Comprehensive Health Planning

AACIA American Association for Clinical Immunology and Allergy

AACN American Association of Colleges of Nursing; American Association of Critical-Care Nurses

AACOM American Association of Colleges of Osteopathic Medicine

AACP American Academy of Cerebral Palsy; American Association of Colleges of Pharmacy; American Association of Community Psychiatrists

AACPDM American Academy for Cerebral Palsy and Developmental Medicine

AACS American Academy of Cosmetic Surgery

AACSH adrenal androgen corticotropic stimulating hormone

AACT American Academy of Clinical Toxicology

AACVPR American Association of Cardiovascular and Pulmonary Rehabilitation

7-AAD 7-amino-actinomycin D

AAD acute agitated delirium; acute aortic dissection; alcohol abuse or dependence; alloxazine adenine dinucleotide; alpha$_1$-antitrypsin deficiency; American Academy of Dermatology; antiarrhythmic drug; antibiotic-associated diarrhea; aromatic acid decarboxylase; average absolute deviation

AADC amino acid decarboxylase; L-aromatic amino acid decarboxylase

AADE American Association of Dental Examiners

AADEJ American Association of Dental Editors & Journalists

AADGP American Academy of Dental Group Practice

AADH alopecia, anosmia, deafness, hypogonadism [syndrome]

AA-DHS African American Diabetes Heart Study

(A−a)D$_{N_2}$ alveolar-arterial nitrogen tension difference

AaDNV *Aedes aegypti* densovirus

aAD$_{O_2}$, (a−A)D$_{O_2}$ arterio-alveolar oxygen tension difference

AADP amyloid A-degrading protease

AADPA American Academy of Dental Practice Administration

AAE active assistive exercise; acute allergic encephalitis; American Association of Endodontists; annuloaortic ectasia

AAEE American Association of Electromyography and Electrodiagnosis

AAEM American Academy of Emergency Medicine; American Academy of Environmental Medicine; American Association of Electrodiagnostic Medicine

AAEV *Aedes aegypti* entomopoxvirus

AA ex active assistive exercise

2-AAF N-2-fluorenylacetamide

AAF acetylaminofluorine; aggregative adherence fimbriae; aortic arch flush; ascorbic acid factor

AAFP American Academy of Family Physicians; American Academy of Family Practice

AAFPRS American Academy of Facial Plastic and Reconstructive Surgery

AAFT amplitude-adjusted Fourier transform

17AAG 17-allylamino-17-demethoxygeldanamycin

AAG 3-alkaladenine deoxyribonucleic acid glycosylase; allergic angiitis and granulomatosis; alpha-1-acid glycoprotein; alveolar arterial gradient; autoantigen

AAGL American Academy of Gynecologic Laparoscopists

AAGP American Association for Geriatric Psychiatry

AAH Academy of Architecture for Health

AAHA American Academy of Hospital Attorneys; American Association of Homes for the Aging

AAHC American Accreditation HealthCare Commission; American Association of Healthcare Consultants; Association of Academic Health Centers

AAHD American Association of Hospital Dentists

AAHE American Association for Health Education

AAHFN American Association of Heart Failure Nurses

AAHN American Association for the History of Nursing

AAHP American Association of Health Plans

AAHPER American Association for Health, Physical Education, and Recreation

AAHPM American Academy of Hospice and Palliative Medicine

AAHRPP Association for the Accreditation of Human Research Protection Programs

AAHS American Association for Hand Surgery

AAHSA American Association of Homes and Services for the Aging

AAHSL Association of Academic Health Sciences Libraries

AAHSLD Association of Academic Health Sciences Library Directors

AAI activator adjusting instrument; acute alveolar injury; Adolescent Alienation Index; American Association of Immunologists; atrial inhibited [pacemaker]

AAIB alpha$_1$-aminoisobutyrate

AAID American Academy of Implant Dentistry

AAIDD American Association on Intellectual and Developmental Disabilities

AAK allo-activated killer

AAKP American Association of Kidney Patients

AAL ambient air level; anterior axillary line

AALAS American Association for Laboratory Animal Science

AALib amino acid library

AALNA American Assisted Living Nurses Association

AALNC American Association of Legal Nurse Consultants

AAM acute aseptic meningitis; American Academy of Microbiology; amino acid mixture

AAm acrylamide

AAMA American Academy of Medical Acupuncture; American Academy of Medical Administrators; American Association of Medical Assistants

AAMC Association of American Medical Colleges

AAMCN American Association of Managed Care Nurses

AAMD American Academy of Medical Directors

AAME acetylarginine methyl ester

AAMFT American Association for Marriage and Family Therapy

AAMI Association for the Advancement of Medical Instrumentation

AAMN American Assembly for Men in Nursing

AAMP American Academy of Maxillofacial Prosthetics

AAMRS automated ambulatory medical record system

AAMS acute aseptic meningitis syndrome; Association of Air Medical Services

AAMSE American Association of Medical Society Executives

AAMSI American Association for Medical Systems and Informatics

AAMT American Association for Medical Transcription

AAMU 5-acetylamino-6-amino-methyluracil

AAN AIDS-associated nephropathy; alpha-amino nitrogen; American Academy of Neurology; American Academy of Nursing; American Academy of Nutrition; American Association of Neuropathologists; amino acid nitrogen; analgesic-associated nephropathy; Associate of Arts in Nursing; attending's admission notes

AANA American Association of Nurse Anesthetists

AANCP American Association of Nurse Life Care Planners

AANE American Association of Nurse Executives

AANEM American Association of Neuromuscular & Electrodiagnostic Medicine

AANM American Association of Nurse-Midwives

AANN American Association of Neuroscience Nurses

AANP American Academy of Nurse Practitioners; American Association of Naturopathic Physicians; American Association of Neuropathologists; American Association of Nurse Practitioners

AAO American Academy of Ophthalmology; American Academy of Optometry; American

Academy of Osteopathy; American Academy of Otolaryngology; American Association of Ophthalmologists; American Association of Orthodontists; amino acid oxidase; ascending aorta; awake, alert, and oriented

AAo ascending aorta

A-a O$_2$ alveolar-arterial oxygen gradient; alveolar-arterial oxygen tension

AAOC antacid of choice

AAOHN American Association of Occupational Health Nurses

AAO-HNS American Academy of Otolaryngology—Head and Neck Surgery

AAOM American Academy of Oral Medicine

AAOMP American Academy of Oral and Maxillofacial Pathology

AAOMR American Academy of Oral and Maxillofacial Radiology

AAOMS American Association of Oral and Maxillofacial Surgeons

AAOO American Academy of Ophthalmology and Otolaryngology

AAOP American Academy of Oral Pathology

AAOS American Academy of Orthopaedic Surgeons; American Association of Osteopathic Specialists; American Association of Orthopaedic Surgeons

AAP acute abdominal pain; acute appendicitis; air at atmospheric pressure; American Academy of Pediatrics; American Academy of Pedodontics; American Academy of Periodontology; American Academy of Psychoanalysis; American Academy of Psychoanalysts; American Academy of Psychotherapists; American Association of Pathologists; Association for the Advancement of Psychoanalysis; Association for the Advancement of Psychotherapy; Association of Academic Physiatrists; Association of American Physicians

AAPA American Academy of Physician Assistants; American Association of Pathologists' Assistants

AAPB American Association of Pathologists and Bacteriologists; Association for Applied Psychophysiology and Biofeedback

AAPBD anomalous arrangement of the pancreaticobiliary duct

AAPC American Academy of Professional Coders; antibiotic-associated pseudomembranous colitis; average annual percent change

AAPCC adjusted annual per capita cost; adjusted average per capita costs; American Association of Poison Control Centers

AaP$_{CO_2}$, (A-a)P$_{CO_2}$ alveolar-arterial carbon dioxide tension difference

AAPD American Academy of Pediatric Dentistry

AAPF antiarteriosclerosis polysaccharide factor

AAPH 2,2′-azobis-(2-amidinopropane) hydrochloride

AAPHD American Association of Public Health Dentistry

AAPHP American Association of Public Health Physicians

AAPL American Academy of Psychiatry and the Law

AAPM American Association of Physicists in Medicine; American Academy of Pain Medicine

AAPMC antibiotic-associated pseudomembranous colitis

AAPM&R American Academy of Physical Medicine and Rehabilitation

AaP$_{O_2}$, (A-a)P$_{O_2}$ alveolar-arterial oxygen tension difference

AAPP American Academy of Physician and Patient

AAPPO American Association of Preferred Provider Organizations

AAPS American Academy of Phalloplasty Surgeons; American Association of Pharmaceutical Scientists; American Association of Physician Specialists; American Association of Plastic Surgeons; Arizona Articulation Proficiency Scale; Association of American Physicians and Surgeons

AAPT Adolescent Alcohol Prevention Trial

AAR active avoidance reaction; acute articular rheumatism; antigen-antiglobulin reaction

aar against all risks

AARC American Association for Respiratory Care

AARE automobile accident, rear end

AARIF arthroscopically assisted reduction and internal fixation

AARNet Australian Academic and Research Network

AAROM active assertive range of motion; active-assisted range of motion

AARP American Association of Retired Persons

AART American Association for Rehabilitation Therapy

AAS Aarskog-Scott [syndrome]; abuse assessment screening; acid aspiration syndrome; acute abdominal series; alcoholic abstinence syndrome; American Academy of Sanitarians; American Analgesia Society;

aneurysm of atrial septum; anthrax antiserum; aortic arch syndrome; Associate of Applied Science; atomic absorption spectrophotometry

AASCIN American Association of Spinal Cord Injury Nurses

AASD American Academy of Stress Disorders

aa seq amino acid sequence

AASH adrenal androgen stimulating hormone; American Association for the Study of Headache

AASK African American Study of Kidney Disease and Hypertension Pilot Study

AASLD American Association for the Study of Liver Diseases

AASM American Academy of Sleep Medicine

AASP acute atrophic spinal paralysis; American Association of Senior Physicians; ascending aorta synchronized pulsation

AASS American Association for Social Security

AAST American Association for the Surgery of Trauma

AAT Aachen Aphasia Test; academic aptitude test; Accolate Asthma Trial; alanine aminotransferase; alkylating agent therapy; alpha-1-antitrypsin; atrial triggered [pacemaker]; auditory apperception test; automatic atrial tachycardia

A1AT α_1-antitrypsin

α_1AT α_1-antitrypsin

AATB American Association of Tissue Banks

AATP American Association for Technology in Psychiatry

AATS American Association for Thoracic Surgery

AAU acute anterior uveitis

AAUT actual amount of use test

AAV adeno-associated virus

AaV *Acherontia atropas* virus; *Allomyces arbuscula* virus

AAVMC Association of American Veterinary Medical Colleges

AAVP American Association of Veterinary Parasitologists

AAW anterior aortic wall

3AB 3-aminobenzamide

AB abdominal; able body; abnormal; abortion; Ace bandage; active bilaterally; aid to the blind; airbag; alcian blue; alertness behavior; antibiotic; antibody; antigen binding; apex beat; asbestos body; asthmatic bronchitis; axiobuccal; Bachelor of Arts [L. *Artium Baccalaureus*]; blood group AB

A/B acid/base ratio

A&B apnea and bradycardia

A>B air greater than bone [conduction]

A-β amyloid beta

Ab abortion; antibiotic; antibody; from [L.]

A_b amount in body

aB azure B

ab aberration; abortion; antibody

ABA abscissic acid; allergic bronchopulmonary aspergillosis; American Board of Anesthesiology; American Burn Association; antibacterial activity; arrest before arrival; autonomic blocking agent

ABACAS Adjunctive Balloon Angioplasty Following Coronary Atherectomy Study

ABAI American Board of Allergy and Immunology

AB/AM antibiotic/antimycotic

ABAT American Board of Applied Toxicology

ABAV Abadina virus

ABB Albright-Butler-Bloomberg [syndrome]; American Board of Bioanalysis

ABBI advanced breast biopsy instrument

ABBQ AIDS Beliefs and Behavior Questionnaire

abbr abbreviated

ABC abacavir; absolute basophil count; absolute bone conduction; acalculous biliary colic; acid balance control; aconite-belladonna-chloroform; adenosine triphosphate binding cassette; airway, breathing, and circulation; alignment, blue, calcium [synovial fluid pearls in gout and pseudogout]; Alpha Beta Canadian [trial]; alternative birth center; alum, blood, and charcoal [purification and deodorizing method]; alum, blood, and clay [sludge deodorizing method]; American Blood Commission; aneurysmal bone cyst; antigen-binding capacity; antigen-binding cell; apnea, bradycardia, cyanosis; aspiration biopsy cytology; assessment of basic competency; atomic, biological, and chemical [warfare]; autism behavior checklist; avidin-biotin complex, avidin-biotin peroxidase complex; axiobuccocervical

A&BC air and bone conduction

ABCA1 adenosine triphosphate−binding cassette A1

ABCC Atomic Bomb Casualty Commission

ABCD airway, breathing, circulation, differential diagnosis (or defibrillate) [in CPR]; amphotericin B colloidal dispersion; appropriate blood pressure control in diabetes; asymmetry, borders are irregular, color variegated, diameter >6 mm [biopsy in melanoma]

ABCDE airway, breathing, circulation, disability, exposure [in trauma patients]; botulinum pentavalent toxoid

ABCDES abnormal alignment, bone periarticular osteoporosis, cartilage-joint space loss, deformities, marginal erosions, soft tissue swelling [radiographic features]; adjust medication, bacterial prophylaxis, cervical spine disease, deep vein thrombosis prophylaxis, evaluate extent and activity of disease, stress-dose steroid coverage [preoperative evaluation]; alignment, bone mineralization, calcifications, distribution of joints, erosions, soft tissue, and nails [radiographic features]; ankylosis, bone osteoporosis, cartilage destruction, deformity of joints, erosions, swelling of soft tissues [radiographic features]

ABCIC airway, breathing, circulation, intravenous crystalloid

ABCIL antibody-mediated cell-dependent immunolympholysis

ABC-M chemical-biological aircraft mask

ABCN American Board of Clinical Neuropsychology

ABCRS American Board of Colon and Rectal Surgery

ABCs active bacterial core surveillance [system]

ABD abdomen; aged, blind, and disabled; aggressive behavioral disturbance; American Board of Dermatology; aortic barodenervated [rat]; automatic border detection; automatic boundary detection; average body dose

Abd, abd abdomen, abdominal; abduct, abduction, abductor

abdom abdomen, abdominal

ABDPH American Board of Dental Public Health

ABE acute bacterial endocarditis; American Board of Endodontics; botulism equine trivalent antitoxin

ABEM American Board of Emergency Medicine

ABEPP American Board of Examiners in Professional Psychology

ABER abducted and externally rotated; abduction and external rotation; auditory brainstem evoked response

aber aberrant

ABF aortic blood flow; aortobifemoral

ABFP American Board of Family Physicians; American Board of Family Practice; American Board of Forensic Psychiatry; American Board of Forensic Psychology

ABG arterial blood gas; axiobuccogingival

ABGC American Board of Genetic Counseling

ABHM Association of Behavioral Healthcare Management

ABHW Association for Behavioral Health and Wellness

ABI Adaptive Behavior Inventory; ankle/brachial index; atherothrombotic brain infarct; auditory brainstem implant

ABIC Adaptive Behavior Inventory for Children; antibody excess immune complex

ABIM American Board of Internal Medicine

ABIMCE American Board of Internal Medicine certifying examination

ABIT assertive behavior inventory tool

ABK aphakic bullous keratopathy

ABL Abelson protooncogene; abetalipoproteinemia; acceptable blood loss; acute basophilic leukemia; African Burkitt lymphoma; allograft-bound lymphocyte; angioblastic lymphadenopathy; antigen-binding lymphocyte; Army Biological Laboratory; automated biological laboratory; axiobuccolingual

Abl ablation

ABLA acute blood loss anemia

ABLB alternate binaural loudness balance

ABLC amphotericin B lipid complex

ABLES Adult Blood Lead Epidemiology and Surveillance

ABM abamectin; adjusted body mass; alveolar basement membrane; attentional bias modification; autologous bone marrow

aBMD areal bone mineral density

ABMG American Board of Medical Genetics

ABMI autologous bone marrow infusion

AbMLV Abelson murine leukemia virus

ABMM American Board of Medical Management

ABMS American Board of Medical Specialties

ABMT American Board of Medical Toxicology; autologous bone marrow transplantation

ABMV Above Maiden virus; Abu Mina virus

AbMV Abutilon mosaic virus

ABN advanced beneficiary notice

AbN antibody nitrogen

Abn, abn abnormal, abnormality(ies)

ABNM American Board of Neurophysiologic Monitoring; American Board of Nuclear Medicine

ABNMP alpha-benzyl-*N*-methyl phenethylamine

ABNO anatomic abnormality

abnor abnormal

ABNS American Board of Neurologic Surgery; American Board of Nursing Specialties

ABO abortion; absent bed occupancy; American Board of Orthodontists; blood group system consisting of groups A, AB, B, and O

ABODM American Board of Disaster Medicine

ABOG American Board of Obstetrics and Gynecology

ABOHN American Board of Occupational Health Nurses

ABOMP American Board of Oral and Maxillofacial Pathology

ABOMS American Board of Oral and Maxillofacial Surgery

ABOP American Board of Oral Pathology

Abor, abor abortion

ABOS American Board of Orthopaedic Surgery

ABOto American Board of Otolaryngology

ABOVE Acute Bleeding Oesophageal Variceal Episodes [study]

ABP actin-binding protein; acute biliary pancreatitis; ambulatory blood pressure; American Board of Pathology; American Board of Pediatrics; American Board of Pedodontics; American Board of Periodontology; American Board of Prosthodontists; aminobiphenyl; androgen-binding protein; antigen-binding protein; arterial blood pressure; automatic systolic blood pressure measurement; avidin-biotin peroxidase

aBP arterial blood pressure

ABPA actin-binding protein, autosomal form; allergic bronchopulmonary aspergillosis

ABPANC American Board of Perianesthesia Nursing Certification

ABPC ampicillin; antibody-producing cell

ABPE acute bovine pulmonary edema

ABPM ambulatory blood pressure monitoring; American Board of Preventive Medicine

ABPMR American Board of Physical Medicine and Rehabilitation

ABPN American Board of Psychiatry and Neurology

ABPS American Board of Physician Specialties; American Board of Plastic Surgery; American Board of Podiatric Surgery

ABQ attitude behavior questionnaire

ABR abortus Bang ring [test]; absolute bed rest; American Board of Radiology; arterial baroreflex; auditory brainstem response

ABr agglutination test for brucellosis

Abr, Abras abrasion

ABRV Abras virus; Arbroath virus

ABS abdominal surgery; acidic ammonium bisulfate; acute brain syndrome; adaptive behavior scale; admitting blood sugar; adult bovine serum; aging brain syndrome; alkylbenzene sulfonate; aloin, belladonna, strychnine; American Board of Surgery; amniotic band sequence; amniotic band syndrome; anti-B serum; Antley-Bixler syndrome; arterial blood sample; at bedside; Australian Bureau of Statistics

Abs absorption

abs absent; absolute

AB-SAAP autologous blood selective aortic arch perfusion

absc abscess; abscissa

abs conf absolute configuration

ABSe ascending bladder septum

abs feb while fever is absent [L. *absente febre*]

ABSITE American Board of Surgery In-Training Examination

absorp absorption

AbSR abnormal skin reflex

ABSSSI acute bacterial skin and skin structure infections

abst, abstr abstract

ABSV Absettarov virus

ABT abstract behavioral type; autologous blood transfusion; lopinavir

abt about

ABTS American Board of Thoracic Surgery

ABU American Board of Urology; asymptomatic bacteriuria

ABV actinomycin D−bleomycin-vincristine; *Agaricus bisporus* virus; Aglaonema bacilliform virus; Aransas Bay virus; arthropod-borne virus

AbV *Agaricus bisporus* virus

ABVD Adriamycin, bleomycin, vinblastine, and dacarbazine

ABW actual body weight; adjusted body weight; average body weight

ABX abciximab; antibiotics

ABY acid bismuth yeast [medium]

AbYV Abutilon yellow virus

5-AC azacitidine

AC abdominal circumference; abdominal compression; ablation catheter; abrupt closure; absorption coefficient; abuse case; acetate; acetylcholine; acidified complement; *Acinetobacter calcoaceticus*; acromioclavicular; activated charcoal; acupuncture clinic; acute; acute cholecystitis; adenocarcinoma; adenylate cyclase; adherent cell; adrenal cortex; adrenocorticoid; Adriamycin/cyclophosphamide; air chamber; air conditioning; air conduction; airway collapse; alcoholic cirrhosis; alternating current; alveolar crest; ambulatory care; anesthesia circuit; angiocellular; anodal closure; antecubital; anterior chamber; anterior column; anterior commissure; antibiotic concentrate; anticholinergic; anticoagulant; anticomplement; antiphlogistic corticoid; aortic closure; aortic compliance; aortocoronary; arm circumference; ascending colon; assist control [ventilation]; atriocarotid; autocorrelation; axiocervical; hydrogen cyanide

A-C acromioclavicular; adult versus child; aortocoronary bypass

A/C albumin/coagulin ratio; anterior chamber of eye; assist control [ventilation]

A2C apical two-chamber [view]

A4C apical four-chamber [view]

Ac accelerator; acetate; acetyl; actinium; anticoagulant, anticoagulation; aortic closure; arabinosyl cytosine

aC abcoulomb; arabinosyl cytosine

ac acceleration; acetyl; acid; acromioclavicular; acute; alternating current; antecubital; anterior chamber; atrial contraction; axiocervical

a.c. before meals [L. *ante cibum*]

ACA abnormal coronary artery; acrodermatitis chronica atrophicans; acute cerebellar ataxia; adenocarcinoma; adult child of an alcoholic; Affordable Care Act; American Certification Agency; American Chiropractic Association; American College of Angiology; American College of Apothecaries; American Council on Alcoholism; American Counseling Association; aminocephalosporanic acid; ammonia, copper, and acetate; amyotrophic choreoacanthocytosis; anisotropic conductive adhesive; anterior cerebral artery; anterior communicating aneurysm/artery; anticapsular antibody; anti-cardiolipin antibody; anti-centromere antibody; anticollagen antibody; anticomplement activity; anticytoplasmic antibody; arrhythmic cardiac arrest; automatic chemical agent alarm; automated clinical analyzer

AC/A accommodative convergence/accommodation [ratio]

ACAAI American College of Allergy, Asthma, and Immunology

ACAC acetyl-coenzyme A cocarboxylase; activated charcoal; artificial cell

ACACN American Council of Applied Clinical Nutrition

ACACT acyl−coenzyme A: cholesterol acyltransferase

ACAD asymptomatic coronary artery disease; atherosclerotic carotid artery disease; Azithromycin in Coronary Artery Disease [study]

Acad academy

ACADA automatic chemical agent detector alarm

ACADEMIC Azithromycin in Coronary Artery Disease Elimination of Myocardial Infarction with Chlamydia [study]

A-CAH autoimmune chronic active hepatitis

ACAM American College for Advancement in Medicine

ACAO acyl−coenzyme A oxidase

ACAPS Asymptomatic Coronary Artery Plaque Study; Asymptomatic Coronary Artery Progression Study

ACAS adaptive cluster analysis system; Asymptomatic Carotid Atherosclerosis Study

ACASI audio computer-assisted self-interview

ACAT acetyl−coenzyme A acetyltransferase; automated computerized axial tomography

ACAV Acara virus; American Committee on Arthropod-Borne Viruses

ACB antibody-coated bacteria; aortocoronary bypass; arterialized capillary blood; asymptomatic carotid bruit

ACBaE air contrast barium enema

ACBC 1-amino-1-cyclobutanecarboxylic acid

AC/BC air conduction/bone conduction

ACBE air contrast barium enema

ACBG aortocoronary bypass graft

ACBS Asymptomatic Cervical Bruit Study

ACC accommodation; acetyl−coenzyme A carboxylase; acinic cell carcinoma; actinomycin C; acute care center; adenoid cystic carcinoma; administrative control center; adrenocortical carcinoma; agenesis of corpus callosum; alveolar cell carcinoma; ambulatory care center; American College of Cardiology; anodal closure contraction; anterior cingulate cortex; antitoxin-containing cell; aplasia cutis congenita; articular chondrocalcinosis; automated cell count; automated cell counter

Acc acceleration; adenoid cystic carcinoma

acc acceleration, accelerator; accident; accommodation

ACCA Advisory Committee on Casualty Assessment; American College of Cardiovascular Administrators

ACC/AHA American College of Cardiology/American Heart Association [Task Force]

ACCE American College of Clinical Engineering

ACCEPT Accupril Canadian Clinical Evaluation and Patient Teaching; American College of Cardiology Electrocardiogram

Proficiency Test; American College of Cardiology Evaluation of Preventive Therapies [study]

ACCESS A Comparison of Percutaneous Entry Sites for Coronary Angioplasty; Acute Candesartan Cilexetil Evaluation in Stroke Survivors; Ambulatory Care Clinic Effectiveness Systems Study; Atorvastatin Comparative Cholesterol Efficacy and Safety Study; automated cervical cell screening system

ACCH Association for the Care of Children's Health

AcCh acetylcholine

AcChR acetylcholine receptor

AcCHS acetylcholinesterase

accid accident, accidental

acc insuff accommodation insufficiency

ACCL, Accl anodal closure clonus

ACCME Accreditation Council for Continuing Medical Education

ACCN accession number

AcCoA acetyl−coenzyme A

accom accommodation

ACCP Alliance for Cervical Cancer Prevention; American College of Chest Physicians; American College of Clinical Pharmacology; American College of Clinical Pharmacy

AcCPV *Arctia caja* cypovirus

ACCR amylase-creatinine clearance ratio

ACCS American-Canadian Cooperative Study

ACCT Amlodipine Cardiovascular Community Trial; aortic cross-clamp time

accum accumulation

accur accurately

ACD absolute cardiac dullness; absolute claudication distance; acid-citrate-dextrose [solution]; actinomycin D; active compression-decompression; adult celiac disease; advanced care directive; allergic contact dermatitis; alopecia, contractures, dwarfism, mental retardation (intellectual disability) [syndrome]; American College of Dentists; ammonium citrate dextrose; anemia of chronic disease; angiokeratoma corporis diffusum; annihilation coincidence detection; anterior chamber depth; anterior chest diameter; anticoagulant citrate dextrose; anticonvulsant drug; area of cardiac dullness; Available Chemicals Directory

AcDB A *Caenorhabditis elegans* Database [gene expression]

AC-DC, ac/dc alternating current/direct current

ACD-CPR active compression-decompression cardiopulmonary resuscitation

ACDF anterior cervical discectomy and fusion

ACD-PCR active compression-decompression postcompression remodeling

ACDV Acado virus

ACE acetonitrile; acetylcholine esterase; acute cerebral encephalopathy; acute coronary event; adrenocortical extract; Adverse Childhood Experience [study]; adverse clinical event; alcohol, chloroform, and ether; analytic continuum electrostatics; angiotensin-converting enzyme; annealed competition of experts [algorithm]; Aspirin and Carotid Endarterectomy [trial]

ace acentric; acetone

ACE2 angiotensin-converting enzyme 2

ACED anhidrotic congenital ectodermal dysplasia

AceDB A *Caenorhabditis elegans* Database [gene expression]

ACEDS angiotensin-converting enzyme dysfunction syndrome

ACEH acid cholesterol ester hydrolase

ACEI angiotensin-converting enzyme inhibitor

ACEIT applied current electrical impedance tomography

ACEP American College of Emergency Physicians

ACES Alternans Cardiac Electrical Safety [study]; Azithromycin and Coronary Events Study

AcEst acetyl esterase

ACET Advisory Committee for the Elimination of Tuberculosis; Azmacort Cost Effectiveness Trial

ACET, acet acetone; vinegar [L. *acetum*]

acetab acetabular, acetabulum

acetyl-CoA acetyl−coenzyme A

ACEV *Anomala cuprea* entomopoxvirus

ACF accessory clinical findings; active case finding; acute care facility; advanced communication function or facility; anisotropic conductive film; anterior cervical fusion; anterior cranial fossa; area correction factor; asymmetric crying facies; autocorrelation function

ACf autocorrelation function

ACFAOM American College of Foot and Ankle Orthopedics and Medicine

ACFAS American College of Foot and Ankle Surgeons

ACG accelerator globulin; adjusted clinical group; alternative care grant; ambulatory care group; American College of Gastroenterology; angiocardiogram, angiocardiography; aortocoronary graft; apexcardiogram

AC-G, AcG, ac-g accelerator globulin

ACGIH American Conference of Governmental Industrial Hygienists

ACGME Accreditation Council for Graduate Medical Education

ACGP American College of General Practitioners

ACGPOMS American College of General Practitioners in Osteopathic Medicine and Surgery

ACGT antibody-coated grid technique

ACH acetylcholine; achalasia; active chronic hepatitis; adrenocortical hormone; air change per hour; amyotrophic cerebellar hypoplasia; arm girth, chest depth, and hip width [index]

ACh acetylcholine; acetylcholinesterase

ACHA American College Health Association; American College of Hospital Administrators

AChA anterior choroidal artery

ACHIEVE Accupril Congestive Heart Failure Investigation and Economic Variable Evaluation

ACHD atherosclerotic coronary heart disease

ACHE American College of Healthcare Executives; American Council for Headache Education

AChE acetylcholinesterase

ACHOO autosomal dominant compelling helioophthalmic outburst [syndrome]

ACHPER Australian Council for Health, Physical Education, and Recreation [survey]

ACHPR Agency for Health Care Policy and Research

ACHR Advisory Committee on Health Research

AChR acetylcholine receptor

AChRAb acetylcholine receptor antibody

AChRP acetylcholine receptor protein

ACHS Australian Council on Healthcare Standards

a.c.h.s./ac&hs before meals and at bedtime

AcHV acciptrid herpesvirus

ACI acceleration index; acoustic comfort index; acute cardiac ischemia; acute coronary infarction; acute coronary insufficiency; adenylate cyclase inhibitor; adrenocortical insufficiency; advancing care information; anticlonus index

ACID Arithmetic, Coding, Information, and Digit Span [ACID subtests]

ACIF acute care index of functions; anterior cervical interbody fusion; anticomplement immunofluorescence

AciHV Acipenserin herpesvirus

AcINH acid labile isonicotinic acid hydrazide

ACIP acute canine idiopathic polyneuropathy; Advisory Committee on Immunization Practices; ambulatory care incentive payment; Asymptomatic Cardiac Ischemia Pilot Study

ACIR Australian Clinical Immunisation Register; Automotive Crash Injury Research

ACIS ambulatory care information system; automated clinical information system

ACIT Asymptomatic Cardiac Ischemia Trial

ACI-TIPI acute cardiac ischemia−time insensitive predictive instrument

ACJ acromioclavicular joint

AcK francium [actinium K]

ACKD acquired cystic kidney disease

ACL access control list; Achievement Check List; acromegaloid features, cutis verticis gyrata, corneal leukoma [syndrome]; American cutaneous leishmaniasis; anterior chamber lens; anterior cruciate ligament; Association for Computational Linguistics

ACl aspiryl chloride

aCL anticardiolipin [antibody]

ACLA American Clinical Laboratory Association

ACLC Assessment of Children's Language Comprehension

ACLD Association for Children with Learning Disabilities

ACLE acute cutaneous lupus erythematosus

ACLF adult congregate living facility

ACLI American Council on Life Insurance; American Council of Life Insurers

ACLM American College of Legal Medicine

ACLP Academy of Consultation-Liaison Psychiatry [formerly Academy of Psychosomatic Medicine]; Association of Child Life Professionals

ACLPS Academy of Clinical Laboratory Physicians and Scientists

ACLR anterior capsulolabral reconstruction

ACLS acrocallosal syndrome; advanced cardiac life support; Assessment of Children's Language Comprehension

AcLV avian acute leukemia virus

ACM access control matrix; acetaminophen; acute cerebrospinal meningitis; adaptive fuzzy C-means algorithm; Adriamycin, cyclophosphamide, methotrexate; albumin-calcium-magnesium; alcoholic cardiomyopathy; alveolar capillary membrane; anticardiac myosin; Arnold-Chiari malformation; asbestos-containing material; Association for Computing Machinery; automated cardiac flow measurement

ACMC Association of Canadian Medical Colleges

ACMD associate chief medical director

ACME Accreditation Commission for Midwifery Education; Advisory Council on Medical Education; Angioplasty Compared to Medicine [study]; assessing changes in medical education; Automated Classification of Medical Entities

ACMF arachnoid cyst of the middle fossa

ACMG American College of Medical Genetics

ACMHV avian carcinoma Mill Hill virus

ACMI age-consistent memory impairment; American College of Medical Informatics

ACML atypical chronic myeloid leukemia

AcMNPV *Autographa californica* multi-capsid nucleopolyhedrovirus

ACMP alveolar-capillary membrane permeability

ACMPH American College of Military Public Health

ACMR Advisory Committee on Medical Research

ACMS American Chinese Medical Society

ACMT artificial circus movement tachycardia

ACMV assist-control mechanical ventilation

ACN acute conditioned neurosis; Ambulatory Care Network; American College of Neuropsychiatrists; American College of Nurse-Midwives; American College of Nutrition; Association of Camp Nurses

ACNM American College of Nuclear Medicine; American College of Nurse-Midwives

ACNN Association of Child Neurology Nurses

ACNP acute care nurse practitioner; American College of Nuclear Physicians

ACO accountable care organization; acute coronary occlusion; alert, cooperative, and oriented; anodal closure odor

ACOA adult child of an alcoholic

ACoA anterior communicating artery

ACODENIC Advisory Committee on Dental Electronic Nomenclature, Indexing, and Classification

ACOEM American College of Occupational and Environmental Medicine

ACOEP American College of Osteopathic Emergency Physicians

ACOEV *Araphia conspersa* entomopoxvirus

ACOFP American College of Osteopathic Family Physicians

ACOG American College of Obstetricians and Gynecologists

ACOHA American College of Osteopathic Hospital Administrators

ACO-HNS American Council of Otolaryngology–Head and Neck Surgery

ACOI American College of Osteopathic Internists

ACOM American College of Occupational Medicine; anterior communicating [artery]

AComA anterior communicating artery

ACOMS American College of Oral and Maxillofacial Surgeons

ACOOG American College of Osteopathic Obstetricians and Gynecologists

ACOP American College of Osteopathic Pediatricians; approved code of practice

ACORDE A Consortium on Restorative Dentistry Education

ACOS American College of Osteopathic Surgeons; associate chief of staff

ACOS/AC associate chief of staff for ambulatory care

ACOSPM American College of Osteopathic Pain Management and Sclerotherapy

Acous acoustics, acoustics

ACOX acetyl–coenzyme A oxidase

ACP accessory conduction pathway; acid phosphatase; acyl carrier protein; advanced care paramedic [Canada]; American College of Pathologists; American College of Physicians; American College of Prosthodontists; American College of Psychiatrists; Animal Care Panel; anodal closure picture; aspirin-caffeine-phenacetin; Association of Clinical Pathologists; Asymptomatic Cardiac Ischemia Pilot (Study); atom class pair

ACPA American Cleft Palate-Craniofacial Association; anticitrullinated protein antibody

AcPase acid phosphatase

ACPC aminocyclopentane carboxylic [acid]

AC-PC anterior commissure–posterior commissure

ACPE American College of Physician Executives

AC-PH, ac phos acid phosphatase

ACPM American College of Preventive Medicine

ACPP adrenocortical polypeptide; prostate-specific acid phosphatase

ACPS acrocephalopolysyndactyly; Advisory Committee for Pharmaceutical Science

ACQUIP Ambulatory Care Quality Improvement Project

ACR abnormally contracting region; absolute catabolic rate; acriflavine; acute-to-chronic ratio; adenomatosis of colon and rectum; adjusted community rate; ambulance call report; American College of Radiology; American College of Rheumatology; anti-constipation regimen; axillary count rate

Acr acrylic

ACRA Associate Commissioner for Regulatory Affairs [FDA designation]

ACRE Appropriateness of Coronary Revascularization [study]

ACRF acute-on-chronic respiratory failure; ambulatory care research facility

ACRM American Congress of Rehabilitation Medicine

ACRN AIDS-Certified Registered Nurse

ACR/NEMA American College of Radiology/National Electrical Manufacturers' Association

ACS abdominal compartment syndrome; access control system; acrocallosal syndrome; acrocephalosyndactyly; acute chest syndrome; acute confusional state; acute coronary syndrome; Alcon Closure System; ambulatory care sensitive; American Cancer Society; American Chemical Society; American College of Surgeons; anodal closure sound; antireticular cytotoxic serum; aperture current setting; Association of Clinical Scientists; automatic corneal shaper

ACs air changes

ACSA adenylate cyclase–stimulating activity

ACSCEPT Assessment for Carotid Stenosis: Correlation with Endarterectomy Specimen Trial

ACS CPS American Cancer Society Cancer Prevention Studies

ACSE association control service element

ACSF artificial cerebrospinal fluid

aCSF artificial cerebrospinal fluid

AC/SIUG ambulatory care special interest user group

ACSM American College of Sports Medicine

ACSML arbitration and control state machine logic

ACSP adenylate cyclase-stimulating protein

ACSSuT ampicillin, chloramphenicol, streptomycin, sulfonamide, and tetracycline

ACST Asymptomatic Carotid Surgery Trial

ACSV aortocoronary saphenous vein

ACSVBG aortocoronary saphenous vein bypass graft

ACT abdominal computed tomography; ablation catheter tip; achievement through counseling and treatment; actin; actinomycin; action class torsion; activated clotting time, activated coagulation time; adaptive current tomography; advanced coronary treatment; Angioplasty Compliance Trial; anterocolic transposition; antichymotrypsin; anticoagulant therapy; anxiety control training; artemisinin combination therapy; Association of Cytogenetic Technologists; asthma care training; atropine coma therapy; Attacking

Claudication with Ticlopidine [study]; Australian Capital Territory [trial]

AcT acceleration time

Act activity

act actinomycin; active, activity

ACTA actin alpha; American Cardiology Technologists Association; automatic computerized transverse axial [scanning]

Act-C actinomycin C

ACTC alpha-actin, cardiac muscle

Act-D actinomycin D

ACT/DB Adaptable Clinical Trials Database

ACTe anodal closure tetanus

ACTG AIDS Clinical Trial Group [study]

ACTH adrenocorticotropic hormone

ACTH-LI adrenocorticotropin-like immunoreactivity

ACTHR adrenocorticotropic hormone receptor

ACTH-RF adrenocorticotropic hormone releasing factor

ACTHR/MC-2 adrenocorticotropin receptor/melanocortin receptor 2

ACTION A Coronary Disease Trial Investigating Outcome with Nifedipine GITS; Assisting Carriers Using Telematics Interventions to Meet Older Persons Needs

ACTIS AIDS Clinical Trials Information Service

activ active, activity

ACTN adrenocorticotropin

ACTOBAT Australasian Clinical Trial of Betamethasone and Thyroid-Releasing Hormone

ACTP adrenocorticotropic polypeptide

ACT/PD actual nursing hours per patient day

ACTS acute cervical traumatic sprain or syndrome; advanced communication technology satellite; advanced computational testing and simulation; American-Canadian Thrombosis Study; American College Testing Services; Auditory Comprehension Test for Sentences

ACTUR Automated Central Tumor Registry

ACTV Acatinga virus; activity

ACU acquired cold urticaria; acute care unit; agar colony-forming unit; ambulatory care unit

ACURP American College of Utilization Review Physicians

ACUTE Analysis of Coronary Ultrasound Thrombolysis Endpoints; Assessment of Cardioversion Utilizing Transesophageal Echocardiography [study]

ACV acute cardiovascular [disease]; acyclovir; assisted controlled ventilation;

atrial/carotid/ventricular; autonomic conduction velocity

ACVB aortocoronary venous bypass

ACVD acute cardiovascular disease, atherosclerotic cardiovascular disease

ACx anomalous circumflex [coronary artery]

AD abductor digiti minimi; above diaphragm; absorbed dose; acceptable daily intake; accident dispensary; accidental death; acetabular depth; acetate dialysis; active disease; active domain; acute dermatomyositis; addict, addiction; adenoid degeneration; adjuvant disease; admitting diagnosis; adrenodoxin; adrenostenedione; adult disease; advanced directive; aerosol deposition; affective disorder; after discharge; alcohol dehydrogenase; Aleutian disease; alveolar diffusion; alveolar duct; Alzheimer dementia; Alzheimer disease; analgesic dose; analog device; anodal duration; anterior division; antigenic determinant; anxiety disorder; appropriate disability; arthritic dose; assistive device; associate degree; atopic dermatitis; attentional disturbance; Aujeszky disease; autistic disorder; autonomic dysreflexia; autosomal dominant; average deviation; average difference; axiodistal; axis deviation; right ear [L. *auris dextra*]

A/D analog-to-digital

A&D admission and discharge; ascending and descending

Ad adenovirus; adrenal; anisotropic disk

ad add; axiodistal; let there be added [up to a specified amount, Lat.]; right ear [L. *auris dextra*]

AD1 Alzheimer disease type 1

ADA adenosine deaminase; American Dental Association; American Dermatological Association; American Diabetes Association; American Dietetic Association; Americans with Disabilities Act; anterior descending artery; antideoxyribonucleic acid antibody; approved dietary allowance; Australian Dental Association

ADAA American Dental Assistants Association

ADACS automatic data acquisition and control system

ADAM adduct detection by acylation with 35S-methionine; adhesion, amniotic deformity, mutilation [syndrome]; A disintegrin and metalloprotease; amniotic deformity; Amsterdam Duration of Antiretroviral Medication [study]

ADAMHA Alcohol, Drug Abuse, and Mental Health Administration

ADAP American Dental Assistants' Program; Assistant Director of Army Psychiatry

ADAPC alcohol and drug abuse prevention and control

ADAPT American Disabled for Attendant Programs Today; Association for Drug and Alcohol Prevention and Treatment; Automated Data Analysis and Pattern Recognition Toolkit

ADAPT-DES Assessment of Dual Antiplatelet Therapy With Drug-Eluting Stents [study]

ADAPTS acute directional atherectomy prior to stenting

ADAS Alzheimer Disease Assessment Scale

ADAS-COG Alzheimer Disease Assessment Scale, cognitive portion

AdASDiM Adaptive Advisory System for Diabetic Management

ADase adenosine deaminase

ADAU adolescent drug abuse unit

ADB accidental death benefit; archival database

ADC adenylate cyclase; adult day care; affective disorders clinic; Aid to Dependent Children; AIDS-dementia complex; albumin, dextrose, and catalase [medium]; ambulance design criteria; analog-to-digital converter; anodal duration contraction; apparent diffusion coefficient; audio-to-digital conversion; automated dispensing cabinets; average daily census; axiodistocervical

AdC adenylate cyclase; adrenal cortex

ADCA autosomal dominant cerebellar ataxia

ADCC acute disorder of cerebral circulation; antibody-dependent cell-mediated cytotoxicity, antibody-dependent cellular cytotoxicity

ADCH autosomal dominant cyclic hematopoiesis

AD-CHF acutely decompensated congestive heart failure

ADCMC antibody-dependent complement-mediated cytotoxicity

AdCMVHSV-TK adenovirus carrying the gene for herpes simplex virus thymidine kinase

ADCP adenosine deaminase complexing protein

AD-CPEO autosomal dominant chronic progressive external ophthalmoplegia

ADCS Argonz−del Castillo syndrome

ADCY adenyl cyclase

ADD acceptable daily dose; adduction; adenosine deaminase; Antiepileptic Drug Development [program]; attention deficit disorder; auditory discrimination in depth; average daily dose

add addition; adductor, adduction; let there be added [L. *addatur*]

ADDA acute dissection of the distal aorta

ADDH attention deficit disorder with hyperactivity

ADD/HA attention deficit disorder/hyperactivity

addict addiction, addictive

AdDNV *Aceta domestica* densovirus

add poll adductor pollicis

ADDS American Digestive Disease Society

ADDU alcohol and drug dependence unit

ADE acute disseminated encephalitis; adaptive delay estimation; adverse drug event; antibody-dependent enhancement; apparent digestible energy

Ade adenine

ADEA American Dental Education Association

ADEAR Alzheimer Disease Education and Referral [center]

AdeCbl adenosyl cobalamine

ADEE age-dependent epileptic encephalopathy

ADEG Antiarrhythmic Drug Evaluation Group [trial]

ADEM academic department of emergency medicine; acute disseminated encephalomyelitis

AdenoCa adenocarcinoma

ADEP Atherosclerotic Disease Evolution by Picotamide [study]

ADEPT Applying Diagnosis, Etiology, Prognosis, and Therapy [program]

adeq adequate

ADF adaptive filter; administrative determination of fault; automatic document feeder; average duration of failures

AD/FHD acetabular depth/femoral head diameter

ADFN albinism-deafness [syndrome]

ADFR activate, depress, free, repeat [coherence therapy]

ADFS alternative delivery and financing system

AD-FSP autosomal dominant familial spastic paraplegia

ADFVd Apple dimple fruit viroid

ADG ambulatory diagnostic group; atrial diastolic gallop; axiodistogingival

ADH Academy of Dentistry for the Handicapped; adhesion; alcohol dehydrogenase; antidiuretic hormone; arginine dihydrolase; atypical ductal hyperplasia

adh adhesion, adhesive; antidiuretic hormone

ADHA American Dental Hygienists Association

ADH/CA atypical ductal hyperplasia with adjacent ductal cancer

ADHD attention-deficit/hyperactivity disorder

ADHDP action-dependent heuristic dual programming

ADHERE Acute Decompensated Heart Failure National Registry

ADHR autosomal dominant hypophosphatemic rickets

ADI Academy of Dentistry International; acceptable daily intake; AIDS-defining illness; allowable daily intake; alternating direction implicit [method]; Alzheimer Disease International; artificial diverticulum of the ileum; atlas-dens interval; autism diagnostic interview; average daily intake; axiodistoincisal

ADI-R autism diagnostic interview-revised

adj adjacent; adjoining; adjuvant

ADK adenosine kinase

ADKC atopic dermatitis with keratoconjunctivitis

ADL active digital library; activities of daily living; adenolymphangitis; advanced distributed learning; Amsterdam Depression List; annual dose limit

ADLAR advanced design linear accelerator radiosurgery

ADLC antibody-dependent lymphocyte-mediated cytotoxicity

ad lib as desired [L. *ad libitum*]

ADLS Activities of Daily Living Survey

ADM abductor digiti minimi; add-drop multiplexer; administrative medicine; admission; Adriamycin; advanced diabetes management

AdM adrenal medulla

adm administration; admission; apply [L. *admove*]

ADMA asymmetric dimethyl arginine

Adm Dr admitting doctor

ADME absorption, distribution, metabolism, and excretion

Admin administration

ADMIRE AMP 579 Delivery for Myocardial Infarction Reduction [study]

ADMIT Arterial Disease Multiple Intervention Trial

AdML adenovirus major late promoter

admov. apply or add

Adm Ph admitting physician

ADMR average daily metabolic rate

ADMS analysis of disorders of masticatory system; atmospheric dispersion modeling system

ADMX adrenal medullectomy

ADN antideoxyribonuclease; aortic depressor nerve; associate degree in nursing

ad naus to the point of producing nausea [L. *ad nauseam*]

ADN-B antideoxyribonuclease B

ADNI Alzheimer's Disease Neuroimaging Initiative

ADO active data object; adenosine; adolescent medicine; allele drop-out; autosomal dominant osteoporosis; axiodistooclusal

Ado adenosine

ADOA autosomal dominant ocular albinism

AdoCbl 5'-adenosylcobalamin

ADOD arthrodentosteodysplasia

AdoDABA adenosyldiaminobutyric acid

AdoHcy *S*-adenosylhomocysteine

adol adolescence, adolescent

AdoMet *S*-adenosylmethionine

ADOPT Accupril Decision on Pharmacotherapy [trial]

ADPD Academy of Dentistry for Persons with Disabilities

ADOS autism diagnostic observation schedule; autosomal dominant Opitz syndrome

ADOTS affective disorder outpatient telephone screening

Adox oxidized adenosine

ADP adenopathy; adenosine diphosphate; adenovirus death protein; administrative psychiatry; approved drug product; approximate dynamic programming; area diastolic pressure; automatic data processing

AdP adductor pollicis

ADPase adenosine diphosphatase

ADPK autosomal dominant polycystic kidney [disease]

ADPKD autosomal dominant polycystic kidney disease

ADPL average daily patient load

ADPR adenosine diphosphate ribose

ADPRT adenosine diphosphate ribosyltransferase

ADQ abductor digiti quinti; adolescent drinking questionnaire

ADR activation, depression, repetition; adrenalin; adrenals; adrenergic receptor; adrenodoxin reductase; Adriamycin; adverse drug reaction; airway dilation reflex; alternative dispute resolution; arrested development of righting response; ataxia, deafness, retardation (intellectual disability) [syndrome]

Adr adrenalin; Adriamycin

adr adrenal, adrenalectomy

ADRA1A alpha-1A adrenergic receptor

ADRA1B alpha-1B adrenergic receptor

ADRA1C alpha-1C adrenergic receptor

ADRA2C alpha-2C adrenergic receptor

ADRAC Adverse Drug Reactions Advisory Committee

ADRAR alpha-2-adrenergic receptor

ADRBK beta-1 adrenergic receptor kinase

ADRBR adrenergic beta receptor

ADRC Alzheimer Disease Research Center

ADRDA Alzheimer's Disease and Related Disorders Association

ADRP adipose differentiation-related protein; autosomal dominant retinitis pigmentosa

ADRT approximate discrete radon transform

ADS acute death syndrome; acute diarrheal syndrome; adenocarcinoma dataset; Alcohol Dependence Scale; alternative delivery system; anatomic dead space; anonymous donor sperm; antibody deficiency syndrome; antidiuretic substance; Army Dental Service

ADSC adipose-derived stem cells; adipose-derived stromal cells; adipose tissue−derived stem cells

ADSD adductor spasmodic dysphonia

ADSL adenylosuccinate lyase; asymmetrical digital single line; asymmetric digital subscription line

ADSP analog-digital signal processor

ADSS adenylosuccinate synthetase

ADSTGD Stargardt-like muscular dystrophy

ADSV Arborea virus

ADT Accepted Dental Therapeutics; adenosine triphosphate; admission, discharge, and transfer; agar gel diffusion test; alternate-day therapy; any desired thing [placebo]; Alzheimer-type dementia; asphyxiating thoracic dystrophy; Auditory Discrimination Test

ADTA American Dental Trade Association

ADTe anodal duration tetanus

ADU alkaline deoxyribonucleic acid unwinding

AD&U acid dissociation and ultrafiltration

ADV adenovirus; adventitia; Aleutian disease virus; Aujeszky disease virus

AdV adenovirus

Adv adenovirus

adv advanced; against [L. *adversum*]

AdvaMed Advanced Medical Technology Association

ADVANCE anxiety reduction, distraction, video modeling and education, adding parents, no excessive reassurance, coaching, and exposure/shaping

ADVIRC autosomal dominant vitreoretino choroidopathy

ADVS activities of daily vision survey

ADW assault with deadly weapon

A5D5W alcohol 5%, dextrose 5%, in water

ADWE adverse drug withdrawl event

ADX adrenalectomized; adrenodoxin

AE above elbow; absolute erythrocytosis; acrodermatitis enteropathica; activation energy;

adaptive equipment, adult erythrocyte; adverse event; aftereffect; agarose electrophoresis; air embolism; air entry; alcoholic embryopathy; aminoethyl; anion exchange; anoxic encephalopathy; antiepileptic; antitoxic unit [Ger. *Antitoxineinheit*]; apoenzyme; aryepiglottic; atherosclerotic encephalopathy; atrial ectopic [heart beat]; avian encephalomyelitis

A&E accident and emergency

A+E accident and emergency; analysis and evaluation

A/E above elbow

AEA acquired epileptic aplasia; alcohol, ether, and acetone

AEB accidental exposure to blood; acute erythroblastopenia; avian erythroblastosis

AEC aminoethylcarbazole; ankyloblepharon, ectodermal defects, and cleft lip [syndrome]; at earliest convenience; Atomic Energy Commission; automatic exposure control

AECB acute exacerbation of chronic bronchitis

AECD allergic eczematous contact dermatitis

AECE-6-AZUMP 5-[2-(aminoethyl) carbamyl]-6-azauridine-5′monophosphate

AECGM ambulatory electrocardiographic monitoring

AECS acute exacerbation of chronic sinusitis

AED academic emergency department; antiepileptic drug; antihidrotic ectodermal dysplasia; anxious ego dissolution; automated external defibrillator

AEDP automated external defibrillator pacemaker

AEE Atomic Energy Establishment

AEF allogenic effect factor; amyloid enhancing factor; aortoenteric fistula

AEFB aerobic endospore-forming bacterium

A$_{EFF}$ effective area

AEFI adverse events following immunization

AEFV acceleration of early flow velocity

AEG acute erosive gastritis; air encephalography, air encephalogram; atrial electrogram

AEGIS Aid for the Elderly in Government Institutions

AEI arbitrary evolution index; arterial elasticity indexes; atrial emptying index; atrial escape interval

AEL acute erythroleukemia

AELV avian entero-like virus

AEM *Academic Emergency Medicine* [journal]; ambulatory electrocardiographic monitoring; analytical electron microscopy; ataxia episodica with myokymia; avian encephalomyelitis

AEMG abdominal electromyography

AEMIS Aerospace and Environmental Medicine Information System

AEMK ataxia episodica with myokymia

A-EMT advanced emergency medical technician

AEN anal epithelial neoplasia; aseptic epiphyseal necrosis

AEP acute edematous pancreatitis; artificial endocrine pancreas; auditory evoked potential; average evoked potential

AEq age equivalent

aeq. equal

AER abduction/external rotation; acoustic evoked response; acute exertional rhabdomyolysis; agranular endoplasmic reticulum; albumin excretion rate; aldosterone excretion rate; apical ectodermal ridge; auditory evoked response; average electroencephalic response; average evoked response

AERE Atomic Energy Research Establishment

Aero *Aerobacter*

AERP aircrew eye and respiratory protection; antegrade effective refractory period; atrial effective refractory period; auditory event–related potential

AERPAP antegrade effective refractory period accessory pathway

AERS acute equine respiratory syndrome

AES acetone-extracted serum; ambulatory encounter system; American Electroencephalographic Society; American Encephalographic Society; American Endocrine Society; American Endodontic Society; American Epidemiological Society; American Epilepsy Society; American Equilibration Society; anterior esophageal sensor; antiembolic stockings; antral ethmoidal sphenoidectomy; aortic ejection sound; Auger electron spectroscopy; autoerythrocyte sensitization

AEs adverse events

AesoNPV *Aedes sollicitans* nucleopolyhedrovirus

AEST aeromedical evacuation support team

AET absorption-equivalent thickness; *S*-(2-aminoethyl) isothiuronium; Antimicrobial Preservative Effectiveness Test [called also APR, PET]

AETT acetylethyltetramethyltetralin

AEV arthritis encephalitis virus; avian encephalomyelitis-like virus; avian erythroblastosis virus

AeV *Antheraea eucalypti* virus

AEZ acrodermatitis enteropathica, zinc deficient

AF abnormal frequency; acid-fast; actin filament; active force; adult female; afebrile; affected female; aflatoxin; albumin free; albumose free; alcoholic female; aldehyde fuchsin; amaurosis fugax; aminofluorine; aminophylline; amniotic fluid; angiogenesis factor; anteflexion; anterior fontanelle; antibody forming; antifog; antifungal; antral follicle; aortic flow; Arthritis Foundation; artificial feeding; ascitic fluid; atrial fibrillation; atrial flutter; atrial fusion; attenuation factor; attributable fraction; audio frequency

aF abfarad

af audio frequency

AFA acromegaloid facial appearance [syndrome]; advanced first aid; alcohol-formaldehyde-acetic acid [fixative]

AFAB assigned female at birth

AFAFP amniotic fluid alpha-fetoprotein

AFAR American Foundation for Aging Research

AFASAK Atrial Fibrillation, Aspirin, Anticoagulation [trial]

AFB acid-fast bacillus; aflatoxin B; aflatoxin biomarker; air fluidized bed; aortofemoral bypass

AFBAC affected family-based control test

AFBG aortofemoral bypass graft

AFC adult foster care; alternative forced choice; amplitude frequency characteristics; antibody-forming cell

AFCAPS Air Force Coronary Atherosclerosis Prevention Study

AFCI acute focal cerebral ischemia

AFCR American Federation for Clinical Research

AFD accelerated freeze drying; acrofacial dysostosis

AFDC Aid to Families with Dependent Children

AFDH American Fund for Dental Health

AFDM adaptive focus deformable model

AFDSM adaptive focus deformable statistical model

AFDW ash-free dry weight

AFE amniotic fluid embolism

afeb afebrile

AFEDI Association Francophone Européene des Infirmiers

AFF atrial fibrillation and flutter; atrial filling fraction

aff afferent

AFFIRM Atrial Fibrillation Follow-Up Investigation of Rhythm Management [study]

AFFN acrofrontofacionasal

AFG abnormal fasting glucose; aflatoxin G; amniotic fluid glucose; arbitrary function generator

aFGF acidic fibroblast growth factor

AFH angiofollicular hyperplasia; anterior facial height

AFI amaurotic familial idiocy; Atrial Fibrillation Investigators [study]

AFIB Atrial Fibrillation Investigation with Bidisomide [trial]

AFib atrial fibrillation

AFIB/FL atrial fibrillation/flutter

AFIP Armed Forces Institute of Pathology

AFIPS American Federation of Information Processing Societies

AFIRME antagonist of the fibrinogen receptor after myocardial events

AFIS amniotic fluid infection syndrome

AFL antifibrinolysin; artificial limb; atrial flutter

AFLNH angiofollicular lymph node hyperplasia

AFLP acute fatty liver of pregnancy; amplified fragment length polymorphism

AFM aflatoxin M; after fatty meal; atomic force microscopy

AFMA automated fabrication of modality aids

AFMC Association of Faculties of Medicine of Canada

AFMR American Federation for Medical Research

AFMU 5-acetylamino-6-formylamino-3-methyluracil

AFN afunctional neutrophil; American Forensic Nurses; antegrade femoral nail

AFNC Air Force Nurse Corps

AFND acute febrile neutrophilic dermatosis

AFO ankle/foot orthotic; ankle-foot orthosis

AFORMED alternating failure of response, mechanical, to electrical depolarization

AFP acute flaccid paralysis; alpha-fetoprotein; anterior faucial pillar; atypical facial pain

AFPP acute fibropurulent pneumonia

AFQ aflatoxin Q

AFR aqueous flare response; ascorbic free radical

AFRAX autism—fragile X [syndrome]

AFRD acute febrile respiratory disease

AFRI acute febrile respiratory illness

AFROC Association of Freestanding Radiation Oncology Centers

AFS acquired/adult Fanconi syndrome; alternative financing system; American Fertility Society; antifibroblast serum

AFSAM Air Force School of Aviation Medicine

AFSCME American Federation of State, County, and Municipal Employees

AFSM adaptive Fourier series modeling

AFSP acute fibrinoserous pneumonia

AFT aflatoxin; agglutination-flocculation test

AFTA American Family Therapy Academy

AFTER Anistreplase Following Thrombolysis Effect on Reocclusion [study]; Aspirin/ Anticoagulants Following Thrombolysis with Eminase in Recurrent Infarction [study]; Aspirin/Anticoagulants Following Thrombolysis with Eminase Results [study]

AFTN autonomously functioning thyroid nodule

AFV amniotic fluid volume; aortic flow velocity; *Aspergillus foetidus* virus

AFV-F *Aspergillus foetidus* virus F

AFV-S *Aspergillus foetidus* virus S

AFX atypical fibroxanthoma

AG abdominal girth; acidophilic granulocyte; agarose; aminoglutethimide; analytical grade; Andersen-Gill [statistical method]; angular gyrus; anion gap; antigen; antigenomic; antiglobulin; antigravity; atrial gallop; attached gingiva; autograft; axiogingival; azurophilic granule

AG, A/G albumin/globulin ratio

Ag antigen; silver [L. *argentum*]

Ag* labeled antigen

ag androgenetic; antigen

AGA accelerated growth area; allergic granulomatosis and angiitis; American Gastroenterological Association; American Genetic Association; American Geriatrics Association; American Goiter Association; antigliadin antibody; antiglomerular antibody; anti-IgG autoantibody; appropriate for gestational age; aspartylglucosamidase

Ag-Ab antigen-antibody complex

AGAC aminoglycoside-aminocyclitol

AGAG acidic glycosaminoglycan

AGAR Australian Group on Antimicrobial Resistance [study]

AGBAD Alexander Graham Bell Association for the Deaf

AG Bell Alexander Graham Bell Association for the Deaf and Hard of Hearing

AGC absolute granulocyte count; anatomically graduated component; atypical glandular cell; automatic gain control

AGC-FN atypical glandular cells favor neoplasia

AGC-FR atypical glandular cells favor reactive

AgCPV *Abraxas grossulariata* cypovirus; *Autographa gamma* cypovirus

AGCT antiglobulin consumption test; Army General Classification Test

AGC-U atypical glandular cells unqualified

AGD Academy of General Dentistry; agar gel diffusion; agarose diffusion; alpha-ketoglutarate dehydrogenase

AGDD agar gel double diffusion

AGE acrylamide gel; acute gastroenteritis; advanced glycation end product; agarose gel electrophoresis; angle of greatest extension; arterial gas embolism

AGED automated general experimental device

AGEG age group

AGE-IEF agarose gel-isoelectric focusing [electrophoresis]

AGEPC acetyl glyceryl ether phosphorylcholine

AGES age, grade, extension, size [tumor]

AGF accelerated graphics port; adrenal growth factor; angiopoietin-related growth factor; angle of greatest flexion

AGG agammaglobulinemia

agg agglutination; aggravation; aggregation

aggl, agglut agglutination

aggrav aggravated, aggravation

aggreg aggregated, aggregation

AGGS anti−gas gangrene serum

AGI adjusted gross income

AGID agar gel immunodiffusion

AGIR autologous gastrointestinal reconstruction

AGIS Advanced Glaucoma Intervention Study

agit agitate [stir or shake]; agitated; agitation

AGIV *Anticarisia gemmatalis* iridescent virus

AGL acute granulocytic leukemia; agglutination; aminoglutethimide; anterior glenoid labrum

AGM absorbent gelling material

AGMK, AGMkK African green monkey kidney [cell]

AgMNPV *Anticarisia gemmatalis* multiple nucleopolyhedrovirus

AGMPyV African green monkey polyoma virus

AGN acute glomerulonephritis; agnosia

agn agnosia

AGNB aerobic gram-negative bacillus

AGNC Association of Genetic Nurses and Counselors

AgNOR silver-staining nucleolar organizer region

AGOS American Gynecological and Obstetrical Society

AGP acid glycoprotein; aerosol-generating procedure; agar gel precipitation; ambulatory glucose profile; azurophil granule protein

AGPA American Group Practice Association; American Group Psychotherapy Association

AGPI agar gel precipitin inhibition

AGPT agar gel precipitation test

AGR aniridia, ambiguous genitalia, mental retardation (intellectual disability) [syndrome]; anticipatory goal res-ponse

agr accessory gene regulator

agri agriculture

AGRP, AgRP agouti-related protein

AGS adrenogenital syndrome; Alagille syndrome; American Geriatrics Society; audiogenic seizures

AGSP Australian Gonococcal Surveillance Programme

AGT abnormal glucose tolerance; activity group therapy; acute generalized tuberculosis; alkylguanine deoxyribonucleic acid alkyltransferase; angiotensin; aniline/glyoxylate aminotransferase; antiglobulin test; Association of Genetic Technologists

agt agent

AGTH adrenoglomerulotropic hormone

AGTr adrenoglomerulotropin

AGTT abnormal glucose tolerance test

AGU aspartylglucosaminuria

AGUS atypia of gland cells of undetermined significance

AGUV aguacate virus

AGV aniline gentian violet

AGVd Australian grapevine viroid

AH abdominal hysterectomy; absorptive hypercalciuria; accidental hypothermia; acetohexamide; acid hydrolysis; acute hepatitis; adrenal hypoplasia; affected hemisphere; afterhyperpolarization; agnathia-holoprosencephaly; alcoholic hepatitis; amenorrhea and hirsutism; aminohippurate; anterior heel; anterior hypothalamus; antihyaluronidase; arcuate hypothalamus; Army Hospital; arterial hypertension; artificial heart; aryl hydrocarbon; ascites hepatoma; assisted hatching; astigmatic hypermetropia; ataxic hemiparesis; atypical hyperplasia; autoimmune hepatitis; autonomic hyperreflexia; axillary hair

A/H amenorrhea-hyperprolactinemia

A+H accident and health

Ah ampere-hours

A·h ampere-hour

aH abhenry

ah hyperopic astigmatism

AHA acetohydroxamic acid; acquired hemolytic anemia; acute hemolytic anemia; American Heart Association; American Hospital Association; anterior hypothalamic area; antiheart antibody; antihistone antibody; area health authority; arthritis, hives, angioedema [syndrome]; aspartyl-hydroxamic acid; autoimmune hemolytic anemia

AHA/ACC American Heart Association/American College of Cardiology [Task Force]

AHB acute hepatitis B; alpha-hydroxybutyric acid

AHC academic health care; academic health center; acute hemorrhagic conjunctivitis; acute hemorrhagic cystitis; adrenal hypoplasia congenita; antihemophilic factor C

AHCA Agency for Health Care Administration; American Health Care Association

AHCD acquired hepatocellular degeneration

AHC/HHG adrenal hypoplasia congenita−hypogonadotropic hypogonadism [syndrome]

aHCl aqueous solution of hydrogen chloride

AHCN American Housecall Network

AHCP allied health care professional

AHCPR Agency for Health Care Policy and Research

AhCPV *Agrochola helvolva* cypovirus

AHCy adenosyl homocysteine

AHD acquired hepatocerebral degeneration; acute heart disease; antihyaluronidase; antihypertensive drug; arteriohepatic dysplasia; arteriosclerotic heart disease; atherosclerotic heart disease; autoimmune hemolytic disease

AHDI Association for Healthcare Documentation Integrity

AHDMS automated hospital data management system

AHDP azacycloheptane diphosphonate

AHDS Allan-Herndon-Dudley syndrome

AHE acute hazardous events; acute hemorrhagic encephalomyelitis

AHEA area health education activity

AHEAD Addiction Health Evaluation and Disease Management; Asset and Health Dynamics

AHEC area health education center

AHEI Alternative Healthy Eating Index

AHES artificial heart energy system

AHF acute heart failure; American Health Foundation; American Hepatic Foundation; American Hospital Formulary; antihemolytic factor; antihemophilic factor; Argentinian hemorrhagic fever; Associated Health Foundation

AHFS American Hospital Formulary Service

AHF SCENE Advanced Heart Failure Shared Clinical Experience Network

AHG aggregated human globulin; antihemophilic globulin; antihuman globulin; arterial hypertension group

AHGG aggregated human gammaglobulin; antihuman gammaglobulin

AHGS acute herpetic gingival stomatitis

AHH alpha-hydrazine analogue of histidine; anosmia and hypogonadotropic hypogonadism [syndrome]; arylhydrocarbon hydroxylase; Association for Holistic Health

AHI acromiohumeral interval; active hostility index; Animal Health Institute; apnea-hypopnea index; applied health informatics

AHIMA American Health Information Management Association

AHIP America's Health Insurance Plans; assisted health insurance plan

AHIS automated hospital information system

AHJ artificial hip joint

AHL apparent half-life

AHLA American Health Lawyers Association

AHLE acute hemorrhagic leukoencephalitis

AHLG antihuman lymphocyte globulin

AHLR actual helium leak rate

AHLS antihuman lymphocyte serum

AHM allied health manpower; ambulatory Holter monitor

AHMA American Holistic Medicine Association; anti–heart muscle autoantibody

AHMC Association of Hospital Management Committees

AHMD alcoholic heart muscle disease

AHN Army Head Nurse; assistant head nurse

AHNA American Holistic Nurses Association

AHNS American Head and Neck Society

AHO acute hematogenous osteomyelitis; Albright hereditary osteodystrophy

AHP accountable health plan/partnership; acute hemorrhagic pancreatitis; after-hyperpolarization; air at high pressure; aminohydroxyphenylalanine; analytic hierarchy process; approved health plan; Assistant House Physician; hyperpolarizing afterpotential

AHPA American Health Planning Association

AHPO anterior hypothalamic preoptic [area]

AHPSR Alliance for Health Policy and Systems Research

AHR antihyaluronidase reaction; aryl hydrocarbon receptor; Association for Health Records; atrial heart rate

aHR adjusted hazard ratio

AhR aryl hydrocarbon receptor

AHRA American Healthcare Radiology Administrators

AHRF acute hypoxemic respiratory failure; American Hearing Research Foundation

AHRQ Agency for Healthcare Research and Quality

AHRTAG Appropriate Health Resources and Technologies Action Group

AHS Academy of Health Sciences; Adventist Health Study; African horse sickness; alveolar hypoventilation syndrome; American Headache Society; American Hernia Society; area health service; assistant house surgeon

AHSA American Health Security Act

AHSDF area health service development fund

AHSG alpha-2HS-glycoprotein

AHSN Assembly of Hospital Schools of Nursing

AHSP AIDS Health Services Program

AHSR Association for Health Services Research

AHSV African horse sickness virus

AHT aggregation half-time; antihyaluronidase titer; augmented histamine test; autogenous hamster tumor

AHTG antihuman thymocyte globulin

AHTP antihuman thymocyte plasma

AHTS antihuman thymus serum

AHU acute hemolytic uremic [syndrome]; air-handling unit; arginine, hypoxanthine, and uracil

AHuG aggregated human immunoglobulin G

AHV Abu Hammad virus; avian herpes-virus

AhV *Atkinsonella hypoxylon* virus

AI accidental injury; accidentally incurred; active ingredient; adiposity index; aggregation index; allergy and immunology; amylogenesis imperfecta; anaphylatoxin inactivator; angiogenesis inhibitor; angiotensin I; anterior insula; anxiety index; aortic incompetence; aortic insufficiency; apical impulse; apnea index; arousal index; articulation index; artificial insemination; artificial intelligence; atherogenic index; atrial insufficiency; autoimmune, autoimmunity; avidity index; axioincisal; first meiotic anaphase

A&I allergy and immunology

ai active ingredient

AIA allylisopropylacetamide; amylase inhibitor activity; antiimmunoglobulin antibody; antiinsulin antibody; aortoiliac aneurysm; aspirin-induced asthma; automated image analysis

AIB aminoisobutyrate; avian infectious bronchitis

AIBA aminoisobutyric acid

AIBS American Institute of Biological Sciences

AIC Akaike information criterion; aminoimidazole carboxamide; Association des Infirmières Canadiennes

A-IC average integrated concentration

AICA anterior inferior cerebellar artery; anterior inferior communicating artery

AI-CAH autoimmune-type chronic active hepatitis

AICAR aminoimidazole carboxamide ribonucleotide

AICD activation-induced cell death; automatic implantable cardioverter-defibrillator

AICE angiotensin I converting enzyme

AICF adaptive impulse correlated filtering; autoimmune complement fixation

AICG appraisal instrument for clinical guidelines

AI/COAG artificial intelligence hemostasis consultant system

AICS acute ischemic coronary syndrome; artery of inferior cavernous sinus

AID acquired immunodeficiency disease; acute infectious disease; acute ionization detector; Agency for International Development; argon ionization detector; artificial insemination by donor; autoimmune deficiency; autoimmune disease; automatic implantable defibrillator; average interocular difference

AIDA automatic interpretation for diagnostic assistance; automatic interpretation of data analysis

AIDCI angle-independent Doppler color imaging

AIDH atypical intraductal hyperplasia

AIDNV *Aedes albopictus* densovirus

AIDP acute idiopathic demyelinating polyneuropathy

AIDS acquired immunodeficiency syndrome

AIDS-KS acquired immunodeficiency syndrome with Kaposi sarcoma

AIDSPIT Artificial Insulin Delivery System Pancreas and Islet Transplantation [study]

AIE acute inclusion-body encephalitis; acute infectious encephalitis; acute infective endocarditis

AIEC adherent invasive *Escherichia coli*

AIEDRP Acute Infection and Early Disease Research Program

AIEP amount of insulin extractable from pancreas

AIF anemia-inducing factor; anti-inflammatory; antiinvasion factor

AIFD acute intrapartum fetal distress

AIFF audio interchange file format

AIG antiimmunoglobulin

AIgE, algE anti−immunoglobulin E antibody

AIH amelogenesis imperfecta, hypomaturation type; American Institute of Homeopathy; artificial insemination, homologous; artificial insemination by husband; autoimmune hemolysis; autoimmune hepatitis; autoimmune-like hepatitis

AIHA American Industrial Hygiene Association; American International Health Alliance; autoimmune hemolytic anemia

AIHC American Industrial Health Conference

AIHD acquired immune hemolytic disease

AIHV alcelaphine herpesvirus

AII acute intestinal infection; angiotensin II; second meiotic anaphase

AIIC Association des Infirmières et Infirmiers du Canada

AIII angiotensin III

AIIR airborne infection isolation room

AIIS anterior inferior iliac spine

AIIT amiodarone-iodine−induced thyrotoxicosis

AIL acute infectious lymphocytosis; angiocentric immunoproliferative lesion; angioimmunoblastic lymphadenopathy

AILA angioimmunoblastic lymphadenopathy; argon ion laser atheroablation

AILD alveolar interstitial lung disease; angioimmunoblastic lymphadenopathy with dysproteinemia

AIM Abridged Index Medicus; acquisition interface module; active ingredient manufacturer; acuity index method; advanced informatics and medicine; all-in medicine; applications integration mechanism; area-of-interest magnification; artificial intelligence in medicine; associate in internal medicine; atypical immature squamous metaplasia

AIMBE American Institute for Medical and Biological Engineering

AIMD abnormal involuntary movement disorder; active implantable medical device

A-IMF areola-to-inframammary fold distance

AIMS abnormal involuntary movement scale; Acylated Plasminogen-Streptokinase Activator Complex [APSAC] Intervention Mortality Study; aid for the impaired medical student; arthritis impact measurement scale; Automated Immunization Management System; automated indexing management system

AIMV alfalfa mosaic virus

AIN acute interstitial nephritis; American Institute of Nutrition; anal intraepithelial neoplasia; anterior interosseous nerve

AINA automated immunonephelometric assay

AINOV Aino virus

AINS anterior interosseous nerve syndrome; antiinflammatory nonsteroidal

AIOD aortoiliac occlusive disease

AION anterior ischemic optic neuropathy

AIOS acute illness observation scale

AIP acute idiopathic pericarditis; acute infectious polyneuritis; acute intermittent porphyria; acute interstitial pneumonia; aldosterone-induced protein; American Institute of Physics; automated immunoprecipitation; average intravascular pressure; integral anatuberculin, Petragnani

AIPE acute interstitial pulmonary emphysema; alcoholism intervention performance evaluation

AIPFP acute idiopathic peripheral facial nerve palsy

AIPRI ACE Inhibition in Progressive Renal Insufficiency [study]

AIPS American Institute of Pathologic Science

AIR acute insulin response; airway responsiveness; American Institutes for Research; amino-imidazole ribonucleotide; aortoiliac reconstruction; automated image registration; average impairment rating

AIRA anti−insulin receptor antibody

AIRE Acute Infarction Ramipril Efficacy [study]; Acute Infarction Ramipril Efficacy [trial]; Acute Infarction Reperfusion Efficacy [study]

AIREX Acute Infarction Ramipril Efficacy Extension [study]

AIRF alterations in respiratory function

AI/RHEUM artificial intelligence rheumatology consultant system

AIRIO Agency for Intramural Research Integrity Officer

AIRS Amphetamine Interview Rating Scale

AIS Abbreviated Injury Scale; absolute increase in survival; acute ischemic stroke; acute ischemic syndrome; adenocarcinoma in situ; administrative information system; adolescent idiopathic scoliosis; aggregate injury score; amniotic infection syndrome; analyzer of interrated sequences [model of a beating ventricle]; androgen insensitivity syndrome; anterior interosseous nerve syndrome; antiinsulin serum; automatic information system; automotive injury score

AISA acquired idiopathic sideroblastic anemia

AISI African Information Society Initiative

AIT acute intensive treatment; aeromedical isolation team

AITD autoimmune thyroid disease

AITIA Aspirin In Transient Ischemic Attacks [study]

AITP autoimmune idiopathic thrombocytopenic purpura

AITT arginine insulin tolerance test; augmented insulin tolerance test

AIU absolute iodine uptake; antigen-inducing unit

AIUM American Institute of Ultrasound in Medicine

AIV Aichi virus

AIVC Australian Influenza Vaccine Committee

AIVR accelerated idioventricular rhythm

AIVV anterior internal vertebral vein

AIX advanced interactive executive

AIx augmentation index

AJ adherens junction; ankle jerk

A/J ankle jerk

AJCC American Joint Committee on Cancer

AJCCS American Joint Committee on Cancer Staging

AJDL arteriojugular venous lactate content difference

AJDO₂ arteriojugular venous oxygen content difference

AJR abdominojugular reflux maneuver; *American Journal of Roentgenology* [formerly *American Journal of Radiology*]

AJS acute joint syndrome

AJT automatic junctional tachycardia

AK above knee; acetate kinase; actinic keratosis; adenosine kinase; adenylate kinase; artificial kidney

A/K, ak above knee

A→K ankle to knee

AKA above-knee amputation; alcoholic ketoacidosis; also known as; antikeratin antibody

aka also known as

AK amp above-knee amputation

AKAV Akabane virus

AKBR arterial ketone body ratio

AKE acrokeratoelastoidosis

A/kg amperes per kilogram

AKP alkaline phosphatase

AKRMLV AKR murine leukemia virus

AKS alcoholic Korsakoff syndrome; auditory and kinesthetic sensation

AKU alkaptonuria

AL absolute latency; acinar lumen; acute leukemia; adaptation level; albumin; alcoholism [and other drug-dependence services]; alignment; amyloid L; amyloidosis; analyzer and loader; anatomic location, anatomic localizer; anterior leaflet; anterolateral;

antihuman lymphocytic [immunoglobulin]; argininosuccinate lyase; avian leukosis; axial length; axillary loop; axiolingual; left ear [L. *auris laeva*]

A$_L$ angiographic area of lateral projection

Al allantoic; allergic, allergy; aluminum

al left ear [L. *auris laeva*]

ALA amebic liver abscess; American Laryngological Association; American Lung Association; aminolevulinate, aminolevulinic acid; axiolabial

ALa axiolabial

Ala, ala alanine

AL-Ab antilymphocyte antibody

ALAD abnormal left axis deviation

ALAD, ALA-D aminolevulinic acid dehydrase; aminolevulinate dehydratase

ALADH aminolevulinate dehydratase

AlaDH alanine dehydrogenase

ALADP aminolevulinic acid dehydrogenase deficiency porphyria

ALAG, ALaG axiolabiogingival

A-LAK adherent lymphokine-activated killer [cell]

ALAL, ALaL axiolabiolingual

A$_{LAO}$ angiographic area of left anterior oblique projection

AlaP, ala-P alafosfalin

ALARA as low as reasonably achievable

ALARM adjustable leg and ankle repositioning mechanism

ALARP as low as reasonably possible

ALAS delta-aminolevulinate synthase

ALASH delta-aminolevulinate synthase, housekeeping type

ALAT alanine aminotransferase

ALB albumin; avian lymphoblastosis

Alb albumin

alb albumin; white [L. *albus*]

ALBC albumin clearance

ALB/GLOB albumin/globulin ratio

ALC absolute lymphocyte count; acute lethal catatonia; aided living center; alternate level of care; Alternative Lifestyle Checklist; approximate lethal concentration; avian leukosis complex; axiolinguocervical

alc alcohol, alcoholic, alcoholism

ALCA anomalous left coronary artery

ALCAPA anomalous origin of left coronary artery from pulmonary artery

ALCAR acetyl-L-carnitine

ALCEQ Adolescent Life Change Event Questionnaire

ALCL anaplastic large cell lymphoma

ALCO Anonymous Fighters Against Obesity

alcoh alcohol, alcoholic, alcoholism

AlCPV *Agrochola lychnidis* cypovirus; *Aporophyla lutulenta* cypovirus

AlCr aluminum crown

AlcR, alcR alcohol rub

ALD adrenoleukodystrophy; alcoholic liver disease; aldehyde dehydrogenase; aldolase; aldosterone; anterior latissimus dorsi; Appraisal of Language Disturbance; approximate lethal dose; assistive listening device

Ald aldolase; aldosterone

ALDA aldolase A

ALDB aldolase B

ALDC afferent lymph dendritic cell; aldolase C

ALDF American Lyme Disease Foundation

ALDH aldehyde dehydrogenase

Aldo aldosterone

ALDOA aldolase A

ALDOC aldolase C

ALDOST aldosterone

ALDP adrenoleukodystrophy protein

ALDR aldose reductase

ALDS albinism-deafness syndrome

ALDUSA Aspirin Low Dosage in Unstable Angina [trial]

ALE active life expectancy; adaptive line enhancer; allowable limits of error; amputated lower extremity

ALEC artificial lung-expanding compound

ALECS acute lower extremity compartment syndrome

ALEP atypical lymphoepithelioid cell proliferation

ALERT Amiodarone vs Lidocaine Inpatient Emergency Resuscitation Trial; Assessment of Lescol in Renal Transplantation [trial]

ALEV Alenquer virus

ALF acute liver failure; advance laser flowmeter; American Liver Foundation; assisted living facilities; automated laser fluorescence

ALFA Assisted Living Federation of America

ALFT abnormal liver function test

ALFV Alfuy virus

ALFW anterolateral free wall

ALG antilymphocytic globulin; axiolinguogingival

alg allergy

ALGOL algorithmic oriented language

ALH angiolymphoid hyperplasia; anterior lobe hormone; anterior lobe of hypophysis

ALHE angiolymphoid hyperplasia with eosinophilia

ALHV alcelaphine herpesvirus

ALI acute lung injury; annual limit of intake; average lobe index

ALICE advanced large-scale integrated computational environment

ALIF anterior lumbar interbody fusion

ALIP abnormal localized immature myeloid precursor

aLIU admission Liver Injury Units

ALIVE Adenosine Lidocaine Infarct Zone Viability Enhancement [trial]; Amiodarone vs. Lidocaine in Prehospital Refractory Ventricular Fibrillation [study]; Azimilide Postinfarction Survival Evaluation [trial]

ALJV Alajuela virus

ALK automated lamellar keratoplasty

ALK, alk alkaline; alkylating

ALK-P, Alk Phos alkaline phosphatase

ALL acute lymphoblastic leukemia; acute lymphocytic leukemia; anterolateral ligament; Antihypertensive and Lipid-Lowering [study]

all allergy, allergic

ALLA acute lymphocytic leukemia antigen

ALLHAT Antihypertensive and Lipid-Lowering Treatment to Prevent Heart Attack Trial

ALLO atypical *Legionella*-like organism

ALM aerial lentiginous melanoma; alveolar living material

ALME acetyl-lysine methyl ester

ALMI anterior lateral myocardial infarct

ALMV Almeirim virus; Almpiwar virus; anterior leaflet of the mitral valve

AlMV alfalfa mosaic virus

ALN allylnitrile; anterior lymph node; axillary lymph node

ALNC advanced legal nurse consultant

ALND axillary lymph node dissection

ALO average lymphocyte output; axiolinguo-occlusal

ALOS average length of stay

ALOSH Appalachian Laboratory for Occupational Safety and Health

ALOX aluminum oxide; arachidonate lipoxygenase

ALOx aluminum oxide

ALP acute leukemia protocol; acute lupus pericarditis; alkaline phosphatase; alveolar proteinosis; anterior lobe of pituitary; antileukoproteinase; antilymphocytic plasma; argon laser photocoagulation; automated linkage preprocessor

AlPase alkaline phosphatase

ALPG alkaline phosphatase, germ-cell

alpha$_2$-AP alpha$_2$-antiplasmin

α$_1$-AT alpha$_1$-antitrypsin

alpha-GLUC alpha-glucosidase

alpha$_2$-M alpha$_2$-macroglobulin

α$_2$-PIPC alpha$_2$-plasmin inhibitor−plasmin complex

ALPL alkaline phosphatase, liver

ALPP alkaline phosphatase, placental

ALPPL alkaline phosphatase−like, placental

ALPS angiolymphoproliferative syndrome; Aphasia Language Performance Scale; attitudinal listening profile system; autoimmune lymphoproliferative syndrome

ALPSA anterior labral periosteal sleeve avulsion; anterior labroligamentous periosteal sleeve avulsion

ALPV aphid lethal paralysis virus

ALR aldehyde reductase

ALRI anterolateral rotatory instability

ALROS American Laryngological, Rhinological, and Otological Society

ALS acute lateral sclerosis; advanced life support; afferent loop syndrome; air leak syndrome; alkali-labile site; amyotrophic lateral sclerosis; angiotensin-like substance; anterolateral sclerosis; anticipated life span; antilymphocyte serum

ALSD Alzheimer-like senile dementia

ALSPAC Avon Longitudinal Study of Pregnancy and Childhood

ALS-PD amyotrophic lateral sclerosis−parkinsonism-dementia [complex]

AlStVa *Alstroemeria* streak virus

AL-SV avian leukosis sarcoma virus

ALT alanine aminotransferase; argon laser trabeculoplasty; autolymphocyte therapy; avian laryngotracheitis

AlT aluminum tartrate

Alt, alt aluminum tartrate; alternate; altitude

ALTB acute laryngotracheobronchitis

ALTE apparent life-threatening event

ALTEE acetyl-L-tyrosine ethyl ester

Alt. hor. every other hour [L. *alternis horis*]

ALTS acute lumbar traumatic sprain/syndrome

ALTV Altamira virus

ALU arithmetic and logic unit

ALV Abelson leukemia virus; adenolike virus; alveolar, alveolus; American latent virus; Arracacha latent virus; ascending lumbar vein; avian leukosis virus

Alv alveolar, alveolus

ALV-A avian leukosis virus A

ALVAD abdominal left ventricular assist device

ALVAL aseptic lymphocyte-dominated vasculitis-associated lesion

ALVF acute left ventricular failure

ALV M alveolar mucosa

ALVT aortic and left ventricular tunnel

alv vent alveolar ventilation
ALVX alveolectomy
ALW arch-loop whorl
ALWMI anterolateral wall myocardial infarct
AM *Academic Medicine* [journal]; actomyosin; acute myelofibrosis; adult male; adult monocyte; aerospace medicine; affected male; akinetic mutism; alcoholic male; alveolar macrophage; alveolar mucosa; amacrine cell; ambulatory; amethopterin; ametropia; ammeter; amperemeter; ampicillin; amplitude modulation; amyl; anovular menstruation; anterior mitral leaflet; antimycotic; arithmetic mean; arousal mechanism; articular manipulation; aviation medicine; axiomesial; meter angle; myopic astigmatism
Am americium; amnion; amyl
A/m amperes per meter
A-m² ampere-square meter
am ametropia; amyl; amplitude; meter angle; myopic astigmatism
AMA against medical advice; alkaline membrane assay; American Management Association; American Medical Association; analog multiplexer array; antimitochondrial antibody; antimyosin antibody; antithyroid microsomal antibody; apocrine membrane antigen; arm muscle area; Australian Medical Association
AMAB assigned male at birth
AMACR α-methylacyl coenzyme A racemase
AMA-DE American Medical Association Drug Evaluation
AMAL Aero-Medical Acceleration Laboratory
AMAN acute motor axonal neuropathy
AMANET, AMA/Net American Medical Association Network
AMAP American Medical Accreditation Program; as much as possible
A-MAT amorphous material
AMAV Amapari virus
AMB amphotericin B; anomalous muscle bundle; anteromedial bundle; avian myeloblastosis
Amb ambulance; ambulatory, ambulation
amb ambient; ambiguous; ambulance; ambulatory
AMBER advanced multiple-beam equalization radiography; assisted model building with energy refinement
ambig ambiguous
AMBL acute megakaryoblastic leukemia
AMbL acute myeloblastic leukemia

AMBRE atraumatic multidirectional bilateral rehabilitation
AMBRI atraumatic, multidirectional bilateral radial instability
ambul ambulatory
AMBV Anhembi virus
AMC academic medical center; acetylmethyl carbinol; Animal Medical Center; antibody-mediated cytotoxicity; antimalaria campaign; arm muscle circumference; Army Medical Corps; arthrogryposis multiplex congenita; ataxia, microcephaly, retardation (intellectual disability) [syndrome]; automated mixture control; axiomesiocervical
AMCAS American Medical College Application Service
AMCB American Midwifery Certification Board
AMCD Aeromedical Certification Division
AMCHA aminomethylcyclohexane-carboxylic acid
aMCI amnestic mild cognitive impairment
AMCN anteromedial caudate nucleus
AmCPV *Antheraea mylitta* cypovirus
AMCRA American Managed Care and Review Association
AMCV avian myelocytomatosis virus
AMD acid maltase deficiency; acromandibular dysplasia; actinomycin D; adrenomy-elodystrophy; advance medical directive; age-related macular degeneration; Aleutian mink disease; alpha-methyldopa; Association for Macular Diseases; axiomesiodistal; S-adenosylmethionine decarboxylase
AMDA American Medical Directors Association
AMDF average magnitude difference function
AMDGF alveolar macrophage-derived growth factor
AMDS Association of Military Dental Surgeons
AMDV Aleutian mink disease virus
AME amphotericin methyl ester; apparent mineralocorticoid excess; aseptic meningo-encephalitis
AMEA American Medical Electroencephalographic Association
AMEAE acute monophasic experimental autoimmune encephalomyelitis
AMED Allied and Complementary Medicine Database; Army Medical Department
AMEDD Army Medical Department
AMEDS Army Medical Service
AMEGL, AMegL acute megakaryoblastic leukemia

AMEND Aiding Mothers and Fathers Experiencing Neonatal Death

AMES age, metastasis, extension, size [thyroid tumor]

AMet adenosyl-L-methionine

AMETHIST Ambroxol Efficacy and Tolerability on Hypersecretion, Italian Study

AMEV *Amsacta moorei* entomopoxvirus

AMF antimuscle factor

Amf amniotic fluid

AMFAR, amfAR American Foundation for AIDS Research

AM/FM automated mapping and facility management

AMFPI active matrix flat-panel imager

AMG alpha-2-macroglobulin; amyloglucosidase; antimacrophage globulin; arterial migraine grinder; axiomesiogingival

A₂MG alpha-2-macroglobulin

AMGA American Medical Group Association

AMH Accreditation Manual for Hospitals; anti-müllerian hormone; automated medical history

Amh mixed astigmatism with myopia predominating over hyperopia

AMHA Association of Mental Health Administrators

AMHIS Alberta Mental Health Information System

AMHT automated multiphasic health testing

AMI acquired monosaccharide intolerance; acute myocardial infarction; advanced medical illness; amitriptyline; anterior my-ocardial−infarction; Argatroban in Myocardial Infarction [study]; Association of Medical Illustrators; Athletic Motivation Inventory; axiomesioincisal

AMIA American Medical Informatics Association

AMIABLE Acute Myocardial Infarction Angioplasty Bolus Lysis Evaluation

AMICUS Austrian Multicenter Isradipine cum Spirapril Study

AMIS Ambulatory Medical Information System; Aspirin in Myocardial Infarction Study; Automated Management Information System

AMISTAD Acute Myocardial Infarction Study of Adenosine

AMKL acute megakaryoblastic leukemia

AML acute monocytic leukemia; acute mucosal lesion; acute myeloblastic leukemia; acute myelocytic leukemia; acute myelogenous leukemia; anatomic medullary locking; angiomyolipoma; anterior mitral leaflet; automated multitest laboratory

AMLB alternate monaural loudness balance

AMLC adherent macrophage-like cell; autologous mixed lymphocyte culture

AMLCD active matrix liquid crystal display

AMLR autologous mixed lymphocyte reaction

AMLS anti−mouse lymphocyte serum

AMLSGA acute myeloblastic leukemia surface glycoprotein antigen

AMM agnogenic myeloid metaplasia; ammonia; antibody to murine cardiac myosin; Association of Medical Microbiologists; World Medical Association [Fr. *Association Médicale Mondiale*]

amm ammonia

AMML acute myelomonocytic leukemia

AMMoL acute myelomonocytic/myelomonoblastic leukemia

ammon ammonia

AMN adrenomyeloneuropathy; alloxazine mononucleotide; aminonucleoside; anterior median nucleus

AMNS aminonucleoside

AMO assistant medical officer; axiomesio-occlusal

AmO alarm object

amo amorphous

A-mod amplitude modulation

A-mode amplitude mode

AMOG adhesion molecule on glia

AMOL, AMoL acute monocytic/monoblastic leukemia

amor amorphous

AMP accelerated mental processes; acid mucopolysaccharide; adenosine monophosphate; Aerospace Medical Panel; 2,3-aminophenazine; 2-amino-2,1-propanol; amphetamine; ampicillin; ampule; amputation; average mean pressure

amp ampere; amplification; amplitude; ampule; amputation, amputee

AMPA alpha-amino-3-hydroxy-5-methyl-4-isoxazolepropionate; American Medical Publishers Association; aminoisopropyl propionic acid

AMPAC American Medical Association Political Action Committee

AMPAR alpha-amino-3-hydroxy-5-methyl-4-isoxazole propionate receptor

AMP-c cyclic adenosine monophosphate

AMPH, amphet amphetamine

amp-hr ampere-hour

AMPI APSAC in Acute Myocardial Infarction Placebo-Controlled Investigation

ampl large [L. *amplus*]

AMPLE allergies, medications, past medical history, last meal, events preceding present condition

A-M pr Austin-Moore prosthesis

Amp-RT amplified reverse transcriptase

AMPS abnormal mucopolysacchariduria; acid mucopolysaccharide

AMPT active mouse protection test; alpha-methylparatyrosine

ampul ampule

AMR acoustic muscle reflex; activity metabolic rate; acute mitral regurgitation; alopecia—mental retardation (intellectual disability) [syndrome]; alternate motion rate; alternating motion reflex; ambulatory medical record

AMRA American Medical Record Association

AMRF American Medical Resources Foundation

AMRI anteromedial rotatory instability

AMRL Aerospace Medical Research Laboratory

AMRNL Army Medical Research and Nutrition Laboratory

AMRO Amsterdam-Rotterdam Trial Comparing Excimer Laser and Percutaneous Transluminal Coronary Angioplasty

AMRS ambulatory medical records system; automated medical record system

AMS ablepharon-microstomia syndrome; accelerator mass spectrometry; act management system; acute mountain sickness; adenosylmethionine synthetase; advanced medical system; aggravated in military service; altered mental status; American Microscopical Society; amount of substance; amylase; antimacrophage serum; Army Medical Service; aseptic meningitis syndrome; Association of Military Surgeons; auditory memory span; automated multiphasic screening

ams amount of a substance

AMSA acridinylamine methanesulfon-*m*-anisidide; American Medical Society on Alcoholism; American Medical Students Association; amsacrine

AMSAODD American Medical Society on Alcoholism and Other Drug Dependencies

AMSC Army Medical Specialist Corps

AMSN Academy of Medical-Surgical Nurses

AMSP Association of Medical School Pharmacology

AMSPC Association of Medical School Pharmacology Chairs

AMSPDC Association of Medical School Pediatric Department Chairs

AMSRDC Army Medical Service Research and Development Command

AMSU ambulatory minor surgery unit

AMSUS Association of Military Surgeons of the United States

AMT acute miliary tuberculosis; Adenosine Scan Multicenter Trial; alpha-methyltyrosine; American Medical Technologists; amethopterin; amitriptyline; amniotic membrane transplantation; amphetamine; anxiety management training; atherogenic metabolic triad

amt amount

AMTV Arumowot virus

amt/vol amount/volume

AMU Army Medical Unit

amu atomic mass unit

AmuLV Abelson murine leukemia virus; amphotrophic murine leukemia virus

AMV alfalfa mosaic virus; apex to mitral valve; assisted mechanical ventilation; asteroid mosaic virus; avian myeloblastosis virus

AMVF additive multiattribute value function

AMVI acute mesenteric vascular insufficiency

aMVL anterior mitral valve leaflet

AMWA American Medical Women's Association; American Medical Writers Association

AMX advanced multiprocessor extension; amoxicillin

AMY, amy amylase

AMyA antimyocardial antibody

AN acanthosis nigricans; acetylnitrile; acne neonatorum; acoustic neuroma; adult, normal; ala nasi; amyl nitrate; aneurysm; anisometropia; anode; anorexia nervosa; antenatal; anterior; antineuraminidase; aseptic necrosis; atmosphere normal; atrionodal; autonomic neuropathy; avascular necrosis

A/N antenatal; as needed

An actinon; anisometropia; anode, anodal; antigen; *Aspergillus niger*; atmosphere normal

A_n atmosphere normal

ANA acetylneuraminic acid; American Narcolepsy Association; American Neurological Association; American Nurses Association; anesthesia; antibody to nuclear antigens; antinuclear antibody; aspartyl naphthylamide

A1-NA A1 area of the nucleus ambiguus

Ana anaplastic

ANAC Association of Nurses in AIDS Care

ANAD anorexia nervosa with associated disorders

ANADA Abbreviated New Animal Drug Application

ANAE alpha-naphthyl acetate esterase

ANAG acute narrow-angle glaucoma

AnalNH anaphylotoxin inhibitor

ANAL, anal analgesia, analgesic; analysis, analytic

ANAM automated neuropsychological assessment metrics

ANAP agglutination negative, absorption positive [reaction]

ANAS anastomosis; auditory nerve activating substance

ANASCD American Nurses Association Steering Committee on Databases

anast anastomosis

ANAT anatomic structure

Anat, anat anatomist, anatomy

ANAV *Anopheles* A virus

ANB alternate nostril breathing; avascular necrosis of bone

ANBN alpha-nitroso-beta-naphthol

ANBP Australian National Blood Pressure [trial]

AN-BP anorexia nervosa with bingeing/purging behaviors

ANBV *Anopheles* B virus

ANC absolute neutrophil count; acid neutralization capacity; active noise control; adaptive noise canceler; adult neuronal ceroid; ancestor; antigen-neutralizing capacity; Army Nurse Corps

ANC₁ ancestor, first level in hierarchy

ANCA antineutrophilic cytoplasmic antibody

ANCC American Nurses Credentialing Center; anodal closure contraction

AnCC anodal closure contraction

ANCHR Access to National Claims History Repository

ANCL adult neuronal ceroid lipofuscinosis

ANCOVA analysis of covariance

ANCR Association of the Nordic Cancer Registries

AND Academy of Nutrition and Dietetics [formerly American Dietetic Association]; algoneurodystrophy; anterior nasal discharge

ANDA Abbreviated New Drug Application

ANDI analytical data interchange

ANDRO, andro androsterone

ANDTE, AnDTe anodal duration tetanus

ANDV Andasibe virus; Andes virus

anes, anesth anesthesia, anesthetic

ANESR apparent norepinephrine secretion rate

AnEx, an ex anodal excitation

ANF alpha-naphthoflavone; American Nurses Foundation; antineuritic factor; antinuclear factor; atrial natriuretic factor

AnfaMNPV *Anagrapha* falciform multiple nucleopolyhedrovirus

ANFO ammonium nitrate fuel oil [explosive]

ANG anagrelide; angiogenin; angiogram, angiography; angiotensin

ANG II, ang II angiotensin II

ang angiogram, angiography; angle, angular

ANGEL a new global environment for learning

ANGFA anti−nerve growth factor antibody

Ang GR angiotensin generation rate

AngHV anguillid herpesvirus

Angio angiogram, angiographic, angiography

ang pect angina pectoris

ANH academic nursing home

anh anhydrous

ANHV Anhanga virus

AnHV anatid herpesvirus

ANI acute nerve irritation

ANIA American Nursing Informatics Association; automated nephelometric immunoassay

ANIM animal

ANIMAL automatic nonlinear image matching and anatomical labeling

ANIS Anorexia Nervosa Inventory for Self-rating

aniso anisocytosis

ANIT alpha-naphthyl-isothiocyanate

ANK, Ank ankyrin

ank ankle

ANL acute nonlymphoblastic leukemia

ANLI antibody negative with latent infection

ANLL acute nonlymphocytic leukemia

ANN Academy of Neonatal Nursing; artificial neural network

Ann annual

ANNA American Nephrology Nurses' Association; antineutrophil nuclear antibody

ann fib annulus fibrosus

ANNP artificial neural network processor

ANOC, AnOC anodal opening contraction

ANOCL anodal opening clonus

ANOCOVA analysis of covariance

ANOP anophthalmia

ANOV, ANOVA analysis of variance

ANP acute necrotizing pancreatitis; adult nurse practitioner; advanced nurse practitioner; ancillary nursing personnel; A-norprogesterone; atrial natriuretic peptide

ANP-A, -B, -C atrial natriuretic peptide A, B, C

A-NPP absorbed normal pooled plasma

ANPR advance notice of public rulemaking

AN-R restricting anorexia nervosa

ANRC American National Red Cross

ANRL antihypertensive neutral renomedullary lipid

ANS acanthion; American National Standards; American Nimodipine Study; American Nutrition Society; 8-anilino-1-naphthalenesulfonic acid; anterior nasal spine; antineutrophilic serum; anti—rat neutrophil serum; Army Nursing Service; arterionephrosclerosis; Associate in Nursing Science; autonomic nervous system

ANSI American National Standards Institute

ANSI-HISPP American National Standards Institute Healthcare Informatics Standards Planning Panel

AN-SIR advice nurse structured implicit review

ANSWER Agency for Toxic Substances and Disease Registry/National Library of Medicine's Workstation for Emergency Response

ANT acoustic noise test; adenine nucleotide translocator; aminonitrothiazole; anterior

ant anterior; antimycin

AntA antimycin A

antag antagonist

ANTENOX Anticoagulant from Enoxaparin [study]

Anth-Gly anthraquinone-glycine

Anth-IDA anthraquinone-iminodiacetate

anti-HB$_c$ antibody to hepatitis B core antigen

anti-HB$_e$ antibody to hepatitis B early antigen

anti-HB$_s$ antibody to hepatitis B surface antigen

anti-PNM Ab anti—peripheral nerve myelin antibody

anti-SSAA(X) anti—silicone surface—associated antigen antibodies

AntLV *Anthriscus* latent virus

ANTOP anorexia nervosa treatment of outpatients

ANTR apparent net transfer rate

ANTU alpha-naphthylthiourea

ANTV Antequera virus

ANT3Y adenine nucleotide translocator 3 Y

ANU artificial neural unit

ANuA antinuclear antibody

ANUG acute necrotizing ulcerative gingivitis

ANUV Ananindeua virus

ANV avian nephritis virus

AnV-S *Aspergillus niger* virus S

ANX annexin

anx anxiety

ANZ Australia and New Zealand [study]

AO abdominal aorta; abdominally obese; achievement orientation; acid output; acridine orange; adult onset; age of onset; ankle orthosis; anodal opening; anterior oblique; antisense oligonucleotide; aorta; aortic opening; arthro-ophthalmopathy; assessment object; atelosteogenesis; atomic orbital; atrioventricular opening; average optical; axio-occlusal

Ao aorta; *Aspergillus ochraceus*

A$_o$ orifice area

A/O atlantooccipital; alert and oriented

A&O alert and oriented

AOA Administration on Aging; Alpha Omega Alpha [Honor Medical Society]; American Optometric Association; American Orthopedic Association; American Orthopsychiatric Association; American Osteopathic Association; ascending aorta

AoA age of acquisition

AOAA amino-oxyacetic acid

AOAC International Association of Official Analytical Collaboration International [previously Association of Official Agricultural Chemists]

AOAP as often as possible

AoArE aortic arch epinephrine

AOAS American Osteopathic Academy of Sclerotherapy

AOB accessory olfactory bulb; alcohol on breath; assignment of benefits

AOBEM American Osteopathic Board of Emergency Medicine

AOBS acute organic brain syndrome

AOC abridged ocular chart; allyloxycarbonyl; amyloxycarbonyl; anodal opening contraction; area of concern; avoidance-oriented coping

AOCA American Osteopathic College of Anesthesiologists

AOCD American Osteopathic College of Dermatology

AOCl anodal opening clonus

AOCN advanced oncology certified nurse

AOCNP advanced oncology certified nurse practitioner

AOCNS advanced oncology certified nurse specialist

AOCP American Osteopathic College of Pathologists

AOCPA American Osteopathic College of Pathologists

AOCPR American Osteopathic College of Proctology

AOCR American Osteopathic College of Radiology; American Osteopathic College of Rheumatology

AOD Academy of Operative Dentistry; Academy of Oral Dynamics; adult-onset diabetes; anesthesiologist on duty; arterial

oxygen desaturation; arteriosclerotic occlusive disease; auriculoosteodysplasia
AODM adult-onset diabetes mellitus
AODME Academy of Osteopathic Directors of Medical Education
AODP alcohol and other drug problems
AOE admission order entry
AoE aortic epinephrine
AOHA American Osteopathic Hospital Association
AoHV aotine herpesvirus
AOI apnea of infancy
AoIR Association of Internet Researchers
AOIVM angiographically occult intracranial vascular malformation
AOL acroosteolysis
AOM acute otitis media; alternatives of management; arthroophthalmopathy; azoxymethane
AOMA American Occupational Medical Association
AOMP, AoMP aortic mean pressure
AON anterior olfactory nucleus
AONE American Organization of Nurse Executives
AOO anodal opening odor; atrial asynchronous [pacemaker]
AOP anodal opening picture; aortic pressure
AoP aortic pressure
AOPA American Orthotic and Prosthetic Association
AOPC adult outpatient psychotherapy clinic
AOPW, AoPW aortic posterior wall
AOR adjusted odds ratio; Alvarado Orthopedic Research; auditory oculogyric reflex
AORN Association of Perioperative Registered Nurses
AOS American Ophthalmological Society; American Otological Society; anodal opening sound; anterior esophageal sensor
A₂-os aortic second sound, opening snap
AOSF adaptive order statistic filter
AOSSM American Orthopedic Society for Sports Medicine
AOT accessory optic tract; acute occlusive thrombus/thrombosis; Anderson Olsson table; anodal opening tetanus; Association of Occupational Therapists
AOTA American Occupational Therapy Association
AOTe anodal opening tetanus
AOTF American Occupational Therapy Foundation
AOU apparent oxygen utilization
AOV aortic valve
AoV aortic valve; *Aspergillus ochraceus* virus

4-AP 4-aminopyridine
AP abdominal pain; abdominal pressure; abdominoperitoneal; accelerated phase; accessory pathway; accounts payable; acid phosphatase; acinar parenchyma; action plan; action potential; activator protein; active pepsin; active pressure; acute pancreatitis; acute phase; acute pneumonia; acute proliferative; adductor pollicis; adenomatous polyposis; adolescent psychiatry; after parturition; agno protein; alkaline phosphatase; alum precipitated; aminopeptidase; aminopyrine; amyloid P-component; amyloid peptide; anatomic profile; angina pectoris; ankle pump; antepartal [L. *ante partum*]; anterior pituitary; anteroposterior; antidromic potential; antiplasmin; antipyrine; antiviral protein; antral peristalsis; aortic pressure; aortopulmonary; apical pulse; apothecary; appendectomy; appendicitis; appendix; apurinic acid; apurinic/apyrimidinic; area postrema; arithmetic progression; arterial pressure; artificial pneumothorax; aspiration pneumonia; assessment and plans; association period; atherosclerotic plaque; atrial pacing; atrioventricular pathway; attending physician; authorized person; axiopulpal; before parturition [L. *ante partum*]
A-P anteroposterior
A&P anterior and posterior; assessment and plans; auscultation and percussion
A/P abdominal/perineal; antepartum; ascites/plasma ratio
A₂ P₂ aortic second sound, pulmonary second sound
Ap apex
A_p amount in plasma
aP acellular pertussis [vaccine]
ap anteroposterior; attachment point
APA action potential amplitude; aldosterone-producing adenoma; Ambulatory Pediatric Association; American Pancreatic Association; American Pharmaceutical Association; American Physiotherapy Association; American Podiatric Association; American Psychiatric Association; American Psychological Association; American Psychopathological Association; American Psychotherapy Association; aminopenicillanic acid; anterior margin of pulmonary artery; antipernicious anemia; antiphospholipid antibody; antiproliferative antibody; arcuate premotor area; aseptic processing area; azidophenacyl
ApA adenylyl (3′-5′) adenosine; azidophenacyl
APAAP alkaline phosphatase-antialkaline phosphatase

APAB, APAb antiphospholipid antibody; azidophenacyl bromide

APACHE Acute Physiology, Age, and Chronic Health Evaluation

APACS analog picture archiving and communication system

APAF antipernicious anemia factor

Apaf-1 apoptotic protease activating factor 1

APAGBI Association of Paediatric Anaesthetists of Great Britain and Ireland

APAMI Asian Pacific Association of Medical Informatics

APAN Asian-Pacific Advanced Network

APAP acetaminophen; adaptive positive airway pressure

APASS Antiphospholipid Antibodies in Stroke Studies

APASTB Asia Pacific Association of Surgical Tissue Banking

APB abductor pollicis brevis; atrial premature beat

APBD adult polyglucosan body disease

APBI accelerated partial breast irradiation

APC acetylsalicylic acid, phenacetin, and caffeine; activated protein C; adenoidal pharyngeal conjunctival; adenomatous polyposis coli; aerobic plate count; allophyocyanin; all-purpose capsule; antigen-presenting cell; antiphlogistic corticoid; aortopulmonary collateral artery; aperture current; apneustic center; argon plasma coagulation; aspirin-phenacetin-caffeine; atrial premature contraction; autologous platelet concentrate

aPC activated protein C

ApCAM aplasia cell adhesion molecule

APCC aspirin-phenacetin-caffeine-codeine

APCD acquired prothrombin complex deficiency [syndrome]; adult polycystic disease

APCF acute pharyngoconjunctival fever

APCG apex cardiogram

Ap4CH apical four-chamber plane

APCKD adult-type polycystic kidney disease

APCO arterial pressure-based cardiac output

ApCPV *Anaitis plagiata* cypovirus; *Antheraea pernyi* cypovirus

APC-R, APCR activated protein-C resistance

APD acquired perforating dermatosis; action potential duration; acute polycystic disease; adult polycystic disease; advanced physical diagnosis; airway pressure disconnect; anteroposterior diameter; antipsychotic drug; articulation-phonologic disorder; atrial premature depolarization; autoimmune progesterone dermatitis; automated peritoneal dialysis; avalanche photodiodes

APD$_{80}$ action potential duration at 80% repolarization

A-PD anteroposterior diameter

APD$_b$ action potential duration, baseline beat

APDF amplitude probability density function

APDI Adult Personal Data Inventory

APDIM Association of Program Directors in Internal Medicine

ApDNV *Aedes pseudoscutellaris* densovirus

APD$_p$ action potential duration, premature stimulus

AP-DRG all patients, diagnosis-related group

APE acetone powder extract; acute polioencephalitis; acute psychotic episode; acute pulmonary edema; airway pressure excursion; aminophylline, phenobarbital, and ephedrine; anterior pituitary extract; asthma of physical effort; avian pneumoencephalitis

APE (test) Antimicrobial Preservative Effectiveness Test [called also AET, PET]

APECED autoimmune polyendocrinopathy-candidiasis–ectodermal dysplasia; autoimmune polyendocrinopathy-candidiasis–ectodermal dystrophy

ApEn approximate entropy

APES aminopropyltriethoxysilane

APEUV Apeu virus

APEX automatic programmable electronic matrix

APF acidulated phosphofluoride; adaptive pattern filtering; American Psychological Foundation; anabolism-promoting factor; animal protein factor; antiperinuclear factor; assigned protection factor

APG acid-precipitated globulin; air plethysmography; ambulatory patient group; animal pituitary gonadotropin; antegrade pyelography

APGAR American Pediatric Gross Assessment Record

APGL alkaline phosphatase activity of granular leukocytes

APGO Association of Professors of Gynecology and Obstetrics

APH alcohol-positive history; alternative pathway hemolysis; aminoglycoside phosphotransferase; antepartum hemorrhage; anterior pituitary hormone; Association of Private Hospitals

Aph aphasia

APHA American Protestant Hospital Association; American Public Health Association

APhA American Pharmacists Association

APHEA Air Pollution in Health, European Approach

APHIS Animal and Plant Health Inspection Service

APHL Association of Public Health Laboratories

APHON Association of Pediatric Hematology and Oncology Nurses

APHP anti-*Pseudomonas* human plasma

API active pharmaceutical ingredient; alkaline protease inhibitor; Analytical Profile Index; annual parasitological index; application program interface; applications programming interface; arterial pressure index; atmospheric pressure ionization; Autonomy Preference Index

APIC Acenocoumarin vs. Pentoxifylline in Intermittent Claudication [trial]; Association for Practitioners in Infection Control; Association for Professionals in Infection Control and Epidemiology

APIE assessment, plan, implementation, and evaluation

APIM Association Professionnelle Internationale des Médecins

APIP additional personal injury protection

APIS Antihypertensive Patch, Italian Study

APIVR artificial pacemaker-induced ventricular rhythm

aPKC atypical protein kinase C

APKD adult-onset polycystic kidney disease

APKH acquired progressive kinking of the hair

APL abductor pollicis longus; accelerated painless labor; acute promyelocytic leukemia; animal placenta lactogen; anterior pituitary—like; anterior pulmonary leaflet

aPL antiphospholipid

A-P&L anteroposterior and lateral

APLA, aPLA antiphospholipid antibody

APLAUD Antiplatelet Useful Dose [trial]

APLAUSE Antiplatelet Treatment After Intravascular Ultrasound Guided Optimal Stent Expansion [trial]

APLP amyloid precursor—like protein

APLPV American plum line pattern virus

APLS advanced pediatric life support; antiphospholipid antibody syndrome

APLV Andean potato latent virus

APM Academy of Physical Medicine; acid precipitable material; admission pattern monitoring; affected pedigree member; alternating pressure mattress; alternative payment models; anterior papillary muscle; anteroposterior movement; apical plasma membrane; aspartame; Association of Professors of Medicine

APMA American Podiatric Medical Association

APML acute promyelocytic leukemia

APMOMS Advisory Panel on the Mission and Organization of Medical Schools

APMoV Andean potato mottle virus

APMV avian paramyxovirus

ApMV apple mosaic virus

APN acute pyelonephritis; advanced practice nurse; Alliance for Psychosocial Nursing; average peak noise

APNA American Psychiatric Nurses Association

APNCU adequacy of prenatal care utilization

APNH antiporter sodium-hydrogen ion

APO abductor pollicis obliquus; acquired pendular oscillation; Adriamycin, prednisone, vincristine; adverse patient occurrence; aphoxide; apolipoprotein; apomorphine; apoprotein

Apo, apo apolipoprotein

APOA, apoA apolipoprotein A

APOB, apoB apolipoprotein B

APOC African Program for Onchocerciasis Control; apolipoprotein C

apoC apolipoprotein C

APOE, apoE apolipoprotein E

APOIV Apoi virus

APOJ, apoJ apolipoprotein J

APORF acute postoperative renal failure

apoth apothecary

APP abdominal perfusion pressure; acute phase protein; alum-precipitated pyridine; aminopyrazolopyrimidine; amyloid peptide precursor; amyloid precursor protein; antiplatelet plasma; aqueous procaine penicillin; automated physiologic profile; average pixel projection; avian pancreatic polypeptide

App, app appendix

APPA American Psychopathological Association; 4-aminophenylacetic acid

appar apparatus

APPC application/advanced program-to-program communication

APPCPT atom and physicochemical property class pair and torsion

APPCR, AP-PCR arbitrarily primed polymerase chain reaction

APPG aqueous procaine penicillin G

APPI Active Persantine in Postischemic Injury [study]

appl appliance; application, applied

APPROACH Alberta Provincial Project for Outcomes Assessment in Coronary Heart Disease

approp appropriate

approx approximate

APPS amyloid precursor protein secretase
APPT Adolescent Pediatric Pain Tool
Appt, appt appointment
appx appendix
appy appendectomy
APR abdominoperineal resection; absolute proximal reabsorption; acute phase reaction/reactant; air-purifying respiratory [particulate respirators, gas masks]; amebic prevalence rate; anatomic porous replacement; annual product review; anterior pituitary reaction; average payment rate
APRAISE Antisense to Prevent Restenosis After Intervention, Stent Evaluation [trial]
aprax apraxia
APRI aspartate aminotransferase/platelet ratio index
APRICOT Antithrombotics in the Prevention of Reocclusion in Coronary Thrombolysis [trial]; Aspirin vs Coumadin Trial; Aspirin vs Coumadin in the Prevention of Reocclusion and Recurrent Ischemia After Successful Thrombolysis Trial
APRL American Prosthetic Research Laboratory
APRN advanced practice registered nurse
AProL acute promyelocytic leukemia
APRP acidic proline-rich protein; acute phase reactant protein
APRT adenine phosphoribosyl transferase
APRV airway pressure release ventilation
APS acute physiology score; adenosine phosphosulfate; advanced photon source; American Pain Society; American Pediatric Society; American Physiological Society; American Proctologic Society; American Prosthodontic Society; American Psychological Society; American Psychosomatic Society; aminopropylsilane; ammonium persulfate; analog processing stage; annual person summary; antiphospholipid antibody syndrome; attending physician's statement; Australian Psychological Society; autoimmune polyglandular syndrome; automated patent system; average pain sensitivity; prostate-specific antigen
APSA American Pediatric Surgical Association
APsaA American Psychoanalytic Association
APSAC acylated plasminogen-streptokinase activator complex; anisoylated plasminogen-streptokinase activator complex
APSD aerodynamic particle size distribution; aorticopulmonary septal defect
ApSDs apical suction devices
APSF Anesthesia Patient Safety Foundation

APSGN acute poststreptococcal glomerulonephritis
APSIS Angina Prognosis Study in Stockholm; Angina Prognosis Study with Isoptin and Seloken [trial]
APSP assisted peak systolic pressure
APSQ Abbreviated Patient Symptom Questionnaire
APSS anterior pull skin stretch; Associated Professional Sleep Societies; Association for the Psychophysiological Study of Sleep
APSU Australian Paediatric Surveillance Unit
APT Ablate and Pace Trial; alum-precipitated toxoid; aminophenylthioether; antiplatelet trials; applied potential tomography; automatic peak tracing
APTA American Physical Therapy Association
APTD Aid to Permanently and Totally Disabled
APTES γ-aminopropyltriethoxysilane
APTF American Physical Therapy Foundation
APTH ambulatory blood pressure monitoring and treatment of hypertension
APTI airway pressure time index
APTT, aPTT activated partial thromboplastin time
APUD amine precursor uptake and decarboxylation
APV abnormal posterior vector; *Acyrthosiphon pisum* virus; amprenavir
aPV acellular pertussis vaccine
APVC anomalous pulmonary venous connection
APVT acute portal vein thrombosis
APW alkaline peptone water
APWS attending physician work station
AQ achievement quotient; acoustic quantification; anthraquinone; any quantity; aphasia quotient; autism-spectrum quotient
aq aqueous; water [L. *aqua*]
AQAB acquired abnormality
AQCESS Automated Quality of Care Evaluation Support System
AQIS Australian Quarantine and Inspection Service
AQL acceptable quality level
AQLQ Asthma Quality of Life Questionnaire
AQMS acute quadriplegic myopathy syndrome
AQP aquaporin
AQS additional qualifying symptoms
AQSIQ Administration of Quality Supervision, Inspection, and Quarantine
aqu aqueous

AR absolute risk; acceptable risk; accounts receivable; achievement ratio; acrosome reaction; actinic reticuloid [syndrome]; active resistance; acute rejection; acute relapse; adherence ratio; admission rate; admitting room; adrenergic receptor; adrenodoxin reductase; airway resistance; alarm reaction; alcohol related; alkali reserve; allergic rhinitis; allowance region; alloy restoration; ambulance report; amphiregulin; amplitude ratio; analytical reagent; androgen receptor; anterior root; aortic regurgitation; apical-radial; Argyll Robertson [pupil]; aromatase; arsphenamine; articulare; artificial respiration; ascorbate reductase; assisted respiration; at risk; atrial rate; atrial reversal; atrophic rhinitis; augmented reality; autoradiography; autoregressive; autosomal recessive

A₁R adenosine A_1 receptor

A/R apical/radial

A&R advised and released

Ar argon; articulare

Aᵣ relative atomic mass

ar aromatic

ARA Academy of Rehabilitative Audiology; Academy of Rehabilitative Audiometry; acetylene reduction activity; adenine regulating agent; American Rheumatological Association; anorectal agenesis; anorectal angle; antireticulin antibody; aortic root angiogram; arabinose; Associate of the Royal Academy; Axenfeld-Rieger (anomaly) syndrome

ara arabinose

ara-A adenine arabinoside

Ara-C arabinosylcytidine

ara-C cytosine arabinose; cytosine arabinoside

ARAL adjustment reaction to adult life

ARAM antigen recognition activation motif

ARAMIS American Rheumatism Association Medical Information System

Aᵣₐₒ angiographic area of right anterior oblique projection

ARAS ascending reticular activating system

ARAT Action Research Arm Test

ara-U arabinosyluracil

ARAV Araguari virus

ARB adrenergic receptor binder; angiotensin receptor blocker

arb arbitrary unit

ARBD alcohol-related birth defects

ARBV Arbia virus

ARC absolute reticulocyte count; accelerating rate calorimetry; Accreditation Review Council; acquired immunodeficiency syndrome [AIDS]; active renin concentration;

American Red Cross; anomalous retinal correspondence; antigen reactive cell; arcuate; Arthritis Rehabilitation Center; arthrogryposis, renal dysfunction, cholestasis [syndrome]; atypical reparative changes; automatic exposure control

ARCA acquired red cell aplasia

ARCD age-related cognitive decline; alcohol-related cognitive disorder

ARCH Amiodarone Reduces Coronary Artery Bypass Grafting Hospitalization [trial]; automated record for child health

ARCI Addiction Research Center Inventory

ARCOS Auckland Region Coronary or Stroke [study]

ARCS Associate of the Royal College of Science; Atherosclerosis Risk in Communities Study

ARC-ST Accreditation Review Council for Educational Programs in Surgical Technology

ARD absolute reaction of degeneration; acute radiation disease; acute respiratory disease; adult respiratory distress; allergic respiratory disease; ancillary report display; anorectal dressing; aortic root diameter; arthritis and rheumatic disease; atopic respiratory disease

AR-DLMD autosomal recessive Duchenne-like muscular dystrophy

ARDMS American Registry of Diagnostic Medical Sonographers

ARDS acute respiratory distress syndrome; adult respiratory distress syndrome

ARE active-resistive exercises; AIDS-related encephalitis; antioxidant response element

AREDS Age-Related Eye Disease Study

AREDYLD acrorenal field defect, ectodermal dysplasia, lipoatrophic diabetes [syndrome]

AREPA acetazolamide-responsive familial paroxysmal ataxia

ARES antireticuloendothelial serum

ARF acute renal failure; acute respiratory failure; acute rheumatic fever; Addiction Research Foundation; ambulance report form; area resource file

ARFC active rosette-forming T-cell; autologous rosette-forming cell

ARFD acrorenal field defect

ARFI acoustic radiation force impulse

ARFI-SWS acoustic radiation force impulse shear wave speed

AR-FSP autosomal recessive familial spastic paraplegia

ARG, Arg arginine

arg arginine; silver [L. *argentum*]

ARGAMI Argatroban Compared with Heparin in Myocardial Infarction Treated with Recombinant Tissue Plasminogen Activator [study]

ARGS antitrypsin-related gene sequence

ArGV *Artogeia rapae* granulovirus

ARI absolute risk increase; activation-recovery interval; acute renal insufficiency; acute respiratory illness or infection; airway reactivity index; aldolase reductase inhibitor; annual rate of infection; anxiety reaction, intense

ARIA acetylcholine receptor—inducing activity; allergic rhinitis and its impact on asthma; automated radioimmunoassay

ARIC acrosome reaction ionophore challenge [test]; Atherosclerosis Risk in Communities [study]

ARIF Aggressive Research Intelligence Facility

ARIMA autoregressive integrated moving average

ARIN Association for Radiologic and Imaging Nursing

ARIS Andrology Research Information System; Anturan Reinfarction Italian Study; autoregulated inspiratory support

ARJ anorectal junction

Ar Kr argon-krypton [laser]

ARKV Arkonam virus

ARL Association of Research Libraries; average remaining lifetime

ARLD alcohol-related liver disease

AR-LGMD autosomal recessive limb-girdle muscular dystrophy

ArLV artichoke latent virus

ArLVM artichoke latent virus M

ArLVS artichoke latent virus S

ARM adrenergic receptor material; advanced respiratory mechanics; aerosol rebreathing method; ambulatory renal monitor; anorectal manometry; anxiety reaction, mild; arginine-rich motif; Armenian [hamster]; artificial rupture of membranes; associations rule mining [algorithm]; atomic resolution microscopy

ARMA autoregressive moving average

ARMD age-related muscle degeneration; age-related macular degeneration

ARMS access by radial artery multilink stent; adverse reaction monitoring system; amplification refractory mutation system

ARMV Arumateua virus

ARN acute renal necrosis; acute retinal necrosis; arcuate nucleus; Association of Rehabilitation Nurses

ARNMD Association for Research in Nervous and Mental Diseases

ARNP Advanced Registered Nurse Practitioner

ARNSHL autosomal recessive non-syndromic hearing loss

ARNT aryl hydrocarbon nuclear translocator; aryl hydrocarbon receptor nuclear translocator

ARNV Aruana virus

ARO adjusted relative odds; Association for Research in Ophthalmology

AROA autosomal recessive ocular albinism

AROAV Aroa virus

AROM active range of motion; artificial rupture of membranes

arom aromatic

ARP absolute refractory period; address resolution protocol; American Registry of Pathologists; American Registry of Pathology; anticipated recovery path; apolipoprotein regulatory protein; assay reference plasma; assimilation regulatory protein; atrial refractory period; at-risk period; automaticity recovery phase

ARPA Advanced Research Projects Agency; anterior lateral retroperitoneal approach

ARPANET Advanced Research Projects Agency Network

ARPC Akaike relative power contribution

ARPD autosomal recessive polycystic disease

ARPES angular resolved photoelectron spectroscopy

ARPKD autosomal recessive polycystic kidney disease

ARPT American Registry of Physical Therapists

ARR absolute risk reduction; aldosterone/renin ratio; aortic root replacement

arr arrest, arrested

ARRC Associate of the Royal Red Cross

ARREST Amiodarone in Out-of-Hospital Resuscitation of Refractory Sustained Ventricular Tachyarrhythmia; Amsterdam Resuscitation Study

ARRP autosomal recessive retinitis pigmentosa

ARRS American Roentgen Ray Society

ARRT American Registry of Radiologic Technologists

ARS acquiescence response scale; acute radiation sickness/syndrome; adult Reye syndrome; alcohol-related seizure; alizarin red S; American Radium Society; American Rhinologic Society; antirabies serum; arsphenamine; arylsulfatase; Atherogenic Risk Study; autonomously replicating sequence

Ars arsphenamine
ARSA arylsulfatase A
ARSAC Administration of Radioactive Substances Advisory Committee
ARSACS autosomal recessive spastic ataxia of Charlevoix-Saguenay
ARSB arylsulfatase B
ARSC arylsulfatase C; Associate of the Royal Society of Chemistry
ARSM acute respiratory system malfunction
ARSPH Associate of the Royal Society for the Promotion of Health
ART absolute retention time; abuse-related technology; Accredited Record Technician; Achilles reflex time; acoustic reflex test; acoustic reflex threshold; adaptive resonance theory; algebraic reconstruction technique; AngioJet Rapid Thrombectomy Catheter [study]; antiretroviral therapy; artery; assisted reproductive technique; automated radiation therapy; automated reagin test; automaticity recovery time
art arterial, artery; articulation; artificial
ARTF artificial
arth arthritis
artic articulated, articulation
artif artificial
ARTIS HIV/AIDS Treatment Information Service
ARTISTIC Angiorad Radiation Technology for In-Stent Restenosis Trial in Coronaries
ARTMAP adaptive resonance theory mapping
Art O₂ arterial oxygen flow
ARTS Arterial Revascularization Therapies Study
ARU arthritis rehabilitation unit
ARUAV Aruac virus
ARV Adelaide River virus; AIDS related virus; anterior right ventricle; antiretroviral; avian orthoreovirus; avian reovirus
ARV-A, to -F Aquareoviruses A to F
ARVC arrhythmogenic right ventricular cardiomyopathy
ARVD arrhythmogenic right ventricular dysplasia
ARVO Association for Research in Vision and Ophthalmology.
ARVP arginine-vasopressin
ARX autoregressive with exogenous input [model]
AS above scale; absence of seizures; access service; acetylstrophanthidin; acidified serum; acoustic schwannoma; acoustic stimulation; active sarcoidosis; active sleep; active surveillance; Adams-Stokes [syndrome]; adolescent suicide; aerosol

sensitivity; aerosol sensitization; allele-specific; Alport syndrome; alveolar sac; amphetamine sulfate; amyloid substance; anabolic steroid; anal sphincter; androsterone sulfate; Angelman syndrome; angiosarcoma; ankylosing spondylitis; anovulatory syndrome; anterior synechia; anteroseptal; anterosuperior; antiserum; antisocial; antistreptolysin; antral spasm; anxiety state; aortic sound; aortic stenosis; approaching significance; aqueous solution; aqueous suspension; archives server; area of stenosis; arteriosclerosis; artificial sweetener; aseptic meningitis; asparagine synthetase; Asperger syndrome; assisted suicide; astigmatism; asymmetric; atherosclerosis; atrial septum; atrial stenosis; atropine sulfate; audiogenic seizure; AutoSuture; left ear [L. *auris sinistra*]
As arsenic; astigmatism; asymptomatic
A(s) asplenia syndrome
A·s ampere second
A/s ampere per second
Aₛ shifted ligand concentration
aS absiemens
as left ear [L. *auris sinistra*]
ASA acetylsalicylic acid; active systemic anaphylaxis; acute severe asthma; Adams-Stokes attack; ambulatory services architecture; American Society of Anesthesiologists; American Standards Association; American Surgical Association; aminosalicylic acid; anterior spinal artery; antibody to surface antigen; argininosuccinic acid; arylsulfatase-A; aspirin-sensitive asthma; asthma—nasal polyps—aspirin intolerance
ASAAC Acetylsalicylic Acid Aorto-Coronary Bypass Surgery; Acetylsalicylic Acid vs. Anticoagulants [study]
ASAAD American Society for the Advancement of Anesthesia in Dentistry
ASABs antisperm antibodies
ASAC acidified serum—acidified complement
ASAH antibiotic-sterilized aortic valve homograft
ASAHP American Society of Allied Health Professions
ASAIO American Society for Artificial Internal Organs
ASAL arginosuccinic acid lyase
ASAM American Society of Addiction Medicine
ASAP Academic Strategic Alliance Program; Acetylsalicylic Acid Persantine [study]; American Society for Adolescent Psychology; apparatus for sensing accuracy

of position; arbitrary signatures from amplification profiles; Areawide Stroke Awareness Program; as soon as possible; Azimilide Supraventricular Arrhythmia Program [trial]

ASAPS American Society of Aesthetic Plastic Surgery

ASAS Anderson Symptom Assessment Scale; argininosuccinate synthetase

ASAT aspartate aminotransferase

ASB American Society of Bacteriologists; anencephaly–spina bifida [syndrome]; anesthesia standby; Anxiety Scale for the Blind; asymptomatic bacteriuria

ASBE Applied Spinal Biomechanical Engineering [techniques]

ASBH American Society for Bioethics and Humanities

ASBMT American Society for Blood and Marrow Transplantation

ASBS American Society for Bariatric Surgery

ASC acetylsulfanilyl chloride; acute suppurative cholangitis; altered state of consciousness; ambulatory surgical center; American Society of Cytopathology; anterior subcapsular cataract; antibody-secreting cell; antigen-sensitive cell; apoptosis-associated speck-like protein with a caspase-recruitment domain; ascorbate, ascorbic acid; asthma symptom checklist; auditory sequence comparison; automatic sensitivity control

asc anterior subcapsular; ascending

ASCA anti–*Saccharomyces cerevisiae* antibody

ASCAD atherosclerotic coronary artery disease

AscAo ascending aorta

ASCB Asymptomatic Cervical Bruit [study]

ASCH American Society of Clinical Hypnosis

ASCI Accelerated Strategic Computing Initiative; acute spinal cord injury; American Society for Clinical Investigation; automated stress relaxation and creep indentation

ASCIA American Spinal Cord Injury Association

ASCII American Standard Code for Information Interchange

ASCIPRO Academy of Spinal Cord Injury Professionals

ASCLS American Society for Clinical Laboratory Science

ASCLT American Society of Clinical Laboratory Technicians

ASCMS American Society of Contemporary Medicine and Surgery

ASCN American Society for Clinical Nutrition

ASCO American Society of Clinical Oncology; American Society of Contemporary Ophthalmology

ASCOT Anglo-Scandinavian Cardiac Outcomes Trial; a severity characterization of trauma

ASCOTA American Student Committee of the Occupational Therapy Association

ASCP American Society for Clinical Pathology; American Society of Consultant Pharmacists

AsCPV *Actias selene* cypovirus; *Agrotis segetum* cypovirus

ASCR American Society of Chiropodical Roentgenology

ASCRS American Society of Colon and Rectal Surgeons

ASCS admissions scheduling system

ASCT American Society for Cytotechnology; autologous stem cell transplantation

ASCUS atypia of squamous cells of undetermined significance

ASCUS-H atypical squamous cell of undetermined significance, high-grade squamous intraepithelial lesion

ASCUS-L atypical squamous cell of undetermined significance, low-grade squamous intraepithelial lesion

ASCVD arteriosclerotic cardiovascular disease; atherosclerotic cardiovascular disease

ASD adaptive seating device; aldosterone secretion defect; Alzheimer senile dementia; antisiphon device; argininosuccinic acid synthetase deficiency; arthritis syphilitica deformans; arthroscopic subacromial decompression; atrial septal defect; autistic spectrum disorder, autism spectrum disorder

ASDA American Sleep Disorders Association

ASDB Active Substance Database; Annotation and Similarity [protein] Database

ASDC American Society of Dentistry for Children; Association of Sleep Disorders Centers

A-SDC anomaly–symptomatic deformity complex

ASDE Accelerated Strategic Computing Initiative [ASCI] Simulation Development Environment

ASDH acute subdural hematoma/hemorrhage

ASDOS Atrial Septal Defect Occlusion System [study]

ASDP anal sphincter dysplasia

ASDS American Society for Dermatological Surgery

ASE acute stress erosion; American Society of Electrocardiography; application service element; axilla, shoulder, and elbow

ASES American Shoulder and Elbow Surgeons

ASEX Arizona Sexual Experiences Scale

ASF African swine fever; aniline-sulfur-formaldehyde

ASFR age-specific fertility rate

ASFV African swine fever virus

ASG advanced cell group; American Society for Genetics; Army Surgeon General; aspermatogenesis

ASGBI Association of Surgeons of Great Britain and Ireland

ASGD American Society for Geriatric Dentistry

ASGE American Society for Gastrointestinal Endoscopy

ASGP asialoglycoprotein

AS/GP antiserum, guinea pig

ASGR asialoglycoprotein receptor

ASH Action on Smoking and Health; aldosterone-stimulating hormone; alkylosing spinal hyperostosis; American Society of Hematology; antistreptococcal hyaluronidase; asymmetric septal hypertrophy

A&Sh arm and shoulder

AsH astigmatism, hypermetropic

ASHA American School Health Association; American Social Health Association; American Speech-Language-Hearing Association

ASHAC AIDS self-help and care

ASHBEAMS American Society of Hospital-Based Emergency Aeromedical Services

ASHBM Associate Scottish Hospital Bureau of Management

ASHCRM American Society of Health Care Risk Managers

ASHCSP American Society for Healthcare Central Service Personnel

ASHCVD atherosclerotic hypertensive cardiovascular disease

ASHD arteriosclerotic heart disease; atrioseptal heart disease

ASHE American Society for Healthcare Engineering

ASHET American Society for Health Manpower Education and Training

ASHFSA American Society for Healthcare Food Service Administrators

ASHG American Society for Human Genetics

ASHHRA American Society for Healthcare Human Resources Administration

ASHI Association for the Study of Human Infertility

ASHL Association of Scottish Health Science Librarians

ASHM Australasian Society for HIV Medicine

ASHN acute sclerosing hyaline necrosis

AS/Ho antiserum, horse

ASHP American Society for Hospital Planning; American Society of Health-System Pharmacists

ASHPA American Society for Hospital Personnel Administration

ASHRM American Society for Healthcare Risk Management

ASHT American Society of Hand Therapists

ASHV Arctic squirrel hepatitis virus

ASI activated stroma index; Addiction Severity Index; anxiety state inventory; anxiety status inventory; arthroscopic screw installation

a-Si amorphous silicon

ASIA American Spinal Cord Injury Association; American Spinal Injury Association

ASIC acid-sensing ion channel; application-specific integrated circuit

aSi/CsI cesium iodide and amorphous silicon

ASIF Association for Study of Internal Fixation

ASII American Science Information Institute

ASIM American Society of Internal Medicine

ASIP American Society for Investigative Pathology; atypical protein kinase C isotype-specific interacting protein

ASIPP American Society of Interventional Pain Physicians

ASIR age-standardized incidence rate

ASIS American Society for Information Science; American Study of Infarct Survival; Angina and Silent Ischemia Study; anterior superior iliac spine; average severity of index score

ASIST Atenolol Silent Ischemia Trial

ASIS&T American Society for Information Science and Technology

ASK anomalous state of knowledge; anti-streptokinase; Australian Streptokinase [trial]

ASKAS Aging Sexual Knowledge and Attitude Scale

ASL angiosarcoma of liver; antistreptolysin; argininosuccinate lyase

ASLIB Association of Special Libraries and Information Bureau

ASLME American Society of Law, Medicine & Ethics

ASLN Alport syndrome–like hereditary nephritis

ASLO antistreptolysin O

ASLT antistreptolysin test

ASLV avian sarcoma and leukosis virus

ASM acid sphingomyelinase; active shape model; age-specific mortality; airway smooth muscle; American Society for Microbiology; angular second moment; anterior scalenus muscle; areola-sparing mastectomy

AsM astigmatism, myopic

asm age-specific mortality

ASMA Aerospace Medical Association; anti−smooth muscle antibody

ASMBS American Society for Metabolic and Bariatric Surgery

ASMC arterial smooth muscle cell

ASMD anterior segment mesenchymal dysgenesis; atonic sclerotic muscle dystrophy

ASME Association for the Study of Medical Education

ASMI anteroseptal myocardial infarct

As/Mk antiserum, monkey

ASMPA Armed Services Medical Procurement Agency

ASMR age-standardized mortality ratio

ASMS archival [imaging] storage management system

ASMSO American Society of Medication Safety Officers [organization name changed to Medication Safety Officers Society, MSOS]

ASMT acetylserotonin methyltransferase; American Society for Medical Technology

ASMTY acetylserotonin methyltransferase Y

ASN abstract syntax notation; alkali-soluble nitrogen; American Society of Nephrology; American Society of Neurochemistry; arteriosclerotic nephritis; asparagine; Associate of Science in Nursing

Asn, asn asparagine

ASO administrative services only; AIDS service organization; allele-specific oligonucleoside; antistreptolysin O; arteriosclerosis obliterans

ASOD anterior segmental ocular dysgenesis

AS ON antisense oligonucleotide

ASOS American Society of Oral Surgeons

ASOT antistreptolysin-O test

ASP abnormal spinal posture; active server page; active server processor; acute suppurative parotitis; acute symmetric polyarthritis; affected sibling pair; African swine pox; aged substrate plasma; alkali-stable pepsin; American Society of Parasitologists; amnesic shellfish poisoning; ankle systolic pressure; ankylosing spondylitis; anorectal malformation, sacral bony abnormality, presacral mass [association]; antibody-specific prediction; antisocial personality; aortic systolic pressure; application service provider; area systolic pressure; asparaginase; aspartic acid; average sales price

Asp asparaginase; aspartic acid

asp aspartame; aspartate; aspartic acid; aspiration; automatic signal processing

ASPA American Society of Physician Analysts; American Society of Podiatric Assistants; aspartoacylase

ASPAC Asia-Pacific [study]

ASPAN American Society of Perianesthesia Nurses

ASPAT antistreptococcal group A polysaccharide test

ASPCR, AS-PCR allele-specific polymerase chain reaction

ASPD anterior superior pancreaticoduodenal artery; antisocial personality disorder

ASPDM American Society of Psychosomatic Dentistry and Medicine

ASPECT Anticoagulants in Secondary Prevention of Events in Coronary Thrombosis; approach to systematic planning and evaluation of clinical trials

ASPEN American Society for Parenteral and Enteral Nutrition

ASPG antispleen globulin

ASP active server processor

AS/PI anterior superior/posterior inferior

ASPIRE Action on Secondary Prevention by Intervention to Reduce Events

ASPM American Society of Paramedics

ASPMA American Society of Podiatric Medical Assistants

ASPMN American Society of Pain Management Nurses

ASPO American Society for Psychoprophylaxis in Obstetrics; American Society of Pediatric Otolaryngology

ASPP American Society of Psychoanalytic Physicians; Association for Sane Psychiatric Practices

ASPREN Australian Sentinel Practice Research Network

ASPRS American Society of Plastic and Reconstructive Surgeons

ASPS advanced sleep phase syndrome; alveolar soft part sarcoma; American Society of Plastic Surgeons

ASPSN American Society of Plastic Surgical Nurses

ASPSOM adaptive structure probabilistic self-organizing map

ASPVD atherosclerotic peripheral vascular disease; atherosclerotic pulmonary vascular disease

ASQ (Connors) Abbreviated Symptom Questionnaire; American Society for Quality; Anxiety Scale Questionnaire
ASR adrenal/spleen ratio; age-standardized rate; air-supplying respirator; aldosterone secretion rate; antistreptolysin reaction; articular surface repair; automated speech recognition
ASRA American Society of Regional Anesthesia
AS/Rab antiserum, rabbit
ASRM American Society for Reproductive Medicine
ASRS Adult ADHD Self-Report Scale
ASRT American Society of Radiologic Technologists; American Society of Registered Technologists
ASS Aarskog-Scott syndrome; acute serum sickness; acute spinal stenosis; acute stroke study; anterior superior spine; argininosuccinate synthetase; Auckland Stroke Study
ASSA, ASSAS aminopterin-like syndrome without aminopterin
ASSC acute splenic sequestration crisis
AS-SCORE age, stage of disease, physiological system involved, complications, response to therapy
ASSENT Assessment of the Safety and Efficacy of a New Thrombolytic Agent
ASSERT Alcohol and Substance Abuse Services and Educating Providers to Refer Patients to Treatment
ASSET Anglo-Scandinavian Study of Early Thrombolysis; Atorvastatin Simvastatin Safety and Efficacy Trial
ASSH American Society for Surgery of the Hand
ASSI Accurate Surgical and Scientific Instruments
ASSIA Applied Social Science Index and Abstracts
assim assimilate, assimilation
ASSIST American Stop Smoking Intervention Study
ASSO American Society for the Study of Orthodontics
Assoc associate; association
ASSP argininosuccinate synthetase pseudogene
ASSQ autism spectrum screening questionnaire
ASSR adult situation stress reaction; auditory steady-state response
ASSURE A Stent vs. Stent Ultrasound Remodeling Evaluation
ASSX argininosuccinate synthetase pseudogene

AST above selected threshold; allele-specific transcript; allergy serum transfer; angiotensin sensitivity test; anterior spinothalamic tract; antimicrobial susceptibility test; antistreptolysin test; aspartate aminotransferase (SGOT); Association of Surgical Technologists; astigmatism; atrial overdrive stimulation rate; audiometry sweep test; Australian Streptokinase Trial
Ast astigmatism
ASTA anti−alpha-staphylolysin
ASTECS Antenatal Steroid Therapy in Elective Cesarean Section [study]
ASTH, Asth asthenopia
ASTHO Association of State and Territorial Health Officials
ASTI antispasticity index
ASTM American Society for Testing and Materials
ASTMH American Society of Tropical Medicine and Hygiene
ASTNA Air and Surface Transport Nurses Association
ASTO antistreptolysin O
as tol as tolerated
ASTPHND Association of State and Territorial Public Health and Nutrition Directors
ASTRO American Society for Radiation Oncology; American Society for Therapeutic Radiology and Oncology
AstV Astrovirus
ASTZ antistreptozyme
ASUB active substance
ASV anodic stripping voltammetry; anti-siphon valve; anti−snake venom; autologous saphenous vein; avian sarcoma virus
ASV-CT10 avian sarcoma virus CT10
ASVO American Society of Veterinary Ophthalmology
ASVPP American Society of Veterinary Physiologists and Pharmacologists
ASVS arterial stimulation venous sampling
ASW artificial sweetener
ASWC averaged spike and wave complex
Asx amino acid that gives aspartic acid after hydrolysis; asymptomatic
asym asymmetric, asymmetry
AT abdominal thrusts; Achard-Thiers [syndrome]; achievement test; Achilles tendon; activity training; acute thrombosis; adaptive thermogenesis; adenine-thymine; adenine-thyronine; adipose tissue; adjunctive therapy; adnexal torsion; air temperature; allergy treatment; amino acid transporter; aminotransferase; aminotriazole; amitriptyline; anaerobic threshold; anaphylotoxin; angiotensin; anterior tibia; antithrombin;

antitrypsin; antral transplantation; applanation tonometry; assistive technology; ataxia-telangiectasia; atmosphere; atraumatic; atresia, tricuspid; atrial tachycardia; atrial tumor; atropine; attenuate, attenuation; autoimmune thrombocytopenia; axonal terminal; old tuberculin [Ger. *alt Tuberkulin*]

A-T ataxia-telangiectasia

AT₁ angiotensin II type 1

AT₁₀ dihydrotachysterol

AT I angiotensin I

AT II angiotensin II

AT III angiotensin III; antithrombin III

At acidity, total; angiotensin; antithrombin; astatine; atrial; atrium

Aₜ amount in tissue

at airtight; atom, atomic; technical atmosphere

ATA advanced technology attachment; alimentary toxic aleukia; American Telemedicine Association; American Thyroid Association; aminotriazole; antithymic activity; antithyroglobulin antibody; anti-*Toxoplasma* antibody; atmosphere absolute; aurintricarboxylic acid

ATACS Antithrombotic Therapy in Acute Coronary Syndromes [trial]

ATAI acute traumatic aortic injury

ATB articulated total body [model]; at the time of the bomb [in Japan]; atrial tachycardia with block

Atb antibiotic

ATBC Alpha-Tocopherol/Beta Carotene [study]

ATC activated thymus cell; alpha-tocopherol; anaplastic thyroid carcinoma; Anatomical Therapeutic Chemical [classification]; around the clock; certified athletic trainer

ATCase aspartate transcarbamoylase

ATCC American Type Culture Collection

ATCL adult T-cell leukemia/lymphoma

ATCM automatic tube current modulation

ATCS anterior tibial compartment syndrome

ATD Alzheimer-type dementia; androstatrienedione; anthropomorphic test dummy; antithyroid drug; aqueous tear deficiency; asphyxiating thoracic dystrophy

ATDNet Advanced Technology Demonstration Network

ATDP Attitude Toward Disabled Persons [scale]

ATE acute toxic encephalopathy; acute toxicity end point; adipose tissue extract; autologous tumor extract

ATEE *N*-acetyl-1-tyrosyl-ethyl ester

ATEM analytic transmission electron microscopy

Aten atenolol

ATEST Atenolol and Streptokinase Trial

ATEV *Aphodius tasmaniae* entomopoxvirus

ATF activating transcription factor; anterior talofibular; ascites tumor fluid

At fib atrial fibrillation

ATG adenine-thymidine-guanine; advanced technology group; antihuman T-lymphocyte immune globulin; antithrombocyte globulin; antithymocyte globulin; antithyroglobulin

AT/GC adenine-thymine/guanine-cytosine ratio

ATH acetyl-tyrosine hydrazide; alkylated thiohydantoin

ATh Associate in Therapy

Athsc atherosclerosis

AtHV ateline herpesvirus

ATI abdominal trauma index; analytical treatment interruption; attitude-treatment interaction

ATIAIS Anturane Transient Ischemic Attack Italian Study

ATIME Accupril Titration Interval Management Evaluation [trial]

ATIP Agricultural Technology Innovation Partnership [USDA affiliate]

ATL Achilles tendon lengthening; active template library; acute T-cell leukemia; adult T-cell leukemia; American tegumentary leishmaniasis; anterior tricuspid leaflet; antitension line; atypical lymphocyte

ATLA adult T-cell leukemia virus-associated antigen; alternatives to laboratory animals

ATLANTIC Angina Treatment, Lasers, and Normal Therapy in Comparison [trial]

ATLANTIS Alteplase Thrombolysis for Acute Noninterventional Therapy in Ischemic Stroke

ATLAS Adolescents Training and Learning to Avoid Steroids; advanced tools for learning anatomic structure; Aspirin and Ticlid vs Anticoagulants for Stents [study]; Assessment of Treatment with Lisinopril and Survival [trial]

ATLAST Antiplatelet Therapy vs. Lovenox Plus Antiplatelet Therapy for Patients with Increased Risk of Stent Thrombosis; Aspirin/Ticlopidine vs. Low-Molecular-Weight Heparin/Aspirin/Ticlopidine Stent Trial

ATLL adult T-cell leukemia/lymphoma

ATLP anterior titanium thoracolumbar locking plate

ATLS acute tumor lysis syndrome; advanced trauma life support

ATLV adult T-cell leukemia virus

ATM abnormal tubular myelin; acute transverse myelopathy; adaptive-template

atm standard atmosphere

ATMA Amiodarone Trials Meta-Analysis; antithyroid plasma membrane antibody

ATMI application transaction manager interface

atmos atmospheric

ATMTN asynchronous transfer mode teleradiology network

ATN acute tubular necrosis; Adolescent Trials Network; augmented transition network

ATNC atraumatic normocephalic

at no atomic number

ATNR asymmetric tonic neck reflex

A-to-D analog-to-digital

ATOS Achievement of Therapeutic Objectives Scale

A$_{TOT}$ total anions

ATP according to protocol; addiction treatment program; adenosine triphosphate; ambient temperature and pressure; annual transmission potential; antitachycardia pacing; Arizona Telemedicine Program; autoimmune thrombocytopenic purpura

A-TP adsorbed test plasma

AT-P antitrypsin-Pittsburgh

AtP attending physician

ATPA 2-amino-3-(hydroxy-5-*tert*-butylisoxazol-4-yl) propanoic acid

AT-PAS aldehyde-thionine—periodic acid Schiff [test]

ATPase adenosine triphosphatase

ATPD dried at ambient temperature and pressure

ATP-2Na adenosine triphosphate disodium

ATPS ambient temperature and pressure, saturated

ATR Achilles tendon reflex; Achilles tendon rupture; acid-tolerance response; alpha-thalassemia mental retardation (intellectual disability) [syndrome]; ataxia-telangiectasia and rad3-related [protein]; attenuated total reflectance; automatic term recognition; axial trunk rotation

atr atrophy

ATR1, ATR2 alpha-thalassemia mental retardation (intellectual disability) [syndrome], type 1, type 2

ATRA all-*trans*retinoic acid

ATRAMI Autonomic Tone and Reflexes After Myocardial Infarction [trial]

ATRAS Adrenal Test Retrieval and Analysis System

Atr fib atrial fibrillation

ATRX, ATR-X X-linked alpha-thalassemia mental retardation (intellectual disability) [syndrome]

ATS Achard-Thiers syndrome; acid test solution; alpha-D-tocopherol acid succinate; American Thoracic Society; American Trauma Society; American Trudeau Society; anti—rat thymocyte serum; antitetanus serum; antithymocyte serum; anxiety tension state; arteriosclerosis; autologous transfusion system

ATS-DLD American Thoracic Society Division of Lung Disease

ATSDR Agency for Toxic Substances and Disease Registry

ATT arginine tolerance test; aspirin tolerance time

att attending

atten attenuated

ATTMH Australian Therapeutic Trial of Mild Hypertension

ATV Abelson virus transformed; *Ambystoma tigrinum stebbinsi* virus; antisense target validation; atazanavir; avian tumor virus

at vol atomic volume

ATVV Auditory, Tactile, Visual, and Vestibular [Multisensory Intervention]

at wt atomic weight

ATX associated expressions

ATx adult thymectomy

atyp atypical

ATZ acetazolamide; atypical transformation zone

AU allergenic unit; Alzheimer unit; Ångström unit; antitoxin unit; arbitrary unit; Australia antigen; azauridine

Au Australia antigen; authorization

a.u. both ears [L. *auris utraque*]

AUA American Urological Association; asymptomatic urinary abnormalities

Au Ag Australia antigen

AUB abnormal uterine bleeding

AUC area under the curve

AUC$_{extra}$ extrapolated area under the curve

AuCPV *Aglais urticae* cypovirus

AUC$_{SS}$ steady-state area under the curve

AUD arthritis of unknown diagnosis

aud auditory

AUDEX automated urologic diagnostic expert [ultrasound]

AUDIT alcohol use disorders identification test

AUDIT-C alcohol use disorders identification test—alcohol consumption questions

aud-vis audiovisual

AUG acute ulcerative gingivitis; adenosine-uracil-guanine

AUGH acute upper gastrointestinal hemorrhage

AuHAA Australia hepatitis-associated antigen

AUI Alcohol Use Inventory; aortouniiliac device

AUL acute undifferentiated leukemia

AUMC area under the first moment curve

AUMC$_{extra}$ extrapolated area under the first moment curve

AUO amyloid of unknown origin

AuP Australian antigen protein

AUPHA Association of University Programs in Health Administration

AUR acute urinary retention; Association of University Radiologists

aur, auric auricle, auricular

AURAV Aura virus

AUROC area under the receiver operating characteristic curve

AURT Association of University Radiologic Technicians

AUS acute urethral syndrome; artificial urinary sphincter

AuS Australia serum hepatitis

aus, ausc auscultation

AuSH Australia serum hepatitis

AUST Australian Urokinase Stroke Trial

AUT authentication

AutoCAD auto—computer assisted diagnosis

Auto-PEEP self-controlled positive end-expiratory pressure

AUV anterior urethral valve

aux auxiliary

AV adeno-associated virus; adenovirus; Adriamycin and vincristine; air velocity; allergic vasculitis; anteroventral; anteversion; anticipatory vomiting; antivirin; aortic valve; arenavirus; arteriovenous; artificial ventilation; ascovirus; assisted ventilation; atrioventricular; audiovisual; augmented vector; average; aviation medicine; avoirdupois

A-V arteriovenous; atrioventricular

A/V ampere/volt; arteriovenous

Av average; avoirdupois

aV abvolt

av air velocity; average; avoirdupois; avulsion

AVA activity vector analysis; anthrax vaccine adsorbed; antiviral antibody; aortic valve annulus; aortic valve area; aortic valve atresia; Arracacha virus A; arteriovenous anastomosis

AvaCPV *Agraulis vanillae* cypovirus

AV/AF anteverted, anteflexed

AVAV Avalon virus

AVB Arracacha virus B; atrioventricular block

AVC aberrant ventricular conduction; Academy of Veterinary Cardiology; aortic valve closure; arteriovenous communication; Association of Vitamin Chemists; associative visual cortex; atrioventricular canal; automatic volume control

AVCN anteroventral cochlear nucleus

AVCO$_2$R arteriovenous carbon dioxide removal

AVCS atrioventricular conduction system

AVCx atrioventricular circumflex branch

AVD aortic valvular disease; apparent volume of distribution; Army Veterinary Department; atrioventricular dissociation

AvDNV *Agraulis vanillae* densovirus

AVDO$_2$ arteriovenous oxygen saturation difference

AVDO$_2$B arteriovenous oxygen saturation difference, basal

AVDP average diastolic pressure

avdp avoirdupois

aVDPV ambiguous vaccine-derived poliovirus

AVE aortic valve echocardiogram

ave average

AVED ataxia with vitamin E deficiency

aver average

AVERT Atorvastatin vs. Revascularization Treatment [trial]

AVEU AIDS Vaccine Evaluation Unit

AVF antiviral factor; arteriovenous fistula

aVF automated volt foot

aV$_F$ unipolar limb lead on the left leg [ECG]

AVG ambulatory visit group; aortic valve gradient

avg average

AVH acute viral hepatitis

AVHD acquired valvular heart disease

AVHS acquired valvular heart syndrome

AVI air velocity index; Association of Veterinary Inspectors; atrioventricular interval; audio-video interleave

AviCPV *Arctia villica* cypovirus

AVID Amiodarone vs. Implantable Defibrillators [trial]; Angiography vs. Intravascular Ultrasound Directed Coronary Stent Placement [trial]; Antiarrhythmics vs. Implantable Defibrillators [study]

AVIR aortic valve replacement

AVJ atrioventricular junction

AVJR atrioventricular junction rhythm

AVJRe atrioventricular junctional reentrant

aV$_K$ unipolar limb lead on the left arm [ECG]

AVL automatic vehicle locator

aVL automated volt left

AVLINE Audiovisuals Online

AVLJ absolute value of logarithm of Jacobian

AVM arteriovenous malformation; atrioventricular malformation; avermectin; aviation medicine

AVMA American Veterinary Medical Association

AVN acute vasomotor nephropathy; atrioventricular node/nodal; atrioventricular node; avascular necrosis

AVNA atrioventricular node artery

AVND atrioventricular node dysfunction

AVNFH avascular necrosis of the femoral head

AVNFRP atrioventricular node functional refractory period

AVNR atrioventricular nodal reentry

AVNRT atrioventricular node reentry tachycardia

AVO aortic valve opening; aortic valve orifice; atrioventricular opening

AVO₂ arteriovenous oxygen ratio

AVOA amorphous vascular occluding agent

AVP abnormal vasopressin; actinomycin-vincristine-Platinol; ambulatory venous pressure; antiviral protein; aortoventriculoplasty; aqueous vasopressin; arginine-vasopressin; arteriovenous passage time

AVP-NPII arginine vasopressin-neurophysin II

AVPU alert, verbal, painful, unresponsive

AVR accelerated ventricular rhythm; antiviral regulator; aortic valve replacement

aVR automated volt right

aVR unipolar limb lead on the right arm [ECG]

AVREO avian reovirus

AVRI acute viral respiratory infection

AVRP atrioventricular refractory period

AVRR antiviral repressor regulator

AVRT atrioventricular reciprocating tachycardia; atrioventricular reentrant tachycardia; atrioventricular reentry

AVS Advanced Visual Systems; aortic valve stenosis; application visualization system; arteriovenous shunt; auditory vocal sequencing

AVSD atrioventricular septal defect

AVSV aortic valve stroke volume

AVT Allen vision test; arginine vasotocin; Aviation Medicine Technician

AVV atrioventricular valve

AvV *Agraulis vanillae* virus

Av3V anteroventral third ventricle

AVVM angiographically visualized vascular malformation

AVY Arracacha virus Y

AVZ avascular zone

AW able to work; above waist; abrupt withdrawal; airways; alcohol withdrawal; alveolar wall; anterior wall; atomic warfare; atomic weight

aW water activity

A&W alive and well

aw airway; water activity

AWAR anterior wall of aortic root

AWBM alveolar wall basement membrane

AWBV Ahlum waterborne virus

AWCR age-weighted citation rate

AWD alive with disease

AWESOME Angina with Extremely Serious Operative Mortality Evaluation

AWFM adaptive Walsh function modeling

AWG American Wire Gauge

AWGN additive white gaussian noise

AWHILES All-Wales Health Information and Library Extension Service

AWHONN Association of Women's Health, Obstetric, and Neonatal Nurses

AWI anterior wall infarction

AWIGS advanced workplace for image-guided surgery

AWL active waiting list

AWM abnormal wall motion

AWMI anterior wall myocardial infarction

AWMN Acid Waters Monitoring Network

AWMV amplitude-weighted mean velocity

AWO airway obstruction

AWP airway pressure; any willing provider; average of wholesale prices; average wholesale price

AWR absolute weighted residual; airway restriction

AWRS anti−whole rabbit serum

AWRU active wrist rotation unit

AWS Alagille-Watson syndrome; alcohol withdrawal syndrome

AWTA aniridia−Wilms tumor association

awu atomic weight unit

ax axial; axillary; axis

AxCPV anti-xanthomista cypovirus

AXD axillary dissection

AXF advanced x-ray facility

AXG adult xanthogranuloma

AXL anexelekto [oncogene]; axillary lymphoscintigraphy

AXR abdominal x-ray

AXT alternating exotropia

AYA acute yellow atrophy

AYF antiyeast factor

AYP autolyzed yeast protein

AYV Anthriscus yellow virus

AZ Aschheim-Zondek [test]; 5-azacytidine; azathioprine

Az nitrogen [Fr. *azote*]
AZA azadirachtin; azathioprine; azelaic acid
AzC azacytosine
AZEV *Acrobasis zelleri* entomopoxvirus
AZF azoospermia factor
AzG, azg azaguanine
AZGP zinc-alpha-2-glycoprotein
AZO two adjacent nitrogen atoms between carbon atoms
AZOA azaorotic acid
AZQ diaziquone
AZR alizarin

AZT Aschheim-Zondek test; azidothymidine; 3'-azido-3'-deoxythymidine; zidovudine (azidothymidine)
AZTEC amplitude zone time epoch coding [ECG]
AZTMP azidothymidine monophosphate
AZT-R azidothymidine resistant
AZT-S azidothymidine susceptible/sensitive
AZTTP azidothymidine trithiophosphate
AZT-TP 3'-azido-3'-deoxythymidine triphosphate
AZU azauracil; azurocidin
AzUr 6-azauridine

B

B bacillus; bands; barometric; base; basophil; basophilic; bath [L. *balneum*]; Baumé scale; behavior; bel; Benoist scale; benzoate; beta; bilateral; biscuspid; black; blood, bloody; blue; body; boils at; Bolton point; bone marrow derived; born; boron; bound; bovine; break; bregma; bronchial, bronchus; brother; *Brucella*; bruit; buccal; Bucky [device]; Bucky factor; bursa cells; burst [pacemaker]; bypass; byte; colorectal tumor extending into adipose tissue; magnetic induction; minimal detectable blurring; supramentale [point]

β anomer of a carbohydrate; buffer capacity; carbon separated from a carboxyl by one other carbon in aliphatic compounds; constituent of a plasma protein fraction; Greek letter beta; probability of type II error; substituent group of a steroid that projects above the plane of the ring

B₀ constant magnetic field in nuclear magnetic resonance

B1 palpable one-lobe prostatic tumor less than 1.5 cm; tumor extending into muscularis propria

B₁ induced field in nuclear magnetic resonance; radiofrequency magnetic field in nuclear magnetic resonance; thiamine

1 − β power of statistical test

B.1.1.529 [includes BA.1/BA.1.1/BA.2/ BA.3/BA.4/BA.5 lineages] Omicron variant of SARS-CoV-2 [also called Botswana variant]

B.1.1.7 [and Q lineages] Alpha variant of SARS-CoV-2 [also called UK variant]

B.1.351 [and descendent lineages] Beta variant of SARS-CoV-2 [also called South Africa variant]

B.1.427/B.1.429 Epsilon variant of SARS-CoV-2 [also called California variant and CAL.20C]

B.1.525 Eta variant of SARS-CoV-2 [also called VUI-21FEB-03]

B.1.526 Iota variant of SARS-CoV-2 [also called New York variant]

B.1.617.1 Kappa variant of SARS-CoV-2

B.1.617.2 [and AY lineages] Delta variant of SARS-CoV-2 [also called India variant]

B.1.621 Mu variant of SARS-CoV-2 [also called Colombia variant]

B2 palpable two-lobe prostatic tumor larger than 1.5 cm; tumor extending into perirectal adipose tissue

B₂ riboflavin

B₆ pyridoxine

B₇ biotin

B₈ adenosine phosphate

B₁₂ cyanocobalamin

b barn; base; boils at; born; brain; branched; [chromosome] break; supramentale [point]; twice [L. *bis*]

b sample regression coefficient

b⁺ positron emission

b⁻ beta emission

BA Bachelor of Arts; bacillary angiomatosis; backache; bacterial agglutination; bactericidal activity; barbituric acid; basion; benzanthracene; benzyladenine; best amplitude; beta-adrenergic; betamethasone acetate; bilateral asymmetric; bile acid; biliary atresia; biologic activity; blocking antibody; blood agar; blood alcohol; bone age; boric acid; bovine albumin; brachial artery; breathing apparatus; bronchial asthma; buccoaxial; buffered acetone

Ba barium; barium enema; basion

ba basion

BAA benzoylarginine amide; bone age assessment; branched amino acid

Baa Bucky amino acid

BAAP bone-anchored auricular prosthesis

BAAPS British Association of Aesthetic Plastic Surgeons

BAATAF Boston Area Anticoagulation Trial for Atrial Fibrillation

BAAV bovine adeno-associated virus

BAB blood agar base

Bab Babinski reflex; baboon

BabK baboon kidney

BAB born after the ban [cases]

BA/BE bioavailability/bioequivalence

BABV Babahoya virus

BAC baclofen; bacterial adherent colony; bacterial antigen complex; bacterial artificial chromosome; blood alcohol concentration; breast arterial calcification; British Association of Chemists; bronchoalveolar carcinoma; bronchoalveolar cells; buccoaxiocervical

Bac, bac *Bacillus*

BACE beta-amyloid converting enzyme

BACT bacterium; best available control technology

Bact, bact bacteria; *Bacterium*, bacterium

BACUS Balloon Angioplasty Compliance Ultrasound Study

BAD biologic aerosol detection; biologically active dose; British Association of Dermatologists

BADE [Thoracic] Bioimpedance as an Adjunct to Dobutamine Echocardiography [study]

BADLs basic activities of daily living

BADS black locks, albinism, deafness syndrome

BAdV bovine adenovirus

BAdV-A, -B, -C bovine adenovirus A, B, C

BAE bounded area elimination; bovine aortic endothelium; bronchial artery embolization

BaE barium enema

BAEC bovine aortic endothelial cell

BAEDP balloon aortic end-diastolic pressure

BAEE benzoylarginine ethyl ester

BaEn barium enema

BAEP brainstem auditory evoked potential

BAER brainstem auditory evoked response

BaEV baboon endogenous virus

BaFBr:Eu europium-activated barium fluorohalide

BAFF B-cell activating factor

BAG buccoaxiogingival

BAGG buffered azide glucose glycerol

BAGV Bagaza virus

BAH biatrial hypertrophy

BAHA bone-anchored hearing aid

BAHAMA Baragwanath Hypertension Ambulatory Blood Pressure Monitoring Multiarm [study]

BA/HPCC biomedical application of high-performance computing and communication

BAHS Boston Area Health Study; butoctamide hydrogen succinate

BAHV Bahig virus

BAI beta-aminoisobutyrate

BAIB beta-aminoisobutyric [acid]

BAIF bile acid independent flow

BAIT bacterial automated identification technique

BAKUV Baku virus

BAKV Bakel virus; Bakau virus

BAL bioartificial liver; biphenotypic acute leukemia; blood alcohol level; British anti-lewisite; bronchoalveolar lavage

bal balance; balsam

BALB binaural alternate loudness balance

BALF bronchoalveolar lavage fluid

bals balsam

BALT bronchial-associated lymphoid tissue, bronchus-associated lymphoid tissue

BAM Bacteriological Analytical Manual [FDA publication]; basilar artery migraine; bilateral augmentation mammoplasty; brachial artery mean [pressure]

BaM barium meal

Bam benzamide

BAME benzoylarginine methyl ester

BAN British Approved Name; British Association of Neurologists

BANPA Bay Area Nurse Practitioner Association

BANS back, arms, neck, and scalp

BANTER Bayesian Network Tutoring and Explanation

BANV Banzi virus

BAO basal acid output; brachial artery output

BAO-MAO basal acid output to maximal acid output [ratio]

BAP bacterial alkaline phosphatase; Behavior Activity Profile; beta-amyloid peptide; blood-agar plate; bovine albumin in phosphate buffer; brachial artery pressure; brightness area product

BAPhysMed British Association of Physical Medicine

BAPI barley alkaline protease inhibitor

BAPN beta-aminoproprionitrile

BAPO British Association of Paediatric Otorhinolaryngologists

BAPP beta-amyloid precursor protein

BAPRAS British Association of Plastic, Reconstructive and Aesthetic Surgeons

BAPS biomechanical ankle platform system; bovine albumin phosphate saline; British Association of Paediatric Surgeons; British Association of Plastic Surgeons

BAPT British Association of Physical Training

BAPTA 1,2-bis(aminophenoxy)ethane-N,N,-N′,N′-tetraacetic acid

BAPV bovine alimentary papillomavirus

BAQ brain-age quotient

BAR bariatrics; barometer, barometric; beta-adrenergic receptor; bright, alert, and responsive [veterinary medicine]

βAR beta-adrenergic receptor

bar barometric

BARASTER Balloon Angioplasty vs. Rotational Atherectomy for Stent Restenosis [registry]

Barb, barb barbiturate, barbituric

BARH bright, alert, responsive, and hydrated [veterinary medicine]

BARI Bypass Angioplasty Revascularization Investigation [trial]

BARK beta-adrenergic receptor kinase

BARN bilateral acute retinal necrosis; Body Awareness Resource Network

BAROCCO Balloon Angioplasty vs. Rotacs for Total Chronic Coronary Occlusion [trial]

BARS behaviorally anchored rating scale

BART blood-activated recalcification time

BARV Barur virus

BAS balloon atrial septostomy; battalion aid station; benzyl antiserotonin; beta-adrenergic stimulation; boric acid solution; Bronx Longitudinal Aging Study

BaS barium swallow

bas basilar; basophil, basophilic

BASA Boston Assessment of Severe Aphasia

BASC Blood Pressure in Acute Stroke Collaboration

BASH body acceleration synchronous with heart rate

BASIC Beginner's All-Purpose Symbolic Introduction Code

BASIS Basel Antiarrhythmic Study of Infarct Survival

BASM biliary atresia splenic malformation [syndrome]

baso basophil

BASOC boundary at the scale of the core

BAstV bovine astrovirus

BAT basic aid training; best available technology; blunt abdominal trauma; bolus arriving time; bright acuity test; brown adipose tissue

BATV Batai virus

BAUP Bovie-assisted uvulopalatoplasty

BAUS brachial artery ultrasound scanning; British Association of Urological Surgeons

BAUV Bauline virus

BAV banana virus; bicuspid aortic valve; Bivens arm virus

BaV Barramundi virus

BAVCP bilateral abductor vocal cord paralysis

BAVFO bradycardia after arteriovenous fistula occlusion

BAW bronchoalveolar washing

BAYV bayou virus

BB bad breath; bed bath; beta-blockade, beta-blocker; biceps brachii; BioBreeding [rat]; blanket bath; blood bank; blood buffer; blow bottle; blue bloaters; bombesin; borderline; Bortfeld-Boyer [radiotherapy]; both bones; breakthrough bleeding; breast biopsy; bronchial blocker; brush border; buffer base; bundle branch; isoenzyme of creatine kinase containing two B subunits

B&B branch and bound [algorithm]

bb Bolton point; both bones

BBA born before arrival

BBB Bad Bug Book [FDA publication]; blood-brain barrier; blood buffer base; bundle branch block

BBBB bilateral bundle-branch block

BBBD blood-brain barrier disruption

BBC bromobenzycyanide; buccal bifurcation cyst

BbCPV *Biston betularia* cypovirus

BBD benign breast disease

BB3DI broad-beam three-dimensional irradiation

BBE *Bacteroides* bile esculin [agar]

BBEP biotechnology, biologics, and environmental protection; brush border endopeptidase

BBF bronchial blood flow

BBI Better Birth Initiatives; Biomedical Business International; Bowman-Birk soybean inhibitor

BBM banked breast milk; brush border membrane

BBMV broad bean mottle virus; brush border membrane vesicle

BBN broadband noise

BBNV broad bean necrosis virus

BBOT 2,5-bis(5-t-butyl-2-benzoxazol-2-yl) thiophene

BBOV Bimbo virus

BBPP Beta-Blocker Pooling Project

BBR bibasilar rate; bundle-branch reentry

BBRS Burks Behavior Rating Scale

BBR-VT bundle-branch reentry-ventricular tachycardia

BBS Bardet-Biedl syndrome; bashful bladder syndrome; benign breast syndrome; bilateral breath sounds; bombesin; borate-buffered saline; brown bowel syndrome; bulletin board software

BBs both bones

BBT basal body temperature

BBTD baby bottle tooth decay

BBV Berkeley bee virus; black beetle virus; Bukalasa bat virus

BB/W BioBreeding/Worcester [rat]

BC Bachelor of Surgery [L. *Baccalaureus Chirurgiae*]; back care; bactericidal concentration; basal cell; basket cell; battle casualty; bicarbonate; biliary colic; bipolar cell; birth control; blastic crisis; blood count; blood culture; Blue Cross; board certified; bone conduction; bowel care; brachiocephalic; brain contour; breast cancer; bronchial carcinoma; buccal cartilage; buccocervical; buffy coat

B&C biopsy and curettage

Bc *Bacillus cereus*

b/c benefit/cost ratio

BCA balloon catheter angioplasty; bell clapper anomaly; bicinchoninic acid; blood color analyzer; Blue Cross Association; branchial cleft anomaly; Breast Cancer Action; breast cancer antigen; bromochloroacetic acid

BCAA branched-chain amino acid

bCaCC bovine calcium-sensitive chloride channel

BCAEC bovine coronary artery endothelial cell

BCAPS Beta-Blocker Cholesterol-Lowering Asymptomatic Plaque Study

BCAT brachiocephalic arterial trunk

BCB blood–cerebrospinal fluid barrier; brilliant cresyl blue

BCBR bilateral carotid body resection

BC/BS Blue Cross/Blue Shield

BCBSA Blue Cross and Blue Shield Association

BCC basal cell carcinoma; bedside communication controller; biliary cholesterol concentration; birth control clinic

bcc blind carbon copy; body-centered cubic

BC-CFC blast cell colony-forming cell

BCCG British Cooperative Clinical Group

BCCP biotin carboxyl carrier protein

BCCV Black Creek Canal virus

BCD binary-coded decimal; bleomycin, cyclophosphamide, dactinomycin

BCDDP Breast Cancer Detection Demonstration Project

BCDF B-cell differentiation factor

BCDL Brachmann–Cornelia de Lange [syndrome]

BCDRS Brief Carroll Depression Rating Scale

BCDS Bulimia Cognitive Distortions Scale

BCDSP Boston-Collaborative Drug Surveillance Program

BCE basal cell epithelioma; benign childhood epilepsy; bone collagen equivalent units; bubble chamber equipment

BCECT benign childhood epilepsy with centrotemporal [spikes]

BCEI breast cancer, estrogen inducible

BCEOP benign partial epilepsy with occipital paroxysms

BCF basic conditioning factor; basophil chemotactic factor; bioconcentration factor; breast cyst fluid

BCFP breast cyst fluid protein

BCG bacillus Calmette-Guérin [vaccine]; ballistocardiogram, ballistocardiography; bicolor guaiac test; bromcresol green

BCGF B-cell growth factor

BCGM biconjugate gradient method

BCH basal cell hyperplasia

BCh Bachelor of Surgery [L. *Baccalaureus Chirurgiae*]

BChD Bachelor of Dental Surgery

BCHE butyrylcholinesterase

BChir Bachelor of Surgery [L. *Baccalaureus Chirurgiae*]

Bchl, bChl bacterial chlorophyll

BCHS Bureau of Community Health Services

BCI behavioral cues index; brain-computer interface

BCIA Biomedical Clinical Instrumentation Association

BCIP 5-bromo-4-chloro-3-inodolyl phosphate

BCIRG Breast Cancer International Research Group

BCIS British Cardiovascular Intervention Society

BCKA branched-chain keto acid

BCKD branched-chain alpha-keto acid dehydrogenase

BCL B-cell leukemia/lymphoma; basic cycle length

BCLD B-cell lymphoproliferative disease

BCLL B-cell chronic lymphocytic leukemia

BCLM below critical length material

BCLP bilateral cleft of lip and palate

BCLS basic cardiac life support

BCM B-cell maturation; beclomethasone; birth control medication; blood-clotting mechanism; body cell mass; body control and movement

BCMA B-cell maturation antigen

BCME bis-chloromethyl ether

BCMF B-cell maturation factor

BCMS Bioethic Citation Maintenance System

BCN basal cell nevus; bilateral cortical necrosis; breast care nursing

BCNS basal cell nevus syndrome

BCNU bis-chlorethylnitrosourea [carmustine]

BCO biliary cholesterol output; biologic cutoff

BCOC bowel care of choice

BCoV bovine coronavirus

BCP basic calcium phosphate; birth control pill; blue cone pigment; Blue Cross Plan; bromcresol purple

BCPD bromcresol purple deoxylate

BCPR bystander cardiopulmonary resuscitation

BCPT Breast Cancer Prevention Trial

BCPV bovine cutaneous papilloma virus

BCQ breast cancer questionnaire

BCR B-cell reactivity; birth control regimen; breakpoint cluster region; bromocriptine; bulbocavernosus reflex

bcr breakpoint cluster region

BCRS brief cognitive rating scale

BCRx birth control drug

BCS battered child syndrome; blood cell separator; bovine calf serum; breast cancer screening; British Cardiovascular Society; Budd-Chiari syndrome

BCSFB blood–cerebrospinal fluid barrier

BCSI breast cancer screening indicator

BCSP Bavarian Cholesterol Screening Project

BCT brachiocephalic trunk; branched-chain amino acid transferase; breast conservation therapy

BCTF Breast Cancer Task Force

BCtg bovine chymotrypsinogen

BCtr bovine chymotrypsin

BCV Batu Cave virus; between class variance; blue crab virus; Bunyip Creek virus

BCVA best corrected visual acuity

BCVd blister canker viroid

BCW biological and chemical warfare

BCYE buffered charcoal yeast extract [agar]

BD barbital dependent; barbiturate dependence; base deficit; base of prism down; basophilic degeneration; Batten disease; behavioral disorder; Behçet disease; belladonna; below diaphragm; Bessel distribution; bicarbonate dialysis; bile duct; binding domain; binocular deprivation; birth date; black death; bladder drainage; block design [test]; blood donor; blue diaper [syndrome]; borderline dull; bound; brain damage; brain dead, brain death; Briquet disorder; bronchodilation, bronchodilator; buccodistal; Byler disease

B-D Becton-Dickinson

Bd board; buoyant density

bd band; bundle

b.d. twice a day [L. *bis in die*]

BDA balloon dilation angioplasty; British Dental Association

BDAC Bureau of Drug Abuse Control

BDAE Boston Diagnostic Aphasia Examination

BDAV Bandia virus

BDC Bazex-Dupré-Christol [syndrome]; bile duct cyst; burn-dressing change

BDD body dysmorphic disorder

BDE balanced differential expression; bile duct examination

BDentSci Bachelor of Dental Science

BDG buccal developmental groove; buffered desoxycholate glucose

BDGF brain-derived growth factor

BDHI Buss-Durkee Hostility Inventory

BDI Baseline Dyspnea Index; Beck Depression Inventory; bile duct injuries

BDIP biomedical digital image processing

BDIS Becton-Dickinson immunocytometry system; Birth Defects Information Service

BDL behaviors of daily living; below detectable limits; bile duct ligation

BDLD big dog/little dog [veterinary medicine]

BDLS Brachmann–de Lange syndrome

BDM 2,3-butanedione 2-monoxime; Becker muscular dystrophy; border detection method

BDMS Bureau of Data Management Strategy

bDNA branched deoxyribonucleic acid

BDNF brain-derived neurotrophic factor

BDO battle dress overgarment

BDOH broad determinants of health

BDP beclomethasone dipropionate; benzodiazepine; bilateral diaphragmatic paralysis; bronchopulmonary dysplasia

BDQ bowel disease questionnaire

BDR background diabetic retinopathy

BDRP Biological Defense Research Program

BDRS Blessed Dementia Rating Scale

BDS Bachelor of Dental Surgery; biologic detection system; Blessed Dementia Scale

BdS blood pressure–depressing substance

BDSc Bachelor of Dental Science

BDT binary distance transformation

BDUR 5-bromodeoxyuridine

BDV border disease virus; Borna disease virus

BDW biphasic defibrillation waveform; buffered distilled water

BE bacillary emulsion; bacterial endocarditis; barium enema; Barrett esophagus; base excess; below elbow; bile esculin [test]; bioequivalence; biologic effect; biologically effective; biologically equivalent; bovine enteritis; brain edema; bread equivalent; breast examination; bronchiectasis; bronchoesophagology

B/E below elbow

B&E brisk and equal

Be beryllium

Bé Baumé scale

BEA below-elbow amputation; bioelectrical activity; bromoethylamine

BEAC Barrett esophagus–associated adenocarcinoma

BEACOPP bleomycin, etoposide, Adriamycin, cyclophosphamide, Oncovin, prednisone, and procarbazine

BEAM brain electrical activity monitoring

BEAP bronchiectasis, eosinophilia, asthma, pneumonia

BEAR biologic effects of atomic radiation

BEB Biomedical Engineering Branch

BEBV Bebaru virus

BEC bacterial endocarditis; behavioral emergency committee; biliary epithelial cells; blood ethyl alcohol content; bromoergocryptine; buccal epithelial cells

BECAIT Bezafibrate Coronary Atherosclerosis Intervention Trial

BECF blood extracellular fluid

BED binge eating disorder; biologically effective dose; biologically equivalent dose
BEE basal energy expenditure
BEFV bovine ephemeral fever virus
beg begin, beginning
BEH benign exertional headache
beh behavior, behavioral
BEHA behavior
BEHAVE-AD Behavioral Pathology in Alzheimer's Disease (scale)
BEI back-scattered electron imaging; biological exposure indexes; butanol-extractable iodine
BEIR biologic effects of ionizing radiation
BEK bovine embryonic kidney
BEL blood ethanol level; bovine embryonic lung
BELIR beta-endorphin−like immunoreactivity
BELTV Belterra virus
BELV Belmont virus
BEM boundary element method
BEMS Bioelectromagnetics Society
BeMV belladonna mottle virus
BEN Balkan endemic neuropathy
bENaC bovine epithelial sodium channel
BENAR blood eosinophilic non-allergic rhinitis
BENEDICT Bergamo Nephrologic Diabetes Complications Trial
BENESTENT Belgian-Netherlands Stent [study]
BENV Benevides virus; Benfica virus
Benz, benz benzene; benzidine; benzoate
BEP basic element of performance; brain evoked potential
B-EP β-endorphin
BEPS Belgian Eminase Prehospital Study
BEPT biliary endoscopic papillotomy
BER base encoding rule; base excision repair; basic electrical rhythm
BERA brainstem evoked response audiometry
BERG balloon-assisted endoscopic retroperitoneal gasless [approach]
BERNWARD building essential concept representations in well-arranged restricted domains
β error type II error
BERT Beneficiary Enrollment Retrieval System [Medicare]; Beta Energy Restenosis Trial
BERV Bertioga virus
BES balanced electrolyte solution; Baltimore Eye Study
BESA brain electric source analysis
BESC bronchitis emphysema symptom checklist

BESM bovine embryonic skeletal muscle
BESMART Bestent in Small Arteries Study
BESP bovine embryonic spleen [cells]
BESS Berlin Pacemaker Study on Syncope; Part B Extract and Summary System [Medicare]
BESSAMI Berlin Stent Study in Acute Myocardial Infarction
BEST Beta-blocker Evaluation of Survival Trial; Beta-blocker Stroke Trial; Beta-Cath System Trial; Bolus Dose Escalation Study of Tissue-Type Plasminogen Activator; Bucindolol Evaluation of Survival Trial
BET benign epithelial tumor; blastocyte embryo transfer; bleeding esophageal varix; Brunauer-Emmet-Teller [method]
BETA Biomedical Electronics Technicians Association
BEV baboon endogenous virus; beam's eye view; Berne virus; bovine enterovirus
BeV, Bev billion electron volts
bev beverage
BF Barmah Forest [virus]; bentonite flocculation; bile flow; biofeedback; black female; blastogenic factor; blister fluid; blood flow; body fat; bouillon filtrate; brain factor; breakfast fed; breastfeeding; buffered; burning feet [syndrome]; butter fat
B/F black female; bound/free [antigen] ratio
B3F band 3 cytoplasmic fragment
bf black female; bouillon filtrate
BFA bifemoral angiography; brefeldin A
BFB biologic feedback; bronchial foreign body
BFC benign febrile convulsion
BFDI bronchodilation following deep inspiration
BFDV beak and feather disease virus; bulk fluid endocytosis
BFE blood flow energy
BFEC benign focal epilepsy of childhood
BFF buried free flap
bFGF basic fibroblast growth factor
BFGS Broyden-Fletcher-Goldfarb-Shanno [algorithm]
BFH benign familial hematuria
BFHD Beukes familial hip dysplasia
BFHI Baby-Friendly Hospital Initiative
BFHR basal fetal heart rate
BFIC benign familial infantile convulsions
BFIRM binary formal inference-based recessive modeling
BFL below functional limit; bird fancier's lung; Börjeson-Forssman-Lehman [syndrome]
BFLS Börjeson-Forssman-Lehmann syndrome
BFM benign familial megalocephaly or macrocephaly

BFNC benign familial neonatal convulsion

BFO balanced forearm orthosis; ball-bearing forearm orthosis; blood-forming organ

BFOD binary frames of discernment

BFP biologic false positive

BFPR biologic false-positive reaction

BFPSTS biologic false-positive serologic test for syphilis

BFR biologic false reaction; blood flow rate; bone formation rate; buffered Ringer [solution]

BFRB body-focused repetitive behaviors

BFS blood fasting sugar

B/F/S blow-fill-seal

BFT bentonite flocculation test; biofeedback training

BFU burst-forming unit

BFU-E burst-forming unit, erythrocytes

BFU-ME burst-forming unit, myeloid/erythroid

BFU-Meg burst-forming unit, megakaryocyte

BFV Barmah Forest virus; bovine feces virus; bovine foamy virus

BG *Bacillus globigii*; basal ganglion; basic gastrin; basophilic granulocyte; Bender Gestalt [test]; beta-galactosidase; beta-glucuronidase; bicolor guaiac [test]; Birbeck granule; blood glucose; bone graft; brilliant green; buccogingival

B-G Bordet-Gengou [agar]

BGA blue-green algae

BGAg blood group antigen

BGAV blue-green algae virus

BGC basal ganglion calcification; blood group class

BGCA bronchogenic carcinoma

BGD blood group degradation

BGE butyl glycidyl ether

BGEM brain gene expression map [mouse]

BGG bovine gamma-globulin

bGH bovine growth hormone

BGIV Bangui virus

Bg^J beige [mouse]

BGLB brilliant green lactose broth

BGlu blood glucose

BGM bedside glucose monitoring

BGMR biological-guided mucosa regeneration

BGNV Bangoran virus

BGO bismuth germanium oxide

BGP beta-glycerophosphatase

BGPS Belgian General Practitioners' Study

BGS balance, gait, and station; Baller-Gerold syndrome; blood group substance; British Geriatrics Society

BGSA blood granulocyte-specific activity

BGTT borderline glucose tolerance test

BGV Bahia Grande virus

BH base hospital; benzalkonium and heparin; bill of health; birth history; Bishop-Harman [instruments]; board of health; boarding home; Bolton-Hunter [reagent]; borderline hypertensive; both hands; brain hormone; Braxton-Hicks [contractions]; breathholding; bronchial hyperreactivity; Bryan high titer; bundle of His

BH4 tetrahydrobiopterin

BHA bound hepatitis antibody; butylated hydroxyanisole

BHAT Beta Blocker Heart Attack Trial

BHAV Bhanja virus

BHB beta-hydroxybutyrate

bHb bovine hemoglobin

BHBA beta-hydroxybutyric acid

BHC benzene hexachloride

BHCDA Bureau of Health Care Delivery and Assistance

β-hCG beta human chorionic gonadotropin

BHF Bolivian hemorrhagic fever; British Heart Foundation

BHFS Benzapril Heart Failure Study

BHI biosynthetic human insulin; brain-heart infusion; British Humanities Index; Bureau of Health Insurance

BHIA brain-heart infusion agar

BHIBA brain-heart infusion blood agar

BHIRS brain-heart infusion and rabbit serum

BHIS beef heart infusion supplemented [broth]

BHK baby hamster kidney [cells]; type-B Hong Kong [virus]

BHL bilateral hilar lymphadenopathy; biologic half-life

bHLH basic helix-loop-helix

bHLH-ZIP basic helix-loop-helix leucine zipper

BHM Bureau of Health Manpower

BHN bephenium hydroxynaphthoate; Brinell hardness number

BHP basic health profile

BHPr Bureau of Health Professions

BHR basal heart rate; benign hypertrophic prostatitis; borderline hypertensive rat; bronchial hyperreactivity

BHRT bioidentical hormone replacement therapy

BHS Bachelor of Health Science; Ballarat Health Services; Beck Hopelessness Scale; beta-hemolytic streptococcus; Bogalusa Heart Study; breathholding spell; Brisighella Heart Study

BHSc Nsg Bachelor of Health Science in Nursing

BHT beta-hydroxytheophylline; breath hydrogen test; bronchial hygiene therapy; butylated hydroxytoluene

BHTE bioheat transfer equation
BHU basic health unit
Bhu *Bordetella* heme utilization
BhuR *Bordetella* heme utilization receptor
BHV bovine herpes virus
BH/VH body hematocrit/venous hematocrit ratio
BHyg Bachelor of Hygiene
BI background interval; bacterial/bactericidal index; base in [prism]; basilar impression; bifunctional inducer; Billroth I [procedure]; biologic indicator; biotechnology infomatics; bodily injury; bone injury; bowel impaction; brain injury; burn index
Bi bismuth
BIA bioelectric impedance analysis; bio-immunoassay; biomechanical impedance analyses
BIAA Brain Injury Association of America
BIAC Bioinstrumentation Advisory Council
BIAD blind insertion airway device
BIB bibliography; biliointestinal bypass; brought in by
BiB balloon in balloon [catheter]
bib, biblio bibliography
bib. drink
BIBRA British Industrial Biological Research Association
B-IBS B-immunoblastic sarcoma
BIC Bayes information criterion; bicoherence; blood isotope clearance; brain imaging center
Bic biceps
BICAO bilateral internal carotid artery occlusion
bicarb bicarbonate
BiCAT bilateral carotid artery traction
BICC Biomedical Information Communications Center
BiCNU bis-chlorethylnitrosourea [carmustine]
BICS Brigham Integrated Computing System
BICS-OE Brigham Integrated Computing System, order entry
BICST biceps skin tone
BID bibliographic information and documentation; brought in dead
bid, b.i.d. twice a day [L. *bis in die*]
BIDA butyliminodiacetic acid
BIDLB block in posteroinferior division of left branch
BIDS biologic integrated detection system; brittle hair, intellectual impairment, decreased fertility, and short stature [syndrome]
BIE Bayes inference engine; bioelectrical impedance; bullous ichthyosiform erythroderma

BIG bone injection gun
BIG 6 analysis of six serum components
BIGGY bismuth glycine glucose yeast
BIGPRO Biguanides and the Prevention of the Risk of Obesity [study]
BIH benign intracranial hypertension
BII beat inclusion index; Billroth II [procedure]; butanol-insoluble iodine
BIL basal insulin level; bilirubin; bodily injury liability
Bil bilirubin
bil bilateral
BILAG British Isles Lupus Assessment Group
BIL/ALB bilirubin/albumin ratio
bilat bilateral
bili bilirubin
bili-c conjugated bilirubin
BilIN biliary intraepithelial neoplasia
bilirub bilirubin
bili T&D bilirubin total and direct
BIM buffered isolation medium
BIMA bilateral internal mammary artery
BIMV Bimiti virus
BIN butylisonitrile
Bin binary
BIND Biological Investigational New Drug
BIO Biotechnology Industry Organization
biochem biochemical, biochemistry
BIOD bony intraorbital distance
bioeng bioengineering
BIOF biologic function
biol biologic, biology
bioLH bioassay of luteinizing hormone
BIOMACS Biochemical Markers of Acute Coronary Syndromes
biophys biophysical, biophysics
BIOS basic input/output system
BIOSIS Biosciences Information Service
biotyping biochemical typing
BIP back-illuminated photo technology; bacterial intravenous protein; Bezafibrate Infarction Prevention [study]; biparietal; bismuth iodoform paraffin; Blue Cross interim payment; brief infertility period
Bip binding protein
BiPAP biphasic positive airway pressure
BIPLED bilateral, independent, periodic, lateralized epileptiform discharge
BIPM International Bureau of Weights and Measures [Fr. *Bureau International des Poids et Mesures*]
BIPP bismuth iodoform paraffin paste
BIR basic incidence rate; British Institute of Radiology
BIRADS Breast Imaging Reporting and Data System

BIRD Bolus Versus Infusion Rescupase Development

BIRLS Beneficiary Identification and Record Locator Subsystem

BIRN Biomedical Informatics Research Network

BIRNH Belgian Interuniversity Research on Nutrition and Health [study]

BIRV Birao virus

BIS bioimpedance spectroscopy; bispectral index; bone cement implantation syndrome; Brain Information Service; British Infection Society; building illness syndrome

B-ISDN broadband—integrated services digital network

BiSP between ischial spines

bisp bispinous

BISTI Biomedical Information Service Technology Initiative

BIT binary digit; bitrochanteric

bit binary digit

BITA bilateral internal thoracic artery

BITE Bulimic Investigatory Test

BIU barrier isolation unit; billion international units

BIV Bohle iridovirus; bovine immunodeficiency virus

BIVAS Body Image Visual Analogue Scale

BJ Bence Jones [protein]; biceps jerk; Bielschowsky-Jansky [disease]; bones and joints

B&J bones and joints

BJE bones, joints, and examination

BJM bones, joints, and muscles

BJP Bence Jones protein/proteinuria

BK below knee; bovine kidney [cells]; bradykinin

B-K initials of two patients after whom a multiple cutaneous nevus was named

B/K below knee

Bk berkelium

bk back

BKA below-knee amputation

BK-A basophil kallikrein of anaphylaxis

BK amp below-knee amputation

BKAT Basic Knowledge Assessment Tool for Critical Care

BKD bacterial kidney disease

bkf breakfast

BKG, Bkg background

BKPyV BK polyomavirus

BKS beekeeper serum

BKTT below knee to toe

BKWP below-knee walking plaster

BL Barré-Lieou [syndrome]; basal lamina; baseline; Bessey-Lowry [unit]; biosafety level; black light; bladder; bleeding; blind loop; blood loss; bone marrow lymphocyte; borderline lepromatous; bronchial lavage; buccolingual; buffered lidocaine; Bullard laryngoscope; Burkitt lymphoma

Bl black

B-l bursa-equivalent lymphocyte

bl black; bleeding, blood; blue

BLA Biologics License Application

BLAD borderline left-axis deviation

blad bladder

BLAS Bronx Longitudinal Aging Study

BLASP Barbados Low-Dose Aspirin Study in Pregnancy

BLAST basic linear/local alignment search tool

BLAT Blind Learning Aptitude Test

BLAV Bobia virus

BLB Baker-Lima-Baker [mask]; Bessey-Lowry-Brock [method, unit]; black light bulb; Boothby-Lovelace-Bulbulian [mask]; bronchoscopic lung biopsy; bulb [syringe]

BL=BS bilateral equal breath sounds

BlC blood culture

BLCL Burkitt lymphoma cell line

B-LCL B-lymphocyte cell line

bl cult blood culture

BLD basal liquefactive degeneration; benign lymphoepithelial disease

bld blood

Bld Bnk blood bank

BLE both lower extremities; buffered lidocaine with epinephrine

BLEL benign lymphoepithelial lesion

BLEO bleomycin

bleph blepharitis

BLEVE boiling liquid expanding vapor explosion

BLFD buccolinguofacial dyskinesia

BLG behavioral leadership group; beta-lactoglobulin

bLH biologically active luteinizing hormone

BLI bombesin-like immunoreactivity

blk black

BLL below lower limit

BLLD British Library Lending Division

BLLV Bloodland Lake virus

BLM basolateral membrane; bilayer lipid membrane; bimolecular liquid membrane; black lipid membrane; bleomycin; Bloom syndrome; buccolinguomasticatory

BLMV Belem virus

BLN bronchial lymph node

BLOB binary large object

BLOBS bladder obstruction

BLOC body location

BLOSUM block substitution matrix [algorithm]

BLOT Bimodality Lung Oncology Trial

BLP beta-lipoprotein

BlP blood pressure

B-LPH beta-lipoprotein hormone

B-LPN beta-lipotropin

bl pr blood pressure

BLQ both lower quadrants

BLRC Biomedical Library Review Committee

BLROA British Laryngological, Rhinological, and Otological Association

BLS bare lymphocyte syndrome; basic life support; B-cell lymphoproliferative syndrome; blind loop syndrome; blood and lymphatic system; blood sugar; Bloom syndrome; Bureau of Labor Statistics

BlS blood sugar

BLSA Baltimore Longitudinal Study of Aging; basic life support ambulance

BLSD bovine lumpy skin disease

BLS-D basic life support defibrillation; Blessed Scale−Dementia

BLT bleeding time; blood-clot lysis time; blood test

BlT bleeding time; blood test; blood type, blood typing

BLU Bessey-Lowry unit

BLV biologic limit value; blood volume; bovine leukemia virus

BlV blood viscosity; blood volume

BLVR biliverdin reductase

Blx bleeding time

BLyS B-lymphocyte stimulator

BM Bachelor of Medicine; Bachelor of Midwifery; barium meal; basal medium; basal metabolism; basement membrane; basilar membrane; betamethasone; biomedical; black male; blood monitoring; body mass; Bohr magneton; bone marrow; bowel movement; breast milk; buccal mass; buccomesial

B/M black male

B2M, β₂m beta-2-microglobulin

bm black male

BMA biologic movement artifacts; bone marrow arrest; bone mineral area; British Medical Association

BmA *Brugia malayi* adult antigen

BMAD Medicare Part B Annual Data

BMAP bone marrow acid phosphatase

B-MAST Brief Michigan Alcoholism Screening Test

BMAV Batama virus

B_max maximum amount bound; maximum binding capacity

BMB biomedical belt; bone marrow biopsy

BMBL benign monoclonal B-cell lymphocytosis; Biosafety in Microbiological and Biomedical Laboratories [CDC publication]

BMBMA bulk motion biologic movement artifacts

BMC blood mononuclear cell; bone marrow cell; bone mineral content

BMCC beta-methylcrotonyl coenzyme A carboxylase

BMCHRD Bureau of Maternal and Child Health and Resources Development

BMD Becker muscular dystrophy; Boehringer Mannheim Diagnostics; bone marrow depression; bone mineral density; bovine mucosal disease

BMDC Biomedical Documentation Center; bone marrow dendritic cell

BMDP biomedical program

BMDSC bone marrow−derived stem cell

BMDW Bone Marrow Donor Worldwide

BME basal medium Eagle; biundulant meningoencephalitis; brief maximal effort

BMed Bachelor of Medicine

BMedBiol Bachelor of Medical Biology

BMedSci Bachelor of Medical Science

BMEI benign myoclonic epilepsy in childhood

BMES Biomedical Engineering Society

BMET biomedical equipment technician

BMF bone marrow failure

BMG benign monoclonal gammopathy

BMH biomechanical heart

BMI body mass index; brief motivational intervention

BMic Bachelor of Microbiology

BMIPP beta-methyliodophenylpentadecanoic acid

BMJ bones, muscles, joints; *British Medical Journal*

bmk birthmark

BML biomedical library; bone marrow lymphocytosis

BMLS billowing mitral leaflet syndrome

BMM bone marrow−derived macrophages

BMM+ bone marrow micrometastasis positive

BMAA beta-methylamino-L-alanine

BMMP benign mucous membrane pemphigoid

BMMS Better Medication Management System

BMN bone marrow necrosis

BMNC blood mononuclear cell

BMOC Brinster's medium for ovum culture

Bmod behavior modification

B-mode brightness modulation

BMP basic metabolic panel; bitmap; bone morphogenetic protein

bmp bone morphogenetic protein

BMPI bronchial mucous proteinase inhibitor

BMPP benign mucous membrane pemphigus; beta-methyliodophenylpentadecanoic acid

BMQA Board of Medical Quality Assurance

BMR basal metabolic rate

BMRC British Medical Research Council

BMS Bachelor of Medical Science; bare-metal stent; Belfast Metoprolol Study; beta-methasone; biomedical monitoring system; biomedical science; bleomycin sulfate; broadcast message server; Bureau of Medical Services; Bureau of Medicine and Surgery; burning mouth syndrome

BMSA British Medical Students Association

BMSP biomedical sciences program

BMST Bruce maximum stress test

BMT Bachelor of Medical Technology; basement membrane thickening; benign mesenchymal tumor; bone marrow transplant/transplantation

BMTd bicyclic monoterpene diols

BMT-GVHD bone marrow transplantation graft-versus-host disease

BMTU bone marrow transplantation unit

BMU basic metabolic unit; basic multicellular unit

BMZ basement membrane zone

BN Bachelor of Nursing; Bayesian network; binucleated; bladder neck; branchial neuritis; bronchial node; brown Norway [rat]; bulimia nervosa

BNA Baromedical Nurses Association; Basle Nomina Anatomica; bronchoscopic needle aspiration

BNAML Brown Norway acute myelocytic leukemia

BNC brain sodium channel

BNCT benign notochord cell tumor; boron neutron capture therapy

BND barely noticeable difference

BNDD Bureau of Narcotics and Dangerous Drugs

BNEd Bachelor of Nursing Education

BNF British National Formulary

BNG Bayesian Network Generation

BNIST National Bureau of Scientific Information [Fr. *Bureau Nationale d'Information Scientifique*]

Bnl branchless

BNML brown Norway rat myelocytic leukemia

BN-NP nonpurging bulimia nervosa

BNO bladder neck obstruction; bowels not opened

bNOS brain nitric oxide synthase

BNP brain natriuretic peptide

BNPA binasal pharyngeal airway

BNR beam nonuniformity ratio [ultrasound]

BN/RN baccalaurate registered nurse

BNS Belfast Nifedipine Study; benign nephrosclerosis

BNSc Bachelor of Nursing Science

BNT Boston Naming Test; brain neurotransmitter

BO Bachelor of Osteopathy; base of prism out; behavior objective; belladonna and opium; body odor; bowel obstruction; bowels opened; bronchiolitis obliterans; buccoocclusal

Bo Bolton point

bo bowels

B&O belladonna and opium

BOA behavioral observation audiometry; born on arrival; British Orthopaedic Association

BOAT back pain outcome assessment team; Balloon vs. Optimal Atherectomy Trial

BOB biorthogonal basis

BOBA beta-oxybutyric acid

BOC blood oxygen capacity; Bureau of Census; butyloxycarbonyl

BOCC biomedical occupation

BoCV bovine enteric calicivirus

BOD biochemical oxygen demand; brachymorphism, onychodysplasia, dysphalangism [syndrome]

Bod Bodansky [unit]

BOE benign occipital epilepsy

BOEA ethyl biscoumacetate

BOEC blood outgrowth epithelial cell

BOF branchiooculofacial [syndrome]

BOFS branchiooculofacial syndrome

BOH board of health

BoHV bovine herpesvirus

BoiHV Boid herpesvirus

BOILER Balloon Occlusive Intravascular Lysis Enhanced Recanalization [strategy]

BOL beginning of life

Bol. bolus

BOLD bleomycin, Oncovin, lomustine, dacarbazine; blood oxygenation−level dependent

BolVX Boletus virus X

BOM bilateral otitis media

BOMA bilateral otitis media, acute

BoNT A to E botulinum neurotoxins A to E

BOOP bronchiolitis obliterans−organizing pneumonia

BOP buffalo orphan prototype [virus]

BOPP boronated protoporphyrin
bOPV bivalent oral poliovirus vaccine
BOR basal optic root; before time of operation; bowels open regularly; branchio-oto-renal [syndrome]
BORR blood oxygen release rate
BORSA borderline resistant *Staphylococcus aureus*
BoRV *Buthus occitanus* reovirus
BOS base of support; Bioethics Online Service; branchio-otic syndrome
BOSC Board of Scientific Counselors
BoSM Bolivian squirrel monkey
BOSS Balloon Optimization vs. Stent Study
BOT botulinum toxin
bot bottle
BOTV Botambi virus
BoTV bovine torovirus
BOU branchio-oto-ureteral [syndrome]
BOUV Bouboui virus
BoV Boolarra virus
BOW bag of waters
BOZOV Bozo virus
1-BP 1-bromopropane
BP Bachelor of Pharmacy; bacillary peliosis; backpassage [culture]; back pressure; back projection; back propagation; barometric pressure; base pairs; basic protein; bathroom privileges; bed pan; before present; behavior pattern; Bell palsy; benzpyrene; beta-protein; binding protein; biochemical pregnancies; biotic potential; biparietal; biphenyl; bipolar; birthplace; bisphosphonate; blood pressure; body plethysmography; boiling point; Bolton point; borderline personality; bowenoid papulosis; breech presentation; British Pharmacopoeia; bronchopleural; bronchopulmonary; buccopulpal; bullous pemphigus/pemphigoid; bypass
B/P blood pressure
BP II bipolar type II disorder
BP180 bullous pemphigoid antigen II
BP230 bullous pemphigoid antigen I
bp base pair; bed pan; boiling point
BPA basic probability assignment; bisphenol A; blood pressure assembly; bovine plasma albumin; British Paediatric Association; bronchopulmonary aspergillosis; burst-promoting activity
BPAEC bovine pulmonary artery endothelial cell
BPAG bullous pemphigoid antigen
BPANN back propagation artificial neural network
B-PAP bilevel positive airway pressure
BPAR body part

BPAS body profile analysis system
BPB biliopancreatic bypass; bromphenol blue
BPC Behavior Problem Checklist; bile phospholipid concentration; blood pressure cuff; British Pharmaceutical Codex
BPCS back pain classification scale
BPD biparental disomy; biparietal diameter; blood pressure decrease; borderline personality disorder; bronchopulmonary dysplasia
BPDE benzo(a)pyrene-diol-epoxide
BPE bacterial phosphatidylethanolamine
BPEAS benign partial epilepsy with affective symptoms
BPEC benign partial epilepsy of childhood; bipolar electrocardiogram; bipolar electrocoagulation
BPED benign proliferative epithelial disorder
BPEG British Pacing and Electrophysiology Group [study]
BPEI blepharophimosis, ptosis, epicanthus inversus
BPES blepharophimosis, ptosis, epicanthus inversus syndrome
BPF bandpass filter; bradykinin-potentiating factor; Brazilian purpuric fever; bronchopulmonary fistula; burst-promoting factor
BPFC Brazilian purpuric fever clone
BPG benzathine penicillin G; D-2,3-bisphosphoglycerate; blood pressure gauge; bypass graft
BPGM bisphosphoglyceromutase
BPH Bachelor of Public Health; benign prostatic hyperplasia; benign prostatic hypertrophy
BPh British Pharmacopoeia; buccopharyngeal
Bph bacteriopheophytin
BPharm Bachelor of Pharmacy
BPHC Bureau of Primary Health Care
BPHEng Bachelor of Public Health Engineering
BPheo bacteriopheophytin
BPHN Bachelor of Public Health Nursing
BPI bactericidal/permeability increasing [protein]; Basic Personality Inventory; beef-pork insulin; Behavior Problem Inventory; bipolar type 1; blood pressure increase; blood pressure index; Brief Pain Inventory
BPIV bovine parainfluenza virus
BPL Beneficiary Program Liability; benign proliferative lesion; benzyl penicilloyl-polylysine; beta-propiolactone
BPLA blood pressure, left arm
BPM beats per minute; best partial match [imaging]; biperidyl mustard; block perfusion monitor; body protein monitor; breaths per minute; brompheniramine maleate

bpm beats per minute

BPMF British Postgraduate Medical Federation

BPMS blood plasma measuring system

BPN bacitracin, polymyxin B, neomycin sulfate; back propagation neural network [algorithm]; brachial plexus neuropathy

BPO basal pepsin output; benzylpenicil-loyl

BPP binding property pair; biophysical profile; bovine pancreatic polypeptide; bradykinin potentiating peptide

BP&P blood pressure and pulse

BPPD Biopesticides and Pollution Prevention Division

BPPN benign paroxysmal positioning nystagmus

BPPV benign paroxysmal positional vertigo; bovine paragenital papillomavirus

BPQ Berne Pain Questionnaire

BPR blood pressure recorder; blood production rate

BPRA blood pressure, right arm

BPROP back propagation neural network

BPRS Brief Psychiatric Rating Scale; Brief Psychiatric Reacting Scale

BPS Basel Prospective Study; beats per second; Behavioral Pharmacology Society; biophysical profile score; bits per second; bovine papular stomatitis; brain protein solvent; breaths per second; bytes per second; systolic blood pressure

Bps, bps bits per second; bytes per second

BPSA bronchopulmonary segmental artery

BPSD behavioral and psychological symptoms of dementia

BPSMC Blood Pressure Study in Mexican Children

BPsTh Bachelor of Psychotherapy

BPSU British Paediatric Surveillance Unit

BPSV bovine papular stomatitis virus

BPT benign paroxysmal torticollis; binding property torsion; bronchial provocation test

BPTI basic pancreatic trypsin inhibitor; basic polyvalent trypsin inhibitor; bovine pancreatic trypsin inhibitor

BPV bat paramyxovirus; bee paralysis virus; benign paroxysmal vertigo; benign positional vertigo; bioprosthetic valve; bovine papillomavirus; bovine parvovirus

BP(Vet) British Pharmacopoeia (Veterinary)

BPXV buffalopox virus

BPyV baboon polyomavirus; bovine polyomavirus

Bq becquerel

BQA Bureau of Quality Assurance

BQSV Barranqueras virus

BR baroreflex; barrier reared [animals]; baseline recovery; bathroom; bed rest; bedside rounds; bilirubin; biologic response; blink reflex; branchial; breathing rate; breathing training; bronchial, bronchitis, bronchus; *Brucella*; brush cytology

Br brain; breech; bregma; bridge; bromine; bronchitis; brown; *Brucella*; brucellosis

bR bacteriorhodopsin

br boiling range; brachial; branch; branchial; breath; brother

BRA bilateral renal agenesis; bone-resorbing activity; brain; brain-reactive antibody; brainstem auditory [response]

BRAC basic rest-activity cycle

Brach brachial

Brady, brady bradycardia

BRAFE brachial, radial, and femoral [approach]

BRAGS Bioelectric Repair and Growth Society

BRAIN-ICU Bringing to Light Risk Factors and Incidence of Neuropsychological Dysfunction in ICU Survivors [study]

BRAINS Biochemical Research and Information Study; Brain Research, Analysis of Images, Networks, and Systems

BRAMS Bech-Rafaelson Melancholia Scale

BRAO branch retinal artery occlusion

BRAP burst of rapid atrial pacing

BrAP brachial artery pressure

BRAT banana, rice, applesauce, and toast [diet]; Baylor rapid autologous transfusion [system]

BRAVE biosense revascularization approach for viable endocardium

BRB blood-retinal barrier; bright red blood

BRBC bovine red blood cell

BRBN blue rubber bleb nevus

BRBNS blue rubber bleb nevus syndrome

BRBPR bright red blood per rectum

BRbx breast biopsy

BRC brain reserve capacity

Brc bromocriptine

BRCA breast cancer

BRCA1, BRCA2 breast cancer susceptibility genes

BRCD breast cancer, ductal

BRCM below right costal margin

BRCS British Red Cross Society

BRCT Brain Resuscitation Clinical Trial

BRD bladder retraining drill; bovine respiratory disease

BrdU, BrdUrd 5-bromodeoxyuridine

BRDV Broadhaven virus

BRE benign rolandic epilepsy

BREASTS bronchopulmonary aspergillosis, radiotherapy, extrinsic allergic alveolitis, ankylosing spondylitis, sarcoidosis, tuberculosis, silicosis

BRESEK brain anomalies, retardation of mentality (intellectual disability), ectodermal dysplasia, kidney dysplasia/hypoplasia [syndrome]

BRESHECK brain anomalies, retardation of mentality (intellectual disability) and growth, ectodermal hypoplasia, Hirschsprung disease, ear deformity and deafness, eye hypoplasia, cleft palate, cryptorchidism, kidney dysplasia/hypoplasia [syndrome]

BRESUS British Hospital Resuscitation Study

BRF bone-resorbing factor

BRFSS Behavioral Risk Factor Surveillance System

BRH benign recurrent hematuria; British Regional Heart [study]; Bureau of Radiological Health

BRHS British Regional Heart Study

BRIC benign recurrent intrahepatic cholestasis

BRIEF Behavioral Rating Inventory of Executive Function

BRILLIANT Blood Pressure, Renal Effects, Insulin Control, Lipids, Lisinopril and Nifedipine Trial

BRIME brief repetitive isometric maximal exercise

BRIN Biomedical Research Infrastructure Network

Brkf breakfast

BRM biologic response modifier; biuret reactive material

BRMS Bannayan-Riley-Myhre-Smith [syndrome]; Bech-Rafaelsen Melancholia Scale

BRMV Berrimah virus

BRN Board of Registered Nursing

brn brown

BRO bronchiolitis obliterans; bronchoscopy

bro brother

brom bromide

Bron, Bronch bronchi, bronchial; bronchoscopy

BRONJ bisphosphonate-related osteonecrosis of the jaw

Broncho bronchoscopy

BRP bathroom privileges; bilirubin production; biologic reference preparation; bronchophony

Brph bronchophony

BRR Bannayan-Riley-Ruvalcaba [syndrome]; baroreceptor reflex response; breathing reserve ratio

BRS baroreflex sensitivity; behavior rating scale; Bibliographic Retrieval Services; British Roentgen Society

BrSM Brazilian squirrel monkey

BRSV bovine respiratory syncytial virus

BRT Brook reaction test

brth breath

BRU bone remodeling unit

5-BrU 5-bromouracil

BrU bromouracil

Bruc *Brucella*

BRUV Bruconha virus

BRV baboon orthoreovirus; bovine rhinovirus; Breda virus

BRVO branch retinal vein occlusion

BRW Brown-Robert-Wells [system]

BS Bachelor of Science; Bachelor of Surgery; *Bacillus subtilis*; Bartter syndrome; base strap; bedside; before sleep; Behçet syndrome; bilateral symmetric; bile salt; Binet-Simon [test]; bismuth sulfite; blood sample; blood sugar; Bloom syndrome; Blue Shield; body system; borderline schizophrenia; bowel sound; breaking strength; breath sound; British Standard; buffered saline; Bureau of Standards; byte structure

B-S Björk-Shiley [valve]

B&S Brown and Sharp [sutures]

B/s, b/s bytes per second

bs bedside; bowel sound; breath sound

b × s brother-sister inbreeding

BSA benzenesulfonic acid; Biofeedback Society of America; bismuth-sulfite agar; bistrimethylsilyl-acetamide; Blind Service Association; Blue Shield Association; body surface area; bovine serum albumin; bowel sounds active

bsa bovine serum albumin

BSAG Bristol Social Adjustment Guide

BSAM basic sequential access method

BSA-NO nitrosated bovine serum albumin

BSAP brief short-action potential; brief, small, abundant potential

BSB body surface burned

BS=BL breath sounds equal bilaterally

BSC bedside care; bedside commode; bench scale calorimeter; best supportive care; bile salt concentration; Biological Stain Commission; biologic safety cabinet; Biomedical Science Corps

BSc Bachelor of Science

BSC-1, BS-C-1 *Cercopithecus* monkey kidney cells

BSCC Björk-Shiley convexo-concave [valve]; British Society for Clinical Cytology

BSCP bovine spinal cord protein

BSD bedside drainage; behavioral symptoms of dementia

BSDAC Biological Sciences Division of Academic Computing

BSDLB block in the superior division of left branch

BSE behavior summarized evaluation; bilateral intranasal sphenoethmoidectomy; bilaterally symmetric and equal; bovine spongiform encephalopathy; brain surface extractor; breast self-examination; bystander effect

BSEP brainstem evoked potential

BSER brainstem evoked response

BSF backscatter factor; B-cell stimulatory factor; benign senescent forgetfulness; busulfan

BSG basigin; biotin streptavidin gold; branchio-skeleto-genital [syndrome]

BSG-DNA biotin streptavidin gold deoxyribonucleic acid

BSH benign sexual headache

BSHAA British Society of Hearing Aid Audiologists

BSI behavior status inventory; bloodstream infection; body substance isolation; borderline syndrome index; bound serum iron; brainstem injury; brief symptom inventory; British Standards Institution

BSID Bayley Scale of Infant Development

BSIF bile salt independent fraction

BSL benign symmetric lipomatosis; biosafety level; blood sugar level

BSM Bachelor of Science in Medicine; Björk-Shiley monostrut [valve]; body surface mapping

BSMC bronchial smooth muscle cell

BSN baccalaureate of science in nursing; Bachelor of Science in Nursing; bowel sounds normal

BSNA bowel sounds normal and active

BSO bilateral sagittal osteotomy; bilateral salpingo-oophorectomy; butathione sulfoximine

BSOFP blood spot on filter paper

BSOP blood spot on filter paper

BSP bone sialoprotein; sulfobromophthalein

BSp bronchospasm

BSPA body space

BSPh Bachelor of Science in Pharmacy

BSPM body surface potential mapping

BSQ behavior style questionnaire

BSQV Bussuquara virus

BSR basal skin resistance; blood sedimentation rate; bowel sounds regular; brain stimulation reinforcement; burst suppression ratio; Buschke selective reminding [test]

BSS Bachelor of Sanitary Science; balanced salt solution; Bernard-Soulier syndrome; black silk suture; buffered salt solution; buffered single substrate

B-SS Bernard-Soulier syndrome

BSSE bile salt−stimulated esterase

bSSFP balanced steady-state free precession

BSSG beta-sitosterol glucoside (sitogluside)

BSSL bile salt−stimulated lipase

BSSO bilateral sagittal split osteotomy

BST bacteriuria screening test; bed nucleus of the striae terminalis; blood serologic test; bovine somatotropin; brief stimulus therapy

BSTFA bis-trifluoroacetamide

BSU Bartholin, Skene, urethral [glands]; basic structural unit; British standard unit

BSUB body substance

BSV banana streak virus; binocular single vision

BS-VLC byte structure variable length coding

BT bacterial translocation; balanced translocation; base of tongue; bedtime; biomedical technology; bitemporal; bitrochanteric; bladder tumor; Blalock-Taussig [shunt]; bleeding time; blood type/typing; blue tetrazolium; blue tongue; body temperature; borderline tuberculoid; bovine turbinate [cells]; brain tumor; breast tumor

Bt *Bacillus thuringiensis*

bt bowel tones

BTA Blood Transfusion Association

BTB breakthrough bleeding; bromthymol blue

BTBL bromothymol blue lactose

BTC basal temperature chart; body temperature chart; butylcholinesterase

BTCG Brain Tumor Cooperative Group

BTD biliary tract disease

BTDG Biological Therapeutics Development Group

BTDS benzoylthiamine disulfide

BTE behind the ear [hearing aid]; biphasic truncated exponential; bovine thymus extract

BTFS breast tumor frozen section

BTG beta-thromboglobulin

BTg bovine trypsinogen

BThU British thermal unit

Bti *Bacillus thuringiensis* var. *israelensis*

Btk Bruton tyrosine kinase

BTKV Boteke virus

BTL bilateral tubal ligation

Btl breathless

BTLS basic trauma life support

BTM benign tertian malaria; blood temperature monitor; body temperature monitor; bone turnover markers

BTMSA bis-trimethylsilacetylene

BTP biliary tract pain; biologic treatment planning; broad terminal phalanges

BTPABA N-benzoyl-L-tyrosyl-*p*-aminobenzoic acid

BTPS at body temperature and ambient pressure and saturated with water vapor

BTR Bezold-type reflex; biceps tendon reflex; bridge to recovery

BTr bovine trypsin

BTRID binomial transform reduced interference distribution

BTRS Belgian Ticlodipine Retinopathy Study

BTS Batten syndrome; blood transfusion service; blue toe syndrome; bradycardia-tachycardia syndrome; British Thoracic Society

BTSG Brain Tumor Study Group

bTSH bovine thyroid-stimulating hormone

BTT bridge to transplant

BTU British thermal unit

BTV blue tongue virus

BTW biologic and toxin weapon

BTWC Biological and Toxin Weapons Convention

BTX botulinum toxin; brevetoxin; bungarotoxin

BTx blood transfusion

BTX-A botulinum toxin serotype A

BTX-B brevetoxin-B

BTZ benzothiazepine

BU base of prism up; Bethesda unit; blood urea; Bodansky unit; bromouracil; burn unit

Bu butyl

bu bushel

BUA blood uric acid; broadband ultrasonic attenuation

BUB budding uninhibited by benzimidazole

Buc, Bucc buccal

BuChE butyrocholinesterase

BUD budesonide

BUDR 5-bromodeoxyuridine

BUDS bilateral upper dorsal sympathectomy

BUE both upper extremities

BUEV Buenaventura virus

BUF buffalo [rat]

BUFUL bumetanide and furosemide on lipid [profile]

BUG buccal ganglion

BUGT bilirubin-uridine diphosphate glucuronosyltransferase

BuHV bubaline herpesvirus

BUI brain uptake index

BUJV Bujaru virus

BULIT bulimia test

BULL buccal or upper lingual of lower

BUMED, BuMed Bureau of Medicine and Surgery

BUMP behavioral regression or upset in hospitalized medical patients [scale]

BUN blood urea nitrogen

bun br bundle branch

BUN/CR blood urea nitrogen/creatine ratio

BUNV Bunyamwera virus

BUO bleeding of undetermined origin; bruising of undetermined origin

BUQ both upper quadrants

BUR bilateral ureteral occlusion

Burd Burdick suction

BUS Bartholin, urethral, and Skene glands; busulfan

BUT break-up time

But, but butyrate, butyric

BV bacilliform virus; bacitracin V; bacterial vaginosis; balloon valvuloplasty; biologic value; blood vessel; blood volume; bronchovesicular

BVA Blind Veterans Association; British Veterinary Association

BVAD biventricular assist device

BVC British Veterinary Codex

BVD bovine viral diarrhea

BVDT brief vestibular disorientation test

BVDU bromovinyldeoxyuridine

BVDV bovine viral diarrhea virus

BVE binocular visual efficiency; blood vessel endothelium; blood volume expander

BVEC bovine valve endothelial cell

BVF bone volume fraction; bulboventricular foramen

BVH biventricular hypertrophy

BVI blood vessel invasion

BVL bilateral vas ligation

BVM bag-valve-mask; bronchovascular markings; Bureau of Veterinary Medicine

BVMGT Bender Visual-Motor Gestalt Test

BVMS Bachelor of Veterinary Medicine and Science

BVO black vinyl overboot; branch vein occlusion

BVP blood vessel prosthesis; blood volume pulse; burst of ventricular pacing

BVR baboon virus replication; Balloon Valvuloplasty Registry

BVS biventricular support; blanked ventricular sense

BVSc Bachelor of Veterinary Science

BV/TV bone volume/trabecular volume ratio

BVU bromoisovalerylurea

BVV bovine vaginitis virus
BW bacteriologic warfare; Beckwith-Wiedemann [syndrome]; bedwetting; below waist; biologic warfare; biologic weapon; birth weight; bladder washout; blood Wasserman [reaction]; body water; body weight
B&W black and white
bw body weight
BWAV Bwamba virus
BWC bladder wash cytology
BWD bacillary white diarrhea
BWFCM bladder wash flow cytometry
BWFI bacteriostatic water for injection
BWG Bland-White-Garland [syndrome]
BWIS Baltimore-Washington Infant Study
BWS battered woman/wife syndrome; Beckwith-Wiedemann syndrome
BWST black widow spider toxin
BWSV black widow spider venom

BWT bilateral Wilms tumor
BWt birth weight
Bwt body weight
BX, bx bacitracin X; biopsy
Bx biopsy
BXO balanitis xerotica obliterans
BXV Bee virus X
ByCPR bystander cardiac pulmonary resuscitation
BYE Barile-Yaguchi-Eveland [medium]
BYP Baeza-Yates/Perleberg [algorithm]
BYV bee virus Y
BZ benzodiazepine
Bz, Bzl benzoyl
BZD benzodiazepine
BZQ benzquinamide
BZRP benzodiazepine receptor peripheral [type]
BZS Bannayan-Zonana syndrome

C

2C two component
3C cranio-cerebello-cardiac syndrome; three component
C about [L. *circa*]; ascorbic acid; bruised [L. *contusus*]; calcitonin forming [cell]; calculus; calorie [large]; *Campylobacter*; *Candida*; canine tooth; capability; capacitance; capsid protein; carbohydrate; carbon; cardiac; cardiovascular disease; carrier; cast; cathode; Caucasian; cell; Celsius; centigrade; central; central electrode placement in electroencephalography; centromeric or constitutive heterochromatic chromosome [banding]; cerebrospinal; certified; cervical; cesarean [section]; chest lead [ECG]; chicken; *Chlamydia*; chloramphenicol; cholesterol; class; clearance; clonus; *Clostridium*; closure; clubbing; coarse; cocaine; coefficient; colorectal tumor with metastases to lymph nodes; color sense; colored [guinea pig]; communicating [pacemaker]; complement; complex; compliance; component; compound; concentration; concept; conditioned, conditioning; condyle; constant; consultation; contamination; contraction; control; conventionally reared [animal]; convergence; correct; cortex; coulomb; count; criteria; *Cryptococcus*; cubic; cubitus; cyanosis; cylinder; cysteine; cytidine; cytochrome; cytosine; gallon [L. *congius*]; horn [L. *cornu*]; hundred [L. *centum*]; molar heat capacity; rib [L. *costa*]; total capacitance; velocity of light; with [L. *cum*]
χ Greek letter chi
χ^2 chi-squared [test, statistic]
χ_m magnetic susceptibility
χ_s electric susceptibility
© cue
°C degree Celsius or centigrade
C' complement
Cγ gamma-chain constant region [immunoglobulins]
Cκ kappa light chain constant region [immunoglobulins]
Cλ lambda light chain constant region [immunoglobulins]
Cμ mu light chain constvant region [immunoglobulins]
C^0 concentration zero
C1 first cervical nerve; first cervical vertebra; first component of complement

C$_1$ first rib
C1–9 complement proteins 1 to 9
C1–9 activated components of complement 1 to 9
C2 prostatic tumor with extracapsular extension and positive margins; second cervical nerve; second cervical vertebra; second component of complement; second concept; tumor with metastases to lymph nodes and extension into perirectal adipose tissue
C^2 community capacity
C$_2$ second rib
3C 3-component; cranio-cerebello-cardiac syndrome
C3 prostatic tumor with seminal vesical involvement; third cervical nerve; third cervical vertebra; third component of complement
C$_3$ Collins' solution; third rib
C4 controlled collapse chip connection; fourth cervical nerve; fourth cervical vertebra; fourth component of complement
C5 fifth cervical nerve; fifth cervical vertebra; fifth component of complement
C6 sixth cervical nerve; sixth cervical vertebra; sixth component of complement
C7 seventh cervical nerve; seventh cervical vertebra; seventh component of complement
C8 eighth component of complement
C9 ninth component of complement
C.37 Lambda variant of SARS-CoV-2 [also called Peru variant]
c about [L. *circa*]; calorie [small]; candle; canine tooth; capacity; capillary; carat; centi-; clinical; complementary [strand]; concentration; contact; cup; curie; cyclic; meal [L. *cibus*]; specific heat capacity; with [L. *cum*]
c' coefficient of partage
c- centi- [10^{-1}]
CA anterior commissure [L. *commissura anterior*]; calcium antagonist; California [rabbit]; cancer; cancer antigen; *Candida albicans*; caproic acid; capsid; capsid protein; carbohydrate antagonist; carbonic anhydrase; carcinoma; cardiac angiography; cardiac apnea; cardiac arrest; cardiac arrhythmia; carotid artery; cast; catecholamine, catecholaminergic; cathode; Caucasian adult; celiac axis; cell automation; cellulose acetate; cerebral aqueduct; cerebral atrophy; certification authority; cervicoaxial; Chemical Abstracts; chemotactic activity; child abuse; chloroamphetamine; cholic acid; chorioamniotic; chromosomal aberration; chronic anovulation; chronologic age; citric acid; clotting assay; coagglutination; coarctation of the aorta; Cocaine Anonymous; coefficient of

absorption; cold agglutinin; colloid antigen; common antigen; compressed air; computer assisted; conceptional age; condyloma acuminatum; coracoacromial; coronary angioplasty; coronary artery; corpora allata; corpora amylacea; corpus albicans; corrected [echo] area; cortisone acetate; cricoarytenoid; cricoid arch; croup associated [virus]; cytosine arabinoside; cytotoxic antibody

C&A Clinitest and Acetest

CA1 carbonic anhydrase I

CA-2 second colloid antigen

CA 15.3 marker for breast carcinoma

CA 19.9 marker for colorectal and pancreatic carcinoma

CA 27.29 marker for breast carcinoma

CA 50 marker for pancreatic or colorectal carcinomas

CA 72.4 marker for gastrointestinal and ovarian carcinomas

CA 125 marker for ovarian and endometrial carcinomas

CA 242 marker for pancreatic and colorectal carcinomas

CA 549 marker for breast carcinoma

Ca calcium; cancer; *Candida albicans*; carcinoma; cathode

ca about [L. *circa*]; candle; carcinoma

CAA carotid audiofrequency analysis; cerebral amyloid angiopathy; circulating anodic antigen; Clean Air Act; computer-assisted assessment; constitutional aplastic anemia; coronary artery aneurysm; crystalline amino acids

CAADAC California Association of Alcohol and Drug Abuse Counselors

CAAH chronic active autoimmune hepatitis

CAAHEP Commission on Accreditation of Allied Health Education Programs

CAAS cardiovascular angiographic analysis system; Commission on Accreditation of Ambulance Services

CAASET Canadian Amlodipine and Atenolol Stress Echo Trial

CAAT computer-assisted axial tomography

CAAV canine adeno-associated virus

CAAX [box] protein segment in which C is cysteine, A is usually but not always an aliphatic amino acid, and X is methionine or serine

CAB captive air bubble; cellulose acetate butyrate; community advisory board; coronary artery bypass

CABBS computer-assisted blood background subtraction

CABF coronary artery blood flow

CABG coronary artery bypass grafting

CABG-Patch Coronary Artery Bypass Graft [trial with/without epicardial] Patch [for automatic implantable cardioverter-defibrillator]

CABGS coronary artery bypass graft surgery

CaBI calcium bone index

Ca²⁺-blocker calcium channel blocker

CABM Center for Advanced Biotechnology and Medicine

CABMET Colorado Association of Biomedical Engineering Technicians

CABP community-acquired bacterial pneumonia

CaBP calcium-binding protein

CABRI Coronary Angioplasty versus Bypass Revascularization Investigation; Coronary Artery Bypass Revascularization Investigation

CABS citric acid—buffered saline; continuous ambulatory blood sampler; coronary artery bypass surgery

CABV Cabassou virus

cabyv cucurbit aphid-borne yellow virus

CAC Carcinogeneity Assessment Committee; cardiac-accelerator center; cardiac arrest code; children's asthma center; circulating anticoagulant; clinical application coordinator

CaCC calcium-sensitive chloride channel; cathodal closure contraction

CAC/CIC chronic active/inactive cirrhosis

CACCN Canadian Association of Critical Care Nurses

CACHET Comparison of Abciximab Complications with Hirulog for Ischemic Events Trial

CACI collagen-covered autologous chondrocyte implantation

CACP cisplatin

CACS cancer anorexia-cachexia syndrome

CaCTe cathodal closure tetanus

CACTIS Comparison of Aspirin with Clopidogrel or Ticlopidine in Stents [trial]

CACV cacao virus

CaCV canine calicivirus

CaCX cancer of cervix

CACY calcyclin

CAD cadaver, cadaveric; Canadian Association of the Deaf; central appointment desk; chronic actinic dermatitis; coenzyme A dehydrogenase; cold agglutinin disease; collisionally activated dissociation; compressed air disease; computer-aided design; computer-aided detection; computer-aided dispatch; computer-assisted design; computer-assisted diagnosis; congenital abduction deficiency; coronary artery disease; coronoradiographic documentation

CaD caldesmon

Cad cadaver, cadaveric

CADA Council on Alcohol and Drug Abuse

CADASIL cerebral autosomal dominant arteriopathy with subcortical infarcts and leukoencephalopathy

CADASILM cerebral autosomal dominant arteriopathy with subcortical infarcts, leukoencephalopathy, and migraine

CAD/CAM computer-aided design/computer-aided manufacturing

CADCCC Central Australia Disease Control Coordinating Committee

CADD computer-aided drug design

CADHYP Coronary Artery Disease in Hypertension [study]

CADI coronary artery disease index

CADILLAC Controlled Abciximab and Device Investigation to Lower Late Angioplasty Complications [study]

CADL communicative abilities in daily living

CADMIO computer-assisted design for medical information objectives

cADPR cyclic adenosinediphosphate-ribose

CADR coronary artery descriptors and restenosis

CADRES Coronary Artery Descriptors and Restenosis [project]

CADS Captopril and Digoxin Study

CaDTe cathodal-duration tetanus

CADV Cano Delgadito virus

CAdV canine adenovirus; caprine adenovirus

CADx computer-aided diagnosis

CAE caprine arthritis-encephalitis; cellulose acetate electrophoresis; childhood absence epilepsy; contingent aftereffects; coronary artery embolism

CaE calcium excretion

CaEDTA calcium disodium ethylene-diaminetetraacetate

CAE-IEF cellulose acetate-isoelectric focusing [electrophoresis]

CAEP Canadian Association of Emergency Physicians; cortical auditory evoked potential

CAER community awareness and emergency response

CAESA computer-assisted estimation of synthetic accessibility

CAESAR Canada, Australia, Europe and South Africa Republic [trial]; computer-assisted ear, nose, and throat surgery using augmented reality; Computer-Assisted Evaluation of Stenosis and Restenosis [system]

CAEV caprine arthritis-encephalitis virus; *Chironomus attenuatus* entomopoxvirus

CAF carcinoma-associated fibroblast; cell adhesion factor; citric acid fermentation; combined acetabular and femoral [navigation]; common assembly format; cortical activation function

Caf caffeine

CAFA Canadian Atrial Fibrillation Anticoagulation [study]

CAFE Coronary Artery Flow Evaluation

CAFS Canadian Atrial Fibrillation Study

CAG Canadian Association of Gerontology; cholangiogram, cholangiography; chronic atrophic gastritis; coronary angiography

CAGA calgranulin A

CAGB calgranulin B

CAGC Canadian Association of Genetic Counsellors

CAGE capillary affinity gel electrophoresis; cerebral arterial gas embolism; cut down, annoyed by criticism, guilty about drinking, "eye-opener" drink in the morning [screening test for alcoholism]

CAH CAS [Chemical Abstracts] Surveyor Hazardous Materials; chronic active hepatitis; chronic aggressive hepatitis; combined atrial hypertrophy; congenital adrenal hyperplasia; cyanacetic acid hydrazide

CAHCIM Consortium of Academic Health Centers for Integrative Medicine

CAHD coronary arteriosclerotic heart disease

CAHEA Committee on Allied Health Education and Accreditation

CAHMR cataract, hypertrichosis, mental retardation (intellectual disability) [syndrome]

CAHPS Consumer Assessment of Health Plans Survey

CAHS central alveolar hypoventilation syndrome

CAHV central alveolar hypoventilation

CaHV canid herpesvirus

CAI celiac artery infusion; cellular adaptive immunotherapy; chemical accident or incident; complete androgen insensitivity; computer-assisted instruction; computer-assisted interview; confluence of informatics

CAID computer-aided implant dentistry

CAIRA chemical accident or incident response and assistance

CAIS complete androgen insensitivity syndrome

CAIUS Carotid Atherosclerosis Italian Ultrasound Study

CAIV Caimito virus

CaIV *Campoletis aprilis* ichnovirus

CAIV-T cold-adapted influenza virus vaccine, trivalent

C(a-jb)O$_2$ arterial-jugular bulb venous oxygen [ratio]

CAK cyclin-dependent kinase-activating kinase

cAK cyclic adenosine monophosphate [cAMP]-dependent protein kinase

CAL café au lait; calcium test; calculated average life; calories; chronic airflow limitation; computer-assisted learning; coracoacromial ligament

Cal caliber; large calorie

cal small calorie

C$_{alb}$ albumin clearance

CALC calcitonin

Calc calcium

calc calculation

calcif calcification

CALCR calcitonin receptor

CALD chronic active liver disease

CALGB cancer and leukemia group B

CALH chronic active lupoid hepatitis

CalHV callitrichine herpesvirus

cALL common null cell acute lymphocytic leukemia

CALLA, cALLA common acute lymphoblastic leukemia antigen

CALM café-au-lait macules

CALP congenital absence of left pericardium

CALS café-au-lait spots

CalV cardamine latent virus

CALYPSO Cylexin as an Adjunct to Lytic Therapy to Prevent Superoxide Reflow Injury [trial]

CAM calf aortic microsome; cell adhesion molecule; cell-associating molecule; chemical agent monitor; chorioallantoic membrane; combined approach matrix; complementary and alternative medicine; compressed adjacency matrix; computer-assisted myelography; confusion assessment method; content-addressable memory; contralateral axillary metastasis; cystic adenomatoid malformation

CaM calmodulin

C$_{am}$ amylase clearance

CaM-A calmodulin-agarose

CAMAC computer-automated measurement and control

CAMAK cataract, microcephaly, arthrogryposis, kyphosis [syndrome]

CAMAT Canadian Amiodarone Myocardial Infarction Arrhythmia Trial

CAMC camera-augmented mobile C-arm; computer application in medical care; computer analysis of mammography phantom images

CAMCAM Center for Assessment and Management of Changes in Academic Medicine

CAMCAT Canadian Multicenter Clentiazem Angina Trial

CAMCOG Cambridge cognitive capacity scale

CAMD computer-aided molecular design

CAMDEX Cambridge mental disorders of the elderly examination

CAMF cyclophosphamide, Adriamycin, methotrexate, fluorouracil

CAMFAK cataract, microcephaly, failure to thrive, kyphoscoliosis [syndrome]

CAMH Centre for Addiction and Mental Health

CAMI Canadian Assessment of Myocardial Infarction [study]; computer-assisted medical intervention

CAMIAT Canadian Amiodarone Myocardial Infarction Arrhythmia Trial; Canadian Myocardial Infarction Amiodarone Trial

CAMIS Center for Applied Medical Information Systems Research

CAMK calmodulin-dependent protein kinase

CaMK calcium-mediated kinase

CAML cystic adenomatoid malformation of the lung

CAMP Christie-Atkins-Munch-Petersen [test]; computer-assisted management protocol; computer-assisted menu planning; concentration of adenosine monophosphate; cyclic adenosine monophosphate; cyclophosphamide, Adriamycin, methotrexate, and procarbazine

cAMP cyclic adenosine monophosphate

CAMPASS Cambridge Database on Protein Alignments Organized as Structural Superfamilies

CAMRT Canadian Association of Medical Radiation Technologists

CAMS computer-assisted monitoring system

CAMT Center for Advanced Medical Technology

CAMTS Commission for Accreditation of Medical Transport Services

CAMV congenital anomaly of mitral valve

CAMVA chorioallantoic membrane vascular assay

CAN cardiac autonomic neuropathy

Can cancer; *Candida*; *Cannabis*

CA/N child abuse and neglect

CANA circulating antineuronal antibody

CaNaEDTA calcium-disodium ethylenediamine tetraacetic acid

CANAHOP Canadian Ambulatory, Home and Office Pressure Study

CANARIE Canadian Network for the Advancement of Research, Industry, and Education

canc cancelled

C-ANCA cytoplasmic antineutrophilic cytoplasmic antibody

c-ANCA antineutrophil antibodies against protease 3 in cytoplasmic granules

CANCERPROJ Cancer Research Projects

CANDA computer-assisted new drug application

CANDELA computer-assisted notification of drug effects on laboratory animals [test]

CANDY Communication Aids Negating Disabilities of Youth

CA*net Canada's High-Performance Network

CANOST Autocanonization System for Organic Structures

CANP calcium-activated neutral protease; Certified Adult Nurse Practitioner

CANPA Central Alabama Nurse Practitioner Association

CANS central auditory nervous system

CAN'T LEAP cyclosporine, alcohol, nicotinic acid, thiazides, lasix, ethambutanol, aspirin, pyrazinamide

CANV Caninde virus

CANX calnexin

CAO Canadian Association of Optometrists; chronic airway obstruction; coronary artery obstruction

CAO₂, CₐO₂ arterial oxygen content

CaOC cathodal opening contraction

CaOCL cathodal opening clonus

CAOD coronary artery occlusive disease

CAOHC Council for Accreditation of Occupational Hearing Conservation

CAOM chronic adhesive otitis media

CAOS computer-assisted orthopedic surgery

CAOT Canadian Association of Occupational Therapists

CaOTe cathodal opening tetanus

CAP camptodactyly, arthropathy, pericarditis [syndrome]; Canada Assistance Plan; capsule; captopril; catabolite gene activator protein; cell attachment protein; cellular acetate propionate; cellulose acetate phthalate; central apical part; chloramphenicol; chronic alcoholic pancreatitis; clinical access program; College of American Pathologists; community-acquired pneumonia; complement-activated plasma; compound action potential; coupled atrial pacing; cyclophosphamide, Adriamycin, and Platinol; cystine aminopeptidase; Canadian Association of Pathologists

Cₐₚ cationic antimicrobial protein; circumference of apex

CaP carcinoma of the prostate

cap capacity; capsule

CAPA cancer-associated polypeptide antigen; Certified Ambulatory Perianesthesia Nurse

CAPARES Coronary Angioplasty Amlodipine in Restenosis [trial]

CAPAS Cutting Balloon Angioplasty vs. Plain Old Balloon Angioplasty Randomized Study

CAPBL computer-assisted problem-based learning

CAPCC Canadian Association of Poison Control Centers

CAPD continuous ambulatory peritoneal dialysis

CAPE Circadian Antiischemia Program in Europe; Clifton assessment procedures for the elderly; computer-assisted patient emulator

CAPERS Computer-Assisted Psychiatric Evaluation and Review System

CapEx capital expenditure

CAPHIS Consumer and Patient Health Information Section

CAPI computer-assisted personal interview; cryptographic applications programming interface

CAP-IT Client Adherence Profiling-Intervention Tailoring [model]

CAPITOL Captopril Postinfarction Tolerance [trial]

CapLV caper latent virus

CAPM continuous airway pressure monitoring

Capox-RT capecitabine and radiotherapy

CAPP Captopril Prevention Project [study]; computer-assisted preoperative planning; Concerted Action Polyp Prevention

CAPPHY Captopril Primary Prevention in Hypertension [study]

CAPPP Captopril Prevention Project

CAPPS Current and Past Psychopathology Scale

CAPR controlled air purifying respirator

CAPRCA chronic, acquired, pure red cell aplasia

CAPRI Cardiopulmonary Research Institute

CAPRICORN Carvedilol Post-Infarct Survival Control in Left Ventricular Dysfunction Study

CAPRIE Clopidogrel vs. Aspirin in Patients at Risk of Ischemic Events

CAPS Cardiac Arrhythmia Pilot Study; care profile system; CIAS1-related autoinflammatory periodic syndromes; community adjustment profile system; computer-aided prototyping system; cryopyrin-associated periodic syndromes

caps capsule

CAPSS columnar alteration with prominent apical snouts and secretions

CAPTIN Captopril Before Reperfusion in Acute Myocardial Infarction [trial]; Captopril Plus Tissue Plasminogen Activator Following Acute Myocardial Infarction [trial]

CAPTISM Captopril Insulin Sensitivity Multicenter [study]

CAPTURE Chimeric 7E3 Antiplatelet Therapy in Unstable Refractory Angina [trial]

CAPV Capim virus

CAQ Certificate of Added Qualifications

CAR Canadian Association of Radiologists; cancer-associated retinopathy; Cardiac Ablation Registry; cardiac ambulation routine; carvedilol; cell adhesion regulator; chronic articular rheumatism; computer-assisted radiology; computer-assisted research; conditioned avoidance response; congenital articular rigidity; constitutive androstane receptor; coping, adaptation, and resilience functions

car carotid

CARA chronic aspecific respiratory ailment

CARAF Canadian Registry of Atrial Fibrillation

CARAFE Cocktail Attenuation of Rotational Ablation Flow Effects [study]

CAR AMP carotid pulse amplitude

CARAT Coronary Angioplasty and Rotablator Atherectomy Trial; coronary artery risk assessment and treatment

CARB carbohydrate; coronary artery bypass graft

carb carbohydrate; carbonate

carbo carbohydrate

CARC chemical agent resistant coating

CARD cardiac automatic resuscitative device; caspase activating and recruiting domain

card cardiac

CARDIA Coronary Artery Risk Development in Young Adults [study]

CARDIAC Cardiovascular Disease and Alimentary Comparison [study]

card insuff cardiac insufficiency

cardiol cardiology

CARDIS Cardiology Information System

CARD PORT Cardiac Arrhythmia and Risk of Death Patient Outcome Research Team

CARE calcium antagonist in reperfusion; cardiac arrhythmias research and education; Carvedilol Atherectomy Restenosis [trial]; Cholesterol and Recurrent Events [study]; comprehensive assessment and referral evaluation; computerized adult and records evaluation [system]; computerized clinical

assessment, research and education; cyclic adenosine monophosphate response element

CAREC Caribbean Epidemiology Centre

CAREID Canada-Asia Regional Emerging Infectious Diseases Project

CARES cancer rehabilitation evaluation system

CARET Beta-Carotene and Retinol Efficacy Trial

CARF Commission on Accreditation of Rehabilitation Facilities

CARG coronary artery [bypass] grafting

CAR_{hd} high-dose carvedilol

CarIV *Casinaria arjuna* ichnovirus

CARMEN Carvedilol Angiotensin Converting Enzyme Inhibitors Remodelling Mild Heart Failure Evaluation

CARN Certified Addictions Registered Nurse

CARP carbonic anhydrase—related polypeptide

CARPORT Coronary Artery Restenosis Prevention on Repeated Thromboxane A_2-Receptor Antagonism Study

CARS Childhood Autism Rating Scale; Children's Affective Rating Scale; Coronary Artery Regression Study; Coumadin Aspirin Reinfarction Study; cysteinyl-transfer ribonucleic acid synthetase

CART classification and regression tree; cocaine-related transcript; Colchicine Angioplasty Restenosis Trial; computer-assisted radiotherapy; constrained access robotic therapy

cART combination antiretroviral therapy

cart cartilage

CARV Caraparu virus

CAS calcarine sulcus; calcific aortic stenosis; Cancer Attitude Survey; carbohydrate-active steroid; Cardiac Adjustment Scale; cardiac surgery; carotid artery stenting; Celite-activated normal serum; Center for Alcohol Studies; central anticholinergic syndrome; cerebral atherosclerosis; Chemical Abstract Service; clinical application suite; clinical assessment score; clinical asthma score; Cognitive Assessment Scale; cold agglutinin syndrome; computer-assisted surgery; congenital alcoholic syndrome; contralateral acoustic stimulation; control adjustment strap; coronary artery spasm; Council of Academic Societies

Cas casualty

cas castration, castrated

CASA cancer-associated serum antigen; Center for Addiction and Substance Abuse; clinical assessment software application;

computer-assisted self-assessment; computer-assisted semen analysis

CASANOVA Coronary Artery Stenosis with Asymptomatic Narrowing: Operation vs. Aspirin [study]

CASCADE Cardiac Arrest in Seattle: Conventional vs. Amiodarone Drug Evaluation; Conventional Arrhythmic vs. Amiodarone in Survivors of Cardiac Arrest Drug Evaluation

CASD computer-assisted synthesis design

CASE Community, Attachment, Structures and Epidemic [study]; computer-aided simulation of clinical encounter; computer-aided systems engineering; coordinated activities, services, and encounters

CASET Carotid Artery Stenting vs. Endarterectomy Trial

CASG Collaborative Antiviral Study Group

CASH Cancer and Steroid Hormone [study]; Cardiac Arrest Study, Hamburg; Caring About Seniors' Health [study]; Commission for Administrative Services in Hospitals; Consensus Action on Salt and Hypertension; corticoadrenal stimulating hormone; cruciform anterior spinal hyperextension

CASHD coronary arteriosclerotic heart disease

CASI cognitive abilities screening instrument; computer-assisted self-interviewing

CASIS Canadian Amlodipine/Atenolol in Silent Ischemia Study; Coronary Artery Stent Implantation Study

CASLPA Canadian Association of Speech-Language Pathologists and Audiologists [former name of (SAC) Speech-Language and Audiology Canada]

CASLPO College of Audiologists and Speech-Language Pathologists of Ontario

CASMD congenital atonic sclerotic muscular dystrophy

CASP Critical Appraisal Skills Programme

CASPER computer-assisted pericardial puncture; computer-assisted pericardial surgery

CasplV *Casinaria* sp. ichnovirus

CASPR contactin-associated protein

CASQ calsequestrin

CASR, CaSR calcium-sensing receptor

CAS-REGN Chemical Abstract Service Registry Number

CASRN Chemical Abstract Service Registry Number

CASRT corrected adjusted sinus node recovery time

CASS cataract, alopecia, sclerodactyly syndrome; Coronary Artery Surgery Study

CASSIS Classification and Search Support Information System; Czech and Slovak Spirapril Intervention Study

CAST calpastatin; Canonical Representation of Stereochemistry [coding]; Cardiac Arrhythmia Suppression Trial; Carotid Artery Stenting Trial; Childhood Autism Screening Test; Children of Alcoholism Screening Test; Chinese Acute Stroke Trial; circumference paraxillary superficial tumescent liposuction; computer-adaptive sequential testing; cyclic amplification and selection of targets

CASTEL Cardiovascular Study in the Elderly

CASTOR Coronary Angioscopic Study of Restenosis

CAT California Achievement Test; cancer after transplantation; capillary agglutination test; Cardiomyopathy Trial; care support terminal; catalase; cataract; catecholamine; Children's Apperception Test; Chinese Angiotensin Converting Enzyme Inhibitor in Acute Myocardial Infarction Trial; chloramphenicol acetyltransferase; chlormerodrin accumulation test; choline acetyltransferase; chronic abdominal tympany; Cognitive Abilities Test; Columbia Center for Advanced Technology; computed abdominal tomography; computed axial tomography; computer-assisted tomography; computer of average transients; coronary angioplasty trial; critically appraised topic

cat catalysis, catalyst; cataract

CAT'ase catalase

CATB catalase B

CAT-CAM contoured adduction trochanteric-controlled alignment method

CATCEC Computer-Supported Assessment and Treatment Consultation for Emotional Crises

CATCH Canadian Association of Teachers of Community Health; Child and Adolescent Trial for Cardiovascular Health; Community Action to Control High Blood Pressure; comprehensive assessment for tracking community health; critically attained threshold of cerebral hypoperfusion

CATCH 22 cardiac defects, abnormal facies, thymic hypoplasia, cleft palate, hypocalcemia [syndrome]

CAT/CLAM Clinical Adaptive Test/Clinical Linguistics Auditory Milestones

Cath cathartic; catheter, catheterize

cath catheterization

CATI computer-assisted telephone interview

CATIE-AD Clinical Antipsychotic Trials of Intervention Effectiveness for Alzheimer Disease

CATIPO Computer-Aided Therapy Planning in Pediatric Oncology

CATIS China Antihypertensive Trial in Acute Ischemic Stroke

CATLINE Catalog Online

CATN-I Course in Advanced Trauma Nursing-Instructor

CATN-P Course in Advanced Trauma Nursing-Provider

CATS Canadian American Ticlopidine Study; Captopril and Thrombolysis Study; Child Abuse Trauma Scale

CAT-S Children's Apperception Test, Supplemental

CAT scan computed axial tomography scan

CATSIM computer case simulation

CATT calcium tolerance test

CATUV Catu virus

CAU central abdomen uptake [finding]

Cauc Caucasian

caud caudal

caut cauterization

CAUV congenital absence of the uterus and vagina

CAV cardiac allograft vasculopathy; *Chara australis* virus; chicken anemia virus; congenital absence of vagina; congenital adrenal virilism; constant angular velocity; croup-associated virus

cav cavity

CAVA Coronary Atherectomy vs. Angioplasty [study]

CAVATAS Carotid and Vertebral Artery Transluminal Angioplasty Study

CAVB complete atrioventricular block

CAVD complete atrioventricular dissociation; completion, arithmetic problems, vocabulary, following directions [test]; congenital aplasia of vas deferens

CAVE cerebroacrovisceral—early lethality [phenotype]

CAVEAT Coronary Angioplasty vs. Excisional Atherectomy Trial

CAVEAT-I Comparison of Directional Atherectomy vs. Coronary Angioplasty Trial

CAVEAT-II Coronary Angioplasty vs. Directional Atherectomy for Patients with Saphenous Vein Bypass Graft Lesions [trial]

CAVG coronary artery vein graft

CAVH continuous arteriovenous hemofiltration

CAVHD continuous arteriovenous hemodialysis

CAVHDF continuous arteriovenous hemodiafiltration

CavHV caviid herpesvirus

CAVLT Children's Auditory Verbal Learning Test

CAVO common atrioventricular orifice

C(a−v)$_{O_2}$ arteriovenous oxygen tension difference

C[a & v̄]O$_2$ arteriovenous gradient of oxygen content

CAVR continuous arteriovenous rewarming

CAVS Conformance Assessment to Voluntary Standards

CAVSD complete atrioventricular septal defect

CAVU continuous arteriovenous ultrafiltration

CAW central airway

C$_{AW}$ airway conductance

CAX central axis

CaYMV canine yellow mottle virus

8CB octylcyanobiphenyl

CB Bachelor of Surgery [L. *Chirurgiae Baccalaureus*]; calcium blocker; cannabinoid; carbenicillin; carotid body; chocolate blood [agar]; chromatin body; chronic bronchitis; circumflex branch; code blue; color blind; compensated base; consensus band; conus branch; Coomassie blue; coprocessor board; coracobrachial

Cb cerebellum; niobium [columbium]

C3b complement component 3b

CBA chronic bronchitis and asthma; Columbia blood agar [test]; cost-benefit analysis

CBAB complement-binding antibody

CBADAA Certifying Board of the American Dental Assistants Association

CBAS carotid bifurcation angioplasty and stenting

CBAVD congenital bilateral absence of vas deferens

CBBEST cutting balloon before stent

CBBM color blindness, blue mono-cone-monochromatic type

CBC carbenicillin; child behavior characteristics; compensatory base change; complete blood cell count

cbc complete blood cell count

CBCL Child Behavior Checklist; cutaneous B-cell lymphoma

CBCL/2−3 Child Behavior Checklist for ages 2 to 3

CBCL-OCS Child Behavior Checklist Obsessive Compulsive Subscale

CBCN carbenicillin

CBCT cone-beam computed tomography

CbCtx cerebellar cortex

CBD carotid body denervation; closed bladder drainage; color blindness, deutan type; common bile duct; Convention on Biological Diversity

CBDC chronic bullous disease of children

CBDE Chemical and Biological Defense Establishment; common bile duct exploration

CBDMP California Birth Defects Monitoring Program

CBDPR computer-based dental patient record

CBDV *Colocasia bobone* disease virus

CBE clinical breast examination

CBER Center for Biologics Evaluation and Research

CBET certified biomedical equipment technician

CBEV *Choristoneura biennis* entomopoxvirus

CBF capillary blood flow; cerebral blood flow; ciliary beat frequency; collagen-binding factor; core-binding factor; coronary blood flow; cortical blood flow

CBFB core-binding factor beta

CBFb beta subunit of core-binding factor

CBFV coronary blood flow velocity

CBG capillary blood gases; coronary bypass graft; corticosteroid-binding globulin; cortisol-binding globulin

CBGv corticosteroid-binding globulin variant

CBH chronic benign hepatitis; cutaneous basophilic hypersensitivity

CbHV cebine herpesvirus

CBI chemical binding index; children's behavior inventory; combined behavioral intervention; continuous bladder irrigation; convergent beam irradiation

CBIC Certification Board of Infection Control and Epidemiology

CBL chronic blood loss; circulating blood lymphocyte; cord blood leukocytes

Cbl cobalamin

CBM capillary basement membrane

CBMMP chronic benign mucous membrane pemphigus

CBN cannabinol; central benign neoplasm; Commission on Biological Nomenclature

CBNB Chemical Business News Database

CBNV Colony B North virus

CBO community-based organization; Congressional Budget Office

CBOC completion bed occupancy care

CBOD chemical and biological oxygen demand

CBOD5 5-day chemical and biological oxygen

CBP calcium-binding protein; carbohydrate-binding protein; cardiopulmonary bypass; chlorobiphenyl; cobalamin-binding protein; color blindness, protan type; convolution back projection; cruciform binding protein; cyclic adenosine monophosphate [cAMP] binding protein

C4BP complement 4 binding protein

CBPR community-based participatory research; computer-based patient record

CBPS chemical and biological protected shelter; congenital bilateral perisylvian syndrome

CBPV chronic bee paralysis virus

CBR carbonyl reductase; case-based reasoning; chemical, biologic, and radiologic [warfare]; chemically bound residue; chronic/complete bed rest; crude birth rate

CBRL contextual bayesian relaxation labeling technique

CBRNE chemical, biological, radiological, nuclear, and high-yield explosives

CBS cervicobrachial syndrome; chronic brain syndrome; clinical behavioral science; conjugated bile salts; culture-bound syndrome; cystathionine beta-synthase

CB3S Coxsackie B3 virus susceptibility

CBSD component-based software development

CBT carotid body tumor; code blue team; cognitive behavioral treatment/therapy; computed body tomography; computer-based testing; computer-based training instruction; cord blood transplant; corticobulbar tract

CBV capillary blood cell velocity; catheter balloon valvuloplasty; central blood volume; cerebral blood volume; circulating blood volume; corrected blood volume; cortical blood volume; Coxsackie B virus

CBVD cerebrovascular disease

CBVI computer-based video instruction

CBW chemical and biologic warfare

CBX computer-based examination

CBZ carbamazepine

CC calcaneal cuboid; calcium cyclamate; calf circumference; cardiac catheterization; cardiac center; cardiac contusion; cardiac cycle; cardiovascular clinic; cascade correlation; cell culture; central compartment; cerebral commissure; cerebral cortex; cervical cancer; chest circumference; chief complaint; cholecalciferol; choledochocholedochostomy; chondrocalcinosis; choriocarcinoma; chronic complainer; circulatory collapse; classical conditioning; clean catch; clinical center; clinical course; clomiphene citrate; closed cup; closing capacity; coefficient of consistency; collagenous colitis; colony count; colorectal cancer; columnar cells; commission certified; common cold; communication client; complicating condition; complications and comorbidity; compound cathartic; computation constant; computer calculated; computer center; concordance; congenital cardiopathy; congenital cataract; consumptive coagulopathy; contrast cystogram; conversion complete; coracoclavicular; cord compression; coronary care; corpus callosum; correlation coefficient; costochondral; Coulter counter; craniocaudal; craniocervical; creatinine clearance; critical care; critical condition; Crohn colitis; Cronkhite-Canada [syndrome]; cross correlation; crus cerebri; cubic centimeter; current complaint; Current Contents

C-C convexo-concave

C&C cold and clammy

Cc concave

cc carbon copy; clean catch; concave; corrected; cubic centimeter

CCA canonical correlation; cephalin cholesterol antigen; chick cell agglutination; chimpanzee coryza agent; cholangiocarcinoma; choriocarcinoma; chromated copper arsenate; circulating cathodic antigen; circumflex coronary artery; common carotid artery; congenital contractural arachnodactyly; constitutional chromosome abnormality

CCAB complex cognitive assessment battery

CCABOT Cornell Coronary Artery Bypass Outcomes Trial

CCAg corpus callosum agenesis

CCAIT Canadian Coronary Atherosclerosis Intervention Trial

CCAM congenital cystic adenomatoid malformation; General Classification of Medical Procedures [Fr. *Classification Commune des Actes Medicaux*]

CCAP Cancer Chromosomal Aberration Project; client-centered accreditation program

C-CAP custom-contoured ablation pattern

CCAT Canadian Coronary Atherectomy Trial; chick cell agglutination test; conglutinating complement absorption test

CCB calcium channel blocker

CCBD central cell-binding domain

CCBV central circulating blood volume

CCC Canadian Cardiovascular Coalition [study]; care-cure coordination; cathodal closure contraction; center for clinical computing; child care center; Children's Communication Checklist; chlorcholine chloride; chronic calculus cholecystitis; chronic catarrhal colitis; citrated calcium cyanamide; comprehensive cancer center; comprehensive care clinic; concentration, clustering, and continuity; concurrent care concern; consecutive case conference;

continuous curvilinear capsulotomy; Council on Clinical Classification; cranio-cerebello-cardiac [dysplasia, syndrome]; critical care complex; cylindrical confronting cisternae

CC&C colony count and culture

CCCC centrifugal countercurrent chromatography

CCCCP Comprehensive Cardiovascular Community Control Program

CCCD cooled charge-coupled device

cccDNA covalently closed circular deoxyribonucleic acid

CCCE cross-cultural cognitive examination

CCCI cathodal closure clonus

CC/CM Current Contents/Clinical Medicine

CCCN Certified Continence Care Nurse; community care coordination network

CCCP carbonyl cyanide *m*-chloro-phenylhydrazone

CCCR closed chest cardiac resuscitation

CCCS condom catheter collecting system; critical care computer system

CCCT closed craniocerebral trauma

CCCU comprehensive cardiac care unit

CCCV *Callistephus chinensis chlorosis* virus

CCD calibration curve data; central collodiaphyseal; central core disease; charge-coupled device; childhood celiac disease; cleidocranial dysplasia; clinical cardiovascular disease; cortical collecting duct; countercurrent distribution; cumulative cardiotoxic dose

CCDC Canadian Communicable Disease Center; consultant in communicable disease control

CCD-CAMPI charge-coupled device computer analysis of mammography phantom images

CCDN Central Council for District Nursing

ccDNA closed circle deoxyribonucleic acid

CCDS case cart delivery system; color-coded duplex sonography

CCE capacitative calcium entry; carboline carboxylic acid ester; chamois contagious ecthyma; cholesterol crystal emboli; clear-cell endothelioma; clubbing, cyanosis, and edema; cornified cell envelope; countercurrent electrophoresis; cruciform cutting endonuclease

CCEHRP Committee to Coordinate Environmental Health and Related Programs

CCEI Crown-Crisp Experimental Index

CCEV *Choristoneura conflicta* entomopoxvirus

CCF cancer coagulation factor; cardiolipin complement fixation; carotid cavernous fistula; centrifuged culture fluid; cephalin-cholesterol flocculation; chronic cardiac failure; compound comminuted fracture; congestive heart failure; cross-correlation function; crystal-induced chemotactic factor

CCFA cefotoxin-cycloserine fructose agar; Crohn's and Colitis Foundation of America

CCFAS compact colony-forming active substance

CCFE cyclophosphamide, cisplatin, fluorouracil, and extramustine

CCFMG Cooperating Committee on Foreign Medical Graduates

CCG cholecystogram, cholecystography; clinically coherent group; costochondral graft

CCGC capillary column gas chromatography

CCGS cell cycle G and S

CCH C-cell hyperplasia; central clinical hospital; chronic chloride hemagglutination; chronic cholestatic hepatitis; cross-correlation histogram

CCHA Canadian Council on Hospital Accreditation

CCHAT Canadian Cozaar, Hyzaar, and Amlodipine Trial

CC-HC coordinated collective homecare

CCHD Caephilly Collaborative Heart Disease [study]; cyanotic congenital heart disease

CCHE Central Council for Health Education

CCHF, C-CHF Crimean-Congo hemorrhagic fever

CCHFA Canadian Council on Health Facilities Accreditation

CCHMS Central Committee for Hospital Medical Services

CCHP Consumer Choice Health Plan; Corpus Christi Heart Project

CCHPR Canadian Consortium for Health Promotion Research; clinical classification of health policy research

CCHS congenital central hypoventilation syndrome; Copenhagen City Heart Study

CCHSA Canadian Council on Health Services Accreditation

CCI Canadian Classification of Health Interventions; Cancer Care International; Cardiovascular Credentialing International; Charlson comorbidity index; cholesterol crystallization inhibitor; chronic coronary insufficiency; common client interface; component communication interface; correct coding initiative; corrected count increment; Cronqvist cranial index; crowded cell index

CCI/F cortico-cortical inhibition and facilitation

CC-IMED California Consortium of Information in Medical Education and Development

CCK cholecystokinin

CCK-8 cholecystokinin octapeptide

CCKLI cholecystokinin-like immunoreactivity

CCK-OP cholecystokinin octapeptide

CCK-PZ cholecystokinin-pancreozymin

CCKRB cholecystokinin receptor B

CCL carcinoma cell line; certified cell line; Charcot-Leyden crystal; continuing care level; continuous cell line; costoclavicular ligament; critical carbohydrate level

CCLE chronic cutaneous lupus erythematosus

CCLI composite clinical and laboratory index

CC/LS Current Contents/Life Sciences

CCM cerebrocostomandibular; Certified Case Manager; chemical cleavage of mismatch; chronic care management; complicated case management; congestive cardiomyopathy; craniocervical malformation; critical care medicine

c cm cubic centimeter

CCMC Committee on the Costs of Medical Care

CCMDS Core Community Minimum Data Set

CCME Coordinating Council on Medical Education

CCMG Canadian College of Medical Geneticists

CCML Comprehensive Core Medical Library

CCMS cerebrocostomandibular syndrome; clean catch midstream; clinical care management system

CCMSU clean catch midstream urine

CCMT catechol methyltransferase

CCMU critical care medical unit

CCN cancer center network; caudal central nucleus; Council on Cardiovascular Nursing; community care network; coronary care nursing; critical care nursing

CCNHP community college nursing home project

CCNS Certified Clinical Nurse Specialist

CCNU N-(2-chloroethyl)-N'-cyclohexyl-N-nitrosourea [lomustine]

CCO continuous cardiac output; cytochrome C oxidase

CcO$_2$ capillary oxygen content

CCOHTA Canadian Coordinating Office for Health Technology Assessment

CCORP Cornell-China-Oxford Research Project

CCOT cervical compression overloading test

CCoV canine coronavirus

CCP Canadian Classification of Diagnostic, Therapeutic, and Surgical Interventions; cephalin-cholesterol flocculation; charge class pair; chronic calcifying pancreatitis;

ciliocytophthoria; columnar cell papilloma; community care plan; comprehensive care plan; cooperative cardiovascular project; coordinated care program; critical control point; cyclic citrullinated peptide; cyclic citrullinated protein; cytidine cyclic phosphate

CCPA California Consumer Privacy Act

CCPD continuous cycling (cyclical) peritoneal dialysis

CCPDS Centralized Cancer Patient Data System

C-CPE C-terminal half of *Clostridium perfringens* enterotoxin

CCPMS Cancer Centre Patient Management System; computer-assisted clinical pathway management system

CCPR closed-chest cardiopulmonary resuscitation; crypt cell production rate

CCPT Chinese Cancer Prevention Trial

CCR Canadian Cancer Registry; complete continuous remission; complex chromosome rearrangement; consistency and concurrency reporting; continuous complex remission; Coriell Cell Repositories; correct classification rate; creatinine clearance

C-CR Computing-Communications Research Division

Ccr, C$_{cr}$ creatinine clearance

CCRC comprehensive care retirement community; continuing care retirement community

CCRD complicated chronic respiratory disease

CCRG Cooperative Cataract Research Group

CCRIS Chemical Carcinogenesis Research Information System

CCRN Critical Care Registered Nurse

CCRS Chemical Carcinogenesis Research Information System; computer-controlled radiotherapy system

CCRS/SP computer-controlled radiotherapy system sequence processor

CCRT Cardiac Catheter Reuse Trial; computer-controlled conformal radiotherapy; computer-controlled radiation therapy; core conflictual relational theme

CcRV-W2 *Carcinus mediterraneus* W2 virus

CCS Canadian Cardiovascular Society; cardiac care system; case-control study; casualty clearing station; cell cycle specific; certified coding specialist; Chinese Cardiac Study; cholecystosonography; chronic cerebellar stimulation; chronic compartment syndrome; clear cell sarcoma; cloudy cornea syndrome; composite cultured skin; concentration camp syndrome; costoclavicular syndrome

CCSCS central cervical spinal cord syndrome

CCSE Cognitive Capacity Screening Examination

CCSG Canadian Cooperative Study Group; Children's Cancer Study Group

CCSK clear cell sarcoma of the kidney

CCSM cervical cancer—specific mortality

CCSP club cell secretory protein; club cell—specific protein

CCSRG Cochrane Collaboration Stroke Review Group

CCST chemical casualty site team

CCT carotid compression tomography; central conduction time; cerebrocranial trauma; charge class torsion; Chinese Captopril Trial; chocolate-coated tablet; coated compressed tablet; combination chemotherapy; combined cortical thickness; composite cyclic therapy; computerized cranial tomography; continuum charge transfer; contrast-enhanced computed tomography; controlled cord traction; conventional computed tomography; coronary care team; cortical collecting tubule; cranial computed tomography; critical care technician; cyclocarbothiamine

CCTA cardiac computed tomographic angiography; coronal computed tomographic arthrography

CCTC Certified Clinical Transplant Coordinator

CCTCC corticocerebellar thalamocortical circuit

CCTe cathodal closure tetanus

CCTG California Cooperative Treatment Group

CC-TGA congenitally corrected transposition of great vessels

CCTN Certified Clinical Transplant Nurse

CC-TOE continuum of care trauma outcome evaluation

CCTP coronary care training program

CCTR Cochrane Controlled Trials Register; common clinical term reference

CCTRN Certified Clinical Care Transportation Nurse

CCTV closed-circuit television

CCU cardiac care unit; Cherry-Crandall unit; clean catch urine; Consulting Committee on Units [Fr. *Comité Consultatif des Unités*]; coronary care unit; critical care unit

ccua clean catch urinalysis

CCUG Culture Collection, University of Göteborg

CCUP colpocystourethropexy

CCV cell culture vaccines; channel catfish virus; closed-circuit voltage; conductivity cell volume; critical closing volume

CCVD chronic cerebrovascular disease

CCVM congenital cardiovascular malformation

CCW counterclockwise; critical care workstation

CCWISB Canadian Chemical Warfare Inter-Service Board

CCX cyclooxygenase

CCyR complete cytogenic response

2CD two-cycle duration

CD cadaver donor; caldesmon; canine distemper [veterinary medicine]; canine dose [veterinary medicine]; carbohydrate dehydratase; carbon dioxide; cardiac disease; cardiac dullness; cardiac dysrhythmia; cardiovascular disease; Carrel-Dakin [fluid]; Castleman disease; cation dependent; caudad, caudal; celiac disease; cell dissociation; cervicodorsal; cesarean delivery; chemical dependency; chlordecone; circular dichroism; *cis*-dioxolane; cluster of differentiation; color Doppler; combination drug; common duct [bile] duct; communicable disease; compact disc; completely denatured; conduct disorder; conduction disorder; conjugata diagonalis; consanguineous donor; conserved domain; contact dermatitis; contagious disease; contrast detail; control diet; controlled drug; conventional dialysis; convulsive disorder; convulsive dose; corneal dystrophy; cortical dysplasia; Cotrel-Dubousset [rod]; Crohn disease; crossed diagonal; curative dose; cutdown; cycle day; cystic duct; cytochalasin D; cytoplasmic domain

C/D cigarettes per day; cup/disk ratio

C&D cystoscopy and dilation

CD4 HIV helper cell count

CD8 HIV suppressor cell count

CD$_{50}$ median curative dose

Cd cadmium; caldesmon; caudal; coccygeal; condylion

cd candela; caudal

c/d cigarettes per day; cycles per degree

CDA Canadian Dental Association; Certified Dental Assistant; chenodeoxycholic acid; chlorproguanil hydrochloride, dapsone, and artesunate; ciliary dyskinesia activity; clinical document architecture; complement-dependent antibody; completely denatured alcohol; compound document architecture; computer diagnostic assistant; congenital dyserythropoietic anemia

CdA chlorodeoxyadenosine

CDAC Clinical Data Abstraction Center

CDAD *Clostridium difficile*–associated disease

CDAE chemical defense aircrew ensemble

CDAI clinical disease activity index; Crohn Disease Activity Index

CDAL clinical data analysis laboratory

CDAP continuous distending airway pressure

CDB communication database

C&DB cough and deep breath

CDC calculated date of confinement; cancer diagnosis center; capillary diffusion capacity; casualty decontamination center; cell division control; cell division cycle; Centers for Disease Control and Prevention; chenodeoxycholate; children's diagnostic classification; Communicable Disease Center; complement-dependent cytotoxicity; Crohn disease of colon

CD-C controlled drinker-control

CDCA chenodeoxycholic acid

CDC-BRFS Centers for Disease Control Behavioral Risk Factor Survey

CDCC complement-dependent cellular cytotoxicity

CDCE constant denaturant capillary electrophoresis

cDCIS comedo-type ductal carcinoma in situ

CDC NAC Centers for Disease Control and Prevention National AIDS Clearinghouse

CDCV Caddo Canyon virus

CDD certificate of disability for discharge; choledochoduodenostomy; chronic degenerative disease; chronic disabling dermatosis; congenital diaphragmatic defect; conserved domain database; contrast-detail dose; craniodiaphyseal dysplasia; current disease descriptions; [poly] chlorinated dibenzo-*p*-dioxin

CDDN Certified Developmental Disabilities Nurse

CDDP cis-diaminedichloroplatinum

CD-DST collagen gel droplet-embedded drug sensitivity test

CDE canine distemper encephalitis; Certified Diabetes Educator; chlordiazepoxide; color Doppler energy; common data element; common duct exploration

CDEC Comprehensive Developmental Evaluation Chart

CDEIS Crohn's Disease Endoscopic Index of Severity

CDER Center for Drug Evaluation and Research

CDEV *Choristoneura diversuma* entomopoxvirus

CDF choledochoduodenal fistula; chondrodystrophia foetalis; class conditional density function; clinical data field; clinical data framework; common data format; cumulative

distribution function; [poly] chlorinated dibenzo-*p*-dioxin

CDFS compact disc file system

CDG central developmental groove; congenital disorder of glycosylation

CDGE constant denaturant gel electrophoresis

CDGG corneal dystrophy Groenouw type, granular

CDGS carbohydrate-deficient glycoprotein syndrome

cDGS complete form of DiGeorge syndrome

CDH ceramide dihexoside; chronic daily headache; congenital diaphragmatic hernia; congenital dislocation of hip; congenital dysplasia of hip

CDHAp calcium-deficient hydroxyapatite

CDH-ECMO congenital diaphragmatic hernia-extracorporeal membrane oxygenation

CDI cell-directed inhibitor; central/chronic diabetes insipidus; Children's Depression Inventory; clinical data interchange; *Clostridium difficile* infection; color Doppler imaging; communicable disease intelligence; cranial diabetes insipidus; cyclin-dependent kinase interactor

CDILD chronic diffuse interstitial lung disease

CDK caldesmon kinase; cell-division kinase; climatic droplet keratopathy; cyclin-dependent kinase

CDL chlordeoxylincomycin; Cornelia de Lange [syndrome]

CDLE chronic discoid lupus erythematosus

CDLS, CdLS Cornelia de Lange syndrome

CDM charges description master; chemically defined medium; clinical decision making; common data model

CDMA code division multiple access

CDMMS chorioretinal dysplasia, microcephaly, mental retardation (intellectual disability) syndrome

CDMNS clinical decision making in nursing scale

CD-MPR cation-dependent mannose-6-phosphate receptor

CDMS Certified Disability Management Specialist

CDN Certified Dialysis Nurse

cDNA circular deoxyribonucleic acid; complementary deoxyribonucleic acid

CDNANZ Communicable Disease Network of Australia and New Zealand

CDNB 1-chloro-2,4-dinitrobenzene

CDONA/LTC Certified Director of Nursing Administration/Long-Term Care

CDP chondrodysplasia punctata; chronic destructive periodontitis; collagenase-digestible protein; continuous distending pressure; coronary drug project; Council on Dental Practice; cytidine diphosphate; cytosine diphosphate

CDPAS Coronary Disease Prevention with Aspirin Study; Coronary Drug Project Aspirin Study

CDPC cytidine diphosphate choline

CDPR chondrodysplasia punctata, rhizomelic

CDPS calcium-dependent protease small subunit

CDPX X-linked chondrodysplasia punctata

CDR calcium-dependent regulator; clinical data repository; clinical dementia rating; close delay ratio; common data repository; complementarity determining region; computerized digital radiography; cup/disk ratio

CD-R compact disc recordable

CDRH Center for Devices and Radiological Health

CD-ROM compact disc—read only memory

CDRP clinical database research program

CDRS Children's Depression Rating Scale

CD-RW compact disc—rewritable

CDS cardiovascular surgery; Care Dependency Scale; catechol-3,5-disulfonate; caudal dysplasia syndrome; Chemical Data System; children's diagnostic scale; clean dataset; clinical decision support; cumulative duration of survival

CdS cadmium sulfide; [gene] coding sequence

CDSA common data security architecture

CDSC Communicable Diseases Surveillance Centre

CDSM Committee on Dental and Surgical Materials

CDSR Cochrane Database of Systematic Reviews

cd-sr candela-steradian

CDSRF chronic disease and sociodemographic risk factor

CDSS clinical decision support system

CD(S)U Communicable Diseases (Scotland) Unit

CDT carbohydrate-deficient transferrin; carbon dioxide therapy; Certified Dental Technician; children's day treatment; *Clostridium difficile* toxin; color discrimination test; combined diphtheria-tetanus [vaccine]

CDTA cyclohexanediaminetetraacetic acid

CDTe cathode duration tetanus

CDTF chemical decontamination training facility

CDU cardiac diagnostic unit; clinical decision unit; color Doppler ultrasound; complete dependence unit

CDUS carotid duplex ultrasonography

CDUV Candiru virus

CDV canine distemper virus; clinical diagnostic validity

cDVH cumulative dose-volume histogram

Cdyn, C$_{dyn}$ dynamic compliance

Cdyn, rs dynamic compliance of the respiratory system

CDYS cell dysfunction

CDZ chlordiazepoxide; conduction delay zone

CE California encephalitis; capillary electrophoresis; capsule endoscopy; carboxylesterase; cardiac enlargement; cardioesophageal; carotid endarterectomy; catamenial epilepsy; cataract extraction; cell extract; center edge [angle]; central episiotomy; chemical energy; chick embryo; chloroform ether; cholesterol ester; cholesteryl ester; chorioepithelioma; chromatoelectrophoresis; ciliated epithelium; cloning efficiency; coded element; coefficient of error; columnar epithelium; conical elevation; conjugated estrogens; constant error; continuing education; contractile element; contrast enhancement; converting enzyme; cornified epithelium; crude extract; cytopathic effect; cytoplasmic extract

C-E chloroform-ether

Ce cerium

C$_e$ effect [compartment] concentration

CEA carcinoembryonic antigen; carotid endarterectomy; cholesterol-esterifying activity; cost-effectiveness analysis; cranial-epidural abscess; crystalline egg albumin; cultured epithelial autograft

CEAC clinical education and assessment center; cost-effectiveness acceptability curve

CEAF cost-effectiveness acceptability frontier

CEAL carcinoembryonic antigen-like [protein]

CEAP class, etiology, anatomy, pathophysiology [classification]; Clinical Efficacy Assessment Project

CEARP Continuing Education Approval and Recognition Program

CEAs cultured epithelial autografts

CEASE Collaborative European Anti-Smoking Evaluation

CEAT chronic ectopic atrial tachycardia

CEB calcium entry blocker

cEBV chronic Epstein-Barr virus [infection]

CEC central echo complex; ciliated epithelial cell; colonic epithelial cells; Commission of the European Community

CECCC confidential enquiry into cardiac catheterization complications

CECR cat-eye syndrome chromosome region

CECT contrast-enhanced computed tomography

CED chondroectodermal dysplasia; clinical engineering department; convection-enhanced delivery

CEDARS Comprehensive Evaluation of Defibrillators and Resuscitative Shock [study]

CeDNV *Casphalia externa* densovirus

CEE Central European encephalitis; chick embryo extract; component execution environment; conjugated equine estrogens

CEEA curved end-to-end anastomosis

CE-EDUS contrast-enhanced endoscopic Doppler ultrasonography

CEEF clinical evaluation encounter form

CEEG computer-analyzed electroencephalography

CEE-MPA conjugated equine estrogen–medroxyprogesterone acetate

CEES chloroethyl ethyl sulfide

CEET chicken enucleated eye test

CEEV Central European encephalitis virus

CEF centrifugation extractable fluid; chick embryo fibroblast; constant electric field

CEFA continuous epidural fentanyl anesthesia

CE-FAST contrast-enhanced fast acquisition in a steady state

CEFMG Council on Education for Foreign Medical Graduates

CEG chronic erosive gastritis

CEH cholesterol ester hydrolase

CEHC calf embryonic heart cell; cost-effective health care

CEHN Children's Environmental Health Network

CEHO Chief Environmental Health Officer

CeHV cercopithecine herpesvirus

CEI character education inquiry; converting enzyme inhibitor

CEI-AMI converting enzyme inhibitor in the treatment of acute myocardial infarction

CEID crossed electroimmunodiffusion

CEJ cement-enamel junction

CEJA Council on Ethical and Judicial Affairs

CEK chick embryo kidney

CEL carboxyl-ester lipase

CelCer1V *Caenorhabditis elegans* Cer1 virus

CELDIC Commission on Emotional and Learning Disorders in Children

CELL Cost-Effectiveness of Lipid Lowering [study]

Cell celluloid

CELO chick embryonal lethal orphan [virus]

CELP code-excited linear prediction

Cels Celsius

CEM care environment management; central extensor mechanism; clinical event monitor; computerized electroencephalographic map; conventional transmission electron microscope

CEMIA Center for Engineering and Medical Image Analysis

CEMIS community-based environmental management information system

CE-MRA contrast-enhanced magnetic resonance angiography

CE-MRI contrast-enhanced magnetic resonance imaging

CeMV cetacean morbillivirus

CEN Certificate for Emergency Nursing; Clinical Experience Network [study]; European Committee for Standardization [Fr. *Comité Européen de Normalisation*]; continuous enteral nutrition

cen centromere; central

CENMR capillary electrophoresis nuclear magnetic resonance

CENOG computerized electroneuroophthalmography

ceNOS constitutional endothelial nitric oxide synthase

CENP centromere protein

CENPA, B, C, D, E centromeric proteins A, B, C, D, E

cent centigrade; central

CENTRAL Cochrane Central Register of Controlled Trials

CEO chick embryo origin; chief executive officer

CEOEECP Clinical Evaluation of Enhanced External Counterpulsation

CEOT calcifying epithelial odontogenic tumor

CEP care evaluation program; centromere evaluation probe; chronic eosinophilic pneumonia; chronic erythropoietic porphyria; clinical evaluation protocol; congenital erythropoietic porphyria; continuing education program; cortical evoked potential; counter-electrophoresis

CEPA chloroethane phosphoric acid

CEPH cephalic; cephalosporin; Council on Education for Public Health

ceph cephalin

CEPH FLOC cephalin flocculation

CEPU cerebellar Purkinje [cell]

CEQ Council on Environmental Quality

CER capital expenditure review; ceramide; ceruloplasmin; comparative-effectiveness research; conditioned emotional response; control electrical rhythm; cortical evoked response

CERAD Consortium to Establish a Registry for Alzheimer's Disease

CERCLA Comprehensive Environmental Response, Compensation, and Liability Act

CERCLIS Comprehensive Environmental Response, Communication, and Liability Information System

CERD chronic end-stage renal disease

CERP complex event-related potential; Continuing Education Recognition Program

CERT Cardiovascular Event Reduction Trial; computer emergency response team

Cert, cert certified

CERTs Center for Education and Research on Therapeutics

Cer1V Cer1 virus

cerv cervical, cervix

CES carboxylesterase; cat-eye syndrome; cauda equina syndrome; Center for Epidemiological Study; central excitatory state; chronic electrophysiologic study; clinical engineering services; conditioned escape response; cumulative embryo score

CESAR Centralised European Studies in Angina Research

CESARZ Clinical European Studies in Angina and Revascularization

CESD cholesterol ester storage disease

CES-D Center for Epidemiological Studies of Depression [scale]

CESG Cerebral Embolism Study Group

CESMA Council for European Specialists Medical Assessment

CESNA Comparative Efficacy and Safety of Nisoldipine and Amlodipine [in hypertension trial]

CESNA II Comparative Efficacy and Safety of Nisoldipine and Amlodipine II [in hypertension with ischemic heart disease trial]

CESS Cooperative Ewing Sarcoma Study

cESS circumferential end-systolic stress

CET capital expenditure threshold; cholesterol-ester transfer; Collaborative Eclampsia Trial; congenital eyelid tetrad

CETE Central European tick-borne encephalitis

CETN Certified Enterostomal Therapy Nurse

CETP cholesteryl-ester transfer protein

CEU congenital ectropion uveae; continuing education unit

CEUS contrast-enhanced ultrasound

CEV California encephalitis virus

CEX clinical evaluation exercise

CEZ cefazolin

CF calcaneal fibular [ligament]; calcium leucovorin; calf blood flow; calibration factor; cancer free; carbol-fuchsin; carbon filtered; carboxyfluorescein; cardiac failure; cardiac fibroblast; carotid foramen; carrier free; cascade filtration; case file; Caucasian female; centrifugal force; cervical fluid; characteristic frequency; chemotactic factor; chest and left leg [ECG]; Chiari-Frommel [syndrome]; chick fibroblast; Christmas factor; chronicity factor; circumflex; citrovorum factor; clotting factor; colicin factor; collected fluid; colonization factor; colony forming; complementary feeding; complement fixation; computed fluoroscopy; constant frequency; contractile force; conversion factor; cord factor; coronary flow; correction factor; cough frequency; count fingers; counting finger; coupling factor; cycling fibroblast; cystic fibrosis; folinic acid [citrovorum factor]

Cf californium

cf centrifugal force; bring together, compare [L. *confer*]; confidence factor

CFA 2-chloro-4-fluoroaniline; cerebro-facio-articular [syndrome]; colonization factor antigen; colony-forming assay; common femoral artery; complement-fixing antibody; complete Freund's adjuvant; configuration frequency analysis; cryptogenic fibrosing alveolitis

CFAE complex fractionated atrial electrograms

CFAG cystic fibrosis antigen

CFAV cell-fusing agent virus

CFB central fibrous body

CFC capillary filtration coefficient; cardio-facio-cutaneous [syndrome]; chlorofluorocarbon; colony-forming capacity; colony-forming cell; continuous-flow centrifugation

CFCN Certified Foot Care Nurse

CfCPV *Choristoneura fumiferana* cypovirus

CFD cephalofacial deformity; color-flow Doppler; computational fluid dynamics; craniofacial dysostosis

CF-DA carboxyfluorescein diacetate

CFDS craniofacial dyssynostosis

CFDU color-flow Doppler ultrasonography/ultrasound

CFEV *Choristoneura fumiferana* entomopoxvirus

CFF critical flicker fusion [test]; critical fusion frequency; cystic fibrosis factor; Cystic Fibrosis Foundation

cff critical flicker fusion; critical fusion frequency

CFFA cystic fibrosis factor activity

CFH complement factor H; Council on Family Health

CFHL complement factor H-like [protein]

CFHP Council on Federal Health Programs

CFI chemotactic-factor inactivator; clenched/closed-fist injury; color flow imaging; community fluorosis index; complement fixation inhibition

CfIV *Campoletis flavicincta* ichnovirus

CFL cofilin

CFM cerebral function monitor; chlorofluoromethane; close-fitting mask; composite filling material; craniofacial microsomia

CFMA Council for Medical Affairs

CFMDB Cystic Fibrosis Mutation Database

CFMG Commission on Foreign Medical Graduates

CfMNPV *Choristoneura fumiferana* multiple nucleopolyhedrovirus

CfMS care flow management system

CFMV constant flow mechanical ventilation

CFN Certified Forensic Nurse

CFND craniofrontonasal dysostosis; craniofrontonasal dysplasia

CFNP Certified Family Nurse Practitioner

CFNS chills, fever, night sweats; craniofrontonasal syndrome

CFO chief financial officer

CfoIV *Casinaria forcipata* ichnovirus

CFOS constrained fast orthogonal search

CFP chronic false positive; ciguatera fish poisoning; Clinical Fellowship Program; Conference for Food Protection; culture filtrate protein; cyclophosphamide, fluorouracil, prednisone; cystic fibrosis of pancreas; cystic fibrosis protein

CFPC College of Family Physicians of Canada

CFPP craniofacial pattern profile

CFPR Canadian Familial Polyposis Registry

CFR case fatality ratio; citrovorum factor rescue; Code of Federal Regulations; complement fixation reaction; coronary flow reserve; correct fast reaction; cyclic flow reduction

CFRN Certified Flight Registered Nurse

CFS cancer family syndrome; Chiari-Frommel syndrome; chronic fatigue syndrome; craniofacial stenosis; crush fracture syndrome; culture fluid supernatant; Cystic Fibrosis Society

CFSAN Center for Food Safety and Applied Nutrition

CFSE carboxyfluorescein succinimidyl ester; crystal field stabilization energy

CFSTI Clearinghouse for Federal Scientific and Technical Information

CFT cardiolipin flocculation test; clinical full time; complement fixation test; crystal field theory

CFTC complication-free tumor control

CFTD congenital fiber type disproportion

CFTR cystic fibrosis transmembrane conductance regulator

CFU colony-forming unit; coupling factor unit

cfu colony-forming unit

CFU-C, CFU$_C$ colony-forming unit—culture

CFU-E, CFU$_E$ colony-forming unit—erythrocyte

CFU-EOS, CFU$_{EOS}$ colony-forming unit—eosinophil

CFU-F, CFU$_F$ colony-forming unit—fibroblastoid

CFU-G, CFU$_G$ colony-forming unit—granulocyte

CFU-GM, CFU$_{GM}$ colony-forming unit—granulocyte macrophage

CFU-GEMM, CFU$_{GEMM}$ colony forming unit—granulocyte, erythrocyte, macrophage, megakaryocyte

CFU-L, CFU$_L$ colony-forming unit—lymphocyte

CFU$_M$ colony-forming unit—megakaryocyte

CFU-MEG, CFU$_{MEG}$ colony-forming unit—megakaryocyte

CFUN cell function

CFU-NM, CFU$_{NM}$ colony-forming unit—neutrophil-monocyte

CFU-S, CFU$_S$ colony-forming unit—spleen; colony-forming unit—stem cells

CFUSA Cystic Fibrosis Foundation USA

CfuT1V *Cladosporium fulvum* T-1 virus

CFUV Corfu virus

CFV chimpanzee foamy virus; continuous-flow ventilation

CFV/HU chimpanzee foamy virus, human

CFVS cerebrospinal fluid flow void sign

CFW Carworth farm [mouse] Webster strain

CFWM cancer-free white mouse

CFX cefoxitin; circumflex coronary artery

CFX-MARG marginal branch of the circumflex artery

CFZ capillary-free zone

CFz clofazimine

CFZC continuous-flow zonal centrifugation

CG calcium gluconate; cardiography; Cardio-Green; caregiver; central gray matter; choking gas [phosgene]; cholecystogram, cholecystography; choriogenic gynecomastia; chorionic gonadotropin; chromogranin; chronic glomerulonephritis; cingulate gyrus; Cockcroft-Gault equation; colloidal gold; continuous-flow ventilation; control group; cryoglobulin; cystine guanine; cytosine-guanine-guanine

Cγ gamma chain constant region

cg center of gravity; centigram; chemoglobulin

CGA catabolite gene activator; color graphics adapter; comprehensive geriatric assessment; contact guard assist

CGAB congenital abnormality

CGAP Cancer Genome Anatomy Project

CGAS Children's Global Assessment Scale

CGAT Canadian Genome and Technology [program]; chromatin granule amine transformer; Constitutional Genetic Array Test

CGB chronic gonadotropin, beta-unit

CGC cumulus-granulosa cell

CGD Cattle Genome Database; chronic granulomatous disease

CGDE contact glow discharge electrolysis

CGE capillary gel electrophoresis

CGF cell-generating factor

CGFH congenital fibrous histiocytoma

CGFNS Commission on Graduates of Foreign Nursing Schools

CGGE constant gradient gel electrophoresis

CGH chorionic gonadotropic hormone; comparative genomic hybridization; congenital generalized hypertrichosis

CGI chronic granulomatous inflammation; Clinical Global Impression [scale]; combustible gas indicator; common gateway interface; computer-generated imagery

CGI-C Clinical Global Impression of Change [scale]

CGI-I Clinical Global Impression of Improvement [scale]

CGI-S Clinical Global Impression of Severity [scale]

cGK cyclic guanosine monophosphate—dependent protein kinase

CGKD complex glycerol kinase deficiency

CGL chronic granulocytic leukemia; clinical guidelines

c gl correction with glasses

CGLV Changuinola virus

CGM Center for Genetics in Medicine; central gray matter

cgm centigram

CGMC Center for Graphic Medical Communication

CGMP current good manufacturing practices

cGMP cyclic guanosine monophosphate; cyclic guanosyl monophosphate

CGN Certified Gastroenterology Nurse; chronic glomerulonephritis

CGNB composite ganglioneuroblastoma

CG/OQ cerebral glucose-oxygen quotient

CGP choline glycerophosphatide; chorionic growth hormone-prolactin; circulating granulocyte pool; circulatory gene pool; *N*-carbobenzoxy-glycyl-l-phenylalanine

CGPM General Conference of Weights and Measures [Fr. *Conférence Générale des Poids et Mesures*]

CGRN Certified Gastroenterology Registered Nurse

CGRP, cGRP calcitonin gene-related peptide

CGRPR calcitonin gene-related peptide receptor

CGS cardiogenic shock; catgut suture; causal genesis syndrome

CGS, cgs centimeter-gram-second

CGT chorionic gonadotropin; cyclodextrin glucanotransferase

CGTT cortisone glucose tolerance test

CGV Chobar Gorge virus

cGVHD chronic graft-versus-host disease

CGW caregiver workstation

cGy centigray

CH case history; Chédiak-Higashi [syndrome]; chiasma; Chinese hamster; chloral hydrate; cholesterol; Christchurch chromosome; chronic hepatitis; chronic hypertension; common hepatic [duct]; communicating hydrocele; community health; community hospital; completely healed; congenital hypothyroidism; Conradi-Hünermann [syndrome]; continuous heparin; cortical hamartoma; crown heel [length]; cycloheximide; cystic hygroma; wheelchair

C_H1, C_H2, C_H3, C_H4 first to fourth constant regions in heavy chains of immunoglobulin molecules

CH_{50} 50% hemolyzing dose of complement

C_H constant region in heavy chain of immunoglobulin molecule

C&H cocaine and heroin; coarse and harsh

Ch chest; Chido [antibody]; chief; child; choline; Christchurch [syndrome]; chromosome

Ch^+ hydrogen ion concentration

ch chest; child; chronic

CHA Canadian Healthcare Association; Catholic Health Association of the United States; Chinese hamster; chronic hemolytic anemia; common hepatic artery; congenital hypoplasia of adrenal glands; congenital hypoplastic anemia; continuously heated aerosol; cyclohexyladenosine; cyclohexylamine

ChA choline acetylase

ChAC choline acetyltransferase

CHAD Cholesterol, Hypertension and Diabetes [study]; cold hemagglutinin disease; cyclophosphamide, hexamethylmelamine, Adriamycin (doxorubicin), and cisplatin

CHADS congestive heart failure, hypertension, age at least 75 years, diabetes, previous stroke or transient ischemic attack

ChAdV chimpanzee adenovirus

CHAF central hyperalimentation nutrition

CHAID chi-squared automatic interaction detection; chi-squared automatic interaction detector

CHAIN Contact Health Advice Information Network for Effective Health Care

CHAMP Cardiac Hospitalization Atherosclerosis Management Program; chemically hardened air-management plant; Children with HIV and Acquired AIDS Model Program; Children's Hospital Automated Medical Program; Combination Hemotherapy and Mortality Prevention [study]

CHAMPUS Civilian Health and Medical Program of Uniformed Services

CHAMPVA Civilian Health and Medical Program of Veterans Administration

CHANDS curly hair, ankyloblepharon, nail dysplasia syndrome

Chang C Chang conjunctiva cells

CHANGE Chronic Heart Failure and Graded Exercise [study]

Chang L Chang liver cells

CHAOS Cambridge Heart Antioxidant Study; Cardiovascular Disease, Hypertension and Hyperlipidemia, Adult-Onset Diabetes, Obesity, and Stroke [study]

CHAP Certified Hospital Admission Program; child health assessment program; Community Health Accreditation Program

CHAPS Carvedilol Heart Attack Pilot Study; 3[3-cholaminopropyl diethylammonio]-1-propane sulfonate

CHAR continuous hyperfractionated accelerated radiotherapy

CHARGE coloboma, heart disease, atresia choanae, retarded growth and retarded development and/or CNS anomalies, genital hypoplasia, and ear anomalies and/or deafness [syndrome]

CHARM Candesartan in Heart Failure Assessment in Reduction of Mortality [trial]

CHARMM Chemistry at Harvard Molecular Mechanics

CHART Continuous Hormones as Replacement Therapy [study]; Continuous Hyperfractionated Accelerated Radiotherapy Trial

CHAS Center for Health Administration Studies; Community Health Assessment Study

CHASE cut holes and sink 'em [operation]

CHAT Checklist for Autism in Toddlers; conversational hypertext access technology

ChAT choline acetyltransferase

CHATH chemically hardened air transportable hospital

CHB chronic hepatitis B; complete heart block; congenital heart block

ChB Bachelor of Surgery [L. *Chirurgiae Baccalaureus*]

CHBA, CHBHA congenital Heinz body hemolytic anemia

CHC chromosome condensation; community health center; community health computing; community health council

CHCIS community health care information system

CHCL congenital healed cleft lip

CHCP correctional health care program

CHCS composite health care system

CHCT caffeine halothane contracture test

CHD Chédiak-Higashi disease; childhood disease; child in semantic hierarchy; chronic hemodialysis; common hepatic duct; congenital heart disease; congenital hip dislocation; congestive heart disease; constitutional hepatic dysfunction; coronary heart disease; cyanotic heart disease

ChD Doctor of Surgery [L. *Chirurgiae Doctor*]

CHDM comprehensive hospital drug monitoring

CHDP Child Health and Disability Prevention [program]

ChE cholinesterase

che a gene involved in chemotaxis

CHEAPER Confirmation that Heparin Is an Alternative to Promote Early Reperfusion in Acute Myocardial Infarction [study]

ChEAT Children's Eating Attitudes Test

CHEC clearinghouse for emergency aid to the community; community hypertension evaluation clinic

CHED congenital hereditary endothelial dystrophy

CHEER Chest Pain Evaluation in Emergency Room [trial]

CHEF Chinese hamster embryo fibroblast; contour-clamped homologous electric field

CHEM chemical

chem chemical, chemistry; chemotherapy

ChemID Chemical Identification; Chemical Identification File

CHEMLINE Chemical Dictionary On-Line

chemo chemotherapy

CHEMTREC Chemical Transportation Emergency Center

CHEP cricohyoidoepiglottopexy

CHEPER Chest Pain Evaluation Registry

CHERSS continuous high-amplitude EEG rhythmic synchronous slowing

CHES chronic hyperplastic eosinophilic sinusitis

CHESS chemical shift selective; Comprehensive Health Enhancement Support System

CHEST chick embryo toxicity screening test; Combined Higher Education Software Team

CHF chick embryo fibroblast; chronic heart failure; congenital hepatic fibrosis; congestive heart failure; Crimean hemorrhagic fever

CHFD controlled high-flux dialysis

CHFDT congestive heart failure data tool

CHF-IES Congestive Heart Failure Italian Epidemiological Study

CHF-STAT Congestive Heart Failure Survival Trial of Antiarrhythmic Therapy

CHFV combined high-frequency ventilation

chg change, changed

CHGA chromogranin A

CHGB chromogranin B

CHH cartilage-hair hypoplasia

CHHS congenital hypothalamic hamartoma syndrome

ChHV chelonid herpesvirus

CHI clinical health informatics; closed head injury; congenital hyperinsulinism; consumer health information; creatinine height index

chi chimera

Chi-A chimpanzee leukocyte antigen

CHIC Cardiovascular Health In Children [study]

CHID Combined Health Information Database

CHIKV Chikungunya virus

CHILD congenital hemidysplasia with ichthyosiform erythroderma and limb defects [syndrome]

CHILI Consumer Health Information Literature

CHIM Center for Healthcare Information Management

CHIME Center for Health Information Management and Evaluation; College of Healthcare Information Management Executives; coloboma, heart anomaly, ichthyosis, mental retardation (intellectual disability), ear abnormality [syndrome]

CHIMR Centre for Health Information Management Research

CHIMS community-based health information system

CHIMV Chim virus

CHIN community health information network

CHINA chronic infectious neurotropic agent

CHIPA community health planning agency

CHIP child health improvement program; Children's Health Insurance Program; comprehensive health insurance plan; Coronary Health Improvement Project

ChIP chromatin immunoprecipitation

CHIPASAT Children's Paced Auditory Serial Addition Task

CHIP catastrophic health insurance plan
CHiQ Centre for Health Information Quality
Chir Doct Doctor of Surgery [L. *Chirurgiae Doctor*]
chirug surgical [L. *chirurgicalis*]
CHIS community health information system; consumer health information system
CHIV Chilibre virus
CHL Chinese hamster lung; chlorambucil; chloramphenicol
Chl chloroform; chlorophyll
CHLA cyclohexyl linoleic acid
Chlb chlorobutanol
CHLD chronic hypoxic lung disease
chlor chloride
CHLS combined heart and lung surgery
ChlVPP chlorambucil, vinblastine, procarbazine, prednisone
ChM Master of Surgery [L. *Chirurgiae Magister*]
CHMD clinical hyaline membrane disease
CHMIS community health management information system
CHMR Centre for Health Information Management Research
CHN carbon, hydrogen, and nitrogen; Certified Hemodialysis Nurse; child health nurse; child neurology; community health nurse
CHNS China Health and Nutrition Survey
CHO carbohydrate; Chinese hamster ovary; chorea; comprehensive health organization
Cho choline
C_H₂O water clearance
choc chocolate
CHOICE Caring for Hypertension on Initiation: Cost and Effectiveness [study]; Congestive Heart Failure Mortality: Investigation on Carvedilol's Efficacy
CHOICES Cancer, Heart Disease, Osteoporosis Interventions, and Community Evaluation Studies
CHOIR Center for Health Outcomes Improvement Research
CHOL, chol cholesterol
c hold withhold
CHOP cyclophosphamide, hydroxydaunomycin, Oncovin, and prednisone
ChoP cell-surface phosphocholine
CHORUS Collaborative Hypertext in Radiology
CHOV Chaco virus
CHP calcineurin homologue protein; capillary hydrostatic pressure; charcoal hemoperfusion; Chemical Hygiene Plan; child psychiatry; Children's Health Project;

community health plan; comprehensive health planning; coordinating hospital physician; cricohyoidopexy; cutaneous hepatic porphyria
ChP chest physician
CHPA community health planning agency; community health purchasing alliance; Consumer Healthcare Products Association
CHPN Certified Hospice and Palliative Nurse
CHPV Chandipura virus; chicken parvovirus
ChPV chipmunk parvovirus
chpx chickenpox
CHQ chloroquinol
CHQCP Cleveland Health Quality Choice Project
CHR cerebro-hepato-renal [syndrome]; chemical hazards regulations; complete hematologic response
Chr *Chromobacterium*
chr chromosome; chronic
c hr candle hour
c-hr curie-hour
ChRBC chicken red blood cell
CHREF Connecticut Healthcare Research and Education Foundation
CHRIS Cancer Hazards Ranking and Information System; Chemical Hazard Response Information System
CHRISTMAS Carvedilol Hibernation Reversible Ischemia Trial: Marker of Success
CHRN Certified Hyperbaric Registered Nurse
CHROMINFO chromosome information [database]
chron chronic
CHRONIC chronic disease, rheumatoid arthritis, neoplasms, infections, cryoglobulinemia
CHRPE congenital hypertrophy of the retinal pigment epithelium
CHRRPE combined hamartoma of the retina and retinal pigment epithelium
CHRS cerebro-hepato-renal syndrome; Christian syndrome
CHRV Chub reovirus
CHS Canada Health Survey; cardiovascular health study; Center for Health Statistics; central hypoventilation syndrome; Charleston Heart Study; Chédiak-Higashi syndrome; Chinese Health Study; cholinesterase; chondroitin sulfate; citizen health system; community health study; compression hip screw; congenital hypoventilation syndrome; contact hypersensitivity; Copenhagen City Heart Study; coronary heart study
CHSD Children's Health Services Division

CHSO total hemolytic serum C activity

CHSP Child Health Surveillance Programme; Clinton Health Security Plan

CHSS Congenital Heart Surgeons Society; cooperative health statistics system

CHSSDC Congenital Heart Surgeons Society Data Center

CHT certified hand therapist; chemotherapy; combined hormone therapy; contralateral head turning

ChTg chymotrypsinogen

ChTK chicken thymidine kinase

ChTX charybdotoxin

CHU centigrade heat unit; closed head unit

CHUSPAN Churg-Strauss Syndrome and Polyarteritis Nodosa [study]

CHV canine herpes virus; Cryphonectria hypovirus

CHVF chemically viewed functionally

CHVS chemically viewed structurally

CHVV Charleville virus

CI calcium ionophore; cardiac index; cardiac insufficiency; cation independent; cell immunity; cell inhibition; cephalic index; cerebral infarction; cervical incompetence; chemical ionization; chemically induced; chemo-immunotherapy; chemotactic index; chemotherapeutic index; chromatid interchange; chronic infection; chronic inflammation; clinical investigator; clomipramine; clonus index; cochlear implant; coefficient of intelligence; colloidal iron; colonization index; color index; Colour Index; competitive index; complete iridectomy; confidence index; confidence interval; conformity index; contamination index; contextual inquiry; continued insomnia; continuous imaging; continuous improvement; continuous infusion; contraindicated, contraindication; convergence insufficiency; coronary insufficiency; corrected count increment; covering index; crystalline insulin; cumulative incidence; cytotoxic index; first concept; first cranial nerve; prostatic tumor with extracapsular extension and negative margins; tumor with metastases to lymph nodes without involvement of perirectal adipose tissue

C^I intercept on concentration

Ci curie

CIA chemiluminescent immunoassay; chymotrypsin inhibitor activity; colony-inhibiting activity; congenital intestinal aganglionosis

CIAC central independent adjudication committee

CIAIT Chinese Infarction Angiotensin Converting Enzyme Inhibitor Trial

CIAS cognitive impairment with schizophrenia

CIBD chronic inflammatory bowel disease

CiBER Centre for Information Behaviour and Analysis Research

CIBHA congenital inclusion body hemolytic anemia

CIBIS Cardiac Insufficiency Bisoprolol Study

CIBMTR Center for International Blood and Marrow Transplant Research

CIBP chronic intractable benign pain

CIBPS chronic intractable benign pain syndrome

CIC cardioinhibitor center; care improvement council; Certified in Infection Control; ciclesonide; circulating immune complex; clean intermittent catheterization; completely in the canal [hearing aid]; computers in cardiology; computing, information, and communication; constant initial concentration; crisis intervention center

Cic cicletanine

CICA cervical internal carotid artery

CICN Center for Integrative and Cognitive Neuroscience [Vanderbilt University]; Colorado Integrated Care Network

CICR calcium-induced calcium release process

CICU cardiac intensive care unit; cardiovascular inpatient care unit; coronary intensive care unit

CID cellular immunodeficiency; Center for Infectious Diseases; charge injection device; chick infective dose; combined immunodeficiency disease; Cosmetic Ingredient Dictionary; cytomegalic inclusion disease

CID$_{50}$ median chimpanzee infective dose

CI$_d$ intercompartmental diffusion

CIDEMS Center for Information and Documentation

CIDEP chemically induced dynamic electron polarization

CIDI composite international diagnostic interview

CIDI-SAM Composite International Diagnostic Interview-Substance Abuse Module

CIDM computerized infectious disease monitor

CIDNP chemically induced dynamic nuclear polarization

CIDP chronic idiopathic polyradiculopathy; chronic inflammatory demyelinating polyradiculoneuropathy; Clinical Initiatives Development Program

CIDR Center for Inherited Disease Research

CIDS Canadian Implantable Defibrillator Study; Canadian Internal Defibrillator Study; cellular immunity deficiency syndrome;

circular intensity differential scattering; continuous insulin delivery system

CIE Canberra Interview for the Elderly; cellulose ion exchange; congenital ichthyosiform erythroderma; countercurrent immunoelectrophoresis; counterimmunoelectrophoresis; crossed immunoelectrophoresis

CIEBOV Côte d'Ivoire Ebola virus

CIEP counterimmunoelectrophoresis; crossed immunoelectrophoresis

CIF cartilage induction factor; cloning inhibitory factor; congenital infantile fibrosarcoma

CIFC Council for the Investigation of Fertility Control

CIG cardiointegram; cold-insoluble globulin; computer-interpretable guidelines

CIg intracytoplasmic immunoglobulin

cIgM cytoplasmic immunoglobulin M

CIGTS Comparison of Initial Glaucoma Treatment Study

CIH carbohydrate-induced hyperglyceridemia; Certificate in Industrial Health; children in hospital

CIHI Canadian Institute for Health Information

CIHR Canadian Institutes of Health Research

ci-hr curie-hour

CIHS central infantile hypotonic syndrome

CiHV ciconiid herpesvirus

CII cancer informatics infrastructure; Carnegie Interest Inventory; continuous intravenous infusion; second cranial nerve

CIIA common internal iliac artery

CIII third cranial nerve

CIIP chronic idiopathic intestinal pseudoobstruction

CIIPX X-linked chronic idiopathic intestinal pseudoobstruction

CIIR Center for Intelligent Information Retrieval

CiIV *Casinaria infesta* ichnovirus

CIK cytokine-induced killer [cells]

CILIP Chartered Institute of Library and Information Professionals

CIM cimetidine; cortically induced movement; Cumulated Index Medicus; cytoimmunologic monitoring

C-IMC circumference of the chest and the inframammary crease

Ci/ml, Ci/mL curies per milliliter

CI-MPR cation-independent mannose-6-phosphate receptor

CIMS chemical ionization mass spectrometry

CIMT carotid intima-media thickness; constraint-induced movement therapy

CIN central inhibition; cervical intraepithelial neoplasia; cervical intraepithelial neoplasm; chromosomal instability; chronic interstitial nephritis; community information network

Cin increased concentration; insulin clearance

CIN 1, CIN I cervical intraepithelial neoplasia, grade 1

CIN 2, CIN II cervical intraepithelial neoplasia, grade 2

CIN 3, CIN III cervical intraepithelial neoplasia, grade 3

CINAHL Cumulative Index to Nursing and Allied Health Literature

Cinahl Cumulative Index to Nursing and Allied Health

CINCA chronic infantile neurologic cutaneous and articular [syndrome]

CINDI Countrywide Integrated Noncommunicable Disease Intervention [study]

CINE chemotherapy-induced nausea and emesis

C1 INH complement 1 inhibitor

C$_1$-INH C$_1$-esterase inhibitor

CINI Computers in Nursing Interactive

CINV cancer chemotherapy-induced nausea and vomiting

CIO chief information officer; corticoid-induced osteoporosis

CIOMS Council for International Organizations of Medical Sciences

CIOSC Canadian Integrated Outbreak Surveillance Center

CIP care information provision; chronic idiopathic polyradiculoneuropathy; chronic intestinal pseudoobstruction; Collection de l'Institut Pasteur

CIPA client interface for professional access; Computer-Aided Identification of Phlebotomine Sandflies of the Americas

CIPC Center for Injury Prevention and Control

CIPD continuous intermittent peritoneal dialysis

CIPF classic interstitial pneumonitis-fibrosis; clinical illness promoting factor

CIPHER Common Information for Public Health Reporting

CIPM International Committee on Weights and Measures [Fr. *Comité International des Poids et Mesures*]

CIPN chronic inflammatory polyneuropathy

CIPOS chronic intestinal pseudoobstruction syndrome

CIPRA Comprehensive International Program of Research on AIDS

CIPSO chronic intestinal pseudoobstruction

CIR constant interval reciprocal

CIRC Ca^{2+}-induced Ca^{2+} release

circ circuit; circular; circumcision; circumference

circ & sens circulation and sensation

CIREN Crash Injury Research and Engineering Network

CIRF clinically insignificant renal fragments; contrast-induced renal failure

CIRSE Cardiovascular and Interventional Radiological Society of Europe

CIRSET Committee on Immunization Registry Standards and Electronic Transactions

CIS capacity information system; carcinoma in situ; catheter-induced spasm; central inhibitory state; Chemical Information Service; clinical information system; clinically isolated syndrome; computer-integrated surgery; computerized information system; continuous interleaved sampler; Coronary Intervention Study; cumulative impairment score

CI-S calculus index, simplified

CiS cingulate sulcus

CISC complex instructional set computing

CISCA$_{II}$B$_{IV}$ Cytoxan, Adriamycin, platinum, vinblastine, bleomycin

cis-DPP cisplatin

CISE Computer and Information Science and Engineering

CISET Committee on International Science, Engineering, and Technology

CISH competitive in situ hybridization

CISMeF Catalog and Index of French-Speaking Resources

CISP chronic intractable shoulder pain

CIS PT cisplatin

13-cis-RA 13-*cis*-retinoic acid

CISS chromosome in situ suppression; Common Internet Scheme Syntax; constructive interference in steady state; Coping Inventory for Stressful Situations

CISST computer-integrated surgical system and technology

CIT citrate; combined intermittent therapy; conjugated-immunoglobulin technique; critical incident technique; crossed intrinsic transfer

cit citrate

CITS Carey Infant Temperament Scale; cerebral infarction with transient symptoms

CITT Chemical Industry Institute for Toxicology

CITTS Central Illinois Thrombolytic Therapy Study

CIV Carey Island virus; ceratitis I virus; continuous intravenous infusion; fourth cranial nerve

CIVI continuous intravenous infusion

CIVII continuous intravenous insulin infusion

CIX ninth cranial nerve

CIXA constant infusion excretory urogram

CJ conjunctivitis

CJA Creutzfeldt-Jakob agent

CJD Creutzfeldt-Jakob disease

CJS Creutzfeldt-Jakob syndrome

CJSV Carajas virus

CjvO$_2$ jugular venous oxygen content

CK calf kidney; casein kinase; chemokine; chicken kidney; cholecystokinin; choline kinase; contralateral knee; creatine kinase; cyanogen chloride; cytokinin

CKII casein kinase II

ck check, checked

C$_K$ kappa light chain constant region

CKB creatine kinase, brain type

CKC cold-knife conization

CKD chronic kidney disease; cone-kernal distribution

CKG cardiokymography

C/kg coulomb per kilogram

CKI cyclin-dependent kinase inhibitor

CKM creatine kinase, muscle type

CKMB creatine kinase, myocardial bound

CKMM creatine kinase, muscle type

CK-PZ cholecystokinin-pancreozymin

CKR chemokine receptor

CKRM clinical knowledge repository manager

CKS classic form of Kaposi sarcoma

CL capillary lumen; cardiolipin; case library; cell line central [venous] line; centralis lateralis; cervical line; chemiluminescence; chest and left arm [ECG]; childhood leukemia; cholelithiasis; cholesterol-lecithin; chronic leukemia; cirrhosis of liver; clavicle; clear liquid; clearance; cleft lip; clinical laboratory; clomipramine; complete linkage; complex loading; composite lymphoma; computational linguistics; confidence level; confidence limit; contact lens; corpus luteum; corrected length; cricoid lamina; criterion level; critical list; cutaneous leishmaniasis; cutis laxa; cycle length; cytotoxic lymphocyte; lung capacity; lung compliance

C-L consultation-liaison

C$_L$ constant region of light chain of immunoglobulin molecule; lung compliance

Cl chloride; chlorine; clavicle; clear; clearance; clinic; *Clostridium*; closure; colistin

cL, cl centiliter

cl clarified; clean; clear; cleft; clinic; clinical; clonus; clotting; cloudy

Cλ lambda light chain constant region [immunoglobulins]

CLA Canadian Lung Association; cerebellar ataxia; Certified Laboratory Assistant; cervicolinguoaxial; closed-loop algorithm; conjugated linoleic acid; contralateral local anesthesia; cutaneous lichen amyloidosis; cutaneous lymphocyte antigen; cyclic lysine anhydride

Cl-α alternative chloride channel

ClAc chloroacetyl

CLAH congenital lipoid adrenal hyperplasia

CLam cervical laminectomy

CLARINET Placebo-Controlled Study of Lanreotide Antiproliferative Response in Patients with Gastroenteropancreatic Neuroendocrine Tumor

CLAS Cholesterol-Lowering Atherosclerosis Study; circulating lupus anticoagulant syndrome; classification; computerized laboratory alerting system; congenital localized absence of skin

CLASP Collaborative Low-Dose Aspirin Study in Pregnancy

CLASS Clomethiazole Acute Stroke Study

class, classif classification

CLASSICS Clopidrogrel Aspirin Stent Interventional Cooperative Study

clav clavicle

CLB chlorambucil; clobazam; configurable logic block; curvilinear body

CLBBB complete left bundle branch block

CLBP chronic low back pain

CLC Charcot-Leyden crystal; Clerc-Levy-Critesco [syndrome]

ClC chloride channel

CLCA compact low-chromatin area

CLCD cleidocranial dysostosis

CLCN chloride channel

ClCN cyanogen chloride

CL/CP cleft lip/cleft palate

Cl$_{cr}$ creatinine clearance

CLCS colchicine sensitivity

CLD central low density; central lung distance; chloride diarrhea; chronic liver disease; chronic lung disease; congenital limb deficiency; crystal ligand field

cld closed

CLDH choline dehydrogenase

cldy cloudy

CLE centrilobular emphysema; congenital lobar emphysema; continuous lumbar epidural [anesthesia]

CLEAR Collaborative Exchange of Antifungal Research

CLED cystine-lactose-electrolyte deficient [agar]

CLEMANTIS clinical engineering management tool and information system

CLEOPAD Clopidogrel in Peripheral Arterial Disease [study]

CLEV *Chironomus luridus* entomopoxvirus

CLF cardiolipin fluorescent [antibody]; ceroid lipofuscinosis; cholesterol-lecithin flocculation

Clf clumping factor

ClfA clumping factor A

CLH chronic lobular hepatitis; cleft limb–heart [syndrome]; congenital lobar hyperinflation; corpus luteum hormone; cutaneous lymphoid hyperplasia

CLI complement lysis inhibitor; corpus luteum insufficiency; critical limb ischemia

CLIA Clinical Laboratory Improvement Amendments

CLIAC Clinical Laboratory Improvement Advisory Committee

CLIBS cation and ligand–induced binding site

CLIF cloning inhibitory factor; *Crithidia luciliae* immunofluorescence

CLIMS clinical laboratory information management system

clin clinic, clinical

CLINPROT Clinical Cancer Protocols

ClinQuery clinical query

CLINT clinical informatics network

Cl$_{int}$ intrinsic clearance

CLIP capitolunate instability pattern; Cholesterol-Lowering Intervention Program; corticotropin-like intermediate lobe peptide

CLIPS C-language integrated production system

CLL cholesterol-lowering lipid; chronic lymphatic leukemia; chronic lymphocytic leukemia; cow lung lavage

CLM capillary-lymphatic malformation

Cl$_M$ metabolic clearance

CLMA Clinical Laboratory Management Association

Cl$_2$MD dichloromethylene diphosphate

CLMF cytotoxic lymphocyte maturation factor

CLML Current List of Medical Literature

CLMS clinical management system

CLN neuronal ceroid lipofuscinosis

CLNC Certified Legal Nurse Consultant

CLO *Campylobacter*-like organism; cod liver oil

Cl$_O$ oral clearance

clo clothing [thermal insulation unit]

CLOB character large object
CLOF clofibrate
CLON clonidine
Clon *Clonorchis*
Clostr *Clostridium*
CLOT Clinical Perspectives on Lysis of Thrombi [study]
CLOUT Clinical Outcomes with Ultrasound Trial; Core Laboratory Ultrasound Analysis Study
CLP cardiac laboratory panel; cecal ligation and puncture; chymotrypsin-like protein; cleft lip with cleft palate; common lymphocyte progenitor; constraining logic programming; paced cycle length
CL/P cleft lip with or without cleft palate
CL(P) cleft lip without cleft palate
ClP clinical pathology
Cl$_R$ renal clearance
CLRA Children's Leukemia Research Association
CLRT continuous lateral rotational therapy
CLRV *Cimex lectularius* reovirus
CLS café-au-lait spot; classical least square; Clinical Laboratory Scientist; Coffin-Lowry syndrome; Cornelia de Lange syndrome
CLSC Centres Locaux de Services Communitaires
CLSE calf lung surfactant extract
CLSF current localization by spatial filtering
CLSH corpus luteum—stimulating hormone
CLSI Clinical and Laboratory Standards Institute
CLSL chronic lymphosarcoma (cell) leukemia
CLSM confocal laser scanning microscope
CLT Certified Laboratory Technician; chronic lymphocytic thyroiditis; Clinical Laboratory Technician; clot lysis time; clotting time; lung-thorax compliance
CL$_{TB}$ total body clearance
CLT(NCA) Certified Laboratory Technician (National Certification Agency for Medical Laboratory Personnel)
CLU clusterin
CLV *Colletotrichum lindemuthianum* virus; common latent virus; constant linear velocity
CLVI complex lower limb vascular injury
CL VOID clean voided specimen
CLZ clozapine
CM California mastitis [test]; calmodulin; capreomycin; carboxymethyl; cardiac monitoring; cardiac murmur; cardiac muscle; cardiomyopathy; carpometacarpal; Caroll/Mackie [radiotherapy]; castrated male; Caucasian male; cause of death [L. *causa mortis*]; cavernous malformation; cell membrane; center of mass; central mentum;

cerebral malaria; cerebral mantle; Certified Midwife; cervical mucosa/mucus; Chick-Martin [coefficient]; chloroquine-mepacrine; chondromalacia; chopped meat [medium]; chronic meningitis; chylomicron; circular muscle; circulating monocyte; circumferential measurement; classification maximization; clindamycin; clinical medicine; clinical modification; coccidioidal meningitis; cochlear microphonic; combined modality; common migraine; complete medium; complications; condition median; conditioned medium; congenital malformation; congestive myocardiopathy; continuous murmur; contrast material; contrast medium; copulatory mechanism; costal margin; cow's milk; cutaneous mastocytosis; cytometry; cytoplasmic membrane; Master of Surgery [L. *Chirurgiae Magister*]; narrow-diameter endosseous screw implant [Fr. *crête manche*]
C-M cardiomyopathy
C/M counts per minute
C&M cocaine and morphine
C$_M$ metabolite clearance
Cm curium; minimal concentration
C$_m$ maximum clearance; membrane capacitance
cM centimorgan
cm centimeter
Cμ mu light chain constant region
cm^2 square centimeter
cm^3 cubic centimeter
CMA Canadian Medical Association; Certified Medical Assistant; chronic metabolic acidosis; cingulate motor area; cow's milk allergy; cultured macrophages
CMAC cerebellar model articulation controller
CMAI Cohen-Mansfield Agitation Inventory
CMAP compound motor/muscle action potential
CMAR cell matrix adhesion regulator
Cmax, C$_{max}$ maximum concentration; peak lidocaine concentration
CMB carbolic methylene blue; Central Midwives' Board; chloromercuribenzoate
CMBC concentration of moving blood cells
CMBES Canadian Medical and Biological Engineering Society
CMC carboxymethylcellulose; care management continuity; carpometacarpal; cell-mediated cytolysis or cytotoxicity; chemical mismatch cleavage; chloramphenicol; chronic mucocutaneous candidiasis; Comprehensive Medicinal Chemistry [database]; critical micellar concentration
cmc critical micelle concentration

CMCC chronic mucocutaneous candidiasis

CMCJ carpometacarpal joint

CMCN Certified Managed Care Nurse

CMCS computer-mediated communication system

CMCT carbodiimide metho-*p*-toluene sulfonate; central motor conduction time

CMCt care management continuity across settings

CMD camptomelic dwarfism; camptomelic dysplasia; cartilage matrix deficiency; cerebromacular degeneration; Certified Medical Densitometrist; chief medical director; childhood muscular dystrophy; common mental disorder; comparative mean dose; congenital muscular dystrophy; corticomedullary differentiation; count median diameter; craniomandibular disorder

CMDD choline and methionine deficient diet

cmDNA cytoplasmic membrane-associated deoxyribonucleic acid

CMDS computer misuse detection system

CMDSC Certified Minimum Data Set Coordinator

CME cervical mediastinal exploration; continuing medical education; Council on Medical Education; crude marijuana extract; cystoid macular edema

CMED central medical emergency dispatch center

CMF calcium-magnesium free; catabolite modular factor; chloromethylfluorescein; chondromyxoid fibroma; Christian Medical Fellowship; cold mitten friction; colonic myofibroblast; cortical magnification factor; craniomandibulofacial; cyclophosphamide, methotrexate, and fluorouracil

CMFDA chloromethylfluorescein diacetate

CMFT cardiolipin microflocculation test

CMFV cyclophosphamide, methotrexate, fluorouracil, and vincristine

CMFVP cyclophosphamide, methotrexate, fluorouracil, vincristine, prednisone

CMG canine myasthenia gravis; congenital myasthenia gravis; case-mix group; chopped meat glucose [medium]; cystometrogram, cystometrography

CMGN chronic membranous glomerulonephritis

CMGS chopped meat–glucose-starch [medium]; Clinical Molecular Genetics Society

CMGT chromosome-mediated gene transfer

CMH cardiomyopathy, hypertrophic; community mental health; congenital malformation of the heart

CMHC community mental health center

C/MHC community migrant health center

CMHIS Community Mental Health Information System

cmH₂O centimeters of water

CMHS center for mental health services; Continuous Medicare History Sample

CMHT community mental health team

CMI carbohydrate metabolism index; care management integration; case-mix index; cell-mediated immunity; cell multiplication inhibition; chronic mesenteric ischemia; circulating microemboli index; colonic motility index; combat medical informatics; combined myocardial infarction; Commonwealth Mycological Institute; computed maxillofacial imaging; computer-managed instruction; Cornell Medical Index

CMID cytomegalic inclusion disease

c/min cycles per minute

CMINET Chinese Medical Information Network

CMIO chief medical information officer

CMIR cell-mediated immune response

CMIS common management information services

CMISP common management information standards/protocol

CMIT Current Medical Information and Terminology

CMJ carpometacarpal joint

CMK chloromethyl ketone; congenital multicystic kidney

CML carboxymethyl lysine; cell-mediated lymphocytotoxicity; cell-mediated lympholysis; central motor latency; chronic myelocytic leukemia; chronic myelogenous leukemia; chronic myeloid leukemia; clinical medical librarian; clinical medical library

c/mL copies per milliliter

CMLNP comprehensive multilevel nursing practice [model]

CMLV camelpox virus

CMM cell-mediated mutagenesis; color Doppler M-mode; Columbia Mental Maturity [scale]; coordinate measuring machine [orthopedic surgery]; cross-modality matching; cutaneous malignant melanoma

cmm cubic millimeter

CMMC cervical myelomeningocele

CMME chloromethyl methyl ether

CMML chronic myelomonocytic leukemia

CMMoL chronic myelomonocytic leukemia

CMMS Columbia Mental Maturity Scale

CMN canine minute virus; caudal mediastinal node; certification of medical necessity; cystic medial necrosis

CMNA complement-mediated neutrophil activation

CMN-AA cystic medial necrosis of ascending aorta

CMO cardiac minute output; chief medical officer; comfort measures only; competitive medical organization; corticosterone methyloxidase

CMO₂ cerebral metabolic oxygen rate

cMO centimorgan

cMOAT canalicular multispecific organic anion transporter

CMOL chronic monocytic leukemia

CMOS compatible monolithic conductivity sensor; complementary metal-oxide semiconductor

CMP cardiomyopathy; cartilage matrix protein; chemical measurement process; chondromalacia patellae; cochlear microphonic potential; competitive medical plan; comprehensive medical plan; cytidine monophosphate

CMPD chronic myeloproliferative disorder

cmpd compound, compounded

CMPGN chronic membranoproliferative glomerulonephritis

cmps centimeters per second

CMR cardiomodulorespirography; cerebral metabolic rate; chief medical resident; child mortality rate; chloroform-methanol residue [vaccine]; chylomicron remnant; common medical record; common mode rejection; computerized medical record; congenital mitral regurgitation; cross-reacting material; crude mortality ratio

CMRG cerebral metabolic rate of glucose

CMRGlc combined metabolic rate of glucose

CMR_Glu, CMRglu cerebral metabolic rate of glucose

CMRI cardiac magnetic resonance imaging

CMRL cerebral metabolic rate of lactate

CMRNG chromosomal control of mechanisms of resistance of *Neisseria gonorrhoeae*

CMRO, CMRO₂ cerebral metabolic rate of oxygen consumption

CMRP cervical magnetic resonance phlebography

CMRR common mode rejection ratio

CMS Centers for Medicare and Medicaid Services; children's medical services; chromosome modification site; chronic myelodysplastic syndrome; circulation, motion, sensation; clinical management system; clofibrate-induced muscular syndrome; Clyde Mood Scale; complement-mediated solubility; content management system; Copenhagen Male Study; cortical magnetic stimulation

cm/s centimeters per second

CMSC computer science

CMSD congenital myocardial sympathetic dysinnervation

cm/sec centimeters per second

CMSRN Certified Medical-Surgical Registered Nurse

CMSS circulation, motor ability, sensation, and swelling; Council of Medical Specialty Societies

CMT California mastitis test; cancer multistep therapy; catechol methyltransferase; certified medical transcriptionist; cervical motion tenderness; Charcot-Marie-Tooth [syndrome]; chemotherapy; circus movement tachycardia; combined modality therapy; complex motor tic; continuous memory test; controlled medical terminology; convergent medical terminology; current medical terminology

CMT1 Charcot-Marie-Tooth [disease or neuropathy] type 1

CMTC cadmium manganese thiocyanate; cutis marmorata telangiectatica congenita; cytoplasmic microtubule complex

CMTD Charcot-Marie-Tooth disease; chronic multiple tic disorder

CMTIA Charcot-Marie-Tooth [disease, neuropathy] type 1A

CMTIB Charcot-Marie-Tooth [disease, neuropathy] type 1B

CMTL computer-mediated tutorial laboratory

CMTS Charcot-Marie-Tooth syndrome

CMTX Charcot-Marie-Tooth [syndrome], X-linked

CMU chlorophenyldimethylurea

CMUA continuous motor unit activity

CMV canine minute virus [veterinary medicine]; continuous mandatory ventilation; controlled mechanical ventilation; controlled medical vocabulary; conventional mechanical ventilation; cool mist vaporizer; cytomegalovirus

CMV-E cytomegalovirus encephalitis

CMV-MN cytomegalovirus mononucleosis

CMV-VE cytomegalovirus ventriculoencephalitis

CMX cefmenoxime

CMYK cyan magenta yellow black

CN caudate nucleus; cellulose nitrate; charge nurse; child nutrition; chloroacetophenone; clinical nursing; cochlear nucleus; condensation nucleus; congenital nystagmus; cranial nerve; Crigler-Najjar [syndrome]; cyanogen; cyanosis neonatorum

C-N circumference of the chest at the nipple

C:N calorie/nitrogen ratio

C/N carbon/nitrogen ratio; carrier/noise ratio; contrast/noise ratio

CN⁻ cyanide anion
CN I first cranial nerve [olfactory]
CN II second cranial nerve [optic]
CN III third cranial nerve [oculomotor]
CN IV fourth cranial nerve [trochlear]
CN V fifth cranial nerve [trigeminal]
CN VI sixth cranial nerve [abducens]
CN VII seventh cranial nerve [facial]
CN VIII eighth cranial nerve [vestibulo-cochlear]
CN IX ninth cranial nerve [glossopharyngeal]
CN X tenth cranial nerve [vagus]
CN XI eleventh cranial nerve [accessory]
CN XII twelfth cranial nerve [hypoglossal]
Cn Copernicium
CNA calcium nutrient agar; Canadian Nurses Association; Certified in Nursing Adminstration; Certified Nursing Assistant
CNAF chronic nonvalvular atrial fibrillation
CNAG chronic narrow-angle glaucoma
CNAP career nurse assistants' programs; compound nerve action potential
CNAV Cananeia virus
CNB cutting needle biopsy
CNBP cellular nucleic acid binding protein
CNC community nursing center
CNCbl cyanocobalamin
CNCC Certified Nurse in Critical Care
CNCD chronic noncommunicable disease
CND care need determination
CNDC chronic nonspecific diarrhea of childhood; chronic nonsuppurative destructive cholangitis
CNDI congenital nephrogenic diabetes insipidus
CNE Certified Nurse Educator; chief nurse executive; chronic nervous exhaustion; concentric needle electrode
C3NeF C3 nephritic factor
CNEMG concentric needle electrode electromyography
CNES chronic nervous exhaustion syndrome
C_NET net compliance
CNF chronic nodular fibrositis; congenital nephrotic syndrome of the Finnish; conjunctive normal form system; cytotoxic necrotizing factor
CNGC cyclic nucleotide gated channel
CNH central neurogenic hyperpnea; community nursing home
CNHD congenital nonspherocytic hemolytic disease
CNI center of nuclear image; chronic nerve irritation; clinical nursing intern; community nutrition institute

CNIDR Clearinghouse for Networked Information Discovery and Retrieval
CNIS clinical nursing information system; computerized nursing information system
CNK cortical necrosis of kidney
CNL cardiolipin natural lecithin; chronic neutrophilic leukemia
CNLCP Certified Nurse Life Care Planner
CNLS complex nonlinear least square
CNM centronuclear myopathy; Certified Nurse-Midwife; combinatorial neural model; computerized nuclear morphometry
CNMDSA community nursing minimum data set, Australia
CNMetHb cyanmethemoglobin
CNMT Certified Nuclear Medicine Technologist
CNN Canadian National Network; Canadian Neonatal Network; Certified in Nephrology Nursing; computational neural network
CNNP Certified Neonatal Nurse Practitioner
CNO chief nursing officer; community nursing organization
CNOR Certified Nurse, Operating Room
cNOS constitutive nitric oxide synthase
CNP Certified Nurse Practitioner; community nurse practitioner; continuous negative pressure; cranial nerve palsy; C-type natriuretic peptide; $2',3'$-cyclic nucleotide $3'$-phosphodiesterase
CNPase $2',3'$-cyclic nucleotide $3'$-phosphohydrolase
CNPB continuous negative pressure breathing
CNPV canarypox virus; continuous negative pressure ventilation
CNQX 6-cyano-7-nitroquinoxaline-2,3-dione
CNR cadherin-related neuronal receptor; cannabinoid receptor; Center for Nursing Research; contrast/noise ratio; Council of Nurse Researchers
C(N,r) combination of N things taken r at a time
CNRC Children's Nutrition Research Center
CNRN Certified Neuroscience Registered Nurse
CNRT corrected sinus node recovery time
CNS central nervous system; clinical nurse specialist; coagulase-negative staphylococci; congenital nephrotic syndrome; cutaneous nerve stimulator; sulfocyanate
CNSHA congenital nonspherocytic hemolytic anemia
CNS-L central nervous system leukemia
CNSLD chronic nonspecific lung disease
CNSN Certified Nutrition Support Nurse

CNST coagulase-negative staphylococci

C$_{Ns}$[t] nonspecific tracer concentration

CNT *Clostridium* neurotoxin; could not test

CNTF ciliary neutrophilic factor

CNTFR ciliary neutrophilic factor receptor

CNTHM conotruncal heart malformation

CNTV Connecticut virus

CNUV Chenuda virus

CNV choroidal neovascularization; contingent negative variation; cutaneous necrotizing vasculitis

CO carbon monoxide; cardiac output; castor oil; casualty officer; centric occlusion; cervical orthosis; cervicoaxial; childhood onset; choline oxidase; coccygeal; coenzyme; compound; control; corneal opacity; cross over; cyclophosphamide and vincristine

C/O, c/o check out; complaining of; complains of; complaints of; in care of

Co cobalt

CO$_2$ carbon dioxide

Co I coenzyme I

Co II coenzyme II

COA Canadian Ophthalmological Association; Canadian Orthopaedic Association; certificate of authority; cervico-oculo-acusticus [syndrome]; coarctation of the aorta; condition on admission

CoA coenzyme A

COACH Canadian Organization for the Advancement of Computers in Health; cerebellar vermis hypoplasia/aplasia, oligophrenia, congenital ataxia, ocular colobomata, hepatic fibrosis [syndrome]

COAD chronic obstructive airway disease; clinician-oriented access to data

COAG chronic open-angle glaucoma

coag coagulated, coagulation

COAL chronic obstructive airflow limitation

COAP cyclophosphamide, cytosine arabinose, vincristine, prednisone

coarct coarctation

COAS clinical observations access service

CoASH uncombined coenzyme A

CoA-SPC coenzyme A—synthesizing protein complex

COAT Children's Orientation and Amnesia Test; Cooperative Osaka Adenosine Trial

COB chronic obstructive bronchitis; coordination of benefits

COBALT Continuous Infusion vs. Bolus Alteplase Trial; Continuous Infusion vs. Double-Bolus Administration of Alteplase

coban cohesive bandage

COBOL common business-oriented language

COBRA Comparison of Balloon-Angioplasty versus Rotational Atherectomy [Study]; computer-operated birth defect recognition aid; Consolidated Omnibus Budget Reconciliation Act

COBS cesarean-obtained barrier-sustained; chronic organic brain syndrome

COBT chronic obstruction of the biliary tract

COC cathodal opening contraction; coccygeal; combination oral contraceptive; commission on cancer; cumulus-oocyte complex

COCI Consortium on Chemical Information

COCl cathodal opening clonus

COCM congestive cardiomyopathy

COCN Certified Ostomy Care Nurse

COCP combined oral contraceptive pill

Co-Cr-Mo cobalt-chromium-molybdenum [alloy]

COCS Cornell-Oxford China Study

COCV cocal virus

COD cause of death; cerebro-ocular dysplasia; chemical oxygen demand; codeine; collaborative organization design; computer-assisted optical densitometry; condition on discharge

cod codeine

CODAS cerebro-oculo-dento-auriculo-skeletal [syndrome]; chronotherapeutic oral drug absorption system

CODATA Committee on Data for Science and Technology

CODEC coder/decoder [device]; compression and decompression

COD-MD cerebroocular dysplasia-muscular dystrophy [syndrome]

CODS Charnes Organizational Diagnosis Survey

coeff coefficient

COEPS cortical originating extrapyramidal system

COER controlled onset, extended release

COF cutoff frequency

CoF cobra factor; cofactor

C of A coarctation of the aorta

COFS cerebro-oculo-facial-skeletal [syndrome]; certificate of free sale

COG center of gravity; Children's Oncology Group; cluster of orthologous groups; cognitive function tests

Cog cognition; cognitive

CoGME Council on Graduate Medical Education

COGTT cortisone oral glucose tolerance test

COH carbohydrate; controlled ovarian hyperstimulation

COHb, CoHb carboxyhemoglobin

CoHgb carboxyhemoglobin

COH-IUI controlled ovarian hyperstimulation before intrauterine insemination

COHN Certified Occupational Health Nurse

COHR computer-based oral health record

COHSE Confederation of Health Service Employees

CoHV Columbid herpesvirus

COI central obesity index; certificate of insurance; conflict of interest; cost of illness

COIF congenital onychodysplasia of the index finger

COIN conformal index

CoIP coimmunoprecipitation

COL central object library; colposcopy

col colicin; collection; collagen; colony; colored; column; strain [L. *cola*]

COLA Commission on Office Laboratory Accreditation

COLD chronic obstructive lung disease

COLD A cold agglutinin titer

COLING computational linguistics

coll collateral; collection, collective; college; colloidal

collat collateral

COLTS Coronary Observational Long-Term Study

CoLV Cole latent virus

COM chronic otitis media; College of Osteopathic Medicine; component object model; computer-output microfilm

com comminuted; commitment

COMA Committee on Medical Aspects

COMAC/HRS/QA Community Concerted Action Programme on Quality Assurance in Health Care

comb combination, combine

COMBIMAN Computerized Biomechanical Man-Model

COMBINE Combined Pharmacotherapies and Behavioral Interventions [study]

COMC carboxymethylcellulose

COME chronic otitis media with effusion

COMET Carvedilol or Metoprolol European Trial; Carvedilol or Metoprolol Evaluation Trial

CoMET concept modeling environment for teachers

comf comfortable

CoMFA comparative molecular field analysis

COMLEX Comprehensive Osteopathic Medical Licensing Examination

comm, commun communicable

CoMMA comparative molecular moment analysis

COMMIT Community Intervention Trial for Smoking Cessation; Comprehensive Multidisciplinary Interventional Trial for Regression of Coronary Heart Disease

COMP cartilage oligomeric matrix protein; cells outside the main population; complication; cyclophosphamide, vincristine, methotrexate, prednisone

comp comparative; compensated, compensation; complaint; complete; composition; compound, compounded; comprehension; compress; computer

COMPACCS Committee on Manpower of Pulmonary and Critical Care Societies

COMPACT computer-optimized parametric analysis for chemical toxicity

COMPASS Comparative Trial of Saruplase vs. Streptokinase; Computerized Online Medicaid Pharmaceutical Analysis and Surveillance System

compd compound, compounded

compl complaint; complete, completed, completion; complicated, complication

complic complicated, complication

compn composition

compr compression

comp stud comparative study

COMS cerebro-oculo-muscular syndrome

CoMSIA comparative molecular similarity index analysis

COMT catecholamine-*O*-methyl transferase; certified ophthalmic medical technologist

COMTRAC computer-based case tracing

COMUL complement-fixation murine leukosis [test]

CON certificate of need; cortisone

Con concanavalin

con against [L. *contra*]; continuation, continue

CON A, Con A concanavalin A

Con A–HRP concanavalin A–horseradish peroxidase

CONC conceptual entity

conc, concentr concentrate, concentrated, concentration

c-onc cellular oncogene

COND cerebro-osteo-nephrodysplasia

cond condensation, condensed; condition, conditioned; conductivity; conductor

conf conference; confined; confinement; confusion

CONFIRM Coronary Computed Tomography Angiography Evaluation for Clinical Outcomes: An International Multicenter Registry

cong congested, congestion; gallon [L. *congius*]

congen congenital

CongHD congenital heart disease

coniz conization

conj conjunctiva, conjunctival

conjug conjugated, conjugation
CONPA-DRI I vincristine, doxorubicin, and melphalan
CONPA-DRI III CONPA-DRI I plus intensified doxorubicin
CONQUEST Computerized Needs-Oriented Quality Measurement Evaluation System
CONS coagulase-negative *Staphylococcus*; consultant, consultation
cons conservation; conservative; consultation
CONSENSUS Cooperative North Scandinavian Enalapril Survival Study
CONSORT Consolidated Standards of Reporting Trials
const constant
constit constituent
consult consultant, consultation
CONSUME Compliance of National Supplements Using Multiform Energy Sources [study]
cont against [L. *contra*]; bruised [L. *contusus*]; contains, contents; continuation, continue
contag contagion, contagious
contr contracted, contraction
contra contraindicated
contralat contralateral
contrib contributory
conv convalescence, convalescent, convalescing; convergence, convergent; convulsions, convulsive
converg convergence, convergent
CONVINCE Controlled Onset Verapamil Investigation for Cardiovascular Endpoints [study]; Controlled Onset Verapamil Investigation of Clinical Endpoints [study]
COO chief operating officer; cost of ownership [analysis]
COOD chronic obstructive outflow disease
COOH carboxy group; carboxy terminus
COOP charts for primary care practices; cooperative
coord coordinated, coordination
COP capillary osmotic pressure; change of plaster; coefficient of performance; colloid oncotic pressure; colloid osmotic pressure; competitive oligonucleotide priming; cryptogenic organizing pneumonitis; cyclophosphamide, Oncovin, and prednisone
COPA Council on Postsecondary Accreditation
COPAD cyclophosphamide, vincristine, Adriamycin, prednisone, cytarabine, asparagine, intrathecal methotrexate
COPC community-oriented primary care
COPD chronic obstructive pulmonary disease
COPE chronic obstructive pulmonary emphysema

COPEM Committee on Pediatric Emergency Medicine
COPERNICUS Carvedilol Prospective Randomized Cumulative Survival [trial]
COP$_i$ colloid osmotic pressure in interstitial fluid
CO/PLL/CG crystal oscillator/phase-lock loop/clock generator
COPMED Council for Postgraduate Medical Deans
COPP cyclophosphamide, Oncovin, procarbazine, prednisone
COP$_p$ colloid osmotic pressure in plasma
COPRO coproporphyrin; coproporphyrinogen
COPS constrained optimal parameter search
COPT circumoval precipitin reaction test; computerized oxygen therapy protocol
COPV canine oral papillomavirus
CoQ coenzyme Q
COR cardiac output recorder; center of rotation; comprehensive outpatient rehabilitation; conditional origin of replication; conditioned orientation reflex; consensual ophthalmotonic reaction; conventional open resection; corrosion, corrosive; cortex; cortisone; crude odds ratio; custodian of records
CoR Congo red
cor body [L. *corpus*]; coronary; corrected, correction
CORA conditioned orientation reflex audiometry
CORALI coronarography and alimentation
CORAMI Cohort of Rescue Angioplasty in Myocardial Infarction
CORD Commissioned Officer Residency Deferment; Council of Emergency Medicine Residency Directors
CORDIS Cardiovascular Occupational Risk Factor Determination in Israel [study]
CORE Center for Organ Recovery and Education; Collaborative Organization for RheothRx Evaluation; comprehensive assessment and referral evaluation; concept reference
CORGENE Coronary Disease and Angiotensin Converting Enzyme I/D Genotype [study]
CORIS Coronary Risk Factor Study
CORLN Certified Otorhinolaryngology Nurse
CorPP coronary perfusion pressure
corr correspondence, corresponding
CORRECT Complete vs. Restrictive Revascularization by Coronary Angioplasty Trial
CORSICA Chronic Occlusion Revascularization with Stent Implantation vs. Coronary Angioplasty [study]
CORT corticosterone
cort bark [L. *cortex*]; cortex

CORTES Clivarin Assessment of Regression of Thrombus: Efficacy and Safety [study]; coordinate reduction time encoding system

CORV Corriparta virus

COS carbon oxysulfide; cheiro-oral syndrome; chief of staff; clinically observed seizures; Clinical Orthopaedic Society

CoS class of service

CoSA comparative spectral analysis

COSATI Committee on Scientific and Technical Information

COSHH Control of Substances Hazardous to Health Regulations

COSMIS Computer System for Medical Information Systems

COSSMHO [National] Coalition of Hispanic Health and Human Services Organizations

COST cardiac output study technology; clinical outcomes of surgical therapy

COSTAR computer-stored ambulatory record

COSTART Coding Symbols for a Thesaurus of Adverse Reaction Terms; Common Standard Thesaurus of Adverse Reaction Terms

COSTED Committee on Science and Technology in Developing Countries

COSTEP Commissioned Officer Student Training and Extern Program

COSY correlated spectroscopy

COT colony overlay test; committee on trauma; content of thought; contralateral optic tectum; critical off-time

COTA Certified Occupational Therapy Assistant; colon-ovary tumor antigen

COTAIM Continuation of Trial Antihypertensive Interventions and Management

COTD cardiac output by thermodilution

COTe cathodal opening tetanus

COTH Council of Teaching Hospitals and Health Systems

COTRANS Coordinated Transfer Application System

COTS commercial off the shelf [product]

COU cardiac observation unit

coul coulomb

COURAGE Clinical Outcomes Using Revascularization vs. Aggressive Strategies; Clinical Outcomes Utilization Revascularization and Aggressive Drug Evaluation

COURT Contrast Media Utilization in High-Risk Percutaneous Transluminal Coronary Angioplasty [trial]

C$_{out}$ outgoing concentration [of blood]

COV covariance; cross-over value

CoV coronavirus

COVER Cover of Vaccination Evaluated Rapidly

COVESDEM costovertebral segmentation defect with mesomelia [syndrome]

CoVF cobra venom factor

COVID coronavirus disease

COVID-19 coronavirus disease 2019 caused by SARS-CoV-2

COVRA Computer Vision in Radiology

COW curse of womanhood (menstruation)

COWS cold to opposite and warm to same side

COX cyclooxygenase; cytochrome oxidase

COYV colony virus

4-CP chlorophenoxyacetic acid

CP candle power; capillary pressure; capsid protein; cardiac pacing; cardiac performance; cardiopulmonary; caudate putamen; cell passage; center of pressure; central pit; cephalic presentation; cerebellopontine; cerebral palsy; ceruloplasmin; cervical position; chemical protection; chemically pure; chest pain; child psychiatry; child psychology; *Chlamydia pneumoniae*; chloropurine; chloroquine-primaquine; chondrodysplasia punctata; choroid plexus; chronic pain; chronic pancreatitis; chronic polyarthritis; chronic prostatitis; chronic pyelonephritis; cicatricial pemphigoid; cleft palate; clinical pathology; clock pulse; closing pressure; coat protein; cochlear potential; code of practice; cold pressor; color perception; combining power; compound; compressed; congenital por-phyria; constant predictor; constant pressure; constrictive pericarditis; coproporphyrin; cor pulmonale; coracoid process; cosine packet; counter propagation [algorithm]; coverage probability [radiotherapy]; C peptide; creatine phosphate; creatine phosphokinase; critical pressure; cross-linked protein; crude protein; current practice; cyclophosphamide; cyclophosphamide and prednisone; cytosol protein

C&P compensation and pension; complete and pain free; cystoscopy and pyelography

C/P cholesterol/phospholipid ratio

C+P cryotherapy with pressure

Cp ceruloplasmin; chickenpox; *Corynebacterium parvum*; peak concentration

C$_p$ concentration in plasma; constant pressure; phosphate clearance

cP centipoise

cp candle power; centipoise; chemically pure; circular plasmid; compare

c$_p$ constant pressure

CPA Canadian Physiotherapy Association; Canadian Psychiatric Association; carboxypeptidase A; cardiophrenic angle; cardiopulmonary arrest; carotid phonoangiography;

cerebellopontine angle; child physical abuse; chlorophenoxyacetic acid; chlorophenylalanine; chronic pyrophosphate arthropathy; circulating platelet aggregate; complement proactivator; control, preoccupation, and addiction; cost per action; costophrenic angle; cyclophosphamide; cyclopiazonic acid; cyproterone acetate

C3PA complement-3 proactivator

C$_{pa}$ cardiac peak amplitude

CPAD chronic peripheral arterial disease

CPAF chlorpropamide-alcohol flushing

C$_{pah}$ para-aminohippurate clearance

CPAM congenital pulmonary airway malformation

CPAN Certified Post Anesthesia Nurse

CP-ANN counterpropagation artificial neural network

CPAP continuous positive airway pressure

CPAS Canadian Prinivil Atenolol Study

CPB carboxypeptidase B; cardiopulmonary bypass; cetylpyridinium bromide; competitive protein binding; controlled position brace

CPBA competitive protein-binding analysis

CPBV cardiopulmonary blood volume

CPC central posterior curve; cerebellar Purkinje cell; cerebral palsy clinic; cerebral performance category; cetylpyridinium chloride; chemical protective clothing; chest pain center; child protection center; Child-Pugh class; chronic passive congestion; circumferential pneumatic compression; clinical-pathologic correlation; clinicopathologic conference; cost per click

CPCI Chronic Pain Coping Inventory

CPCL congenital pulmonary cystic lymphangiectasia

CPCP chronic progressive coccidioidal pneumonitis

CPCR cardiopulmonary cerebral resuscitation; Center for Primary Care Research

CPCRA Community Programs for Clinical Research on AIDS

CPCS circumferential pneumatic compression suit; computer-based patient case simulation system

CPCV Cacipacore virus

CPD calcium pyrophosphate deposition; cephalopelvic disproportion; cerebelloparenchymal disorder; childhood or congenital polycystic disease; chorioretinopathy and pituitary dysfunction; chronic peritoneal dialysis; chronic protein deprivation; citrate-phosphate-dextrose; contact potential difference; contagious pustular dermatitis; critical point drying; cyclobutane pyrimidine dimer; cyclopentadiene

cpd cigarettes per day; compound; cycles per degree

CPDA citrate-phosphate-dextrose-adenine

CPDD calcium pyrophosphate deposition disease; *cis*-platinum-diamine dichloride; College on Problems of Drug Dependence

cpd E compound E

CP DEPMEDS chemically protected deployable medical system

cpd F compound F

CPDL cumulative population doubling level

CPDN Certified Peritoneal Dialysis Nurse

CPDX cefpodoxime

CPDX-PR cefpodoxime proxetil

CPE capillary parenchymal element; carbon paste electrode; cardiac pulmonary edema; chronic pulmonary emphysema; clinical progress exercise; *Clostridium perfringens* enterotoxin; collective protection equipment; compensation, pension, and education; complete physical examination; complicated pleural effusion; corona-penetrating enzyme; cryopreserved embryo transfer; cryptogenic partial epilepsy; cytopathogenic effect

CPEO chronic progressive external ophthalmoplegia

CPEP Chicago Coronary Prevention Evaluation Program; clinical practice enhancement project

CPE-R *Clostridium perfringens* enterotoxin receptor

CPEV *Chironomus plumosus* entomopoxvirus

CPF center point of force; clot-promoting factor; complication probability factor; contraction peak force; current patient file

C$_{pf}$ cardiac peak frequency

CPFC chemically protective footgear cover

CPG capillary blood gases; cardiopneumographic recording; carotid phonoangiogram; central pattern generator; clinical practice guidelines; computerized pattern generator

CPGN chronic proliferative glomerulonephritis

CPGs clinical practice guidelines

CPH Certificate in Public Health; chronic paroxysmal hemicrania; chronic persistent hepatitis; chronic primary headache

CPHA Canadian Public Health Association; Commission on Professional and Hospital Activities

CPHA-PAS Commission on Professional and Hospital Activities—Professional Activity Study

CPHL Central Public Health Laboratory

CPHLN Canadian Public Health Laboratory Network

CPHQ certified professional in health care quality

CPHRP Coronary Prevention and Hypertension Research Project

CPHS Centre for Public Health Sciences

CPHSS Center for Public Health Systems Science

CPhT Certified Pharmacy Technician

CpHV caprine herpesvirus

CPI California Personality Inventory; Cancer Potential Index; common patient index; congenital palatopharyngeal incompetence; constitutional psychopathic inferiority; conventional planar imaging; coronary prognosis index; cysteine proteinase inhibitor

CPIB chlorophenoxyisobutyrate

CPIJH compass proximal interphalangeal joint hinge

CPIP chronic pulmonary insufficiency of prematurity

CPIR cephalic-phase insulin release

CPK cell population kinetic [model]; creatine phosphokinase

cPK cytosolic protamine kinase

CPK-BB creatine phosphokinase, brain type

cPKC classical protein kinase C

CPKD childhood polycystic kidney disease

CPL caprine placental lactogen; conditioned pitch level; congenital pulmonary lymphangiectasia; cost per lead

C/PL cholesterol/phospholipid ratio

cpl complete, completed

CPLM cysteine-peptone-liver infusion medium

CPLS cleft palate—lateral synechia syndrome

CPM calorie-protein malnutrition; central pontine myelinosis; Certified Professional Midwife; chlorpheniramine maleate; confidence profile method; confined placental mosaicism; continuous passive motion; cost per 1000 impressions; critical path method; cyclophosphamide

C$_{PM}$ circumference of papillary muscle

cpm counts per minute; cycles per minute

CP-MCT chirp pulse microwave computed tomography

CPMG Carr-Purcell-Meiboom-Gill [sequence]

CPMP Committee for Proprietary Medicinal Products; complete patient management problems

CPMS chronic progressive multiple sclerosis

CPN causal probabilistic network; celiac plexus neurolysis; central parenteral nutrition; Certified Pediatric Nurse; chronic polyneuropathy; chronic pyelonephritis; community pediatric nurse; community psychiatric nurse

CPNA Certified Pediatric Nurse Associate

CPNE clinical performance nursing examination

CPNL Certified Practical Nurse, Long-Term Care

CPNM corrected perinatal mortality

CPNP Certified Pediatric Nurse Practitioner

CPO cleft palate only; contract provider organization; coproporphyrinogen oxidase

CPOE computerized physician order entry; computerized provider order entry

CPOG chemically protective overgarment

CPON Certified Pediatric Oncology Nurse

CPOPR computerized problem-oriented patient record

C-PORT Cardiovascular Patient Outcomes Research Team [trial]

CPOS chest pain order sheet

CPOTHA chest pain onset to hospital arrival

CPOU chest pain observation unit

CPP cancer proneness phenotype; canine pancreatic polypeptide; cerebral perfusion pressure; chest pain policy; $(\pm)$-2[3-(2′-chlorophenoxy)phenyl] propionic [acid]; chronic pelvic pain; chronic pigmented purpura; coronary perfusion pressure; cyclopentenophenanthrene

CPPB continuous positive-pressure breathing

CPPD calcium pyrophosphate dihydrate deposition [syndrome]; chest percussion and post drainage; cisplatin; cost per patient day

CPPT Coronary Primary Prevention Trial

CPPV continuous positive pressure ventilation

CPQA certified professional in quality assurance

CPR cardiopulmonary reserve; cardiopulmonary resuscitation; centripetal rub; cerebral cortex perfusion rate; chlorophenyl red; computerized patient record; cortisol production rate; cumulative patency rate; customary, prevailing, and reasonable

c-PR cyclopropyl

cpr computerized patient record

CPRAM controlled partial-rebreathing anesthesia method

CPRCA constitutional pure red cell aplasia

CPRD Committee on Prosthetics Research and Development

CPRG Coronary Prevention Research Group

CPRI Computerized Patient Record Institute

CPRO coproporphyrinogen oxidase

CPRP chemical personnel reliability program

CPRS Children's Psychiatric Rating Scale; Comprehensive Psychopathological Rating Scale; computerized patient record system

CPS Caerphilly Prospective Study; Cancer Prevention Study; carbamoylphosphate synthetase; cardioplegic perfusion solution; cardiopulmonary support; center for preventive services; centipoise; cervical pain syndrome; characters per second; chest pain syndrome; Child Personality Scale; Child Protective Services; chloroquine, pyrimethamine, and sulfisoxazole; chronic prostatitis syndrome; classroom performance system; clinical performance score; Clinical Pharmacy Services; coagulase-positive *Staphylococcus*; complex partial seizures; concurrent planning system; constitutional psychopathic state; contagious pustular stomatitis; coronary perfusate solution; C-polysaccharide; cumulative probability of success; current population survey

cps counts per second; cycles per second

CPSA charged particle surface area

CPSC congenital paucity of secondary synaptic clefts [syndrome]; Consumer Product Safety Commission

CPSD carbamyl phosphate synthetase deficiency

CPSE complex partial status epilepticus

CPSF cleavage and polyadenylation specificity factor

CPSM Council for Professions Supplementary to Medicine

CPSMP chronic pain self-management program

CPSN Certified Plastic Surgical Nurse

CPSO College of Physicians and Surgeons of Ontario

CPSP central poststroke pain

CPSTS Chinese Poststroke Treatment Study

CPT camptothecin; carnitine palmityl transferase; carotid pulse tracing; chest physiotherapy; child protection team; ciliary particle transport; cold pressor test; combining power test; complex physical therapy; computer psychometric test; conditional probability table; conjunctival provocation test; continuous performance task; continuous performance test; current procedural terminology

CPT-11 irinotecan

CPTA Center for Practice and Technology Assessment

CPTH chronic posttraumatic headache

CPTN culture positive toxin negative

CPTP culture positive toxin positive

CPTX chronic parathyroidectomy

CPU caudate putamen; central processing unit

CPUE chest pain of unknown etiology

CPV canine parvovirus [veterinary medicine]; Coastal Plains virus; Cotia virus; cypovirus; cytoplasmic polyhedrosis virus

CpV *Calliteara pudibunda* virus; cypovirus; cytoplasmic polyhedrosis virus

CPVC common pulmonary venous channel

CPVD congenital polyvalvular disease

CPX cleft palate, X-linked; clinical practice examination; complete physical examination

CPXD chondrodysplasia punctata, X-linked dominant

CPXR chondrodysplasia punctata, X-linked recessive

CPZ cefoperazone; chlorpromazine; Compazine

CQ chloroquine [phosphate]; chloroquine-quinine; circadian quotient; conceptual quotient

CQI continuous quality improvement

CQIN clinical quality improvement network

CQI/TQM continuous quality improvement/total quality management

CQIV Calchaqui virus

CQM chloroquine mustard

CQMS cost quality management system

CQOLC caregiver quality-of-life index-cancer

CQS central query system

CqV *Callimorpha quadripunctata* virus

CR cadherin-specific repeat; calculation rate; calculus removed; calorie-restricted; cardiac rehabilitation; cardiac resuscitation; cardiac rhythm; cardiorespiratory; cardiorrhexis; caries resistant; cathode ray; cellular receptor; central ray; centric relation; chemoradiation; chest and right arm [ECG]; chest roentgenogram/roentgenography; chief resident; child resistant; chimeric receptor; choice reaction; chromium; chronic rejection; chrysene; clinical record; clinical remission; clinical research; clot retraction; coefficient of fat retention; colon resection; colonization rate; colonization resistance; colony reared; colorectal; complement receptor; complete remission; complete response; compression ratio; computed radiography; computerized record; conditioned reflex, conditioned response; confidence region; congenital rubella; Congo red; contractile reserve; controlled release; controlled respiration; conversion rate; cooling rate; correlation; correlation ratio; corticoresistant; creatinine; cremaster reflex; cresyl red; critical ratio; crown-rump [measurement]; cruciate retaining [arthroplasty]

CR1, 2, 3, 4, 5 complement receptor types 1 to 5

C&R convalescence and rehabilitation

Cr chromium; cranial, cranium; creatinine; crown

CRA central retinal artery; Chinese restaurant asthma; chronic rheumatoid arthritis; clinical research associate; constant relative alkalinity

CRABP cellular retinoic acid-binding protein

CRAC calcium release-activated channel; compliance-related acute complication

CRADA Cooperative Research and Development Agreement

CRAF computer rod and frame test

CRAFT Catheterization Rescue Angioplasty Following Thrombolysis [trial]; Controlled Randomized Atrial Fibrillation Trial

CRAG *Cryptococcus* antigen

CRAHCA Center for Research in Ambulatory Health Care Administration

CRALBP cellular retinaldehyde-binding protein

CRAM common random access memory

CRAMS circulation, respiration, abdomen, motor, speech

cran cranium, cranial

CRAO central retinal artery occlusion

CRASH corpus callosum hypoplasia, retardation, adducted thumbs, spastic paraplegia, hydrocephalus [syndrome]

CraV Cynara virus

CRAW computed tomography acquisition workstation

CRB chemical, radiologic, and biologic; congenital retinal blindness; Cramer-Rao bound

CrB Creola bodies

CRBBB complete right bundle branch block

CRBC chicken red blood cell

CRBP cellular retinol-binding protein

CRC calcium release channel; cancer research campaign; cardiovascular reflex clinical research center; cardiovascular reflex conditioning; class responsibilities collaboration; colorectal cancer; colorectal carcinoma; concentrated red blood cells; contrast recovery coefficient; corrected reticulocyte count; creatinine clearance; cross-reacting cannabinoids; cyclic redundancy check

CrCl creatinine clearance

CRCS cardiovascular reflex conditioning system

CRD carbohydrate-recognition domain; child restraint device; childhood rheumatic disease; chorioretinal degeneration; chronic renal disease; chronic respiratory disease; complete reaction of degeneration; complex repetitive discharge; cone-rod retinal dystrophy; congenital rubella deafness; crown-rump distance

CRDC Central Research and Development Committee

CRDEC Chemical Research Development and Engineering Center

CR-DIP chronic relapsing demyelinating inflammatory polyneuropathy

CRDS Charles River Data System; client response documentation system

CRE cumulative radiation effect; creatinine; cyclic adenosine monophosphate response element

creat creatinine

CREATE Cholesterol Research Education and Treatment Evaluation

CREB cyclic adenosine monophosphate responsive element binding [protein]

CREDO Clopidogrel Reduction of Events During Extended Observation [study]

CREG cross-reactive antigen group

CREM center for rural emergency medicine; cyclic adenosine monophosphate response element modulator

crem cremaster

CREOG Council on Resident Education in Obstetrics and Gynecology

crep crepitation, crepitus

CREST calcinosis, Raynaud phenomenon, esophageal involvement, sclerodactyly, and telangiectasia [syndrome]; Carotid Revascularization and Endarterectomy vs. Stent Trial

CREW Coronary Regression with Estrogen in Women [study]

CRF cardiorespiratory function; case report form; chronic renal failure; chronic respiratory failure; circulating recombinant form; coagulase-reacting factor; complex reduction forceps; continuous reinforcement; coronary reserve flow; corticotropin-releasing factor; cytokine receptor family

CRFK Crandell feline kidney cells

CRFR corticotropin-releasing factor receptor

CRG cardiorespirogram; central respiratory generator; collaborative review group

CRH corticotropin-releasing hormone

CRHBP corticosterone-releasing hormone binding protein

CRHL Collaborative Radiological Health Laboratory

CRHV cottontail rabbit herpesvirus

CrHV cricetid herpesvirus

CRI Cardiac Risk Index; catheter-related infection; chronic renal insufficiency; chronic respiratory insufficiency; Composite Risk Index; congenital rubella infection; contact ratio index; corneal relaxing incision; Craniofacial Risk Index; cross-reaction idiotype

C-RI corecessive inheritance

CRIB clinical risk index for babies

CRIE crossed radioimmunoelectrophoresis

CRIP cysteine-rich intestinal protein

CRIS Calcium Antagonist Reinfarction Italian Study; clinically related information system

CRISP Cholesterol Reduction in Seniors Program; Computer Retrieval of Information on Scientific Projects; Consortium Research in Systems Performance; Consortium Research on Indicators of System Performance

CRISPR clustered regularly interspaced short palindromic repeats

Crit, crit critical; hematocrit

CRIYFS Cardiovascular Risk in Young Finns Study

CRKL v-crk sarcoma virus CT10 oncogene homologue

CRL cell repository line; central right lung; Certified Record Librarian; clinical reasoning learning; complement receptor location; complement receptor lymphocyte; crown-rump length

CRLM colorectal liver metastases

CRM Certified Reference Materials; coding recognition module; counting rate meter; cross-reacting material; crown-rump measurement; customer relationship management

CRM⁺ cross-reacting material—positive

CRMO chronic recurrent multifocal osteomyelitis

CR-MVB Cramer-Rao minimum variance bound

CRN Certified Radiologic Nurse; complement requiring neutralization

CRNA Certified Registered Nurse Anesthetist

CRNF chronic rheumatoid nodular fibrositis

CRNFA Certified Registered Nurse First Assistant

CRNI Certified Registered Nurse Infusion

CRNL Certified Registered Nurse, Long-term Care

Cr Nn, cr nn cranial nerves

CRNO Certified Registered Nurse in Ophthalmology

CRNP Certified Registered Nurse Practitioner

CRO cathode ray oscilloscope; centric relation occlusion; contract research organization

CROM cervical range of motion

CROME congenital cataracts, epileptic fits, mental retardation (intellectual disability) [syndrome]

C-ROMS comprehensive radiation oncology management system

CROP compliance, rate, oxygenation, and pressure

CROS contralateral routing of signals [hearing aid]

CRP chronic relapsing pancreatitis; corneal-retinal potential; coronary rehabilitation program; C-reactive protein; cross-reacting protein; cyclic adenosine monophosphate receptor protein; cysteine-rich protein

CrP creatine phosphate

CRPA C-reactive protein antiserum

CRPC castration-resistant prostate cancer

CRPD chronic restrictive pulmonary disease

CRPF chloroquine-resistant *Plasmodium falciparum*; closed reduction and percutaneous fixation; contralateral renal plasma flow

CRPG central respiratory pattern generator

CRPS complex regional pain syndrome

CRPV cottontail rabbit papillomavirus; crowpox virus

CRQ-M Chronic Respiratory Questionnaire Mastery Subscale

CRRMP Committee on Radiation from Radioactive Medicinal Products

CRRN Certified Rehabilitation Registered Nurse

CRRT continuous renal replacement therapy

CrRT cranial radiotherapy

CRS Carroll rating scale for depression; catheter-related sepsis; caudal regression syndrome; cervical spine radiography; Chinese restaurant syndrome; *cis*-acting repressive sequence; colon and rectum surgery; compliance of the respiratory system; congenital rubella syndrome; craniosynostosis; cryptidin-related sequence

C_{RS+} respiratory system compliance

CRSM cherry red spot myoclonus

CRSP comprehensive renal scintillation procedure

CRS-R Coma Recovery Scale-Revised

CRST calcinosis, Raynaud phenomenon, sclerodactyly, telangiectasia [syndrome]; corrected sinus recovery time

CRT cadaver renal transplantation; calreticulin; cardiac resuscitation team; cardiac resynchronization therapy; cathode-ray tube; central reaction time; certified; Certified Radiologic Technologist [California license]; certified record techniques; Certified Respiratory Therapist; chemoradiation therapy; choice reaction time; chromium release test; complex reaction time; computed renal tomography; conformal radiation therapy; conformal radiotherapy; copper reduction test; corrected; corrected retention time; cortisone-resistant thymocyte; cranial radiation therapy

CrT crista terminalis

crt hematocrit

CRT-D cardiac resynchronization therapy-defibrillator

CRTM cartilage matrix protein

CRTP Consciousness Research and Training Project

CRTS Certified Recreational Therapy Specialist

CRTT Certified Respiratory Therapy Technician

CRU cardiac rehabilitation unit; clinical research unit

CRUISE Can Routine Ultrasound Influence Stent Expansion? [study]

CRUSADE Coronary Reserve Utilization for Stent and Angiography: Doppler Endpoint [study]; Coronary Revascularization Ultrasound Angioplasty Device [trial]

CRV Channel catfish reovirus; central retinal vein; Cowbone Ridge virus; Nile crocodile poxvirus

CRVF congestive right ventricular failure

CRVO central retinal vein occlusion

Cry crystal

CRYG gamma-crystallin gene

CRYM mu-crystallin

cryo cryogenic; cryoglobulin; cryoprecipitate; cryosurgery; cryotherapy

Cryoppt cryoprecipitate

CRYP cryptospiridiosis

crys, cryst crystal, crystalline

CS calf serum; campomelic syndrome; canalicular system; Capgras syndrome; carcinoid syndrome; cardiogenic shock; caries susceptible; carotid sheath; carotid sinus; cat scratch; celiac sprue; central service; central supply; cerebral scintigraphy; cerebrospinal; cervical spine; cervical stimulation; cesarean section; chest strap; chief of staff; cholesterol stone; cholesterol sulfate; chondroitin sulfate; chorionic somato-mammotropin; chronic schizophrenia; cigarette smoke; cigarette smoker; circumsporozoite; citrate synthase; climacteric syndrome; clinical laboratory scientist; clinical stage; clinical status; clinic scheduling; Cockayne syndrome; Cogan syndrome; complete stroke; compression syndrome; concentrated strength; conditioned stimulus; congenital syphilis; conjunctival secretion; connection service; conscious, consciousness; conscious sedation; conservative surgery; constant spring; contact sensitivity; continue same; contrast sensitivity; control

serum; control subjects; convalescence, convalescent; coordinate system; coronary sclerosis; coronary sinus; corpus striatum; corticoid sensitive; corticosteroid; cortico-subcortical; countershock; crush syndrome; current smoker; current strength; Cushing syndrome; cyclic somatostatin; cycloserine; cyclosporine; cytology sample

C4S chondroitin-4-sulfate

C/S cesarean section; cycles per second

C&S calvarium and scalp; conjunctiva and sclera; culture and sensitivity

Cs case; cell surface; cyclosporine; static compliance

C_s standard clearance; static compliance; static respiratory compliance

cS centistoke

cs catalytic subunit; chromosome; consciousness

CSA Cambridge Scientific Abstracts; Canadian Standards Association; canavaninosuccinic acid; carbonyl salicylamide; cell surface antigen; certified surgical assistant; chemical shift anisotropy; child sexual abuse; chondroitin sulfate A; chorionic somato-mammotropin A; classical simulated annealing; client server architecture; clinical skills assessment; colony-stimulating activity; colony survival array; compressed spectral array; computerized spectral analysis; Controlled Substances Act; cross-section area; cyclosporin A

CsA cyclosporin A

CSAA Child Study Association of America

CSAD corporate services administration department

CSAT cell substratum attachment; center for substance abuse treatment

CSAVP cerebral subarachnoid venous pressure

CSB contaminated small bowel; craniosynostosis, Boston type

csb chromosome break

CSBF coronary sinus blood flow

CSBS contaminated small bowel syndrome

CSC blow on blow [Fr. *coup sur coup*]; chondroitin sulfate C; cigarette smoke condensate; collagen sponge contraceptive; corticostriatocerebellar; cryogenic storage container; cytokine-secreting cell

CSCC circuits, systems, communications, and computers; cross-sectional case control; cutaneous squamous cell carcinoma

CSCD Center for Sickle Cell Disease

CSCE Committee on Scientific Conduct and Ethics

CSCHDS Caerphilly and Speedwell Collaborative Heart Disease Studies

CSCI corticosterone side-chain isomerase

CSCL computer-supported collaborative learning

CSCR Central Society for Clinical Research

CSCV critical serum chemistry value

CSCW computer-supported collaborative work

CSD cardiac support device; carotid sinus denervation; cat scratch disease; collimator-skin distance; combined-system disease; computerized severity index; conditionally streptomycin dependent; conduction system disease; cortical spreading depression; craniospinal defect; critical stimulus duration

CSDB cat scratch disease bacillus

CSDH chronic subdural hematoma

CSDMS Canadian Society of Diagnostic Medical Sonographers

CSDS Cardiovascular System Dynamics Society

CSE cardiac source of embolus; clinical-symptom/self-evaluation; common standards for quantitative electrocardiography; cone-shaped epiphysis; conventional spin-echo; cross-sectional echocardiography

C sect, C-section cesarean section

CSEP clinical sepsis; conducted somatosensory evoked potential; cortical somatosensory evoked potential

CSEPP chemical stockpile emergency preparedness program

CSER cortical somatosensory evoked response

CSERIAC Crew System Ergonomics Information Analysis Center

CSES Chronic Obstructive Pulmonary Disease [COPD] Self-Efficacy Scale

CSF cancer family syndrome; cerebrospinal fluid; cold stability factor; colony-stimulating factor; coronary sinus flow; critical success factor

CS-F colony-stimulating factor

CSFH cerebrospinal fluid hypotension

CSFII Continuing Survey of Food Intakes by Individuals

CSF-IR colony-stimulating factor I receptor

CSFP cerebrospinal fluid pressure; coronary slow-flow phenomenon

CSFQ Changes in Sexual Functioning Questionnaire

CSFR colony-stimulating factor receptor

CSFV cerebrospinal fluid volume; classic swine fever virus

CSF-WR cerebrospinal fluid Wassermann reaction

CSG cell surface glycoprotein; central sympathetic generator; cholecystogram, cholecystography; clinical study group; collaborative study group; *Coronaviridae* [or Coronavirus] Study Group

csg chromosome gap

CSGBI Cardiac Society of Great Britain and Ireland

CSGBM collagenase soluble glomerular basement membrane

CSGE conformational sensitive gel electrophoresis

CSGTEI Collaborative Study Group Trial on the Effect of Irbesartan

CSH carotid sinus hypersensitivity; chronic subdural hematoma; combat support hospital; cortical stromal hyperplasia

CSHA Canadian Study of Health and Aging

CSHCN children with special health care needs

CSHE California Society for Healthcare Engineering

CSHH congenital self-healing histiocytosis

CSHL Cold Spring Harbor Laboratory

CSHN children with special health needs

CSHS Canadian Smoking Health Survey

CSI calculus surface index; cancer serum index; cavernous sinus infiltration; cervical spine injury; chemical safety inspection; chemical shift imaging; chemical surety inspection; cholesterol saturation index; computerized severity of illness [index]; continuous subcutaneous infusion; coronary sinus intervention; craniospinal irradiation

CSICU cardiac surgical intensive care unit

CSI-D Community Screening Instrument for Dementia

CSIF cytokine synthesis inhibitory factor

CSII continuous subcutaneous insulin infusion

CSIIP continuous subcutaneous insulin infusion pump

CSIN Chemical Substances Information Network

CSIRO Commonwealth Scientific and Industrial Research Organisation

CSIS clinical supplies and inventory system

CS IV clinical stage 4

CsIV *Campoletis sonorensis* ichnovirus

CSL cardiolipin synthetic lecithin; corticosteroid liposome

CSLM confocal scanning laser microscopy

cSLO confocal scanning laser ophthalmoscope

CSLP cervical spine locking plate

CSLT Canadian Society of Laboratory Technology

CSLU chronic stasis leg ulcer

CSM cardiosynchronous myostimulator; care systems management; carotid sinus massage; cerebrospinal meningitis; circulation, sensation, motion; Committee on Safety of Medicines; confined space medicine; Consolidated Standards Manual; corn-soy milk

CSMA chronic spinal muscular atrophy

CSMA/CD carrier sense multiple access and collision detection

CSMAP celiac—superior mesenteric artery portography

C-SMART Cardiomyoplasty-Skeletal Muscle Assist Randomized Trial

CSMB Center for the Study of Multiple Birth

CSMLS Canadian Society for Medical Laboratory Science

CSMMG Chartered Society of Massage and Medical Gymnastics

CSMP chloramphenicol-sensitive microsomal protein

CSMSS Collaborative Social and Medical Services System

CSMT chorionic somatomammotropin

CSN cardiac sympathetic nerve; carotid sinus nerve; Chemical Safety Newsbase; cycloserine

CSNA congenital sensory neuropathy with anhidrosis [syndrome]

CSNB congenital stationary night blindness

CS(NCA) Clinical Laboratory Scientist certified by the National Certification Agency for Medical Laboratory Personnel

CSNDB Cell Signaling Network Database

CSNK casein kinase

CSNRT, cSNRT corrected sinus node recovery time

CSNS carotid sinus nerve stimulation

CSNU cystinuria

CSO claims services only; common source outbreak; craniostenosis; craniosynostosis; ostium of coronary sinus

CSOM chronic suppurative otitis media

CSOP coronary sinus occlusion pressure

CSP carotid sinus pressure; cavum septi pellucidi; cell surface protein; central silent period; cerebrospinal protein; Chartered Society of Physiotherapy; chemistry screening panel; chondroitin sulfate protein; circumsporozoite protein; complications screening program; Cooperative Statistical Program; criminal sexual psychopath; cutaneous silent period; cyclosporin; cytosarcoma phyllodes

Csp cervical spine

CSPAMM complementary spatial modulation of magnetization [imaging]

CSPG chondroitin sulfate proteoglycan

CSPI Center for Science in the Public Interest; certified specialist in poison information

CSPINE corticosteroid use, seropositive rheumatoid arthritis, peripheral joint destruction, involvement of cervical nerves, nodules (rheumatoid), established disease [mne-monic]

C-spine cervical spine

CsplV *Campoletis* sp. ichnovirus

CSPR cell-specific perfusion rate

CSPS continual skin-peeling syndrome

CSpT corticospinal tract

CSQ Coping Strategies Questionnaire

CSR Center for Scientific Review; central supply room; chart-stimulated recall [test]; Cheyne-Stokes respiration; continued stay review; continuous speech recognition; corrected sedimentation rate; corrected survival rate; cortisol secretion rate; cumulative survival rate

CSRA cardio-surgical recovery area

CSRM case-specific reference model

CSRP cysteine-rich protein

CSRS cardiac surgery reporting system

CSRT Canadian Society of Respiratory Technology; Canadian Society of Respiratory Therapists; continuous speech recognition technology

CSS Canadian Stroke Scale; Cancer Surveillance System; carotid sinus stimulation; carotid sinus syndrome; cavernous sinus syndrome; central sterile section; central sterile supply; chewing, sucking, swallowing; chronic subclinical scurvy; Churg-Strauss syndrome; client satisfaction scale; clinical support system; Copenhagen Stroke Study; cranial sector scan; critical care system

C^{ss} [plasma] concentration at steady state

CSSA Carotid Stent-Supported Angioplasty [trial]

CSSAE Communication Skills Self-Assessment Exam

CSSCD Cooperative Study of Sickle Cell Disease

CSSD central sterile supply department

CSSRD Cooperative Systematic Study of Rheumatic Diseases

CSSSI complicated skin and skin structure infections

CSSU central sterile supply unit

CST cardiac stress test; cardiovascular self-assessment tool; cavernous sinus thrombosis; certified surgical technologist; chemostatin; Christ-Siemens-Touraine [syndrome]; compliance, static; computer scatter tomography; contraction stress test; conversational speech task; convulsive shock therapy; corticospinal tract; cosyntropin stimulation test; cystatin

cSt centistoke

C$_{st}$, C$_{stat}$ static compliance

CSTB Computer Science and Telecommunications Board

CSTD chronic single tic disorder

CSTE Council of State and Territorial Epidemiologists

CstF cleavage stimulation factor

CSTI Clearinghouse for Scientific and Technical Information

CSTM cervical prevertebral soft tissue measurement

c-STM cervical specimen transport medium

CSTP Committee for Scientific and Technological Policy

Cst,rs static compliance of respiratory system

CSTT cold-stimulation time test

CSU cardiac surgery unit; casualty staging unit; catheter specimen of urine; central statistical unit; clinical specialty unit

CSUF continuous slow ultrafiltration

CSV chick syncytial virus

CSVD coughing, sneezing, vomiting, and diarrhea [veterinary medicine]

CSVT central splanchnic venous thrombosis

CSW Certified Social Worker; commercial sex worker; current sleepwalker

CSWG Clinical Systems Working Group

CSWSS continuous spike waves of slow sleep

CT calcitonin; calf testis; carboxyl terminal; cardiac tamponade; cardiothoracic [ratio]; carnitine transporter; carotid tracing; carpal tunnel; cell therapy; cerebral thrombosis; cerebral tumor; cervical traction; cervicothoracic; chemotaxis; chemotherapy; chest tube; chicken tumor; *Chlamydia trachomatis*; chlorothiazide; cholera toxin; cholesterol, total; chordae tendineae; chronic thyroiditis; chymotrypsin; circulation time; classic technique; clinical trial; closed thoracotomy; clotting time; coagulation time; coated tablet; cobra toxin; cognitive therapy; coil test; collecting tubule; colon, transverse; combined tumor; community transmission; compressed tablet; computed tomography; connective tissue; continue treatment; continuous-flow tube; contraceptive technique; contraction time; controlled temperature; Coombs test; corneal transplant; coronary thrombosis; corrected transposition; corrective therapy; cortical thickness; corticospinal tract; cough threshold; crest time; crista terminalis; cystine-tellurite; cytotechnologist; cytotoxic therapy; unit of attenuation

C/T compression/traction ratio

C&T color and temperature

C$_T$ total compliance

C$_{T-1824}$ T-1824 (Evans blue) clearance

Ct carboxyl terminal; concentration

ct carat; chromatid; count

CTA Canadian Tuberculosis Association; center for total access; chemotactic activity; chromotropic acid; Committee on Thrombolytic Agents; computed tomography of the abdomen; computed tomographic angiography; congenital trigeminal anesthesia; cosmetic tissue augmentation; cuff tear arthropathy; cyanotrimethyl-androsterone; cystine-trypticase agar; cytoplasmic tubular aggregate; cytotoxic assay

CTAB cetyltrimethyl-ammonium bromide

CTAC Cancer Treatment Advisory Committee

CTAF Canadian Trial of Atrial Fibrillation; conotruncal anomaly face [syndrome]

CTAFS conotruncal anomaly face syndrome

cTAL cortical thick ascending limb

CTAP computed tomography in arterial portography; connective tissue activating peptide; Coronavirus Treatment Acceleration Program

CTAT computed transaxial tomography

CTB ceased to breathe; cholera toxin B

ctb chromated break

CTC chlortetracycline; circulating tumor cells; Clinical Trial Certificate; Common Toxicity Criteria; computed tomographic colography; computed tomography-based virtual colonoscopy; computer-aided tomographic cisternography; consent to continue; cultured T cells

CTCL cutaneous T-cell lymphoma

ctCO$_2$ carbon dioxide concentration

CTD carboxy-terminal domain; chest tube drainage; carpal tunnel decompression; congenital thymic dysplasia; connective tissue disease; cumulative trauma disorder

CT&DB cough, turn, and deep breathe

CTDI computed tomography dose index

ctDNA chloroplast deoxyribonucleic acid

CTE calf thymus extract; chronic traumatic encephalopathy; cultured thymic epithelium

CTEM conventional transmission electron microscopy

CTEP Cancer Therapy Evaluation Program

CTEV *Camptochironomus tentans* entomopoxvirus

CTF cancer therapy facility; certificate; Colorado tick fever; contrast transfer function; cytotoxic factor

ctf certificate

CTFE chlorotrifluoroethylene

CTFS complete testicular feminization syndrome

CTFV Colorado tick fever virus

CTG cardiotocography; cervicothoracic ganglion; chymotrypsinogen; control technique guidelines

C/TG cholesterol/triglyceride ratio

ctg centigray; chromated gap

CTGA complete transposition of great arteries

CTGF connective tissue growth factor

CTGFN Convergent Terminology Group for Nursing

CTH ceramide trihexoside; chronic tension headache; computer-assisted tomographic holography; cystathionase

CTh carrier-specific T-helper [cell]

C$_{Th}$ thoracic compliance

CTHA computed tomographic hepatic angiography

CTHD chlorthalidone; conotruncal heart defect

CTI cardiac troponin I; coffee table injury; computers in teaching initiatives; computer-telephony integration

CTIBL castration treatment—induced bone loss

CTL cervicothoracolumbar; computational tree logic; control; cytolytic T lymphocyte; cytotoxic T lymphocyte

CTLA cytotoxic T-lymphocyte antigen

CTLL cytotoxic lymphoid line

CTLp cytotoxic T-lymphocyte precursor

CTLSO cervicothoracolumbosacral orthosis

CTM calibration of test material; cardiotachometer; central tendency measure; Chlortrimeton; computed tomographic myelography; cricothyroid membrane; cricothyroid muscle

CTMC connective tissue mast cell

CTMM computed tomographic metrizamide myelography

CTMM-SF California Test of Mental Maturity-Short Form

CTMR clinical treatment and medical research

CT/MRI computed tomography/magnetic resonance imaging

CTN calcitonin; Certified Transcultural Nurse; clinical trials notification; computer tomography number; continuous noise

cTn cardiac troponin

cTn-I cardiac troponin I

cTNM clinical classification of primary tumors, regional nodes, and metastases

CTO cervicothoracic orthosis; chronic total occlusion

CTOPP Canadian Trial of Physiological Pacing

CTP California Test of Personality; Child-Turcotte-Pugh [classification]; citrate transport protein; clinical terms project; composite theoretic performance; comprehensive treatment plan; cytidine triphosphate; cytosine triphosphate

C-TPN cyclic total parenteral nutrition

CTPP cerebral tissue perfusion pressure

CTPVO chronic thrombotic pulmonary vascular obstruction

CTQ Child Trauma Questionnaire

CTQ-SF Childhood Trauma Questionnaire-Short Form

CTR cardiothoracic ratio; carpal tunnel release; central tumor registry; click-through rate; Connecticut Tumor Registry

ctr central; center; centric

CTRB chymotrypsinogen B

CTRD Cardiac Transplant Research Database

CTRL chymotrypsin-like [protease]

CTRN Certified Transport Registered Nurse

CTRS certified therapeutic recreation specialist

CTRX ceftriaxone

CTS cardiothoracic surgery; cardiotonic steroids; carpal tunnel syndrome; clinical trials support [program]; Collaborative Transplant Study; composite treatment score; computed tomographic scan; conflict tactics scales; contralateral threshold shift; corticosteroid

CTSB cathepsin B

CTSD cathepsin D

CTSE cathepsin E

CTSG cathepsin G

CTSH cathepsin H

CTSI computed tomography severity index

CTSL cathepsin L

CTSNFR corrected time of sinoatrial node function recovery

CTSP Cooperative Triglyceride Standardization Program

CTSPC Conflict Tactics Scale: Parent-Child Version

CTSS cathepsin S; closed tracheal suction system

CTT cefotetan; central tegmental tract; central transmission time; classic test theory; colonic transit time; compressed tablet triturate; computed transaxial tomography; critical tracking time

CTTAC clinical trials and treatment advisory committee

CTU cardiac-thoracic unit; centigrade thermal unit; constitutive transcription unit

CTV cervical and thoracic vertebrae; clinical target volume; clinical tumor volume

CTVDR conformal treatment verification, delivery, and recording

CTW central terminal of Wilson; combined testicular weight

CTX cefotaxime; ceftriaxone; cerebrotendinous xanthomatosis; chemotaxis; ciguatoxin; clinical trials exemption scheme; costotendinous xanthomatosis; cytoxan

CTx cardiac transplantation; conotoxin

CTZ cetirizine; chemoreceptor trigger zone; chlorothiazide

CU cardiac unit; casein unit; cause undetermined; cause unknown; chymotrypsin unit; clinical unit; color unit; contact urticaria; convalescent unit

C$_u$ urea clearance

cu cubic

CUA Certified Urologic Associate; cost-utility analysis

CUAVD congenital unilateral absence of vas deferens

CuB copper band

CUBA Cutting Balloon vs. Conventional Balloon Angioplasty [study]

CUC chronic ulcerative colitis

cu cm cubic centimeter

CUCNS Certified Urologic Clinical Nurse Specialist

CUD cause undetermined; congenital urinary deformity

CuD copper deficiency

CUE confidential unit exclusion; cumulative urinary excretion

CUG Computer-Stored Ambulatory Record User's Group; cystidine, uridine, and guanidine; cystourethrogram, cystourethrography

CUI character-based interface; concept unique identifier; Cox-Uphoff International [tissue expander]

cu in cubic inch

cult culture

cum cumulative

cu m cubic meter

CUMITECH Cumulative Techniques and Procedures in Clinical Microbiology

cu mm cubic millimeter

CUNP Certified Urologic Nurse Practitioner

CUP carcinoma unknown primary

CUR cystourethrorectal

cur curative, cure; current

CURE Clopidogrel in Unstable Angina to Prevent Recurrent Ischemic Events [trial]; Columbia University Restenosis Elimination [trial]

CURL compartment of uncoupling of receptors and ligands

CURN Certified Urologic Registered Nurse; Conduct and Utilization of Research in Nursing

CurrMIT Curriculum Management and Information Tool

CUS carotid ultrasound examination; catheterized urine specimen; contact urticaria syndrome

CuS copper supplement

CUSA Cavitron ultrasonic aspirator

CUSSN computer use in social service network

CuTS cubital tunnel syndrome

CV calicivirus; canker virus; cardiac volume; cardiovascular; care vigilance; carotenoid vesicle; cell viability; cell volume; central venous; cephalic vein; cerebrovascular; cervical vertebra; Chikungunya virus; Chlorella virus; chlorosis virus; chorionic villi; circovirus; closing volume; clump virus; coefficient of variation [statistics]; color vision; concentrated volume; conducting vein; conduction velocity; conjugata vera; contrast ventriculography; conventional ventilation; corpuscular volume; costovertebral; cresyl violet; cross validation; cryptic virus; crystal violet; cultivar; cutaneous vasculitis; cyclic voltamogram; cyclic voltometry; fifth cranial nerve

C/V coulomb per volt

Cv specific heat at constant volume

C$_v$ coefficient of variation; constant volume

cv coefficient of variability; cultivar

CVA cardiovascular accident; cerebrovascular accident; Certified Vascular Nurse; chronic villous arthritis; common variable agammaglobulinemia; costovertebral angle; cyclophosphamide, vincristine, and Adriamycin

CV-A1 to A22 human coronaviruses A1 to A22

CVAH congenital virilizing adrenal hyperplasia

CVAP cerebrovascular amyloid peptide

CVAT costovertebral angle tenderness

CVB chorionic villi biopsy

CV B1 to B6 human coxsackieviruses B1 to B6

CVBS congenital vascular bone syndrome

CVC calcifying vascular cell; central venous catheter

CV cath central venous catheter

CVCT cardiovascular computed tomography

CVD cardiovascular disease; Center for Vaccine Development; chemical vapor deposition; chronic venous disease; collagen vascular disease; color-vision deviant; common variable immunodeficiency; congenital vascular disorder

CVELTP Comox Valley Electronic Lab Transfer Project

CVF cardiovascular failure; central visual field; cervicovaginal fluid; cobra venom factor

CVFn cardiovascular function

CVFS computerized visual feedback system

CVG composite valve graft; contrast ventriculography; coronary venous graft; cutis verticis gyrata

CVG/MR cutis verticis gyrata/mental retardation (intellectual disability) [syndrome]

CVGV Csiro Village virus

CVH cerebroventricular hemorrhage; cervicovaginal hood; chronic viral hepatitis; combined ventricular hypertrophy; common variable hypogammaglobulinemia

cVDPV circulating vaccine-derived poliovirus

CVHD chronic valvular heart disease

CvHV cervid herpesvirus

CVI cardiovascular incident; cardiovascular insufficiency; cerebrovascular incident; cerebrovascular insufficiency; Children's Vaccine Initiative; chronic venous insufficiency; common variable immunodeficiency; content validity index; sixth cranial nerve

CVICU cardiovascular intensive care unit

CVID common variable immunodeficiency

CVII seventh cranial nerve

CVIII eighth cranial nerve

CVIS cardiovascular imaging system

CVK computerized videokeratography

CVL central venous line

CVLM caudal ventrolateral medulla; caudoventrolateral medulla

CVLP chimeric viruslike particle

CVLT California Verbal Learning Test; clinical vascular laboratory

CVM cardiovascular monitor; Center for Veterinary Medicine; cerebral venous malformation; congenital vascular malformation; contingent valuation method; cyclophosphamide, vincristine, and methotrexate

CVMP Committee on Veterans Medical Problems

CVO central vein occlusion; central venous oxygen; chief veterinary officer; circumventricular organ; credentialing verification organization

CVO$_2$ central venous oxygen content; central venous oxygen saturation

CVOD cerebrovascular obstructive disease

CVP cardioventricular pacing; cell volume profile; central venous pressure; chlorfenvinphos; cyclophosphamide, vincristine, and prednisone

cvPO$_2$, cvPo$_2$ cerebral venous partial pressure of oxygen

CVPR computer vision and pattern recognition

CVR cardiovascular-renal; cardiovascular-respiratory; cephalic vasomotor response; cerebrovascular resistance

CVRD cardiovascular-renal disease

CVRMED computer vision, virtual reality, and robotics in medicine

CVRR cardiovascular recovery room

CVRS cardiovascular and respiratory elements of trauma score

CVS cardiovascular surgery; cardiovascular system; challenge virus strain; chorionic villi sampling; clean voided specimen; coronavirus susceptibility; current vital signs; cyclical vomiting syndrome

CVSMC cultured vascular smooth muscle cells

CVST cerebral venous sinus thrombosis; computerized visual search task

CVST-T Cerebral Venous Sinus Thrombosis Trial

CVT cardiovascular technologist; central venous temperature; cerebral venous thrombosis; congenital vertical talus

CVTR charcoal viral transport medium

CVU chronic venous ulceration

CVV Cache Valley virus; ceratitis V virus

CVVH continuous venovenous hemofiltration

CVVHD continuous venovenous hemodialysis

CVVHDF continuous venovenous hemodiafiltration

CVX code for vaccines administered

CW cardiac work; case work; cell wall; chemical warfare; chemical weapon; chest wall; children's ward; clinical workbench; clockwise; continuous wave; crutch walking

Cw crutch walking

C/W compare with; consistent with

CWA cognitive work analysis

CWBTS capillary whole blood true sugar

CWC Chemical Weapons Convention; chest wall compliance

CWCN Certified Wound Care Nurse

CWD cell wall defect; Choi-Williams distribution; continuous-wave Doppler

CWDF cell wall—deficient form

CWD/NAF cell wall—deficient, non—acid fast [*Mycobacterium tuberculosis*]

CWEQ Conditions of Work Effectiveness Questionnaire

CWF Cornell Word Form

CWG Communications Working Group

CWH cardiomyopathy and wooly hair-coat [syndrome]

CWHB citrated whole human blood
CWI cardiac work index
CWIS campus-wide information system
CWISH Council of Women's and Infants' Specialty Hospitals
CWL cutaneous water loss
CWM cardiologic workspace manager
CWMS color, warmth, movement, sensation
CWOCN Certified Wound, Ostomy, Continence Nurse
CWOP childbirth without pain
CWP childbirth without pain; coal worker's pneumoconiosis
CWPEA Childbirth Without Pain Education Association
CWR chest wall recurrence
CWRUNET Case Western Reserve University Network
CWS cell wall skeleton; Chemical Warfare Service; chest wall stimulation; child welfare service; children's clinical workstation; clinician's workstation; cold water soluble; cotton wool spots
CWT circuit weight training; cold water treatment; continuous wavelet transform
Cwt, cwt hundredweight
CWV Cape Wrath virus
CWW clinic without walls
CWXSP Coal Workers' X-ray Surveillance Program
CX cervix; chest x-ray; connexin; critical experiment; phosgene oxime; tenth cranial nerve
Cx cervix; circumflex; clearance; complaint; complex; connexin; convex
cx cervix; complex; connexin; culture; cylinder axis
CXB3S Coxsackie B3 virus susceptibility
CxCor circumflex coronary [artery]
CXEV *Chorizagrotis auxiliaris* entomopoxvirus
CXI eleventh cranial nerve
CXII twelfth cranial nerve
CXMD canine X-linked muscular dystrophy
CXR, CxR chest x-ray
CY casein-yeast autolysate [medium]; cyclophosphamide
Cy cyanogen; cyclophosphamide; cyst; cytarabine
cy cyanosis
Cy3 cyanine 3
Cy5 cyanine 5
cyan cyanosis

CyA cyclosporine A
CYBOCS Children's Yale-Brown Obsessive Compulsive Scale
CYC cyclophosphamide; cytochrome C
cyc cyclazocine; cycle; cyclotron
CYCAZAREM Cyclophosphamide vs. Azathioprine during Remission of Systemic Vasculitis [trial]
CYCLO, Cyclo cyclophosphamide; cyclopropane
Cyclo C cyclocytidine hydrochloride
CYCLOPS cyclically ordered phase sequence; Cyclophosphamide in Systemic Vasculitis
Cyd cytidine
CYE charcoal yeast extract [agar]
CYH chymase
CyHV cyprinid herpesvirus
CYL casein yeast lactate
cyl cylinder; cylindrical lens
CYM chymase, mast cell
CYMP chymosin, pseudogene
CYN cyanide
CYP cyclophilin; cyproheptadine; cytochrome P
CYPA cyclophilin A
CYPC cyclophilin C
CypCV *Cypripedium calceolus* virus
CYPH cyclophilin
CYS cystoscopy
Cys cyclosporine; cysteine
Cys-Cys cystine
CysLT1 cysteinyl leukotriene 1
CySNO nitrosated L-cysteine
CYSTO cystogram
cysto cystoscopy
CYT cytochrome
Cyt cytolytic
Cyt cytoplasm; cytosine
cyt cytochrome; cytologic, cytology; cytoplasm; cytosine
Cyto cytotechnologist
cytol cytologiv, cytology
CY-VA-DIC cyclophosphamide, vincristine, Adriamycin, and dacarbazine
CZ carzinophilin; cefazolin
Cz central midline placement of electrodes [EEG]
CZB Catot-Ziomek-Bavister [medium]
CZE capillary zone electrophoresis
CZI crystalline zinc insulin
C$_{zn}$ zinc clearance
CZP clonazepam

D

D absorbed dose aspartic acid; cholecalciferol; coefficient of diffusion; dacryon; dalton; date; daughter; day; dead; dead air space; debye; deceased; deciduous; decimal reduction time; degree; density; dental; dependent; dermatologic, dermatologist, dermatology; deuterium; deuteron; development; deviation; dextro; dextrose; diabetic; diagnosis; diagonal; diameter; diaphorase; diarrhea; diastole; diathermy; died; difference; diffusing, diffusion; diffusion coefficient; dihydrouridine; dilution; diopter; diplomate; dipyridamole; disease; dispense; displacement; distal; distance; diuresis; diurnal; divergence; diversity; diverticulum; divorced; doctor; dog; donor; dorsal; double; drive; drug; dual; duct; duodenal, duodenum; duration; dwarf; electric displacement; mean dose; right [L. *dexter*]; unit of vitamin D potency

Δ uppercase Greek letter delta
1D, 1-D one-dimensional
D1 prostatic tumor with microscopic involvement of pelvic lymph nodes
D₁ diagonal one; first dorsal vertebra
2D, 2-D two-dimensional
2D FTICR-MS two-dimensional Fourier transform ion cyclotron resonance mass spectrometry
D₂ diagonal two; second dorsal vertebra
2,4-D 2,4-dichlorophenoxyacetic acid
3D, 3-D three-dimensional
D/3 distal third
D₃₋₁₂ third to twelfth dorsal vertebrae
4D, 4-D four-dimensional
D4 domain 4; fourth digit
D₁₀ decimal reduction time
D50 50% dextrose solution
D mean dose
d atomic orbital with angular momentum quantum number 2; dalton; day; dead; deceased; deci-; decrease, decreased; degree; density; deoxy; deoxyribose; dextro-; dextrorotatory; diameter; diastasis; died; diopter; distal; distance; diurnal; dorsal; dose; doubtful; duration; dyne; right [L. *dexter*]
δ lowercase Greek letter delta; immunoglobulin D
d- deci- [10^{-1}]
1/d once a day
2/d twice a day
d mean difference of samples observations

DA dark adaptation; dark agouti [rat]; daunomycin; decision analysis; decontaminating agent; decision analysis; decontaminating agent; degenerative arthritis; degree of anisotropy; delayed action; dental assistant; deoxyadenosine; descending aneurysm; descending aorta; detrusor areflexia; developmental age; dextroamphetamine; diabetic acidosis; differential amplifier; differential analyzer; differentiation antigen; digital angiography; digital to analog; diphenylchlorarsine; Diploma in Anesthetics; direct agglutination; disability assistance; disaggregated; discriminant analysis; dissecting aneurysm; distal arthrogryposis; dopamine; drug addict/addiction; drug administration; ductus arteriosus

D-A donor-acceptor
D/A date of accident; date of admission; digital to analog; discharge and advise
D&A dilation and aspiration; drugs and allergy
DA1 distal arthrogryposis type 1
DA2 distal arthrogryposis type 2
2,4-DA 2,4-diaminoanisole
Da dalton
d(A) primary donor
da daughter; day; deca-
da- deka- [10^1]
DAA database access agreement; decompensated autonomous adenoma; dementia associated with alcoholism; dialysis-associated amyloidosis; diaminoanisole
DAAF deoxyribonucleic acid amplification fingerprinting; Digoxin in Acute Atrial Fibrillation [study]
DAAO diaminoacid oxidase
D(A−a)O₂ alveolar arterial oxygen gradient
DAB 3,3'-diaminobenzidine; days after birth; dysrhythmic aggressive behavior
DABA 2,4-diaminobutyric acid
DABP D-site albumin promoter binding protein
DABV Dabakala virus
DAC derived air concentration; digital acquisition; digital-to-analog converter; disaster assistance center; division of ambulatory care
dac dacryon
DACCM department of anesthesiology and critical care medicine
DACL Depression Adjective Check List
DACM N-(7-diamethylamino-4-methyl-3-coumarinyl) maleimide
DACMD deputy associate chief medical director
DACS data acquisition and control system

DACT dactinomycin; daily activity

DAD delayed afterdepolarization; diffuse alveolar damage; Disability Assessment in Dementia; discharge abstract databank; dispense as directed

DADA dichloroacetic acid diisopropylammonium salt

DADDS diacetyldiaminodiphenylsulfone

DADS Director of Army Dental Service

DAdV duck adenovirus

DAdV-1 egg drop syndrome virus

DAE differential algebraic equation; diphenylanthracene endoperoxide; diving air embolism; dysbaric air embolism

DA/ES data analysis expert system

DAEV *Dermolepida albohirtum* entomopoxvirus

DAF decay-accelerating factor; delayed auditory feedback; drug-adulterated food

DAFV Desulfurolobus virus

DAG diacylglycerol; dianhydrogalactitol; directed acyclic graph; dystrophin-associated glycoprotein

DAGK diacylglycerol kinase

DAGL diacylglycerol lipase

DAGT direct antiglobulin test

DAGV D'Aguilar virus

DAH diffuse alveolar hemorrhage; disordered action of the heart

DAHEA Department of Allied Health Education and Accreditation

DAHM Division of Allied Health Manpower

DAI diffuse axonal injury; drug attitude inventory

DAIDS Division of Acquired Immunodeficiency Syndrome

DAIS Diabetes Atherosclerosis Intervention Study

DAISY Diabetes Autoimmunity Study in the Young

DAIT Division of Allergy, Immunology, and Transplantation

DaIV *Diadegma acronyctae* ichnovirus

Dal, dal dalton

DALA delta-aminolevulinic acid

DALE disability-adjusted life expectancy; Drug Abuse Law Enforcement

DALM dysplasia with associated lesion or mass

DALT dalton

DALY disability-adjusted life-year

DAM data-associated message; database access module; degraded amyloid; diacetyl monoxime; diacetylmorphine

dam decameter

DAMA discharged against medical advice

DAMAD Diabetic Microangiopathy Modification with Aspirin vs. Dipyridamole [study]

DAMET Diet and Moderate Exercise Trial

DAMOS drug application methodology with optical storage

DAMP damage-associated molecular pattern

dAMP deoxyadenosine monophosphate; deoxyadenylate adenosine monophosphate

DAN data acquisition in neurophysiology; diabetic autonomic neuropathy; diaminonaphthalene

DANAMI Danish Multicenter Study of Acute Myocardial Infarction

DANB Dental Assisting National Board

DANC decontaminating agent, noncorrosive

D and C dilation and curettage

DANS 1-dimethylaminonaphthalene-5-sulfonyl chloride

DANTE delays altered with nutation for tailored excitation

DAO diamine oxidase

DAo descending aorta

DAOM depressor anguli oris muscle

DAP data acquisition processor; data architecture project; depolarizing afterpotential; diabetes-associated peptide; diaminopimelic acid; diaminopyridine; diastolic aortic pressure; diastolic arterial pressure; dihydroxyacetone phosphate; dipeptidylaminopeptidase; direct latex agglutination pregnancy [test]; dose area product; Draw-a-Person [test]; Drug Action Programme; Duke Autoimmunity in Pregnancy [registry]

D-AP5 d-2-amino-5-phosphonovaleric acid

D-AP7 d-2-amino-7-phosphonoheptanoic acid

DAP&E Diploma of Applied Parasitology and Entomology

DAPI 4,6-diamino-2-phenylindole

DAPPAF Dual-Site Atrial Pacing for Prevention of Atrial Fibrillation [trial]

DAPRE daily adjustable progressive resistive exercise

DAPRU Drug Abuse Prevention Resource Unit

DAPs Database Access Project

DAPT diaminophenylthiazole; direct agglutination pregnancy test

DAQ data acquisition; Diagnostic Assessment Questionnaire; digital acquisition

DAR daily activity record; daily effective rhythm; death after resuscitation; diacereine; differential absorption ratio; dual asthmatic reaction

DA-R dopamine receptor

DARE Database of Abstracts of Reviews of Effectiveness; Drug Abuse Resistance Education

DARP drug abuse rehabilitation program

DARPA Defense Advanced Research Project Agency

DART Developmental and Reproductive Toxicology; Diet and Reinfarction Trial; Dilation vs. Ablation Revascularization Trial

D/ART Depression Awareness, Recognition, and Treatment

DARTS Diabetes Audit and Research in Tayside, Scotland; Drug and Alcohol Rehabilitation Testing System

DAS data acquisition system; dead air space; Death Anxiety Scale; delayed anovulatory syndrome; dextroamphetamine sulfate; 4,15-diacetoxyscripenol; diallyl sulfide; Dietary Alternatives Study; digital angiography segmentation; disability assessment scale; double addition of serum; Dyadic Adjustment Scale

DASA distal articular set angle

DASD direct access storage device

DASH Delay in Accessing Stroke Healthcare [trial]; Dietary Approaches to Stop Hypertension [trial]; Distress Alarm for the Severely Handicapped

DASI Duke activity status index

DASM data acquisition system management

DASS Dilazep Aspirin Stroke Study

DAST diethylaminosulfur trifluoride; drug abuse screening test; drug and alcohol screening test

DAstV duck astrovirus

DAT delayed-action tablet; dementia, Alzheimer type; dental aptitude test; diacetylthiamine; diet as tolerated; differential agglutination titer; Differential Aptitude Tests; diphtheria antitoxin; direct agglutination test; direct antiglobulin test; disaster action team; divided attention; dopamine transporter

DATA Diltiazem as Adjunctive Therapy to Activase [study]

DATE dental auxiliary teacher education

DATF Difficult Airway Task Force

DATOS Diet and Antismoking Trial of Oslo Study

DATP deoxyadenosine triphosphate

dATP deoxyadenosine monophosphate

DATTA diagnostic and therapeutic technology assessment

DAU 3-deazauridine; Dental Auxiliary Utilization

dau daughter

DAU drug abuse testing and urine

DAV data valid; Disabled American Veterans; disease-associated virus; duck adenovirus

DAVF dural arteriovenous fistula

DAVIT Danish Verapamil Infarction Trial

DAVM dural arteriovenous malformation

DAvMED Diploma in Aviation Medicine

DAVP deamino-arginine vasopressin

DAW digital audio workcenter; dispense as written

DAWN Drug Abuse Warning Network

DAZ deleted in azoospermia

DB database; date of birth; deep breath; dense body; dextran blue; diabetes, diabetic; diagonal band; diet beverage; direct bilirubin; disability; distobuccal; double blind; double buffer; duodenal bulb; Dutch belted [rabbit]

Db diabetes, diabetic

D$_b$ database; body density

dB, db decibel

db database; date of birth; diabetes, diabetic

DBA database administrator; Diamond-Blackfan anemia; dibenzanthracene; *Dolichos biflorus* agglutinin

DBAE dihydroxyborylaminoethyl

DBB diagonal band of Broca

DBC dibencozide; distal balloon catheter; dye-binding capacity

DB&C deep breathing and coughing

DBCL dilute blood clot lysis

DBCP dibromochloropropane

DBD definite brain damage; deoxyribonucleic acid−binding domain; dibromodulcitol; dynamic beam delivery

DBDC distal bile duct carcinoma

DBDG distobuccal developmental groove

DBDO decabromodiphenyl oxide; desert battle dress overgarment

DBDS database definition structure

DB/DS database of datasets

dB/dt change of magnetic flux with time

DBE deep breathing exercise; dibromoethane; double-balloon enteroscopy

DbE dobutamine echocardiography

DBED N,N'-dibenzyl ethylenediaminediacetic acid

dbEST database expressed sequence tag; Database of Expressed Sequence Tags

DBEV Demodema entomopoxvirus

dbGSS database genome survey sequence; Database on Genome Survey Sequences

DBH dopamine beta-hydroxylase

DbH diagnosis by hybridization

DBI development at birth index; phenformin hydrochloride

DBil direct bilirubin

DBIOC database input/output control

DBIR Directory of Biotechnology Information Resources

dBk decibels above 1 kilowatt

DBL desbromoleptophos

DBLE Double Bolus Lytic Efficacy [trial]

DBM database management; dibromomannitol; dobutamine

dBm decibels above 1 milliwatt

dBMAN database manager

DBMS database management system

DBN dynamic bayesian network

DBNN decision-based neural network

DBO distobucco-occlusal

db/ob diabetic obese [mouse]

DBP deoxyribonucleic acid−binding peptide; diastolic blood pressure; dibutylphthalate; distobuccopulpal; Döhle body panmyelopathy; vitamin D−binding protein

DBPOFC double-blind placebo-controlled oral food challenge

DBP-PEG/DNA deoxyribonucleic acid−binding peptide-polyethylene glycol/deoxyribonucleic acid

DBR distorted breathing rate

DBRI dysfunctional behavior rating instrument

DBRPC double-blind randomized placebo-controlled

DBS deep brain stimulation; Denis Browne splint; despeciated bovine serum; Diamond-Blackfan syndrome; dibromosalicil; diminished breath sounds; direct bonding system; Division of Biological Standards; double-blind study; double-burst stimulus; dysgenesis of corpus callosum

dbSNP Database of Single Nucleotide Polymorphisms

DBSP dibromosulphthalein

dbSTS Database of Sequence Tagged Sites; database sequence target site

DBSV deconvolution based on shape variation

DBT dry bulb temperature

DBV Dakar bat virus; *Dioscorea* bacilliform virus

DBW desirable body weight; desired breast width

dBW decibels above 1 watt

DBZ dibenzazepine

DC daily census; data communication; data conversion; decrease; deep compartment; defining characteristic; dendritic cell; dendritic core; Dental Corps; deoxycholate; descending colon; dextran charcoal; diagnostic center; diagnostic cluster; diagnostic code; diagonal conjugate; differentiated cell; diffusion capacity; digit copying; digital computer; dilatation and curettage; dilation catheter; diphenylcyanoarsine; direct Coombs [test]; direct current; discharge, discharged; discontinue, discontinued; distal colon; distocervical; Doctor of Chiropractic; donor cells; dopachrome; dorsal column; dressing change; duodenal cap; Dupuytren contracture; duty cycle; dyskeratosis congenita; electric defibrillator using direct current discharge

D/C discharge; discontinue

D&C dilation and curettage; drugs and cosmetics

Dc critical dilution rate

D/c discontinue; discharge

DC65 Darvon compound 65

dC deoxycytidine

dc decrease; direct current; discharge; discontinue

DCA deoxycholate-citrate agar; deoxycholic acid; desoxycorticosterone acetate; dichloroacetate; directional color angiography; directional coronary atherectomy

DCα deoxycortisone acetate

DCABG double coronary artery bypass graft

DCAF dilated cardiomyopathy and atrial fibrillation

2D-CAG two-dimensional coronary angiography

DCAld dichloroacetaldehyde

DCB 3,4-dichlorobenzamil

DCBE double contrast barium enema

DCBF dynamic cardiac blood flow

DCbN deep cerebellar nucleus

DCC day care center; deleted in colorectal cancer; desquamated cornified cells; device communication controller; dextran-coated charcoal; diameter of cylindrical collimator; N,N'-dicyclohexylcarbodiimide; digital compact cassette; disaster control center; dorsal cell column; double concave; dysgenesis of corpus callosum

2DCC two-dimensional cross-correlation

DCCMP daunomycin, cyclocytidine, 6-mercaptopurine, and prednisolone

DC$_{CO_2}$ diffusing capacity for carbon dioxide

DCCT Diabetes Control and Complications Trial

DCCV direct current cardioversion

DCD developmental coordination disorder; differential current density; Diploma in Chest Diseases; disorders of cortical development; donation (after) cardiac death; dynamic cooling device

D/c'd, dc'd discontinued

D/CDK D-type cyclin-dependent kinase

DCE desmosterol-to-cholesterol enzyme; distributed computing environment; dynamic contrast enhanced

DCE-MRI dynamic contrast-enhanced magnetic resonance imaging

DCET dicarboxyethoxythiamine

DCF 2′-deoxycoformycin; dichlorofluorescein; direct centrifugal flotation; dopachrome conversion factor

DCFDA 2′,7′-dichlorofluorescein diacetate

DCFH dichlorofluorescein

DCFH-DA dichlorofluorescein diacetate

DCG dacryocystography; deoxycorticosterone glucoside; diagnosis cost-related group; disodium cromoglycate; dynamic electrocardiography

DCGE denaturation gradient gel electrophoresis

DCH delayed cutaneous hypersensitivity; Diploma in Child Health

DCh Doctor of Surgery [L. *Doctor Chirurgiae*]

DCHA docosahexaenoic acid

DCHEB dichlorohexafluorobutane

DCHN dicyclohexylamine nitrite

DChO Doctor of Ophthalmic Surgery

DCI dichloroisoprenaline; dichloroisoproterenol; digital cardiac imaging; Doppler color imaging; duplicate coverage inquiry

DCIA deep circumflex iliac artery

DCIEM Defense and Civil Institute for Environmental Medicine

DCIM digital camera images

DCIP dichlorophenolindophenol

DCIS ductal carcinoma in situ

DCK, dCK deoxycytidine kinase

DCL data control language; dicloxacillin; diffuse/disseminated cutaneous leishmaniasis; digital case library

DCLHb diaspirin cross-linked hemoglobin

DCLS deoxycholate citrate lactose saccharose

DCM dichloromethane; dichloromethotrexate; dilated cardiomyopathy; Doctor of Comparative Medicine; dyssynergia cerebellaris myoclonica

DCMADS District of Columbia Metropolitan Area Drug Study

DCML dorsal column medial lemniscus

3D-CMM three-dimensional coordinate measuring machine

DCMP daunomycin, cytosine arabinoside, 6-mercaptopurine, and prednisolone

dCMP deoxycytidine monophosphate

DCMS data creation and maintenance system

DCMT Doctor of Clinical Medicine of the Tropics

3D-CMT three-dimensional computed microtomography

DCMX 2,4-dichloro-*m*-xylenol

DCN data collection network; deep cerebral nucleus; delayed conditioned necrosis; depressed, cognitively normal; document control number; dorsal cochlear nucleus; dorsal column nucleus; dorsal cutaneous nerve

DCNB 1,2-dichloro-4-nitrobenzene

DCNU chlorozotocin

DCO death certificate only; Diploma of the College of Optics

D$_{CO}$ diffusing capacity for carbon monoxide

dCO$_2$ dissolved carbon dioxide

DCOG Diploma of the College of Obstetricians and Gynaecologists

DCOP distal coronary occlusion pressure

DCOR Dialysis Clinical Outcomes Revisited [trial]; dopachrome oxidoreductase

DCP des-γ-carboxy prothrombin; dicalcium phosphate; Diploma in Clinical Pathology; Diploma in Clinical Psychology; district community physician; dual-chamber pacemaker; dynamic compression plate

DCPA chlorthal-dimethyl

DCPP Disease Control Priorities Project

DCR dacryocystorhinostomy; data conversion receiver; digitally composited radiograph; direct cortical response

DCRT Division of Computer Research and Technology

3DCRT, 3D CRT three-dimensional conformal radiation therapy; three-dimensional conformal radiotherapy

DCS decompression sickness; dense canalicular system; diffuse cortical sclerosis; discharge summary; distal coronary sinus; dorsal column stimulation, dorsal column stimulator; dynamic condylar screw; dynamic contrast-enhanced subtraction; dynamic contrast-enhanced tomography; dynamic control system; dyskinetic cilia syndrome

dcSSc diffuse cutaneous systemic sclerosis

DCSWS dementia with continuing spike wave during slow-wave sleep

DCT detached ciliary tuft; direct Coombs test; discrete cosine transform; distal convoluted tubule; diurnal cortisol test; dynamic computed tomography

3DCT, 3D-CT three-dimensional computed tomography

DCTMA desoxycorticosterone trimethylacetate

dCTP deoxycytidine triphosphate

DCTPA desoxycorticosterone triphenylacetate

DCTS dynamic carpal tunnel syndrome

DCV diagnostic content validity; distribution of conduction velocities

D$_{2CV}$ Doppler 2-chamber view

D$_{4CV}$ Doppler 4-chamber view

DCVC dichlorovinyl cystine

DCVMN Developing Country Vaccine Manufacturers' Network

DCX double charge exchange

DCx double convex

DD dangerous drug; Darier disease; data definition; data dictionary; day of delivery; D-dimer; death domain; degenerated disk; degenerative disease; delusional disorder; depth dose; detrusor dyssynergia; developmental disability; diastrophic dysplasia; died of the disease; differential diagnosis; differential display; digest and discharge; digestive disorder; Di Guglielmo disease; discharge diagnosis; discharged dead; disk diameter; dog dander; double diffusion; double dummy; drug dependence; dry dressing; Duchenne dystrophy; Dupuytren disease

D&D design and development

D6D delta-6-desaturase

dd dideoxy

DDA Dangerous Drugs Act; dideoxyadenosine; digital differential analysis

ddA 2′,3′-dideoxyadenosine

DDase deoxyuridine diphosphatase

ddATP dideoxyadenosine triphosphate

DDAVP, dDAVP 1-deamino-8-d-arginine vasopressin

DDB dosimetric databank

DDBJ DNA Data Bank of Japan

DDC dangerous drug cabinet; dideoxycytidine; 3,5-diethoxycarbonyl-1,4-dihydrocollidine; diethyl-dithiocarbamate; dihydroxyphenylalanine decarboxylase; direct display console; diverticular disease of the colon

DDc double concave

ddC dideoxycytidine; zalcitabine

DDD AV universal [pacemaker]; Dali domain dictionary; defined daily dose; degenerative disk disease; dehydroxydinaphthyl disulfide; dense deposit disease; Denver dialysis disease; dichlorodiphenyl-dichloroethane; dihydroxydinaphthyl disulfide; dorsal dural deficiency; double dose delay; Dowling-Degos disease; dual mode, dual pacing, dual sensing

DDD CT double dose delay computed tomography

DDDD-CAT Drug Delivery Device Dispatch in Coronary Angioplasty Trial

DDDi infant defined daily dose

DDE dichlorodiphenyldichloroethylene; dynamic data exchange

DDEB dominantly inherited dystrophic epidermolysis bullosa

DDF demographic data form; difficulty describing feelings

Δdf differences between degrees of freedom

ddF dideoxy fingerprinting

DDFP dodecafluoropentane

DDG deoxy-d-glucose

ddGTP dideoxyguanidine triphosphate

DDH developmental dysplasia of the hip; dihydrodiol dehydrogenase; Diploma in Dental Health; dissociated double hypertropia

ddH$_2$O double-distilled water

DDI dideoxyinosine; Division of Drug Information; dynamic data icon

ddI didanoside; dideoxyinosine

DDIB Disease Detection Information Bureau

DDKase deoxynucleoside diphosphate kinase

DDL data definition language

DDM differential diagnosis manager; Diploma in Dermatological Medicine; Doctor in Dental Medicine; Dyke-Davidoff-Masson [syndrome]

DDMR dam-directed mismatch repair

DDNA Developmental Disabilities Nurses Association

dDNA denatured deoxyribonucleic acid

DDNTP, ddNTP dideoxynucleotide triphosphate

DDO Diploma in Dental Orthopaedics

DDP cisplatin; density-dependent phosphoprotein; difficult denture patient; digital data processing; distributed data processing

DDPA Delta Dental Plans Association

DD-PCR, DDPCR differential display polymerase chain reaction

DDQ database directed query

2D DQFC NMR two-dimensional double quantum filtered correction nuclear magnetic resonance spectroscopy

DDR diastolic descent rate; Diploma in Diagnostic Radiology; DNA damage response; double data rate

DDRB Doctors' and Dentists' Review Body

DDRP DNA damage-responsive protein

DDRT diseases, disorders, and related topics

DDS damaged disk syndrome; dapsone; data definition structure; dendrodendritic synaptosome; dental distress syndrome; Denys-Drash syndrome; depressed DNA synthesis; dialysis disequilibrium syndrome; diaminodiphenylsulfone; directional Doppler sonography; Director of Dental Services;

dirty data set; disability determination service; Disease-Disability Scale; Doctor of Dental Surgery; dodecyl sulfate; double decidual sac; dystrophy-dystocia syndrome
DDSc Doctor of Dental Science
DDSI digital damage severity index
DDSO diaminodiphenylsulfoxide
DDSS Defense Dental Standard System; diagnostic decision support system; double decidual sac sign
DDST Denver Developmental Screening Test
DDST-R Denver Developmental Screening Test-Revised
DDT diastolic deceleration time; dichlorodiphenyltrichloroethane; ductus deferens tumor; dynamic data table
Ddt deceleration time
DDTC diethyldithiocarbamate
DDTN dideoxy-didehydrothymidine
ddTTP dideoxythymidine triphosphate
DDU data deficit unit; data definition unit; dermo-distortive urticaria; duplex Doppler ultrasound
dDVH differential dose-volume histogram
DDW Digestive Diseases Week
D/DW dextrose in distilled water
D 5% DW 5% dextrose in distilled water
DDx differential diagnosis
DE data encoder; dendritic expansion; deprived eye; design effect; diagnostic error; dialysis encephalopathy; diesel exhaust; digestive energy; direct excitation; donor egg; dose equivalent; dream element; drug evaluation; duodenal exclusion; duration of ejection
D&E diet and elimination; dilation and evacuation
D=E dates equal to examination
2DE two-dimensional echocardiography
3DE three-dimensional echocardiography
dE differential in energy
DEA dehydroepiandrosterone; diethanolamine; Drug Enforcement Administration
DEAD Dying Experience at Dartmouth
DEAE diethylaminoethyl
DEAE-D diethylaminoethyl dextran
DEAFF detection of early antigen fluorescent foci
DEALE declining exponential approximation of life expectancy
DEATH Dying Experience at the Hitchcock
DEB diepoxybutane; diethylbutanediol; Division of Environmental Biology; doxorubicin-eluting beads; drug-eluting balloon; dystrophic epidermolysis bullosa
deb debridement

DEBA diethylbarbituric acid
DEBATE Doppler Endpoints Balloon Angioplasty Trial, Europe
debil debilitation
DEBRA Dystrophic Epidermolysis Bullosa Research Association
DEBS dominant epidermolysis bullosa simplex
DEC decrease; deoxycholate citrate; diagnostic episode cluster; diethylcarbamazine; dynamic environmental conditioning
Dec, dec decant
dec deceased; deciduous; decimal; decompose, decomposition; decrease, decreased
DECA Demographic and Economic Characteristics of the Aged
decd deceased
DECG differentiated electrocardiogram
decoct decoction
DECODE Diabetes Epidemiology, Collaborative Analysis of Diagnostic Criteria in Europe
DECOMP decomposition
decomp decompensation; decompose, decomposition
decr decrease, decreased
D-ECST Dutch-European Cerebral Sinus Thrombosis [trial]
DECU decubitus
decub lying down [L. *decubitus*]
DED date of expected delivery; death effector domain [cell]; defined exposure dose; delayed erythema dose
DEE daily energy expenditure
DEEDS Data Elements for Emergency Department Systems
DEEG depth electroencephalogram/electroencephalography
DEER Diet and Exercise in Elevated Risk [trial]
DEERS Defense Enrollment Eligibility Reporting System
DEET *N,N*-diethyl-*m*-toluamide
DEF decayed primary teeth requiring filling, decayed primary teeth requiring extraction, and primary teeth successfully filled; dose-effect factor
def defecation; deferred; deficiency, deficient
DEFIANT Doppler Flow and Echocardiography in Functional Cardiac Insufficiency Assessment of Nisoldipine Therapy [trial]
defib defibrillation
DEFIBRILAT Defibrillator as Bridge to Later Transplantation [study]
defic deficiency, deficient
DEFN Danubian endemic familial nephropathy

DEF$_{NT}$ dose-effect factor for normal tissue

deform deformed, deformity

DEFT direct epifluorescent filter technique

DEF$_T$ dose-effect factor for tumor

DEFV deceleration of early flow velocity

DEG degenerin; diagnostic evaluation group; diethylene glycol

Deg, deg degeneration, degenerative; degree

degen degeneration, degenerative

DEH dysplasia epiphysealis hemimelica

DEHP di(2-ethylhexyl)phthalate

DEHR distributed electronic health record

DEHS Division of Emergency Health Services

DEHT developmental hand function test

dehyd dehydrated, dehydration

DEI dual-energy indices

DEJ, dej dentinoenamel junction; dermo-epidermal junction

del deletion; delivery; delusion

DELFIA dissociated enhanced lanthanide fluoroimmunoassay

deliq deliquescence, deliquescent

DELIRIUM drugs, electrolytes, low temperature, lunacy-intoxication and intracranial processes, retention of urine or feces, infection, unfamiliar surroundings, myocardial infarction [causes of delirium]

Delt deltoid

DELTA Descriptive Language for Taxonomy; Dietary Effects on Lipoproteins and Thrombogenic Activity

DEM Demerol; diethylmaleate; diffusion equation method

Dem Demerol

DEMO dynamic essential modeling

demo demonstrate, demonstration

DEN denervation; dengue; dermatitis exfoliativa neonatorum; Device Experience Network; diethylnitrosamine

denat denatured

DENT Dental Exposure Normalization Technique

Dent, dent dental; dentist, dentistry; dentition

DENTALPROJ Dental Research Projects

DENV dengue virus

DEP depression emulation program; dielectrophoresis; diethylpropanediol; dilution end point

dep dependent; deposit

DEPA diethylene phosphoramide

DEPC diethyl pyrocarbonate

depr depressed, depression

DEPS distal effective potassium secretion

DEP ST SEG depressed ST segment

DEPT distortionless enhancement by polarization transfer

dept department

DEQ Depression Experiences Questionnaire

DER disulfiram-ethanol reaction; dual energy radiography

DeR degeneration reaction

der derivative

DERI Diabetes Epidemiology Research International [study]

deriv derivative, derived

Derm, derm dermatitis; dermatologic, dermatologist, dermatology; dermatome

DERS dependent error regression smoothing

DES Danish Enoxaparin Study; data encryption standard; dementia rating scale; dermal-epidermal separation; descendant; desmin; dialysis encephalopathy syndrome; diethylstilbestrol; diffuse esophageal spasm; disequilibrium syndrome; dissociative experience scale; doctor's emergency service; drug-eluting stent

DES$_1$ descendant, first level in hierarchy

desat desaturated

desc descendant; descending

DescAo descending aorta

DESIRE Debulking and Stenting in Restenosis Elimination [trial]

desq desquamation

DESS double-echo steady state

DEST Denver Eye Screening Test; dichotic environmental sounds test; differentially expressed sequence tag

DESTINI Doppler Endpoint Stent International Investigation; Duke University Clinical Cardiology Study Elective Stent Trial: A Cost Containment Initiative

DeSyGNER Decision Systems Group Nucleus of Extensible Resources

DET diethyltryptamine; dipyridamole echo-cardiography test; double embryo transfer

DETC diethyldithiocarbamate

Det-6 detroid-6

determ determination, determined

detn detention

detox detoxification

DEUC direct electronic urethrocystometry

DEV deviant, deviation; duck embryo vaccine; duck embryo virus

dev development; deviation

devel development

DevPd developmental pediatrics

DEW diagnostic encyclopedia workstation

DEX blood sugar; dexamethasone

Dex dextrose

dex dexterity; dextrorotatory; right [L. *dexter*]

DEXA dual-energy x-ray absorptiometry

DF decapacitation factor; decontamination factor; deferoxamine; defibrillation; deficiency factor; defined flora; degree of freedom; diabetic father; dietary fibers; digital fluoroscopy; diphase fix; discriminant function; disseminated foci; distribution factor; dominant frequency; dorsiflexion; dysgonic fermenter

D&F Diamond and Forrester [analysis]

Df *Dermatophagoides farinae;* discrimination factor; duodenal fluid

df degrees of freedom

DF-2 dysgonic fermenter 2 [obsolete]

DFA detrended fluctuation analysis; direct fluorescent antibody; discriminant function analysis; dorsiflexion angle; dorsiflexion assistance

DFB dinitrofluorobenzene; dysfunctional bleeding

DFC developmental field complex; dry-filled capsule

DFD data flow diagram; defined formula diets; developmental field defect; diisopropyl phosphorofluoridate

DFDB demineralized freeze-dried bone

dFdCTP difluorodeoxycytidine triphosphate

DFDT difluoro-diphenyl-trichloroethane

DfDx, Df/Dx, df/dx differential diagnosis

DFE diffuse fasciitis with eosinophilia; distal femoral epiphysis

DFECT dense fibroelastic connective tissue

3DFEM three-dimensional finite element method

2D-FFT two-dimensional fast Fourier transform

DFG direct forward gaze

DFHom Diploma of the Faculty of Homeopathy

DFHS Department of Family and Health Services

DFI disease-free interval; dye fluorescence index

DFIB defibrillation

DFL digital film library

DFM decreased fetal movement

DFMC daily fetal movement count

DFMO difluoromethylornithine

DFMR daily fetal movement record

DFN distal femoral nail

DFO, DFOM deferoxamine

DFP deferiprone; diastolic filling period; diisopropyl-fluorophosphate

DF^{32}P radiolabeled diisopropylfluorophosphate

DFPP double-filtration plasmapheresis

DFR designated family respondent; diabetic floor routine; digital fluororadiography; distal femoral replacement

DFS disease-free survival; distraction-flexion staging; distributed file system

DFSP dermatofibrosarcoma protuberans

DFT defibrillation threshold; dementia of frontal type; diagnostic function test; discrete Fourier transform

DFT$_3$ dialyzable fraction of triiodothyronine

DFT$_4$ dialyzable fraction of thryoxine

2DFT two-dimensional Fourier transform

3DFT three-dimensional Fourier transform

DFTS digital flashing tomosynthesis

DFU dead fetus in utero; diabetic foot ulcer; dideoxyfluorouridine

DFV diarrhea with fever and vomiting

DFW dog fight wounds [veterinary medicine]

DG data gathering; dentate gyrus; deoxyglucose; desmoglein; diacylglycerol; diagnosis; diastolic gallop; DiGeorge [anomaly, syndrome]; diglyceride; distogingival

2DG 2-deoxy-d-glucose

Dg dentate gyrus

dg decigram; diagnosis

DGA DiGeorge anomaly

DGAC Dietary Guidelines Advisory Committee

DGAP DNA-guided assembly of proteins

DGAT diacylglycerol transferase

DGAVP desglycinamide-9-[Arg-8] vasopressin

DGBG dimethylglyoxal bisguanylhydrazone

DGC density gradient centrifugation

DGCR DiGeorge chromosome region; DiGeorge critical region

DGE delayed gastric emptying; diglycidyl ether

dge drainage

2D-GEMS two-dimensional gel electrophoresis mass spectrometry

DGF duct growth factor

DGGE denaturing gradient gel electrophoresis

DGI dentinogenesis imperfecta; disseminated gonococcal infection

dGI dorsal giant interneuron

DGIM Division of General Internal Medicine

DGKV Dera Ghazi Khan virus

DGLA dihomo-gamma-linolenic acid

dGMP deoxyguanosine monophosphate

DGMS Division of General Medical Sciences

DGN diffuse glomerulonephritis

DGNA delayed gamma neutron activation

DGO Diploma in Gynaecology and Obstetrics

DGP 2,3-diglycerophosphate; Dutch General Practices Study; dynamic graciloplasty
DGPG diffuse proliferative glomerulonephritis
DGR duodenogastric reflux
DGS developmental Gerstmann syndrome; diabetic glomerulosclerosis; DiGeorge sequence; DiGeorge syndrome; disease guidance systems; dysplasia-gigantism syndrome
DGSCR DiGeorge syndrome critical region
DGSX X-linked dysplasia-gigantism syndrome
dGTP deoxyguanosine triphosphate
DGU uracil deoxyribonucleic acid glycosylase
DGV dextrose-gelatin-Veronal [buffer]
DG/VCF DiGeorge/velocardiofacial [syndrome]
DH daily habits; day hospital; dehydrocholate; dehydrogenase; delayed hypersensitivity; department of health; dermatitis herpetiformis; developmental history; diaphragmatic hernia; disseminated histoplasmosis; dominant hand; dorsal horn; drug history; ductal hyperplasia; Dunkin-Hartley [guinea pig]
D&H distributed and heterogeneous
D/H deuterium/hydrogen ratio
DHA dehydroacetic acid; dehydroascorbic acid; dehydroepiandrosterone; dihydroacetic acid; dihydroxyacetone; district health authority
DHAD mitoxantrone hydrochloride
DHAOS Dutch Hypertension and Offspring Study
DHAP dihydroxyacetone phosphate
DHAP-AT dihydroxyacetone phosphate acyltransferase
DHAS dehydroandrostenedione
DHB dihydroxybenzoate; duck hepatitis B
DHBE dihydroxybutyl ether
DHBG dihydroxybutyl guanine
DHBS dihydrobiopterin synthetase
DHBV duck hepatitis B virus
DHC dehydrocholate; dehydrocholesterol; delivery of health care
DHCA deep hypothermia and circulatory arrest; dihydroxycholestanoic acid
DHCC dehydroxycholecalciferol
DHCCP Department of Health and Social Security Hypertension Care Computing Project
DHCP decentralized/distributed hospital computer program; dental health care provider; dynamic host configuration protocol
DHCS Department of Health and Community Services

DHD district health department
DH-DATA Department of Health Library Database
DHE dihematoporphyrin ether; dihydroergocryptine; dihydroergotamine; distributed health care environment
DHEA dehydroepiandrosterone
DHEAS, DHEA-S dehydroepiandrosterone sulfate
DHEC dihydroergocryptine
DHES Division of Health Examination Statistics
DHESN dihydroergosine
DHEW Department of Health, Education, and Welfare
DHF dengue hemorrhagic fever; dihydrofolate; dorsihyperflexion
DHF/DSS dengue hemorrhagic fever/dengue shock syndrome
DHFR dihydrofolate reductase
DHFRase dihydrofolate reductase
DHFRP dihydrofolate reductase pseudogene
DHFS Diet-Heart Feasibility Study
DHg Doctor of Hygiene
DHGG deaggregated human gammaglobulin
DHHS Department of Health and Human Services
DHI Dental Health International; dihydroxyindole
DHIA dehydroisoandrosterol
DHIAP Defense Healthcare Information Assurance Program
DHIC dihydroisocodeine
DHICA 5,6-dihydroxyindole-2-carboxylic acid
DHIS distributed health care information system; district health information system; Duke Hospital Information System
DHL diffuse histiocytic lymphoma
DHLA haloalkane dehalogenase
DHLD dihydrolipoamide dehydrogenase
DHM dihydromorphine
DHMA 3,4-dihydroxymandelic acid
DHMO dental health maintenance organization
DHO dihydro-orotate
dH₂O distilled water
DHODH dihydro-orotate dehydrogenase
DHOV Dhori virus
DHP dehydrogenated polymer; dihydroprogesterone; 1,4-dihydropyridine; dual heuristic programming
DHPA dihydroxypropyl adenine
DHPCCB dihydropyrimidine calcium channel blocker
DHPDH dihydropyrimidine dehydrogenase

DHPG dihydroxyphenylglycol; dihydroxypropoxymethylguanine

DHPR dihydropteridine reductase

DHR delayed hypersensitivity reaction; Department of Human Resources; disk−large homologous region

DHS dehydrated hereditary stomatocytosis; delayed hypersensitivity; demographic and health survey; diabetic hyperosmolar state; document handling system; duration of hospital stay; dynamic hip screw

D-5-HS 5% dextrose in Harman's solution

DHSM dihydrostreptomycin

DHSS Department of Health and Social Security; dihydrostreptomycin sulfate

DHT dehydrotestosterone; dihydroergotoxine; dihydrotachysterol; dihydrotestosterone; dihydrothymine; dihydroxytryptamine; discrete Hartley transform

5,7-DHT 5,7-dihydroxytryptamine

DHTP dihydrotestosterone propionate

DHTR dihydrotestosterone receptor

DHU dihydroxyuracil

DHUA Division of Health and Utilization Analysis

DHV duck hepatitis virus

DHWD decompressive hemicraniectomy with duraplasty

DHy, DHyg Doctor of Hygiene

DHZ dihydralazine

DI date interviewed; date of injury; defective interfering [particle]; dental index; dental informatics; dentinogenesis imperfecta; deoxyribonucleic acid index; depression inventory; desorption ionization; deterioration index; detrusor instability; diabetes insipidus; diagnostic imaging; dialyzed iron; diastolic interval; digital imaging [technologist]; disability insurance; dispensing information; distoincisal; document index; donor insemination; dorsoiliac; dose intensity; double indemnity; drug information; drug injection; drug interactions; duct injection; dyskaryosis index

3DI developmental, dimensional, and diagnostic interview; three-dimensional imaging

5′DI 5′-deiodinase

DIA depolarization-induced automaticity; diabetes; diaphorase; diazepam; Drug Information Association

DiA Diego antigen

dia diakinesis; diathermy

diab diabetes, diabetic

DIACOMP Diabetes Complications [study]

DiaComp diabetes computer-aided [management]

DIAG diagnostic procedure

Diag diagnosis

diag diagnosis; diagonal; diagram

diam diameter

DIAMOND Danish Investigation of Arrhythmia and Mortality on Dofetilide

DIAMOND-CHF Danish Investigation of Arrhythmia and Mortality on Dofetilide in Congestive Heart Failure

DIAMOND-MI Danish Investigation of Arrhythmia and Mortality on Dofetilide in Myocardial Infarction

diaph diaphragm

dias diastole, diastolic

diath diathermy

DIB diagnostic interview for borderlines; difficulty in breathing; disability insurance benefits; dot immunobinding; duodenoileal bypass

DIBAL diisobutylaluminum

diBr-HQ 5,7-dibromo-8-hydroxy-quinidine

DIC dicarbazine; differential interference contrast microscopy; diffuse intravascular coagulation; direct isotope cystography; disseminated intravascular coagulation; drip infusion cholangiography; drug information center

dic dicentric

DICA diagnostic interview of children and adolescents

DICD death in intercurrent disease; dispersion-induced circular dichroism

DICO diffusing capacity of carbon monoxide

DICOM Digital Imaging and Communications in Medicine

DICOM-RT digital image communications in medicine−radiation therapy

DICPM distributed information, computation, and process management

DID dead of intercurrent disease; Dictionary of Drugs; dissociative identity disorder; double immunodiffusion

DIDA diethyl iminodiacetic acid

DIDD dense intramembranous deposit disease

DiDi Diltiazem in Dilated Cardiomyopathy [trial]

DIDMOA diabetes insipidus, diabetes mellitus, optic atrophy [syndrome]

DIDMOAD diabetes insipidus, diabetes mellitus, optic atrophy, deafness [syndrome]

DIDS 4,4′diisothiocyanostilbene-2,2-disulfonate

DIE died in emergency department; difference in electronegativity

DIEA diisopropylethylamine

diEMG diaphragmatic electromyography

DIEP deep inferior epigastric perforator

DIET Dietary Intervention: Evaluation of Technology [study]

DIEV *Dicentrarchus labrax* encephalitis virus

DIF difficulty identifying feelings; diffuse interstitial fibrosis; direct immunofluorescence; dose increase factor

DIFF, diff difference, differential; diffusion

diff diagn differential diagnosis

diff Dx differential diagnosis

DIFP diffuse interstitial fibrosing pneumonitis; diisopropyl fluorophosphonate

dif-PIPE diffuse persistent interstitial pulmonary emphysema

DIG digitalis; Digitalis Investigation Group; digoxigenin; digoxin; drug-induced galactorrhea

dig digitalis; digoxigenin; digoxin

DIGAF Digoxin in Atrial Fibrillation [study]

DIGAMI Diabetes Mellitus, Insulin Glucose Infusion in Acute Myocardial Infarction [study]

DIH digoxin-induced hyperkalemia; Diploma in Industrial Health

DIHE drug-induced hepatic encephalopathy

diHETE dihydroxyeicosatetraenoic acid

DIHPPA diiodohydroxyphenylpyruvic acid

DII dynamic invocation interface

D$_{ii}$ input delay

DiIV *Diadegma interruptum* ichnovirus

D$_{ij}$ transfer delay

DIL Dilantin; drug-induced lupus

Dil Dilantin; dilation, dilated; drug-induced lupus

dil dilute, diluted, dilution

dilat dilation

DILCACOMP Diltiazem Captopril Comparative Study

DILD diffuse infiltrative lung disease; diffuse interstitial lung disease

DILDURANG Diltiazem Duration in Angina [study]

DILE drug-induced lupus erythematosus

DILI drug-induced liver injury

DILIN Drug-Induced Liver Injury Network

DILPLACOMP Diltiazem Placebo Comparative Trial

DILS diffuse infiltrative lymphocytosis syndrome

DIM divalent ion metabolism; domain information model; median infective dose [L. *dosis infectionis media*]

dim dimension; diminished

DIMFP differential inverse mean free path

DIMIT 3,5-dimethyl-3′-isopropyl-1-thyronine

DIMM dual in-line memory module

DIMOAD diabetes insipidus, diabetes mellitus, optic atrophy, deafness

DIMS disorder in initiating and maintaining sleep

DIMSE DICOM message service element

DIMT Dutch Ibopamine Multicenter Trial

DIN damage inducible; digital imaging network; dissolved inorganic nitrogen; ductal intraepithelial neoplasia

din damage inducible

DIN/PACS digital imaging network/picture archiving communications system

DIOS distal intestinal obstruction syndrome

DIP desquamative interstitial pneumonitis; diffuse interstitial pneumonitis; digital imaging processing; diisopropylamine; diisopropyl phosphate; diphtheria; dissolved inorganic phosphate; distal interphalangeal; drip infusion pyelogram; dual-in-line package; dynamic integral proctography

Dip diplomate

dip diploid; diplotene

DIPA diisopropylamine

DIPAP Dipyridamole in Peripheral Arteriopathy [study]

DipBact Diploma in Bacteriology

DIPC diffuse interstitial pulmonary calcification

DipChem Diploma in Chemistry

DipClinPath Diploma in Clinical Pathology

DIPF diffuse interstitial pulmonary fibrosis; diisopropylphosphofluoridate

DIPG diffuse intrinsic pontine glioma

diph diphtheria

diph-tet diphtheria-tetanus [toxoid]

diph-tox AP alum precipitated diphtheria toxoid

DIPI defective interfering particle induction

DIPJ distal interphalangeal joint

DIPS-PCR detection of integrated papillomavirus sequences by polymerase chain reaction

Dipy dipyridamole

DIR double inversion recovery; double isomorphous replacement

Dir, dir direction, directions; director

DIRD drug-induced renal disease

DIRECT Diabetes Intervention: Reaching and Educating Communities Together; Direct Myocardial Revascularization in Regeneration of Endomyocardial Channels Trial

DIRLINE Directory of Information Resources Online

DIRS Dutch Invasive Reperfusion Study

DIS Department of Information Services; departmental information system; Diagnostic

Interview Schedule; Diagnostic Interview Survey; draft international standard; drug information system

DI-S debris index, simplified

dis disability, disabled; disease; dislocation; distal; distance

DISC Diagnostic Interview Schedule for Children; Dietary Intervention Study in Children; digital interchange standards for cardiology

disc discontinue

disch discharge, discharged

DISC-HSV disabled infectious single-cycle herpes simplex virus

DISCO diagnostic interview for social and communication disorders

dis eval disability evaluation

DISF-SR Derogatis Interview for Sexual Functioning-Short Report

DISH Dietary Intervention Study of Hypertension; diffuse idiopathic skeletal hyperostosis; disseminated idiopathic skeletal hyperostosis

DISI dorsal intercalated segment instability

DISIDA diisopropyl iminodiacetic acid

disinfect disinfection

disl, disloc dislocated, dislocation

disod disodium

disp dispensary, dispense

DISS disease or syndrome; distributed image spreadsheet

diss dissolve, dissolved

dissem disseminated, dissemination

DIST Dutch Iliac Stent Trial

dist distal; distance; distill, distillation, distilled; distribution; disturbance, disturbed

DISTRESS Dispatch Stent Restenosis Study

DIT deferoxamine infusion test; defining issues test; diet-induced thermogenesis; diiodotyrosine; drug-induced thrombocytopenia

dit dictyate

dITP deoxyinosine triphosphate

D$_{iv}$ intravenous dose

div divergence, divergent; divide, divided, division

DIVBC disseminated intravascular blood coagulation

DIVC disseminated intravascular coagulation

DJ duodenal juice

DJD degenerative joint disease

DJJ duodenojejunal junction

DJOA dominant juvenile optic atrophy

DJS Dubin-Johnson syndrome

DK dark; decay; diabetic ketoacidosis; diet kitchen; diseased kidney; dog kidney [cells]

dk deka

dk- deka- [10^1]

DKA diabetic ketoacidosis

DKB deep knee bends

DKC dyskeratosis congenita

dkg dekagram

DKI dextrose potassium insulin

DKIE decontaminating kit, individual equipment

dkL, dkl decaliter

dkm dekameter

DKP dikalium phosphate

DKS Damus-Kaye-Stansel [anastomosis]

DKTC dog kidney tissue culture

DKV deer kidney virus

DL danger list; data language; deep lobe; De Lee [catheter]; description language; description logic; developmental level; diagnostic laparoscopy; difference limen; digital library; dipole layer; direct laryngoscopy; disabled list; dissimilarity level; distolingual; equimolecular mixture of the dextrorotatory and levorotatory enantiomorphs; lethal dose; lung diffusion

DL, D-L Donath-Landsteiner [antibody]

D$_L$ diffusing capacity of the lungs

dL, dl deciliter

DLA dermatolymphangioadenitis

D$_{LA}$ diameter of left atrium

DLa distolabial

DLaI distolabioincisal

DLaP distolabiopulpal

DLB dementia with Lewy body

DL&B direct laryngoscopy and bronchoscopy

DLBD diffuse Lewy body disease

DLC Dental Laboratory Conference; differential leukocyte count; downloadable content; dual-lumen catheter

DLCL diffuse large cell lymphoma

DLCO, DL$_{CO}$ carbon monoxide diffusion in the lung

DL$_{CO_2}$ carbon dioxide diffusion in the lungs

DL$_{CO}{}^{SB}$ single-breath carbon monoxide diffusing capacity of the lungs

DL$_{CO}{}^{SS}$ steady-state carbon monoxide diffusing capacity of the lungs

DLD dihydrolipoamide dehydrogenase

dld d-lactate dehydrogenase [gene]

D-LDH d-lactate dehydrogenase

DLE deep lamellar endothelial [keratoplasty transplant surgery]; delayed light emission; dialyzable leukocyte extract; discoid lupus erythematosus; disseminated lupus erythematosus

D$_1$LE diagonal 1 lower extremity

D$_2$LE diagonal 2 lower extremity

DLF Disabled Living Foundation; dorsolateral funiculus

DLG distolingual groove
Dlg, dlg disk large
Dlg-R disk large, related
DLH domestic long-haired cat [veterinary medicine]
DLI Digital Libraries Initiative; distolinguoincisal; donor lymphocyte infusion; double-label index
DLIS digoxin-like immunoreactive substance
DLK diffuse lamellar keratitis
DLL dihomo-gamma-linoleic acid; dynamic link library
DLLI dulcitol lysine lactose iron
DLM dipole localization method
DLMD Duchenne-like muscular dystrophy
DLMO dim light melatonin onset
DLMP date of last menstrual period
DLN draining lymph nodes
DLNMP date of last normal menstrual period
DLO Diploma in Laryngology and Otology; distolinguo-occlusal
Dl$_{O_2}$ diffusing capacity of the lungs for oxygen
DLP delipidized serum protein; direct linear plotting; dislocation of patella; distolinguopulpal; dose length product; dysharmonic luteal phase
DLPFC dorsolateral prefrontal cortex
DLR digital luminescence radiography
D/LR dextrose in lactated Ringer solution
D$_5$LR dextrose in 5% lactated Ringer solution
DLST dihydrolipoamide *S*-succinyltransferase
DLT digital library technology; dihydroepiandrosterone loading test; direct linear transformation; dose-limiting toxicity; double-lumen endotracheal tube; double lung transplantation
DLV defective leukemia virus; delavirdine
DLW dry lung weight
DM defined medium; dermatomyositis; Descemet's membrane; differentiation medium; design manager; dextromaltose; dextromethorphan; diabetes mellitus; diabetic mother; diastolic murmur; distal metastases; dopamine; dorsomedial; double minute; duodenal mucosa; dry matter; dystrophia myotonica; phenarsazine chloride [diphenylaminechloroarsine]
D$_M$ membrane component of diffusion
dm decimeter; diabetes mellitus; dorsomedial
dm^2 square decimeter
dm^3 cubic decimeter

DMA department of medical assistance; Dietary Managers Association; dimethylamine; dimethylaniline; dimethylarginine; dimethylarsinic acid; direct memory access; director of medical affairs; distributed multiple analysis
dMA dominant motor area
DMAA dimethylarsinic acid; Disease Management Association of America
DMAB dimethylaminobenzaldehyde
DMAC *N,N*-dimethylacetamide; disseminated *Mycobacterium avium* complex
DMAD dimethylaminodiphosphate
DMAE dimethylaminoethanol
DMAEM, DMAEMA *N,N'*-dimethylaminoethyl methacrylate
DMAP dimethylaminophenol; dimethylaminopyridine
DMAPN dimethylaminopropionitrile
DMARD disease-modifying antirheumatic drug
D$_{max}$ maximum denaturation; maximum diameter; maximum dose
DMB diffuse microvascular bleeding; diffusional microburet
DMBA 7,12-dimethylbenz[a]anthracene
DMC demeclocycline; di(*p*-chlorophenyl)methylcarbinol; direct microscopic count; duration of muscle contraction; Dyggve-Melchior-Clausen [syndrome]
DMCC direct microscopic clump count
DMCL diffuse mixed cell lymphoma; dimethylclomipramine
DMCM methyl-6,7-dimethoxy-4-ethyl-beta-carboline-3-carboxylate
DMCO Disease Management and Clinical Outcomes
DMCS Diagnostic Marker Cooperative Study
DMCT, DMCTC dimethylchlortetracycline
DMD disease-modifying drug; Doctor of Dental Medicine; Duchenne muscular dystrophy; dystonia musculorum deformans
DMD/BMD Duchenne/Becker muscular dystrophy
DMDC 2'-deoxy-2'-methylidenecytidine; dimethyldithiocarbamate
DMDD disruptive mood dysregulation disorder
DMDT dimethoxydiphenyl trichloroethane
DMDZ desmethyldiazepam
DME degenerative myoclonus epilepsy; dimethyl diester; dimethyl ether; diphasic meningoencephalitis; direct medical education; director of medical education; Division of Medical Education; dropping mercury

electrode; drug-metabolizing enzyme; Dulbecco modified Eagle [medium]; durable medical equipment

DMEM Dulbecco modified Eagle medium

DMF decayed, missing, and filled [teeth]; dimethyl fluoride; diphasic milk fever; *N,N*-dimethylformamide

DmFb dermal fibroblast

DMFS decayed, missing, filled surfaces

DMFT decayed, missing, and filled teeth

DMG dimethylglycine

DMGBL dimethyl-gammabutyrolactone

DMGT deoxyribonucleic acid-mediated gene transfer

DMH 1,2-dimethylhydrazine; diffuse mesangial hypercellularity; domestic medium-haired cat [veterinary medicine]; dorsal medial hypothalamic [nucleus]

DMHD dimenhydrinate

DMI Defense Mechanism Inventory; Diagnostic Medical Instruments; diaphragmatic myocardial infarction; direct migration inhibition

DMID Division of Microbiology and Infectious Diseases

DMIM Defense Medical Information Management

D$_{min}$ minimum diameter

dmin double minute

DMIS Defense Medical Information System

DMJ Diploma in Medical Jurisprudence

DMKA diabetes mellitus ketoacidosis

DMKase deoxynucleoside monophosphate kinase

DML data manipulation language; distal motor latency

DMLP Dutch Medical Language Processor

DMM dimethylmyleran; disproportionate micromelia

DMN desmuslin; dimethylnitrosamine; dorsal motor nucleus; dysplastic melanocytic nevus

DMNA dimethylnitrosamine

DMNL dorsomedial hypothalamic nucleus lesion

DMNX dorsal motor nucleus of the vagus nerve

DMO 5,5-dimethyl-2,4-oxazolidinedione (dimethadione)

D$_{mo2}$ membrane diffusing capacity for oxygen

DMOA diabetes mellitus−optic atrophy [syndrome]

DMOD disease model

DMOOC diabetes mellitus out of control

DMP data map publication; diabetes mellitus program; diffuse mesangial proliferation; dimercaprol; dimethylphthalate

DMPA depot medroxyprogesterone acetate

DMPC dimyristyl phosphatidyl choline

DMPE, DMPEA 3,4-dimethoxyphenylethylamine

DMPP dimethylphenylpiperazinium

DMPS dysmyelopoietic syndrome

DMPTU dimethylphenylthiourea

DMR depolarizing muscle relaxant; differentially methylated region; Diploma in Medical Radiology; direct myocardial revascularization; distributed medical record; dose monitoring rate

DM-R decayed plus missing teeth, minus replaced teeth

DMRD Diploma in Medical Radiodiagnosis

DMRE Diploma in Medical Radiology and Electrology

DMRF dorsal medullary reticular formation

dMRI diffusion tensor magnetic resonance imaging

3D-MRI three-dimensional magnetic resonance imaging

DMRT Diploma in Medical Radiotherapy

DMS delayed match to sample; delayed microembolism syndrome; demarcation membrane system; department of medicine and surgery; dermatomyositis; diagnostic medical sonographer; diffuse mesangial sclerosis; dimethylsulfate; dimethylsulfoxide; Doctor of Medical Science; drug misuse statistics; dysmyelopoietic syndrome

DMSA dimercaptosuccinic acid; dimethylsuccinic acid

DMSO dimethyl sulfoxide

DMSS data mining surveillance system

DMT [3-(2-dimethylamino)ethyl] indole; dermatophytosis; disease-modifying therapy; District Management Team; Doctor of Medical Technology; dynamometer muscle testing; *N,N*-dimethyltryptamine

DMTU dimethylthiourea

DMU dimethanolurea; dual method of use

DMV diurnal mood variations; Doctor of Veterinary Medicine; dorsal motor nucleus of the vagus nerve; dwarf mosaic virus

DMWP distal mean wave pressure

DN Deiter's nucleus; dextrose-nitrogen; diabetic neuropathy; dibucaine number; dicrotic notch; DiFrancesco-Noble [equation]; dinitrocresol; Diploma in Nursing; Diploma in Nutrition; District Nurse; do not [resuscitate]; Doctor of Nursing; dominant negative; duodenum

D/N dextrose/nitrogen ratio

D&N distance and near

Dn dekanem

dn decinem

DNA deoxyribonucleic acid; Dermatology Nurses Association; did not answer

DNA DSB DNA double-strand break

DNAP DNA phosphorus

DNA-PK DNA-protein kinase

DNAR do not attempt resuscitation

DNASE, DNAse, DNase deoxyribonuclease

DNB dinitrobenzene; Diplomate of the National Board [of Medical Examiners]; dorsal nonadrenergic bundle

DNBP dinitrobutylphenol

DNBS 2,4-dinitrobenzene sulfonate

DNC did not come; dinitrocarbanilide; dinitrocresol; disaster nursing chair

DNCB dinitrochlorobenzene

DNCM cytoplasmic membrane−associated DNA

DND died a natural death; Drugs for Neglected Diseases

DNE director of nursing education; Doctor of Nursing Education

DNET dysembryoplastic neuroepithelial tumor

DNF distinctive normal form system

DNFB dinitrofluorobenzene

DNH do not hospitalize

DNIC diffuse noxious inhibitory control

DNK did not keep

DNKA did not keep appointment

DNLL dorsal nucleus of lateral lemniscus

DNM descending necrotizing mediastinitis; dynamin

dNMP deoxynucleotide monophosphate

1D NMR one-dimensional nuclear magnetic resonance

2D NMR two-dimensional nuclear magnetic resonance

DNMS delayed nonmatch to sample; director of Naval Medical Services

DNMT DNA methyltransferase

Dnmt DNA methyltransferase gene

DNO district nursing officer

DNOC dinitroorthocresol

DNP deoxyribonucleoprotein; dinitrophenol; dinitropyrene; Doctor of Nursing Practice; dynamic nuclear polarization

2,4-DNP 2,4-dinitrophenol

DNPH dinitrophenylhydrazine

DNPM dinitrophenol-morphine

DNQX 6,7-dinitroquinoxaline-2,3-dione

DNR daunorubicin; do not resuscitate; dorsal nerve root

DNS deviated nasal septum; diaphragmatic nerve stimulation; did not show; Dietitians in Nutrition Support; director of nursing services; Doctor of Nursing Science; dysplastic nevus syndrome

D/NS dextrose in normal saline

D5NS 5% dextrose in normal saline [solution]

D$_5$NSS 5% dextrose in normal saline solution

DNT dermonecrotic toxin; did not test; 2,4-dinitrotoluene; dysembryoplastic neuroepithelial tumor

DNTM disseminated nontuberculous mycobacterial [infection]

dNTP deoxyribonucleoside triphosphate

DNTT terminal deoxynucleotidyltransferase

DNV densovirus, dorsal nucleus of vagus nerve; double-normalized value

DO diamine oxidase; digoxin; Diploma in Ophthalmology; Diploma in Osteopathy; directly observed; dissolved oxygen; distoocclusal; distraction osteogenesis; Doctor of Ophthalmology; Doctor of Optometry; Doctor of Osteopathy; doctor's orders; drugs only

D$_O$ oxygen diffusion

D$_{O_2}$ oxygen delivery

DOA date of admission; dead on arrival; Department of Agriculture; depth of anesthesia; differential optical absorption; dominant optic atrophy

DOAC Dubois oleic albumin complex

DOB date of birth; 1-(2,5-dimethoxy-4-bromophenyl)-2-aminopropane; doctor's order book

Dob dobutamine

DObstRCOG Diploma of the Royal College of Obstetricians and Gynaecologists

DOBV Dobrava-Belgrade virus; double outlet, both ventricles

DOC date of conception; deoxycholate; deoxycorticosterone; diagnostically operative causal [graph]; died of other causes; disorders of cornification; dissolved organic carbon; distributed object computing; doctor on call; Doctors Ought to Care

doc doctor; document, documentation

DOCA deoxycorticosterone acetate

DOCG deoxycorticosterone glucoside

DOCLINE Documents On-Line

DO$_{2crit}$ critical oxygen delivery

DOCS deoxycorticosteroids

DOcSc Doctor of Ocular Science

DOCUSER Document Delivery User

DOD date of death; dementia syndrome of depression; depth of discharge; Dictionary of Organic Compounds; died of disease; dissolved oxygen deficit

DoD Department of Defense

DoDCPR Department of Defense computerized patient record

DOE date of examination; desoxyephedrine; direct observation evaluation; dyspnea on exertion

DOES disorder of excessive sleepiness

DOF, dof degrees of freedom

DOFCOSY double quantum filtered correlated spectroscopy

DOFISK Dose Finding of Streptokinase [trial]

DOFOS disturbance of function occlusion syndrome

DOG deoxyglucose; derivative of gaussian [function]; difference of gaussians; distraction osteogenesis

DoG difference of gaussians

DOH, DoH department of health

DOHyg Diploma in Occupational Hygiene

DOI date of injury; died of injuries; digital object identifier; document object identifier

DO$_2$I oxygen delivery index

DOIA Dermatological Online Atlas

Dol dolichol

dol pain [L. *dolor*]

DOLLS double-loop locking suture

DOLV double-outlet left ventricle

DOM deaminated *O*-methyl metabolite; department of medicine; dimethoxymethylamphetamine; dissolved organic matter; document object model; dominance, dominant

dom dominant

DOMA dihydroxymandelic acid

DOMBL distal, occlusal, mesial, buccal, lingual

DOMF 2′,7′-dibromo-4′-(hydroxymercuri) fluorescein

DOMIOS Determinants of Myocardial Infarction Onset [study]

DOMS Diploma in Ophthalmic Medicine and Surgery

DON deoxynivalenol; diazooxonorleucine; director of nursing; dissolved organic nitrogen

DONALD dissection of neck arteries, longterm follow-up determination

DOOR deafness, onycho-osteodystrophy, mental retardation (intellectual disability) [syndrome]

DOP dioctyl phthalate; directory of physicians; dissolved organic phosphate

DOPA, dopa dihydroxyphenylalanine

DOPAC dihydrophenylacetic acid

dopamine dihydroxyphenylethylamine

dopase dihydroxyphenylalanine oxidase

DOPC determined osteogenic precursor cell; dioleoyl-phosphatidyl choline

DOPE dioleoyl-phosphatidyl ethanolamine

DOph Doctor of Ophthalmology

DOPP dihydroxyphenylpyruvate

DOPS diffuse obstructive pulmonary syndrome; dihydroxyphenylserine; dioleoyl-phosphatidyl serine

DOPS-DL threodihydroxyphenylserine [DL-threo-DOPS]

DO-PT directly observed preventive therapy

dor dorsal

DORA double-outlet right atrium

DORNA desoxyribonucleic acid

Dors dorsal

DOrth Diploma in Orthodontics; Diploma in Orthoptics

DORV double-outlet right ventricle

DoRV *Dacus oleae* reovirus

DOS date of service; day of surgery; deoxystreptamine; Doctor of Ocular Science; Doctor of Optical Science; dysosteosclerosis

dos dosage, dose

DOSC Dubois oleic serum complex

DOSPO documentation system for pediatric oncology

DOSS dioctyl sodium sulfosuccinate; distal over-shoulder strap; docusate sodium

DOT date of transfer; date of travel; Dictionary of Occupational Titles; directly observed therapy

DOTA tetraazacyclododecanetetraacetic acid

DOTC Dameshek's oval target cell

DOTES dosage record and treatment-emergent symptoms

DOTF Document Oncology Task Force

DOTMA di-oleoyloxopropyl-trimethylammonium chloride

DOTS directly observed therapies; directly observed treatment, short course

DOUBLE Double Bolus Lytic Efficacy [trial]

DOUBTFUL double quantum transition for finding unresolved lines

DOUBTLESS Doppler and Ultrasound-Guided Balloon Therapeutics for Coronary Lesions [study]

DOUV Douglas virus

DOV dolphin poxvirus

DOVE deoxyverrucarol

DOX doxorubicin

Dox doxorubicin

dOxo 2′-deoxyaxanosine

DOX-SL stealth ribosomal doxorubicin

DP data processing; deep pulse; definitive procedure; degradation product; degree of polymerization; dementia praecox; dementia pugillistica; dendritic peptide; dental prosthesis, dental prosthesis; *Dermatophagoides pteronyssimus;* desmoplakin; dexamethasone pretreatment; diabetic patient; diastolic pressure; diazepam; diffuse precipitation; diffusion pressure; digestible protein; diphosgene; diphosphate; dipropionate; directional preponderance; disability pension; discrimination power; distal pancreatectomy; distal phalanx; distal pit; distopulpal; docking protein; Doctor of Pharmacy; Doctor of Podiatry; donor plasma; dorsalis pedis

ΔP change in pressure

D/P dialysate/plasma ratio

Dp duplication; dyspnea

D$_p$ pattern difference

3DP three-dimensional printing

DPA Department of Public Assistance; diphenylalanine; diphenylamine; dipicolinic acid; dipropylacetic acid; direct provider agreement; D-penicillamine; dual photon absorptiometry; dynamic physical activity

DPAHC durable power of attorney for health care

DpAV *Diadromus pulchellus* ascovirus

DPB days post burn; differential pencil beam [radiotherapy]; diffuse panbronchiolitis

DPBP diphenylbutylpiperidine

DPC delayed primary closure; desaturated phosphatidylcholine; diethylpyrocarbonate; direct patient care; discharge planning coordinator; distal palmar crease; DNA probe chromatography; DNA protein crosslinks

dpc days post coitum

DPCM differential pulse code modulation

DpCPV *Danaus plexippus* cypovirus; *Dasychira pudibunda* cypovirus

DPCRT double-blind placebo-controlled randomized clinical trial

DPD Department of Public Dispensary; depression pure disease; desoxypyridoxine; diffuse pulmonary disease; diffusion pressure deficit; diphenamid; Diploma in Public Dentistry; direct patient dose

DPDCH dedicated physical data channel

DPDL diffuse poorly differentiated lymphocytic lymphoma

dP/dt first derivative of pressure measured over time

dpdt double-pole double-throw

dP/dV pressure per unit change in volume

DPE dipalmitoyl phosphatidyl ethanolamine; dipiperidinoethane; downstream promoter element

DPEP dipeptidase

DPF Dental Practitioners' Formulary; diisopropyl fluorophosphate; probability density function

DPFC distal palmar flexion crease

DPFR diastolic pressure-flow relationship

DPG 2,3-diphosphoglycerate; displacement placentogram

2,3-DPG 2,3-diphosphoglycerate

2,3-DPGM 2,3-diphosphoglycerate mutase

DPGN diffuse proliferative glomerulonephritis

DPGP diphosphoglycerate phosphatase

DPH Department of Public Health; diphenhydramine; diphenylhexatriene; diphenylhydantoin; Diploma in Public Health; Doctor of Public Health; Doctor of Public Hygiene; dopamine beta-hydrolase; ductal papillary hyperplasia

DPhC Doctor of Pharmaceutical Chemistry

DPhc Doctor of Pharmacology

DPHN Doctor of Public Health Nursing

DPhys Diploma in Physiotherapy

DPhysMed Diploma in Physical Medicine

DPI daily permissible intake; days post inoculation; dietary protein intake; diphtheria-pertussis immunization; disposable personal income; dots per inch; drug prescription index; dry powder inhaler; Dynamic Personality Inventory

DPJ dementia paralytica juvenilis

DPKC diagnostic problem-knowledge coupler

DPL diagnostic peritoneal lavage; dipalmitoyl lecithin; distopulpolingual

DPLa distopulpolabial

DPLN diffuse proliferative lupus nephritis

DPLS differentially polarized light scattering

DPM Diploma in Psychological Medicine; discontinue previous medication; Doctor of Physical Medicine; Doctor of Podiatric Medicine; Doctor of Preventive Medicine; Doctor of Psychiatric Medicine; dopamine

dpm disintegrations per minute

DPN dermatosis papulosa nigra; diabetic peripheral neuropathy; diabetic polyneuropathy; diphosphopyridine nucleotide; disabling pansclerotic morphea; dorsal parabrachial nucleus

DPNB dorsal penile nerve block

DPNH reduced diphosphopyridine nucleotide

DPO days postovulation; dimethoxyphenyl penicillin; disabled people's organization

D$_{po}$ oral [per os] dose

DPP Diabetes Prevention Program; differential pulse polarography; digital pulse plethysmography; dimethylphenylpenicillin; dipeptidylpeptidase; distal photoplethysmography; document pattern processing

dpp decapentaplegic

DPPC dipalmitoylphosphatidylcholine; double-blind placebo-controlled trial

DPPD diphenylphenylenediamine

DpPHR duodenum-preserving pancreatic head resection

DPPITC diphenyl diphosphoroisothiocyanate

DPPO Data Privacy and Protection Office; Dental Preferred Provider Organization

DPR dietary prevention of recurrent myocardial infarction; drug price review; dynamic perception resolution; dynamic planar reconstructor

DpRV *Diadromus pulchellus* reovirus

DPS deep pericardial stitch; delayed primary suture; descending perineum syndrome; dimethylpolysiloxane; Division of Provider Studies; dysesthetic pain syndrome

dps decay per second

dpst double-pole single-throw

DPSWF discrete prolate spheroidal wave function

DPT Demerol, Phenergan, and Thorazine; dermatopontin; Diabetes Prevention Trial; dichotic pitch discrimination test; diphtheria-pertussis-tetanus [vaccine]; diphtheritic pseudotabes; dipropyltryptamine; Doctor of Physical Therapy; dual platform technique; dumping provocation test

Dpt house dust mite [*Dermatophagoides pteronyssinus*]

DPTA diethylenetriamine pentaacetic acid

DPTI diastolic pressure time index

DPTP domain protein tyrosine phosphatase

DPTPM diphtheria-pertussis-tetanus-poliomyelitis-measles [vaccine]

Dptr diopter

DPTU diphenylthiourea

DPUF Doppler ultrasound flowmeter

DPV *Dasychira pudibunda* virus; deer papillomavirus; disabling positional vertigo; mule deer poxvirus

DPVS Denver peritoneovenous shunt

DPW Department of Public Welfare; distal phalangeal width

DQ deterioration quotient; developmental quotient

D$_q$ quasithreshold dose

3DQCT three-dimensional quantitative computed tomography

DQE degradation of image quality; detective quantum efficiency

DQFC double−quantum filtered correlation spectroscopy

DQFC NMR double−quantum filtered correlation spectroscopy nuclear magnetic resonance

DQO data quality objective

DQP data quality probe

3D-QSAR three-dimensional quantitative structure-activity relationship

DR death receptor; degeneration reaction; delayed rectifier; delivery room; deoxyribose; diabetic retinopathy; diagnostic radiology; dietary recall; digital radiography; direct repeat; distal recurrence; distribution ratio; doctor; dopamine receptor; dorsal raphe; dorsal root; dose ratio; drug receptor; dynamic range; dynamic resistance

ΔR additional resistance

Dr doctor

dR deoxyriboside; dextroribose

dr dorsal root; drain; dram; dressing

DRA dextran-reactive antibody; digital rotational angiography; distal rectal adenocarcinoma; distal reference axis

3d-RA three-dimensional rotational angiography

DRACOG Diploma of Royal Australian College of Obstetricians and Gynaecologists

DRACR Diploma of Royal Australasian College of Radiologists

DRAP dorsal root action potential

dr ap dram, apothecary

DRASIC dorsal root ganglion cells acid-sensing ion channel

DRASTIC Dutch Renal Artery Stenosis Intervention Cooperative Study

DRAT differential rheumatoid agglutination test

DRB daunorubicin; dynamic reference basis

DRBC denatured red blood cell; dog red blood cell; donkey red blood cell

DRC damage risk criterion; daunorubicin; dendritic reticulum cell; diagnostic reporting console; digitorenocerebral [syndrome]; DNA repair capacity; dorsal root, cervical; dose-response curve; dynamic range compression; dynamic range control

DRCOG Diploma of Royal College of Obstetricians and Gynaecologists

DRCPath Diploma of Royal College of Pathologists

DRCR.net Diabetic Retinopathy Clinical Research Network

DRD dihydroxyphenylalanine-responsive dystonia; dorsal root dilator; dystrophia retinae pigmentosa-dysostosis [syndrome]

DRD$_2$ dopamine D$_2$ receptor

DRD$_3$ dopamine D$_3$ receptor

DRD$_4$ dopamine D$_4$ receptor

DRE damage response element; digital rectal examination; dioxin-responsive elements; dioxin-responsive enhancer; direct response element

DREF dose rate effectiveness factor

DREN Department of Defense Research and Engineering Network

DRES dynamic random element stimuli

DRESS depth-resolved surface-coil spectroscopy

DREZ dorsal root entry zone

DRF daily rating form; daily replacement factor; Deafness Research Foundation; digestive-respiratory fistula; dose reduction factor; dynamic reference frame

DR-FFP donor-retested fresh frozen plasma

DRFS Dundee Rank Factor Score

DRG diagnosis-related group; Division of Research Grants; dorsal respiratory group; dorsal root ganglion; duodenal-gastric reflux gastropathy

drg drainage

DrHyg Doctor of Hygiene

DRI defibrillation response interval; discharge readiness inventory; Doppler resistive index; dynamic response index

dRib deoxyribose

DRID double radial immunodiffusion; double radioisotope derivative

DRIN direct reconstructor interface

DRIP delirium and drugs, restricted mobility and retention, infection, inflammation and impaction, polyuria [mnemonic]; delirium, restricted mobility, infection, impaction, pharmaceuticals

ΔR,L additional resistance, lung

DRL dorsal root, lumbar; drug-related lupus

D5RL 5% dextrose in Ringer lactate

DRM digital rights management

DRME Division of Research in Medical Education

Dr Med Doctor of Medicine

DRMF directional recursive median filtering

DRMS drug reaction monitoring system

DrMT Doctor of Mechanotherapy

DRN dorsal raphe nucleus

DRNDP diribonucleoside-3′,3′-diphosphate

DrNP Doctor of Nursing Practice

DRnt diagnostic roentgenology

DRO differential reinforcement of other behavior; disablement resettlement officer

DRP digoxin reduction product; dorsal root potential; drug-related problems; dystrophin-related protein

dRp deoxyribose-phosphate

dRPase,
dRpase deoxyribophosphodiesterase

DrPH Doctor of Public Health; Doctor of Public Hygiene

DRPLA dentorubral-pallidoluysian atrophy

DRQ discomfort relief quotient

DRR digitally reconstructed radiograph; dorsal root reflex; dysjunction regulator region

ΔR,rs additional resistance, respiratory system

DRS descending rectal septum; diagnostic review station; diffuse reflectance spectroscopy; Diltiazem Reinfarction Study;

disability rating scale; drowsiness; Duane retraction syndrome; dynamic renal scintigraphy; Dyskinesia Rating Scale

drsg dressing

DRSP drug-resistant *Streptococcus pneumoniae*

DRST Delayed Recognition Span Test

DRT dorsal root, thoracic

3DRT three-dimensional radiotherapy

3-DRTP three dimensional radiation treatment planning

DRUGS Doctor, Recreational User, Gynaecological Sensitivities [study]

DRUJ distal radioulnar joint

DrV *Diplocarpon rosae* virus

dRVVT dilute Russell viper venom time

ΔR,w additional resistance, chest wall

DRY donryu [rat]

DS Dahl strain [rat]; dataset; dead air space; dead space; decontaminating solution; deep sedative; deep sleep; defined substrate; dehydroepiandrosterone sulfate; delayed sensitivity; dendritic spine; density standard; dental surgery; dermatan sulfate; dermatology and syphilology; desmosome; desynchronized sleep; Devic syndrome; dexamethasone-spermine; dextran sulfate; dextrose-saline; diameter stenosis; diaphragm stimulation; diastolic murmur; differential stimulus; diffuse scleroderma; dilute strength; dioptric strength; direct sequencing; disaster services; discrimination score; disoriented; disseminated sclerosis; dissolved solids; Doctor of Science; donor serum; Doppler sonography; double-stranded; double strength; double stringency; Down syndrome; Dravet syndrome; drug store; dry swallow; Duane syndrome; dumping syndrome; duplex scan; duration of systole

D&S dermatology and syphilology

D/S dextrose/saline

%DS percent diameter stenosis

D1S first year dental student

D2S second year dental student

DS2 decontaminating solution 2

D3S third year dental student

D4S fourth year dental student

D-5-S 5% dextrose in saline solution

Ds darmstadtium

ds double stranded

DSA Defense Security Agency; density spectral array; destructive spondyloarthropathy; digital subtraction angiography; dynamic scalable architecture

DSACT, D-SACT direct sinoatrial conduction time

DSAF Decision Support Access Facility

DSAP disseminated superficial actinic porokeratosis
DSAS discrete subaortic stenosis
DSB, dsb double-strand break
Dsb single-breath diffusion capacity
DSBL disabled
DSBR double-strand break repair
DSBT donor-specific blood transfusion
DSC de Sanctis–Cacchione [syndrome]; desmocollin; differential scanning calorimetry; digital scan converter; disodium chromoglycate; Doctor of Surgical Chiropody; Down syndrome child; dynamic susceptibility contrast
DSc Doctor of Science
Dsc desmocollin
DSCA double-strand conformation analysis
DSCCL diffuse small cleaved cell lymphoma
DSCF Doppler-shifted constant frequency
DSCG disodium chromoglycate
DSC-MRI dynamic susceptibility contrast magnetic resonance imaging
DsCPV *Dendrolimus spectabilis* cypovirus
DSCR developmental self-care requisites
DSCT dorsal spinocerebellar tract
DSCU dementia special care unit
DSD Déjerine-Sottas disease; depression spectrum disease; discharge summary dictated; disorders of sex development; disorders of sex differentiation; disorders of sexual development; dry sterile dressing
DS-DAT Discomfort Scale for Dementia of the Alzheimer Type
DSDDT double sampling dye dilution technique
dsDNA double-stranded deoxyribonucleic acid
DsDNV *Diatraea saccharalis* densovirus
DSE dobutamine stress echocardiography; Doctor of Sanitary Engineering
DSG decision system group; desmoglein; dry sterile gauze
Dsg desmoglein
DSH deliberate self-harm; dexamethasone-suppressible hyperaldosteronism; disproportionate share hospital; domestic short-haired cat [veterinary medicine]; dyschromatosis symmetrica hereditaria
DSHEA Dietary Supplements Health and Education Act
DSHEFS Division of Surveillance, Hazard Evaluations, and Field Studies
DSHR delayed skin hypersensitivity reaction
DSI deep shock insulin; Depression Status Inventory; desmocollin-specific insertion; disulfide isomerase; Down Syndrome International; dynamic skeleton interface

DSIM Doctor of Science in Industrial Medicine
DSIP delta sleep-inducing peptide
DSL digital subscriber line; distal sensory latency
DSLAM digital subscriber line access multiplier
DSLL diffuse small lymphocytic lymphoma
DSL MU distal sensory latency, median-ulnar
dslv dissolve
DSM dextrose solution mixture; Diagnostic and Statistical Manual [of Mental Disorders]; digital standard MUMPS [Massachusetts General Hospital Utility Multi-Programming System]; Diploma in Social Medicine; drink skim milk
DSM, dsm disease-specific mortality
DSM-III-R Diagnostic and Statistical Manual [of Mental Disorders], Third Edition, Revised
DSM-IV Diagnostic and Statistical Manual [of Mental Disorders], Fourth Edition
DSM-5 Diagnostic and Statistical Manual [of Mental Disorders], Fifth Edition
DSMA Diet and Stress Management in Angina; disodium monomethanearsonate
DSMB Data Safety Monitoring Board
DSMC data and safety monitoring committee
DSN data source name
DSNI deep space neck infection
DSO digital storage oscilloscope; distal subungual onychomycosis
DSORT discrete stochastic optimization of radiation therapy
DSP decreased sensory perception; delayed sleep phase; desmoplakin; diarrheic shellfish poisoning; dibasic sodium phosphate; digital signal processing; digital subtraction phlebography; display; distal sensory polyneuropathy; Doppler signal processor
DSPC disaturated phosphatidylcholine
DSPCR, DS-PCR double stringency polymerase chain reaction
DsplV *Dusona* spp. ichnovirus
DSPN distal sensory polyneuropathy; distal symmetric polyneuropathy
DSR digital subtraction analysis; distal splenorenal; double simultaneous recording; dynamic spatial reconstructor
DSRCT desmoplastic small round cell tumor
dsRNA double-stranded ribonucleic acid
DSRS Dementia Severity Rating Scale; distal splenorenal shunt
DSS decision support system; Dejerine-Sottas syndrome; demographic surveillance site; dengue shock syndrome; dextran sulfate sodium; digital signature standard; digital storage system; dioctyl sodium sulfosuccinate;

Disability Status Scale; discrete subaortic stenosis; docusate sodium; dosage-sensitive sex [reversal]; double simultaneous stimulation

DSSc Diploma in Sanitary Science

DSS/DH digital signature standard/Differ-Hellman

DSSEP dermatomal somatosensory evoked potential

DSSI Duke social support index

DSST digital symbol substitution test

DST desensitization test; desiccate, sequester, and transport; dexamethasone suppression test; dihydrostreptomycin; disproportionate septal thickening; donor-specific transfusion; drug susceptibility test; dural sinus thrombosis

D$_{st+}$ Dice's similarity coefficient

DS-TRIEL Decision Support Trial Eligibility

DSTY derived semantic type

DSUH directed suggestion under hypnosis

DSur Doctor of Surgery

DSV dermal sarcoma virus; Desert Shield virus

DSVP downstream venous pressure

DSWI deep surgical wound infection

DT database tomography; deceleration time; decision table; decision tree; defibrillation threshold; definitive type; delirium tremens; dental technician; depression of transmission; dietetic [services]; dietetic technician; differential technique; digitoxin; diphtheria-tetanus [toxoid]; discharge tomorrow; dispensing tablet; distance test; dorsalis tibialis; double tachycardia; duration of tetany; dye test

D/T date of treatment; total ratio of deaths

dT deoxythymidine

dt due to; dystonic

d/t due to

D3T 1,2-dithiole-3-thione

d4T stavudine

DTA decision to abort; Dental Trade Alliance; descending thoracic aorta; differential thermal analysis; diphtheria toxin A

DTaP diphtheria and tetanus toxoids and acellular pertussis [vaccine]

DTB dedicated time block

DTBC d-tubocurarine

DTBM demineralized trabecular bone matrix

DTBN di-*tert*-butyl nitroxide

DTC day treatment center; differential thyroid carcinoma; direct to consumer; differential thyroid carcinoma; dithiocarb sodium

dTc d-tubocurarine

DTCD Diploma in Tuberculosis and Chest Diseases

DTCH Diploma in Tropical Child Health

DTD delivered total dose; desmoglein terminal domain; diastrophic dysplasia; document type definition

DTDase deoxyuridine triphosphate diphosphohydrolase

DTDES dynamic template-driven data entry system

dTDP deoxythymidine diphosphate

DTE desiccated thyroid extract

DTF deep temporal fascia; detector transfer function

D-TGA dextraposed transposition of great arteries

DTH delayed-type hypersensitivity; Diploma in Tropical Hygiene

DTH-T delayed-type hypersensitivity T cell

DTI diffusion tensor imaging; dipyridamole-thallium imaging; direct thrombin inhibitor; Doppler tissue imaging

DTIA Doppler tissue imaging acceleration

DTIC dacarbazine; dimethyltriazenyl imidazole carboxamide

DTICH delayed traumatic intracerebral hematoma; delayed traumatic intracerebral hemorrhage

DTIE Doppler tissue imaging energy

D time dream time

DTIV Doppler tissue imaging velocity

DtIV *Diadegma terebrans* ichnovirus

DTLA Detroit Test of Learning Aptitudes

DTM dermatophyte test medium; Diploma in Tropical Medicine

DTM&H Diplomate of Tropical Medicine and Hygiene

DTMP deoxythymidine monophosphate

DTMS Drug Therapy Monitoring System

dTMS double-pulse transcranial magnetic stimulation

DTN diphtheria toxin, normal

DTNB 5,5'-dithiobis-(2-nitrobenzoic) acid

DTO data terminal operator; deodorized tincture of opium

DtoA digital to analog

DTP Demerol, Thorazine, Phenergan; diphtheria-tetanus-pertussis [vaccine]; distal tingling on percussion

DTPA diethylenetriaminepentaacetic acid

DTPa diphtheria−tetanus−acellular pertussis [vaccine]

DTPBw diphtheria−tetanus−whole-cell pertussis [vaccine]

DTPH Diploma in Tropical Public Health

dTPM deoxythymidine monophosphate

DTR deep tendon reflex; dietetic technician, registered

DTRTT digital temperature recovery time test

DTS dense tubular system; diphtheria toxin sensitivity; distributed time service; donor transfusion, specific; Duke treadmill score

DTs delirium tremens

DTT diagnostic and therapeutic team; diphtheria tetanus toxoid; direct transverse traction; dithiothreitol

DTTCI 3,3-diethylthiatricarbocyanamide iodide

dTTP deoxythymidine triphosphate

DTUS diathermy, traction, and ultrasound

DTV desktop videoconferencing; *Dioscorea trifida* virus

DtV *Darna trima* virus

DT-VAC diphtheria-tetanus vaccine

DTVM Diploma in Tropical Veterinary Medicine

DTVMI developmental test of visual motor integration

DTVP developmental test of visual perception

DTwP diphtheria and tetanus toxoids and whole-cell pertussis vaccine

DTX dendrotoxin; detoxification; dinophysitoxin

DTZ diatrizoate

DU decubitus ulcer; density unknown; deoxyuridine; dermal ulcer; diagnosis undetermined; diagnostic unit; diazouracil; dog unit; duodenal ulcer; duplex ultrasound; duroxide uptake; Dutch [rabbit]

dU deoxyuridine

du dial unit; duplication

DUA dorsal uterine artery

DUB dysfunctional uterine bleeding

DUCCS Duke University Clinical Cardiology Study

DUDP Drug Use and Drug Prevention [study]

dUDP deoxyuridine diphosphate

DUE drug use evaluation

D₁UE diagonal 1 upper extremity

D₂UE diagonal 2 upper extremity

DUET Dispatch Urokinase Efficacy Trial

DUF Doppler ultrasonic flowmeter; drug use forecast

DUFSS Duke University of North Carolina Functional Social Support [questionnaire]

DUGV Dugbe virus

DUH dyschromatosis universalis hereditaria

DUHP Duke University Health Profile

DUI driving under the influence

DUL diffuse undifferentiated lymphoma

dulc sweet [L. *dulcis*]

dUMP deoxyuridine monophosphate

duod duodenal, duodenum

dup duplication

DU-PAN-2 marker for pancreatic cancer

DUQUES Duke University quantitative/qualitative evaluation system

DUR drug use/utilization review

Dur, dur duration, durating

DURAC duration of anticoagulation

DURS Duane retraction syndrome

DUS diagnostic ultrasonography; Doppler flow ultrasound; dynamic ultrasound of shoulder

3D-US three-dimensional ultrasonography

DUSN diffuse unilateral subacute neuroretinitis

DUSOCS Duke Social Support and Stress scale

DUSOI Duke University Severity of Illness [index]

dut deoxyuridine triphosphatase

DUTCH-TIA Dutch Transient Ischemic Attack [study]

dUTP deoxyuridine triphosphate

dUTPase deoxyuridine triphosphatase

DUV damaging ultraviolet

DUVV Duvenhage virus

DV *Datura* virus; dependent variable; diagnostic variable; difference in volume; digital vibration; digital video; dilute volume; distemper virus; domestic violence; domiciliary visit; dorsoventral; double vibration; double vision; ductus venosus; dwarf virus

ΔV change in volume

3-DV three dimensional visualization

D&V diarrhea and vomiting

dv double vibrations

DVA Department of Veterans Affairs; developmental venous anomaly; distance visual acuity; duration of voluntary apnea; vindesine

DVB divinylbenzene

DVC divanillylcyclohexane; dorsal vagal complex

DVCC Disease Vector Control Center

DVCV Diodia vein chlorosis virus

DVD dissociated vertical deviation

DV&D Diploma in Venereology and Dermatology

dVDAVP 1-deamine-4-valine-D-arginine vasopressin

DVE duck virus enteritis

DVH Diploma in Veterinary Hygiene; Division for the Visually Handicapped; dose volume histogram

DVI AV sequential [pacemaker]; deep venous insufficiency; device independent; diastolic velocity integral; digital vascular imaging; digital video interface; Division on Visual Impairments; Doppler velocity index

DVIS digital vascular imaging system

DVIU direct-vision internal urethrotomy
DVL deep vastus lateralis
DVM digital voltmeter; Doctor of Veterinary Medicine
DVMS Doctor of Veterinary Medicine and Surgery
DVN dorsal vagal nucleus
2D-VNQ two-dimensional N-Quoit filter [imaging]
3D-VNQ three-dimensional N-Quoit filter [imaging]
DVNV Dendrobium vein necrosis virus
DVP deep venous pressure; digital volume pulse; Doppler velocity profile
DVR digital vascular reactivity; digital video recorder; direct volume rendering; Doctor of Veterinary Radiology; double valve replacement; double ventricular response
DVS Doctor of Veterinary Science; Doctor of Veterinary Surgery
DVSc Doctor of Veterinary Science
DVT Danish Verapamil Trial; deep venous thrombosis
DVT/PE deep venous thrombosis/pulmonary embolism
DW daily weight; data warehouse; deionized water; dextrose in water; diffusion weighted [imaging]; distilled water; doing well; dry weight
D/W dextrose in water
D5W, D₅W 5% dextrose in water
D10W 10% aqueous dextrose solution
dw dwarf [mouse]
DWA died from wounds by the action of the enemy
DWCE density-weighted contrast enhancement
DWD died with disease
DWDL diffuse well-differentiated lymphocytic lymphoma
DWDM dense wave division multiplexing
DWECNP Dr. Welford's Electronic Chart Notes Program
DWI diffusion-weighted imaging; driving while impaired; driving while intoxicated
DWL dry weight liver

DWM Dandy-Walker malformation
DWML deep white matter lesion
DWS Dandy-Walker syndrome; demonstrator workstation; disaster warning system
DWT dichotic word test; discrete wavelet transform; dyadic wavelet transform
dwt pennyweight
DWV Dandy-Walker variant
DX dextran; diagnosis code; dicloxacillin; DNA region X chromosome
Dx, dx diagnosis
D&X dilation and extraction
DXA dual [energy] absorptiometry
dx cath diagnostic catheterization
DXD discontinued
DXM, DXMS dexamethasone
DXP digital x-ray prototype
DxPLAIN Massachusetts General Hospital's expert diagnostic system
DXPNET Digital X-Ray Prototype Network
DXR deep x-ray
DXRT deep x-ray therapy
DXT deep x-ray therapy; dextrose
dXTP deoxyxanthine triphosphate
D$_{xx}$ input delay
D$_{xy}$ transfer delay
DY dense parenchyma
Dy dysprosium
dy dystrophia muscularis [mouse]
DYLOMMS dynamic lattice-oriented molecular modeling system
dyn dynamic; dynamometer; dyne
DYNAMO dynamic decision modeling [system]
dyne/cm dyne per centimeter
DYS dysautonomia
dysfx dysfunction
dysp dyspnea
DZ diazepam; dizygotic; dizziness
dZ impedance change
dz disease; dozen
dZ/dt time-dependent impedance change
DZM dorsal zone of membranelle
DZP diazepam
DZPIAR disordered zona pellucida−induced acrosome reaction

E

E air dose; cortisone [compound E]; each; eating; edema; effects variable; elastance; electric charge; electric field vector; electrode potential; electromotive force; electron; embyro; emmetropia; encephalitis; endangered [animal]; endogenous; endoplasm; enema; energy; Entamoeba; enterococcus; enzyme; eosinophil; epicondyle; epinephrine; epithelial, epithelium; error; erythrocyte; erythroid; erythromycin; *Escherichia*; esophagus; ester; estradiol; ethanol; ethyl; examination; exhalation; expectancy; expected frequency; experiment, experimenter; expiration; expired air; exposure; external control [pacemaker]; extract, extracted, extraction; extraction fraction; extralymphatic; eye; glutamic acid; internal energy; kinetic energy; mathematical expectation; redox potential; unit [Ger. *Einheit*]

E- exa- [10^{18}]

E- stereodescriptor to indicate the configuration at a double bond [Ger. *entgegen*, opposite]

E* lesion on the erythrocyte cell membrane at the site of complement fixation

E° standard electrode potential

Ē average beta energy

E₀ baseline effect; electric affinity

E1 ubiquitin-activating enzyme

E₁ estrone

E-1 to E-33 Human echoviruses 1 to 33

E2 ubiquitin-conjugating enzyme

E₂ 17β-estradiol

E3 ubiquitin-protein ligase

E₃ estriol

E₄ estetrol

4E four-plus edema

e base of natural logarithms; egg transfer; ejection; electric charge; electron; elementary charge; exchange

e⁺ positron

e⁻ negative electron

ε lowercase Greek letter epsilon; heavy chain of IgE; permittivity; specific absorptivity

η lowercase Greek letter eta; absolute viscosity

EA early antigen; educational age; egg albumin; electric affinity; electrical activity; electroacupuncture; electroanesthesia; electronic patient record [EPR] attributes; electrophysiological abnormality; embryonic antibody; endocardiographic amplifier; Endometriosis Association; enteral alimentation; enteroanastomosis; enzymatically active; epiandrosterone; episodic ataxia; erythrocyte antibody; erythrocyte antiserum; esophageal atresia; estivoautumnal; ethacrynic acid

E/A early/late diastolic filling ratio; emergency admission

E&A evaluate and advise

Ea kinetic energy of alpha particles

Eₐ energy of aggregation

ea each

EAA electroacupuncture analgesia; Epilepsy Association of America; essential amino acid; excitatory amino acid; extraalveolar air; extrinsic allergic alveolitis

EAAC excitatory amino acid carrier

EAAV equine adeno-associated virus

EAB elective abortion; Ethics Advisory Board

EABV effective arterial blood volume

EAC early arthritis clinic; Ehrlich ascites carcinoma; electroacupuncture; endocrine-active compound; epithelioma adenoides cysticum; erythema annulare centrifugum; erythrocyte, antibody, complement; external auditory canal

EACA epsilon-aminocaproic acid

EACD eczematous allergic contact dermatitis

EACH essential access community hospital

EACL European Chapter of the Association for Computational Linguistics

EACSS European and Australian Cooperative Stroke Study

EACT educational activity

EAD early afterdepolarization; enteral access device; Enterprise Access Directory; extracranial arterial disease

EA-D early antigen, diffuse

E-ADD epileptic attention deficit disorder

EaDNV *Euxoa auxiliaris* densovirus

EADS early amnion deficit spectrum/syndrome

EAdV equine adenovirus

EAdV-B equine adenovirus B

EAE ethylaminoethanol; experimental allergic encephalomyelitis; experimental autoimmune encephalitis; experimental autoimmune encephalomyelitis

EAEC enteroadherent/enteroaggregative *Escherichia coli*

EAF eosinophilic angiocentric fibrosis

EAFT European Atrial Fibrillation Trial

EAG electroarteriography

EAGAR Estrogen and Graft Atherosclerosis Research Trial

EAggEC enteroaggregative *Escherichia coli*

EAGLES Expert Advisory Group on Language Engineering Standards

EAHF eczema, asthma, and hay fever

EAHIL European Association for Health Information and Libraries

EAHLG equine antihuman lymphoblast globulin

EAHLS equine antihuman lymphoblast serum

EAI Emphysema Anonymous, Inc.; erythrocyte antibody inhibition

EAK ethyl amyl ketone

EAM episodic ataxia with myokymia; external acoustic meatus

EAMG experimental autoimmune myasthenia gravis

EAMI exercise training in anterior myocardial infarction

EAN experimental allergic neuritis

EAO experimental allergic orchiitis

EAP electric acupuncture; electroactive polymer; employee assistance program; epiallopregnanolone; Epstein-Barr–associated protein; erythrocyte acid phosphatase; evoked action potential

EAPV early/atrial peak velocity ratio

EAQ eudismic affinity quotient

EAR European Association of Radiology

EA-R early antigen, restricted

Ea R reaction of degeneration [Ger. *Entartungs-Reaktion*]

EARHA East Anglian Regional Health Authority

EARR extended aortic root replacement

EARS European Atherosclerosis Research Study

EAS Edinburgh Artery Study; emergency ambulance service; endarterectomized aortic segment; European Atherosclerosis Society

EASI eczema area and severity index; emotionality, activity, sociability, impulsivity [scale]; European Antiplatelet Stent Investigation; European applications in surgical interventions; extraamniotic saline infusion

EAST Eastern Association for the Surgery of Trauma; elevated-arm stress test; Emory Angioplasty vs. Surgery Trial; external rotation, abduction stress test

EASY European Prototype for Integrated Care [EPIC] assessment system

EAT Eating Attitudes Test; Ehrlich ascites tumor; electroaerosol therapy; epidermolysis acuta toxica; experimental autoimmune thymitis; experimental autoimmune thyroiditis

EATB European Association of Tissue Banks

EATC Ehrlich ascites tumor cell

EAV entity-attribute-value [model]; equine abortion virus; equine arteritis virus

EAVC enhanced atrioventricular conduction

EAVM extramedullary arteriovenous malformation

EAVN enhanced atrioventricular nodal [conduction]

EB elective abortion; electron beam; elementary body; embryoid body; emotional behavior; endometrial biopsy; epidermolysis bullosa; Epstein-Barr [virus]; esophageal body; estradiol benzoate; Evans blue

E$_b$ binding energy

EBA early bacterial activity; epidermolysis bullosa acquisita; epidermolysis bullosa atrophicans; extrahepatic biliary atresia; orthoethoxybenzoic acid

EBAA Eye Bank Association of America

EBC esophageal balloon catheter

EBCDIC Extended Binary Coded Decimal Interchange Code

EBCP evidence-based clinical practice

EBCT electron-beam computed tomography

EBD epidermolysis bullosa dystrophica

EBDA effective balloon dilated area

EBDC ethylene bisdithiocarbamate; evidence-based health care

EBDCT epidermolysis bullosa dystrophica, Cockayne Touraine [type]

EBDD epidermolysis bullosa dystrophica, dominant

EBDR epidermolysis bullosa dystrophica, recessive

EBE Excluder bifurcated endoprosthesis

EBER Epstein-Barr–encoded RNA

EBF erythroblastosis fetalis; exclusive breast-feeding

E-BFU erythroid blood-forming unit

EBG electroblepharogram, electroblepharography

EBH epidermolysis bullosa hereditaria; evidence-based health care

EBHC evidence-based health care

EBI emetine bismuth iodide; erythroblastic island; estradiol binding index; European Bioinformatics Institute; external beam irradiation

EBIF emotional behavioral index form

EBIORT, EB-IORT electron beam intraoperative radiotherapy

EBK embryonic bovine kidney

EBL erythroblastic leukemia; estimated blood loss

eBL endemic Burkitt lymphoma

EBL/S estimated blood loss during surgery

EBLV European bat lyssavirus

EBM electrophysiologic behavior modification; epidermal basement membrane; epidermolysis bullosa, macular type; evidence-based medicine; expressed breast milk

EBMS Engineering and Biology in Medicine Society

EBMT European Group for Blood and Marrow Transplantation

EBMTR European Bone Marrow Transplantation Registry

EBMWG Evidence-Based Medicine Working Group

EBN evidence-based nursing

EBNA Epstein-Barr virus—associated nuclear antigen

EBO Ebola [disease, virus]

EBOB 4'-ethynyl-4-n-propyl-bicycloorthobenzoate

E/BOD electrolyte biochemical oxygen demand

EBO-R Ebola Reston virus

EBOV Ebola virus

EBP error-back propagation; estradiol-binding protein

EbpS elastin-binding protein of *Staphylococcus aureus*

EBRI Employee Benefit Research Institute

EBRT electron beam radiotherapy; external beam radiation therapy

EBS elastic back strap; electric brain stimulation; Emergency Bed Service; epidermolysis bullosa simplex

EBSS Earle's balanced salt solution

EBT electron beam tomography; external beam therapy

EBV effective blood volume; Egypt bee virus; Epstein-Barr virus; estimated blood volume

EBv Epstein-Barr virus

EBVS Epstein-Barr virus susceptibility

EBZ epidermal basement zone

EC effective concentration; ejection click; electrochemical; electron capture; embryonal carcinoma; emergency center; emergency contraception; endemic cretinism; endocrine cells; endothelial cell; energy charge; enteric coating; entering complaint; enterochromaffin; entorhinal cortex; Enzyme Commission; epidermal cell; epirubicin/cyclophosphamide; epithelial cell; epithelial component; equalization-cancellation; error correction; *Escherichia coli*; esophageal carcinoma; ethics committee; ethyl chloride; excitation-contraction; experimental control; expiratory center; extended care; exterior coat; external carotid [artery]; external conjugate; extracellular; extracellular concentration; extracorporeal; extracranial; eye care; eyes closed

E-C ether-chloroform

E/C endocystoscopy; enteric-coated; estrogen/creatinine ratio

EC$_{50}$ median effective concentration

Ec ectoconchion; entorhinal cortex

e/c enteric coated

ECA electrical control activity; electrocardioanalyzer; endothelial cell antibody; endothelial cytotoxic activity; enterobacterial common antigen; epidemiologic catchment area; esophageal carcinoma; ethacrynic acid; ethylcarboxylate adenosine; external carotid artery

E$_{Ca}$ calcium reversal potential

ECAA European Concerted Action on Anticoagulation [study]

E-CABG endarterectomy and coronary artery bypass graft

ECAC epidermoid carcinomas of the anal canal; European Collection of Animal Cell Cultures; expiratory central airway collapse

ECaC epithelial calcium channel

E-CAD E-cadherin

ECAF extension corner avulsion fracture

ECAO enteric cytopathogenic Avian orphan [virus]

ECAP European Concerted Action Project

ECAQ Elderly Cognitive assessment Questionnaire

ECASS European Cooperative Acute Stroke Study

ECAT emission computer-assisted tomography; European Concerted Action on Thrombosis and Disabilities [study]

ECAT AP European Concerted Action on Thrombosis: Angina Pectoris [study]

ECBD exploration of common bile duct

ECBO enteric cytopathogenic bovine orphan [virus]

ECBS Expert Committee on Biological Standardization

ECBT enhanced cognitive behavior therapy

ECBV effective circulating blood volume

ECC electrocorticogram, electrocorticography; electronic claim capture; embryonal cell carcinoma; emergency cardiac care; emergency care center; encoding combinatorial chemistry; endocervical cone; endocervical curettage; Erlangen Cancer Center; error correction code; estimated creatinine clearance; external cardiac compression; extracorporeal circulation

ECCE Effects of Captopril on Cardiopulmonary Exercise [study]; extracapsular cataract extraction

ECCI electronic clinical communication implementation

ECCL encephalocraniocutaneous lipomatosis

ECCLS European Committee for Clinical Laboratory Standards

ECCO enteric cytopathogenic cat orphan [virus]; European Culture Collection Organisation

ECCO$_2$ extracorporeal carbon dioxide

ECCOMAC European Concerted Community Action Programmes

ECCO$_2$R extracorporeal carbon dioxide removal

ECD early child development; ectrodactyly; electrochemical detection, electrochemical detector; electron capture detector; emergency call device; endocardial cushion defect; enzymatic cell dispersion; equivalent current dipole; Erdheim-Chester disease; ethylcysteinate dimer; extended criteria donor; external cardioverter-defibrillator; external continence device; extracellular domain; extracranial Doppler sonography

ECDC *Escherichia coli* Database Collection

ECDEU Early Clinical Drug Evaluation Unit [manual]

E/CDK cyclin E−dependent kinase

ECDO enteric cytopathic dog orphan [virus]

ECE equine conjugated estrogen; extracapsular extension

ECEO enteric cytopathogenic equine orphan [virus]

ECETOC European Centre for Ecotoxicity and Toxicology of Chemicals

ECF effective capillary flow; eosinophilic chemotactic factor; enhanced tuberculosis case finding; erythroid colony formation; *Escherichia coli* filtrate; ethyl chloroformate; extended care facility; extracellular fluid; extracytoplasmic function

ECFA, ECF-A eosinophilic chemotactic factor of anaphylaxis

ECFC eosinophilic chemotactic factor complement

ECFMG Educational Commission for Foreign Medical Graduates; Educational Council for Foreign Medical Graduates

ECFMS Educational Council for Foreign Medical Students

E-CFU erythroid colony-forming unit

ECFV extracellular fluid volume

ECFVD extracellular fluid volume depletion

ECG electrocardiogram, electrocardiography

ECGF endothelial cell growth factor

ECGS endothelial cell growth supplement

ECH educator contact hour

ECHO echocardiography; enteric cytopathic human orphan [virus]; Etoposide, cyclophosphamide, Adriamycin, and vincristine

EchoCG echocardiography

Echo-Eg echoencephalography

Echo-VM echoventriculometry

ECHRA electronic health care record architecture

ECHSCP Exeter Community Health Services Computer Project

ECI electrocerebral inactivity; eosinophil chemotaxis index; eosinophilic cytoplasmic inclusions; extracorporeal irradiation

ECIB extracorporeal irradiation of blood

EC/IC extracranial/intracranial

ECICD European Consortium for Intensive Care Data

ECIL extracorporeal irradiation of lymph

ECIS equipment control information system

ECK extracellular potassium

ECL electrochemiluminescent; emitter-coupled logic; enterochromaffin-like [cell]; euglobin clot lysis

ECLAP European Collaboration on Low-Dose Aspirin in Polycythemia Vera

ECLAT European Community and Latin American Network on Biology and Control of Triatomines

ECLiPS encoded combinatorial libraries on polymeric support

ECLRS electronic clinical laboratory reporting system

ECLS extracorporeal life support

ECM electronic claims management; embryonic chick muscle; erythema chronicum migrans; experimental cerebral malaria; expression of extracellular matrix; external cardiac massage; extracellular material; extracellular matrix

ECML extracellular membrane layer

ECMO enteric cytopathic monkey orphan [virus]; extracorporeal membrane oxygenation

ECN equipment control number

ecNOS endothelial cell nitric oxide synthase

ECO Pan-American Center for Human Ecology and Health

E co *Escherichia coli*

ECochG electrocochleography

E Codes external codes

ECOG Eastern Cooperative Oncology Group

ECoG electrocorticogram, electrocorticography

E COLI eighth nerve action potential, cochlear nucleus, olivary complex (superior), lateral lemniscus, inferior colliculus [hearing test]

E coli *Escherichia coli*

ECP ectrodactyly−cleft palate [syndrome]; effective conduction period; effector cell precursor; electronic claims processing; emergency care provider; endocardial potential; endoscopic calcaneoplasty; entry control point; eosinophil cationic protein; erythrocyte coproporphyrin; erythroid committed precursor; *Escherichia coli* polypeptide; estradiol cyclopentane propionate; external cardiac pressure; external counterpulsation; extracellular protein; extracorporeal photochemotherapy; free cytoporphyrin of erythrocytes

ECPA Electronic Communication Privacy Act

ECPO enteric cytopathic porcine orphan [virus]

ECPOG electrochemical potential gradient

ECPR external cardiopulmonary resuscitation

ECR effectiveness/cost ratio; electrocardiographic response; emergency care research; emergency chemical restraint; European Congress of Radiology; extensor carpi radialis

ECRB extensor carpi radialis brevis

ECRHS European Community Respiratory Health Survey

ECRI Emergency Care Research Institute

ECRL extensor carpi radialis longus

ECRLAB extracorporeal right-to-left atrium bypass

ECRO enteric cytopathogenic rodent orphan [virus]

ECR-SCSI European Committee for Recommendation−Standard on Computer Aspects of Diagnostic Imaging

ECS elective cosmetic surgery; electrocerebral silence; electroconvulsive shock; electroshock; endocannabinoid system; endocervical swab; endothelial cells; extracapsular spread; extracellular solids; extracellular space

ECSG European Cooperative Study Group

ECSO enteric cytopathic swine orphan [virus]

ECSP epidermal cell surface protein

ECSS European Coronary Surgery Study

ECST European Carotid Surgery Trial

ECSURF economic evaluation of surfactant

ECSYSVAS European Community Systemic Vasculitis [trials]

ECT electroconvulsive therapy; emission computed tomography; enteric coated tablet; euglobulin clot test; European compression technique

ect ectopic, ectopy

ECTA esophageal gastric tube airway; Everyman's Contingency Table Analysis

EC-TEOLA epichlorohydrin-triethanolamine

ECTR endoscopic carpal tunnel release

ECTV ectromelia virus

ECU environmental control unit; extended care unit; extensor carpi ulnaris

ECV endocardial volume; enteric calicivirus; epithelial cell vacuolization; extracellular volume; extracorporeal volume

EcV *Euploea corea* virus

ECVA extracranial vertebral artery

ECVAM European Centre for the Validation of Alternative Methods

ECVD extracellular volume of distribution

ECW extracellular water

ED early death; early decision; early differentiation; ectodermal dysplasia; ectopic depolarization; effective dose; Ehlers-Danlos [syndrome]; elbow disarticulation; electrodialysis; electron density; electron diffraction; elemental diet; embedding dimension; embryonic death; emergence delirium; emergency department; emotional disorder, emotionally disturbed; end diastole; endocrine disruptor; energy diversive [radiology]; enteric drainage; entering diagnosis; Entner-Doudoroff [pathway]; enzyme deficiency; epidural; epileptiform discharge; equine dermis [cells]; erectile dysfunction; erythema dose; ethyl dichlorarsine; ethynodiol; event definition; evidence of disease; exertional dyspnea; exponential distribution; extensive disease; extensor digitorum; external diameter; extra-low dispersion

E-D ego defense; Ehlers-Danlos [syndrome]

ED$_{01}$ effective dose, 1% response

ED$_{50}$ median effective dose

ED$_{99}$ effective dose, 99% response

E$_d$ depth dose

ed edema

EDA ectodermal dysplasia, anhidrotic; electrodermal activity; electrodermal audiometry; electrolyte-deficient agar; electron donor acceptor; electronic design automation; end-diastolic area; exploratory data analysis

EDAC 1-ethyl-3-diethylaminopropyl carbodiimide; excessive dynamic airway collapse

EDAM electron-dense amorphous material

EDAP emergency department approved for pediatrics

EDAX energy dispersive x-ray analysis

EDB early dry breakfast; electron-dense body; Enrollment Database; ethylene dibromide; expert database; extended definition beta; extensor digitorum brevis

EDBP erect diastolic blood pressure

EDC electronic data capture; emergency decontamination center; end-diastolic count;

endocrine-disrupting chemical; endocrine-disrupting compound; estimated date of conception; ethylene dichloride; expected date of confinement; expected delivery, cesarean; extensor digitorum communis

ED&C electrodesiccation and curettage

EDCF endothelium-derived contracting factor

EDCI energetic dynamic cardiac insufficiency

EDCP eccentric dynamic compression plate

EDCS end-diastolic chamber stiffness; end-diastolic circumferential stress

EDc(V) extrapolated dose converted (volume)

EDD effective drug duration; electron dense deposit; end-diastolic dimension; esophageal detection device; estimated due date; expected date of delivery

EDDA expanded duty dental auxiliary

EDDS electronic development delivery system

EDE effective dose equivalent

EDECS emergency department expert charting system

edent edentia, edentulous

EDF edge response function; eosinophil differentiation factor; erythroid differentiation factor; extradural fluid

EDG electrodermography

EDGE Evaluation of Dispatch Catheter for Vein Graft Revascularization

EDH epidural hematoma

EDHEP European Donor Hospital Education Program

EDHF endothelium-derived hyperpolarizing factor

EDI eating disorder inventory; electronic data interchange; estimated daily intake

EDIC Echocardiography Dobutamine International Cooperative Study; Epidemiology of Diabetes Intervention and Complications

EDIM epizootic diarrhea of infant mice

E-diol estradiol

EDIT Early Defibrillator Implantation Trial; Early Diabetes Intervention Trial

EDJT endoluminal duodenojejunal tube

EDK energy deposition kernel

EDL end-diastolic length; end-diastolic load; Essential Drug List; estimated date of labor; extensor digitorum longus

ED/LD emotionally disturbed and learning disabled

ED LOS emergency department length of stay

EDM early diastolic murmur; electro-discharge machining; electron density map; esophageal Doppler monitoring; Essential Drugs and Medicines; extramucosal duodenal myotomy

EDMA ethylene glycol dimethacrylate; Euclidean distance matrix analysis

EDMD emergency physician; Emery-Dreifuss muscular dystrophy

EDN electrodesiccation; eosinophil-derived neurotoxin

EDNA Emergency Department Nurses Association

EDNF endogenous digitalis-like natriuretic factor

EDNOS eating disorder not otherwise specified

EDOC estimated date of confinement

EDOU emergency department observation unit

EDP electron dense particle; electronic data processing; end-diastolic pressure

EDQ extensor digiti quinti

EDR early diastolic relaxation; effective direct radiation; electrodermal response; electronic death reporting; endothelium-dependent relaxation; equianalgesic dose ratio

EDRES Effects of Debulking on Restenosis [trial]

EDRF endothelium-derived relaxing factor

EDRM emergency department readmission monitor

EDS edema disease of swine; egg drop syndrome; Ehlers-Danlos syndrome; electronic decision support; Emery-Dreifuss syndrome; energy-dispersive spectrometry; epigastric distress syndrome; essential dataset; excessive daytime sleepiness; extradimensional shift

EDSR electronic document storage and retrieval

EDSS expanded disability status scale

EDT end-diastolic thickness; erythrocyte density test

EDTA ethylenediamine tetraacetic acid

EDTMP ethylenediamine tetramethylene phosphoric acid

EDTR emergency department—based trauma response

EDTU emergency diagnostic and treatment unit

Educ education

EDV end-diastolic volume; endothelium-dependent vasodilation; epidermodysplasia verruciformis

ED(V) extrapolated dose (volume)

EDVI end-diastolic volume index

EDVX X-linked epidermodysplasia verruciformis

EDWTH end-diastolic wall thickness

EDX, EDx electrodiagnosis

EDXA energy-dispersive x-ray analysis

Edyn,l dynamic elastance, lung

Edyn,rs dynamic elastance, respiratory system

Edyn,w dynamic elastance, chest wall

EE electronic encyclopedia; embryo extract; end to end; end expiration; energy expenditure; *Enterobacteriaceae* enrichment; eosinophilic esophagitis; equine encephalitis; ethinyl estradiol; expressed emotion; external ear; eye and ear

E-E erythema-edema

E&E eye and ear

EEA electroencephalic audiometry; end-to-end anastomosis; expanded endonasal approach

EE$_{act}$ energy expenditure due to physical activity

EEC ectrodactyly, ectodermal dysplasia, clefting [syndrome]; enteropathogenic *Escherichia coli*

EECD endothelial-epithelial corneal dystrophy

EECG electroencephalography

EECP enhanced external counterpulsation

EED experimental emergency department

EEE eastern equine encephalitis; eastern equine encephalomyelitis; experimental enterococcal endocarditis; external eye examination

EEEP end-expiratory esophageal pressure

EEEV eastern equine encephalitis virus

EEG electroencephalogram, electroencephalography

EEGA electroencephalographic audiometry

EEG-CSA electroencephalography with computerized spectral analysis

EEGL emergency exposure guidance level; low-voltage electroencephalography

EEGV1 electroencephalographic variant pattern 1

EEHS emergency evacuation hyperbaric stretcher

EEL environmental exposure limit

EELS electron energy loss spectroscopy

EELV end-expiratory lung volume

EEM ectodermal dysplasia, ectrodactyly, macular dystrophy [syndrome]; erythema exudativum multiforme

EEMCO European Group for Efficacy Measurements on Cosmetics and Other Topical Products

EEME, EE3ME ethinylestradiol-3-methyl ether

EEMG evoked electromyogram

EENT eye, ear, nose, and throat

EEP end-expiratory pressure; epidemiology elective program; equivalent effective photon

EEPI extraretinal eye position information

EER electroencephalographic response; extended entity relationship; extraesophageal reflex

EES erythromycin ethylsuccinate; ethyl ethanesulfate

EESG evoked electrospinogram

EET epoxyeicosatrienoic [acid]

EEV endocardial ventriculotomy; equine encephalitis virus; equine encephalosis virus; extracellular enveloped virus

EEV 1 to 7 equine encephalosis viruses 1 to 7

EF ectopic focus; edema factor; ejection fraction; elastic fibril; electric field; elongation factor; embryo-fetal; embryo fibroblasts; emergency facility; encephalitogenic factor; endothoracic fascia; endurance factor; eosinophilic fasciitis; epithelial focus; equivalent focus; erythroblastosis fetalis; erythrocyte fragmentation; escalation factor; executive function; exposure factor; extended field; extra fine; extrinsic factor

E$_f$ free enzyme

EF-1α elongation factor 1-alpha

EFA Epilepsy Foundation of America; essential fatty acid; extrafamily adoptee

EFAD essential fatty acid deficiency

EFAP employee and family assistance program

EFAS embryofetal alcohol syndrome

EFC elastin fragment concentration; endogenous fecal calcium; ephemeral fever of cattle

EFCC European Federation of Coding Centres

EFD estimated fluid deficit

EFDA expanded function dental assistant

EFE endocardial fibroelastosis

EFERF Enalapril Felodipine Extended Release Factorial Study

EFF electromagnetic field focusing

eff effect; efferent; efficiency; effusion

effect effective

effer efferent

EFFU epithelial focus-forming unit

EF-G elongation factor G

EFH explosive follicular hyperplasia

EFICAT Ejection Fraction in Carvedilol-treated Transplant Candidates [study]

EFL effective focal length

EFM elderly fibromyalgia; electronic fetal monitoring; electrostatic force microscopy; external fetal monitor

EFMI European Federation for Medical Informatics

EFORT exogenous follicle-stimulating hormone ovarian reserve test

EFP early follicular phase; effective filtration pressure; endoneural fluid pressure

EFPO Educating Future Physicians for Ontario

EFR effective filtration rate

EFRT extended field radiotherapy

EFS earliest finishing shift; electric field stimulation; European Fraxiparin Study; event-free survival

EFSA European Food Safety Authority

EFT electronic funds transfer; Embedded Figures Test; emotional freedom technique

EFTR endoscopic full-thickness skin graft resection

EF-Tu [prokaryotic] elongation factor Tu

EFV extracellular fluid volume

EFVC expiratory flow-volume curve

EFW estimated fetal weight

EFZ efavirenz

EG electrogram; enteroglucagon; eosinophilic granuloma; Erb-Goldflam [syndrome]; esophagogastrectomy; esophagogastric; ethylene glycol; external genitalia

eg, e.g. for example [L. *exempli gratia*]

EGA enhanced graphics adaptation; estimated gestational age

EGAD Expressed Gene Anatomy Database

EGALITÉ Ensuring Global Access to Links, Information and Technology to Promote Equity in Health

EGBUS external genitalia, Bartholin, urethral, Skene glands

EGC early gastric cancer; epithelioid-globoid cell

EGD esophagogastroduodenoscopy

EGDF embryonic growth and development factor

EGDT early goal-directed therapy

EGF early graft failure; endothelial growth factor; epidermal growth factor

EGFP, eGFP extended green fluorescent protein

EGFR, EGF-R epidermal growth factor receptor

eGFR estimated glomerular filtration rate

EGF-URO epidermal growth factor, urogastrone

EGG electrogastrogram, electrogastrography; electroglottogram

EGH equine growth hormone

EGHIN Ellen Gartenfeld Health Information Network

EGHP employer group health plan

EGIR European Group for the Study of Insulin Resistance

EGJ esophagogastric junction

EGL eosinophilic granuloma of the lung

EGLT euglobin lysis time

EGM electrogram; extracellular granular material

EGME ethylene glycol monomethyl ether

EGN experimental glomerulonephritis

EGNB enteric gamma-negative bacteria

EGOT erythrocytic glutamic oxaloacetic transaminase

EGPA eosinophilic granulomatosis with polyangiitis

EGR early growth response; erythema gyratum repens

E-GR erythrocyte glutathione reductase

EGR-2 early growth response protein 2

EGRA equilibrium-gated radionuclide angiography

EGRAC erythrocyte glutathione reductase activity coefficient

EGRP Epidemiology and Genomics Research Program

EGS electrogalvanic stimulation; electron gamma shower; external guide sequence

EGT ethanol gelation test

EGTA esophageal gastric tube airway; ethyleneglycol-bis-(β-aminoethylether)-N,N,N',N'-tetraacetic acid

EGTCSA epilepsy with generalized tonic-clonic seizures on awakening

EGTM European Group on Tumor Markers

EG-VEGF/Prok-1 endocrine gland−derived vascular endothelial growth factor/prokineticin-1

EH eligible hospital; enlarged heart; epidermal hyperplasia; epidermolytic hyperkeratosis; epidural hematoma; epoxide hydratase; esophageal hiatus; essential hypertension; external hyperalimentation

E/H, E&H environment and heredity

E$_h$ redox potential

eh enlarged heart

EHA Emotional Health Anonymous; Environmental Health Agency

EHAA epidemic hepatitis−associated antigen

EHB elevate head of bed

EHBA extrahepatic biliary atresia

EHBD extrahepatic bile duct

EHBF estimated hepatic blood flow; exercise hyperemia blood flow; extrahepatic blood flow

EHC enterohepatic circulation; enterohepatic clearance; essential hypercholesterolemia; ethylhydrocupreine hydrochloride; extended health care; extrahepatic cholestasis

EHCR electronic health care record

EHCW emergency health care worker

EHD electrohemodynamics; epizootic hemorrhagic disease

EHDP ethane-1-hydroxy-1,1-diphosphate

EHDV epizootic hemorrhagic disease virus

EHEC enterohemorrhagic *Escherichia coli*

EHF epidemic hemorrhagic fever; exophthalmos-hyperthyroid factor; extremely high frequency

EHFR elastomeric half-facepiece respirator

EHG electrohysterogram, electrohysterography

EHH esophageal hiatal hernia

EHI employer's health insurance; environmental health indicator

EHIA environmental health impact assessment

EHIBCC European Health Industry Business Communications Council

EHIV exposure to human immunodeficiency virus

EHK epidermolytic hyperkeratosis

EHL effective half-life; electrohydraulic lithotripsy; endogenous hyperlipidemia; Environmental Health Laboratory; essential hyperlipemia; extensor hallucis longus

EHM extrahepatic metastases

EHME employee health maintenance examination

EHMS electrohemodynamic ionization mass spectometry

EHNA 9-erythro-2-(hydroxy-3-nonyl) adenine

EHNV epizootic hematopoietic necrosis virus

EHO environmental health officer; extrahepatic obstruction

EHP di-(2-ethylhexyl) hydrogen phosphate; electron hole pair; Environmental Health Perspectives; excessive heat production; extrahigh potency

EHPAC Emergency Health Preparedness Advisory Committee

EHPH extrahepatic portal hypertension

EHPT Eddy hot plate test

EHQ Eating Habits Questionnaire

EHR electronic health care record; extended-high rate

EHS environmental health and safety

EHSDS experimental health services delivery system

EHT electrohydrothermoelectrode; essential hypertension

EHV Edge Hill virus; electric heart vector; epidermal hyperplasia virus; equid herpesvirus

EHVT Edinburgh Heart Valve Trial

EI earliness index; Edmonton injector; electrical injury; electrolyte imbalance; electron impact; electron ionization; emotionally impaired; energy index; energy intake; enzyme inhibitor; eosinophilic index; Evans index; excretory index; exercise induced

E/I expiration/inspiration ratio

E$_I$ ionic reversal potential

e-I early inspiratory

EIA electroimmunoassay; enzyme immunoassay; enzyme-linked immunosorbent assay; equine infectious anemia; erythroimmunoassay;

excessive inappropriate aggression; exercise-induced anaphylaxis; exercise-induced asthma; external iliac artery

EIAB extracranial-intracranial arterial bypass

EIAV equine infectious anemia virus

EIB electrophoretic immunoblotting; eosinophilic intracytoplasmic inclusion body; exercise-induced bronchospasm

EIC elastase inhibition capacity; enzyme inhibition complex; extensive intraductal carcinoma; extensive intraductal component

EICESS European Intergroup Cooperative Ewing Sarcoma Study

EID ecological interface design; egg infectious dose; electroimmunodiffusion; emergency infusion device

EIDE enhanced integrated drive electronics

EIEC enteroinvasive *Escherichia coli*

EIEE early infantile epileptic encephalopathy

EIES Electronic Information Exchange System

EIF, eIF erythrocyte initiation factor; eukaryotic initiation factor

eIF4E eukaryotic initiation factor 4E

EIHDW Evaluation of Ischemic Heart Disease in Women [study]

EII electrical impedance imaging

EIM elastic image matching; equity implementation model; excitability-inducing material

EIMS electron ionization mass spectrometry

EIN employee identification number

EINECS European Inventory of Existing Commercial Chemical Substances

EINet Emerging Infections Network

EIO European Institute of Oncology

EIP Emerging Infections Program; end-expiratory pause; ethylisopropylamiloride; extensor indicis proprius

EIPS endogenous inhibitor of prostaglandin synthase

eIPV enhanced inactivated poliomyelitis vaccine

EIRnv extra incidence rate of nonvaccinated groups

EIRP effective isotropic radiated power

EIRv extra incidence in vaccinated groups

EIS Environmental Impact Statement; Epidemic Intelligence Service; European Infarction Study

EIT electrical impedance tomography; erythroid iron turnover

EIU enzyme immunoassay unit

EIV equine influenza virus; external iliac vein

EIW electronic information warehouse

EJ elbow jerk; external jugular

EJB ectopic junctional beat

EJM epilepsy, juvenile myoclonic

EJP excitation junction potential

EJV external jugular vein

EK enterokinase; erythrokinase

E$_K$ potassium equilibrium potential; potassium reversal potential

E$_k$ kinetic energy

EKC epidemic keratoconjunctivitis

EKF extended Kalman filtering

EKG electrocardiogram, electrocardiography

EKLF erythroid Krüppel-like factor

EKS epidemic Kaposi sarcoma

EKV erythrokeratodermia variabilis

EKY electrokymogram, electrokymography

EL early latent; elbow; electroluminescence; erythroleukemia; exercise limit; external lamina

El elastase; explanation library

el elixir

ELA elastase; elastomer-lubricating agent; endotoxin-like activity

ELAD extracorporeal liver assist device

ELAM endothelial leukocyte adhesion molecule

ELAS extended lymphadenopathy syndrome

ELAT Embolism in Left Atrial Thrombi [study]

ELAV embryonic lethal, abnormal vision

ELB early, light breakfast; elbow

elb elbow

ELBW extremely low birth weight

ELCA Excimer Laser Coronary Angioplasty [registry]

ElCPV *Eriogaster lanestris* cypovirus

ELD egg lethal dose

ELDH extraforaminal lumbar disk herniation

elec electric, electricity

elect elective; electuary

ELECTZ electrosurgical loop excision of the cervical transformation zone

ELEM equine leukoencephalomalacia

elem elementary

elev elevated, elevation, elevator

ELF elective low forceps; extremely low frequency

ELG eligibility

ELH egg-laying hormone

ELHE Evaluation of Losartan in Hemodialysis [study]

ElHV elephantid herpesvirus

ELI exercise lability index

ELIA enzyme-linked immunoassay

eLib electronic library

ELICT enzyme-linked immunocytochemical technique

ELIEDA enzyme-linked immunoelectron diffusion assay

ELIOT electron intraoperative therapy

ELIRA enzyme-linked immunoreceptor assay

ELISA enzyme-linked immunosorbent assay

ELISK excimer laser intrastromal keratomileusis

ELITE Evaluation of Losartan in the Elderly [study]

ELIV Ellidaey virus

elix elixir

ELL elongation factor homologous to mixed lineage leukemia

ELLV Ellidaey virus

ELM external limiting membrane; extravascular lung mass

ELMCV El Moro Canyon virus

ELMP expertise-led medical protocol

ELN elastin; electronic noise

ELND elective lymph node dissection

ELOD expected average load [score]

ELOP estimated length of program

ELOS estimated length of stay

ELP elastaselike protein; endogenous limbic potential; exogenous lipoid pneumonia

ELPS excessive lateral pressure syndrome

ELR electronic laboratory reporting

ELRA European Language Resources Agency

ELS Eaton-Lambert syndrome; electron loss spectroscopy; emergency life support; enzymatic labile site; extended least squares; extensive limb swelling; extralobar sequestration; extremely low frequency

ELSA European Lacidipine Study on Atherosclerosis; European Longitudinal Study on Aging

ELSI ethical, legal, and social issues

ELSS emergency life support system

ELST endolymphatic sac tumor

ELT endless loop tachycardia; euglobulin lysis time

ELV enterolike virus; environmental limit value; erythroid leukemia virus

ELVD Exercise in Left Ventricular Dysfunction [trial]

ELVD-CHF Exercise in Left Ventricular Dysfunction and Chronic Heart Failure [trial]

elx elixir

EM early memory; ejection murmur; electromagnetic; electron micrograph; electron microscope, electron microscopy; electrophoretic mobility; Embden-Meyerhof [pathway]; emergency management; emergency medicine; emmetropia; emotional disorder, emotionally disturbed; end of memory; ergonovine maleate; erythema migrans; erythema multiforme; erythrocyte mass; erythromycin; esophageal manometry; esophageal motility; estramusine; expectation maximization [algorithm]; extensive metabolizer; extracellular matrix

E-M expectation maximization

E/M electron microscope, electron microscopy; evaluation and management

E&M endocrine and metabolic; evaluation and management

Em emmetropia

E_m midpoint redox potential

EMA electronic microanalyzer; emergency management agency; emergency medical assistance; emergency medical assistant; emergency medical attendant; endothelial monocyte antigen; epithelial membrane antigen; extramural absorber

EMAB endothelial monocyte antigen B

EMAP Environmental Monitoring and Assessment Program; evoked muscle action potential

E_{max} maximum effect; maximum energy

EMB embryology; endomyocardial biopsy; engineering in medicine and biology; eosin-methylene blue; ethambutol; explosive mental behavior

emb embolism; embryo; embryology

EMBASE Excerpta Medica Database

EMBL European Molecular Biology Laboratory

EMBO European Molecular Biology Organization

embryol embryology

EMBS Engineering in Medicine and Biology Society

EMC electromagnetic compatibility; electron microscopy; emergency medical care; emergency medical communication; emergency medical condition; emergency medical coordinator; encephalomyocarditis; enzyme mismatch cleavage; essential mixed cryoglobulinemia

EMCR electronic medical care record

EMC&R emergency medical care and rescue

EMCRO Experimental Medical Care Review Organization

EMCV encephalomyocarditis virus

EMD electromechanical dissociation; emergency medical dispacher; emergency medical doctor; Emery-Dreifuss muscular dystrophy; esophageal mobility disorder

EMDIS European Marrow Donor Information System

EMDR eye movement desensitization and reprocessing

EME electromechanical energy

EMEA European Agency for the Evaluation of Medicinal Products

EMEDI European Medical Electronic Data Interchange [group]

EMEM Eagle minimal essential medium

EMER electromagnetic molecular electron resonance

emer emergency

EMF electromagnetic field; electromagnetic flow; electromagnetic flowmeter; electromotive force; Emergency Medicine Foundation; endomyocardial fibrosis; equivalent molecules of immunofluorescence; erythrocyte maturation factor; evaporated milk formula

emf electromotive force

EMG electromyogram, electromyography; eye movement gauge; exomphalosmacroglossia-gigantism [syndrome]

EMGBF electromyographic biofeedback

EMG(int) integrated electromyographic [value]

EMGN extramembranous glomerulonephritis

EMG/NCV electromyography/nerve conduction velocity [test]

EMI electromagnetic immunity; electromagnetic interference; emergency medical information

EMIAT European Myocardial Infarction Amiodarone Trial; European Myocardial Infarction Arrhythmia Trial

EMIC emergency maternal and infant care; Environmental Mutagen Information Center

EMICBACK Environmental Mutagen Information Center Backfile

EM/IM extramedullary/intramedullary

EMIP European Myocardial Infarction Project

EMIP-FR European Myocardial Infarction Project-Free Radicals

EMIR envelope mastectomy and immediate reconstruction

EMIT enzyme multiplied immunoassay technique; European Mivazerol Trial

EmIV *Enytus montanus* ichnovirus

EMJH Ellinghausen-McCullough-Johnson-Harris [medium]

EML erythema nodosum leprosum

EMLA eutectic mixture of local anesthetics

EMM erythema multiforme major

EMMA eye movement measuring apparatus

EMO Epstein-Macintosh-Oxford [inhaler]; exophthalmos, myxedema circumscriptum praetibiale, and osteoarthropathia hypertrophicans [syndrome]

emot emotion, emotional

EMP electric membrane property; electromagnetic pulse; Embden-Meyerhof pathway; emergency medicine providers; European Myocardial Infarction Project; external membrane potential; external membrane protein; extramedullary plasmacytoma; malignant proliferation of eosinophils

EMPAR Enoxaparin MaxEPA Prevention of Angioplasty Restenosis [study]

EMPIRE Economics of Myocardial Perfusion Imaging in Europe [study]

EMPS exertional muscle pain syndrome

EMPSGC endocrine mucin-producing sweat gland carcinoma

EMQ exercise motivation questionnaire

EMR electromagnetic radiation; electronic medical record; emergency mechanical restraint; emergency medicine resident; endoscopic mucosal resection; essential metabolism ratio; eye movement record

EMRA Emergency Medicine Residents Association

EMRC European Medical Research Council

EMRD emergency medicine residency director

E-MRI extremity magnetic resonance imaging

EMRS electronic medical record system

EMRSA epidemic strain of methicillin-resistant *Staphylococcus aureus*

EMS early morning specimen; early morning stiffness; electrical muscle stimulation; Electronic Medical Service; emergency management of stroke; emergency medical services; endometriosis; environmental management system; eosinophilia-myalgia syndrome; ethyl methane-sulfonate; European Multicenter Study

EMSA electrophoretic mobility shift assay; Emergency Medical Services Agency

EMSC emergency medical services for children

EMSS emergency medical services system

EMSU epidemiology and medical statistics unit

EMT emergency medical tag; emergency medical team; emergency medical technician; emergency medical treatment; endocardial mapping technique; epithelial-mesenchymal transition

EMTA endomethylene tetrahydrophthalic acid

EMT-A emergency medical technician-ambulance; emergency medical technician providing basic life support or cardiopulmonary resuscitation

EMTAC Enhanced Metabolic Testing Activity Chamber

EMTALA Emergency Medical Treatment and Active Labor Act

EMT-B emergency medical technician-basic

EMTD estimated maximum tolerated dose

EMT-D emergency medical technician providing basic life support or defibrillation

EMT-I emergency medical technician-intermediate

EMT-M emergency medical technician mining

EMT-P emergency medical technician-paramedic

EMTS electromagnetic tracking system

EMT-W emergency medical technician-wilderness

EMU early morning urine; energy-mode ultrasound

emu electromagnetic unit

emul emulsion

EMV equine morbillivirus; eye, motor, voice

EmV *Eucocytis meeki* virus

EMVC early mitral valve closure

EMY emergency medicine resident year

EMZL extranodal marginal zone B-cell lymphoma

EN endoscopy; enrolled nurse; enteral nutrition; epidemic nephritis; erythema nodosum

En, en enema

ENA Emergency Nurses Association; epithelial neutrophil-activating [protein]; extractable nuclear antigen

E$_{Na}$ sodium reversal potential

ENaC epithelial sodium channel

ENACT enzyme activity in chemical toxicity; Expanding Nilotinib Access in Clinical Trials

ENASA Enoxaparin and/or Aspirin in Unstable Angina [trial]

ENB esthesioneuroblastoma

ENC encounter; encryption; endotoxin neutralizing capacity; environmental control

ENCODE Encyclopedia of DNA Elements

ENCORE Evaluation of Nifedipine and Cerivastatin on Recovery of Endothelial Function [trial]

END early neonatal death; elective neck dissection; endocrinology; endorphin; endothelin; endurance

end endoreduplication

ENDIT European Nicotinamide Diabetes Intervention Trial

Endo endocardial, endocardium; endocrine, endocrinology; endodontics; endonuclease; endotracheal

endo endoscopy

EndoCAM endothelial cell adhesion molecule

Endo-M endocardium and M region

ENDOR electron nuclear double resonance

Endo X endonuclease X

ENDPT end point of flow velocity after angioplasty; evaluation of Doppler parameters during percutaneous transluminal coronary angioplasty

ENDR endothelin receptor

ENDRB endothelin receptor B

ENDT electroneurodiagnostic technologist

ENE ethylnorepinephrine

ENeG electroneurography

enem enema

ENF enfuvirtide

ENG electroneurograph, electroneurography; electronystagmogram, electronystagmography

Eng English

ENHR Essential National Health Research

ENI elective neck irradiation; elective nodal irradiation

ENIAC Electronic Numerical Integrator and Computer

ENK enkephalin

ENL equivalent number of looks [echocardiography]; erythema nodosum leproticum

ENMG electroneuromyography

ENN environmental noise

ENO, Eno enolase

ENOG, ENoG electroneuronography

eNOS endothelial nitric oxide synthase

ENOXART enoxaparin in arterial surgery

ENP emergency nurse practitioner; ethyl-*p*-nitrophenylthiobenzene phosphate; excellence for nursing practice; extractable nucleoprotein

ENPC emergency nursing pediatric course

E-NPI end nuclear polymorphism index

ENR eosinophilic nonallergic rhinitis; extra-thyroid neck radioactivity

ENRICAD Enhancing Recovery in Coronary Heart Disease [trial]

ENRICHD Enchancing Recovery in Coronary Heart Disease Patients [trial]

ENS empty nose syndrome; enteral nutritional support; enteric nervous system; epidermal nevus syndrome; ethylnorsuprarenin

ENSV Enseada virus

ENT ear, nose, and throat; enzootic nasal tumor; extranodular tissue

ent enterotoxin

ent A enterotoxin A

ENTICES Enoxaparin and Ticlopidine After Elective Stenting [study]

Entom entomology

ENTV *Entamoeba* virus; Entebbe virus

ENTY entity

ENU *N*-ethyl-nitrosourea

Env envelope

env, environ environment, environmental

ENVR environmental effect

ENX endonexin

enz enzyme, enzymatic

EO early onset; eosinophil; ethylene oxide; eyes open

E$_o$ skin dose

EOA effective orifice area; erosive osteoarthritis; esophageal obturator airway; examination, opinion, and advice

EOAD early-onset Alzheimer disease

EOB edge of bed; emergency observation bed; explanation of benefits

EOC emergency observation center; emergency operations center; epithelial ovarian cancer

EoC episode of care

EOCA early-onset cerebellar ataxia

EOCAD early-onset coronary artery disease

EO-CFC eosinophil-leukocyte colony forming cell

EOD entry on duty; every other day; explosive ordnance disposal

EoE eosinophilic esophagitis

EOF end of file

E of M error of measurement

EOG electrooculogram, electrooculography; electroolfactogram, electroolfactography; eosinophilic gastroenteritis; ethylene oxide gas

EOGBS early-onset group B streptococcal

EOJ extrahepatic obstructive jaundice

EOL end of life

EOM electrooptic modulator; end of message; equal ocular movement; external otitis media; extraocular movement; extraocular muscle

EoM equation of motion

EOMA emergency oxygen mask assembly

EOMB explanation of Medicare benefits

EOMI extraocular muscles intact

EOM NL extraocular eye movements normal

EOP efficiency of plating; emergency outpatient

EOR European Organization for Research; exclusive operating room

EORTC European Organisation for Research and Treatment of Cancer

EOS end of saturated bombardment; end of service [pacemaker]; end of study; eosinophil; European Orthodontic Society

eos, eosin eosinophil

Eosm effective osmolarity

EOT effective oxygen transport; externally oriented thinking

EOTD early-onset torsion dystonia

EOU epidemic observation unit

EOx eye oximeter

EP echo planar; ectopic pregnancy; edible portion; electronic palpation; electrophoresis; electrophysiologic; electroprecipitin; emergency physician; emergency procedure; endocochlear potential; endogenous pyrogen;

endoperoxide; endorphin; end plate; end point; enteropeptidase; environmental protection; enzyme product; eosinophilic pneumonia; epicardial electrogram; epirubicin; epithelial, epithelium; epoxide; erythrocyte protoporphyrin; erythrophagocytosis; erythropoietic porphyria; erythropoietin; esophageal pressure; estramustine phosphate; European Pharmacopoeia; evoked potential; evolutionary programming; excretory phase; exophytic papilloma; expert panel; extreme pressure

E$_p$ primary etiology; proton energy

EPA eicosapentaenoic acid; empiric phrase association; Environmental Protection Agency; erect posterior–anterior; erythroid potentiating activity; extrinsic plasminogen activator

EPAP expiratory positive airway pressure

EPAQ Extended Personal Attitudes Questionnaire

EPA/RCRA Environmental Protection Agency Resource Conservation and Recovery Act

EPAS evolution of physiologic analysis systems

EPB extensor pollicis brevis

EPBF effective pulmonary blood flow

EPC endothelial progenitor cell; end plate current; epilepsia partialis continua; evidence-based practice center; external pneumatic compression

EPCA external pressure circulatory assistance

EPCG endoscopic pancreatocholangiography

EPCOT European Prospective Cohort on Thrombophilia

EPCRLS European Pancreatic Cancer Reference Library System

EPCS emergency portacaval shunt

EPD embolic protection device; energy-protein deficit; etiologic potentials display

EPDC epicardially derived cell

EPDML epidemiologic, epidemiology

EPE erythropoietin-producing enzyme

EPEC enteropathogenic *Escherichia coli*

EPEG etoposide

EPESE Established Populations for Epidemiologic Studies of the Elderly

EPF early pregnancy factor; endocarditis parietalis fibroplastica; endothelial proliferating factor; established program financing; estrogenic positive feedback; exophthalmos-producing factor

ePFT endoscopic pancreatic function test

EPG eggs per gram; electropalatography; electropneumogram, electropneumography; ethanolamine phosphoglyceride

EPH edema-proteinuria-hypertension; episodic paroxysmal hemicrania; extensor proprius hallucis

EPHIP education program for health informatics professionals

EPhMRA European Pharmaceutical Market Research Association

EpHV elapid herpesvirus

EPHX epoxide hydrolase

EPI echo planar imaging; electronic portal imaging; Emotion Profile Index; epilepsy; epinephrine; epirubicin; epithelial, epithelium; Estes Park Institute; evoked potential index; Expanded Programme of Immunization; extrapyramidal involvement; extrinsic pathway inhibitor

Epi epidemic [as in Epi-curve]

epi epinephrine

EPIC Echocardiography Persantine International Cooperative Study; Echo Persantine Italian Cooperative Study; European Prevalence of Infection in Intensive Care Study; European Prospective Investigation into Cancer and Nutrition Study; European Prototype for Integrated Care; Evaluation of 7E3 for the Prevention of Ischemic Complications

EPICORE Epidemiology Coordinating and Research Centre

EPICS Early Postmenopausal Intervention Cohort Study

EPID electronic portal imaging device; epidemiology

epid epidemic

EPIDS Early Post–Myocardial Infarction Intravenous Dipyridamole Study

epil epilepsy, epileptic

EPILOG Evaluation of Percutaneous Transluminal Coronary Angioplasty to Improve Long-Term Outcome with Abciximab Glycoprotein IIb/IIIa Blockade [trial]

epineph epinephrine

epis episiotomy

EPISODE Evaluation Peripheral Intramuscular Sonography on Dotter Effect

EPI/STAR echo planar imaging with signal targeting and alternating radiofrequency

EPISTENT Epilog Stent Trial; Evaluation of IIb/IIIa Platelet Inhibitor for Stenting

epith epithelium

EPIV enhanced potency inactivated polio vaccine

EPIX Emergency Preparedness Information Exchange

Epi-X Epidemic Information Exchange

EPL early pregnancy loss; effective path length; effect of patient's life; equivalent path length; essential phospholipid; extensor pollicis longus; extracorporeal piezoelectric lithotriptor

EPM electron probe microanalysis; electrophoretic mobility; energy-protein malnutrition
EPMR progressive epilepsy with mental retardation (intellectual disability)
EPN emphysematous pyelonephritis
EPNP 1,2-epoxy-3(4′-nitrophenoxy)propane
EPO eosinophil peroxidase; epidemiology program office; erythropoiesis; erythropoietin; evening primrose oil; exclusive provider organization; expiratory port occlusion
Epo erythropoietin
EPOB employee per occupied bed
EPOC excess post-exercise oxygen consumption
EPOCH Erythropoietin in Chinese Hamster Ovary [study]
EPOR erythropoietin receptor
EPOX epoxygenase
EPP end plate potential; equal pressure point; erythropoietic protoporphyria; extrapleural pneumonectomy
epp end plate potential
EPPB end positive-pressure breathing
EPPS Edwards Personal Preference Schedule
EPQ Eysenck Personality Questionnaire
EPR early phase reaction; early progressive resistance; effective poor radius; electron paramagnetic resonance; electronic patient record; electrophrenic respiration; emergency physical restraint; enhanced permeability and retention; Epidemic and Pandemic Alert and Response; epitympanic recess; estimated protein requirement; estradiol production rate; evoked potential response; extraparenchymal resistance; extrapyramidal reaction
EPRCSS European Prospective Randomized Coronary Surgery Study
EpRE/ARE electrophile/antioxidant response element
EPROM erasable programmable read-only memory
EPROU Electronic Patient Record System at Osaka University Hospital
EPRS electronic patient record system; European Prospective Randomized Study
EPS ear-patella-short stature [syndrome]; early progressing stroke; elastosis perforans serpiginosa; electrophysiologic study; endoscopic pancreatic sphincterectomy; enzyme pancreatic secretion; exhaustion syndrome; exophthalmos-producing substance; expressed prostatic secretions; extracellular polysaccharide; extracellular protein secretion; extrapyramidal side effects; extrapyramidal symptom; extrapyramidal syndrome

EPs eligible professionals [Medicaid designation]
ep's epithelial cells
EPSC excitatory postsynaptic current
EPSDT early and periodic screening diagnosis and treatment program
EPSE extrapyramidal side effects
EPSEM equal probability of selection method
EPSI echo planar spectroscopic imaging
EPSP excitatory postsynaptic potential
EPSS E point to septal separation
EPT early pregnancy test; endorectal pull-through
EPTE existed prior to enlistment
EPTFE, ePTFE expanded polytetrafluoroethylene
EPTS existed prior to service
EPV encephaloclastic proliferative vasculopathy; entomopoxvirus
EPXMA electron probe x-ray microana-lyzer
EQ educational quotient; empathy quotient; encephalization quotient; energy quotient; equal to
Eq, eq equation; equivalent
EQA external quality assessment
EQAM Ervin quality assessment measure
EQLIPSE Evaluation and Quality in Library Performance System for Europe
EQOL economics and quality of life
EQP extensor quinti proprius
EqPV equine picornavirus
EQS electroquasistatic
EqTV equine torovirus
EQuIP Evaluation and Quality Improvement Program
equip equipment
EQUIPP Evaluation of Quinapril in Primary Practice [trial]
equiv equivalency, equivalent
ER efficiency ratio; ejection rate; electroresection; emergency room; endoplasmic reticulum; enhanced reactivation; enhancement ratio; entity relationship; environmental resistance; enzyme reactor; epigastric region; equine rhinopneumonia; equivalent roentgen; erythematotelangiectatic rosacea; erythrocyte receptor; estradiol receptor; estrogen receptor; etretinate; evoked response; expiratory reserve; extended release; extended resistance; external resistance; external rotation
E-R, E/R entity relationship
ER⁺ increased estrogen receptor
ER⁻ decreased estrogen receptor
Er erbium; erythrocyte

E$_r$ repulsive energy

er endoplasmic reticulum

ERA early [electronic] referrals application; echo record access [study]; electrical response activity; electroencephalic response audiometry; electronic remittance advice; energy return ability; Enoxaparin Restenosis After Angioplasty [study]; entity relationship attribute; estradiol receptor assay; estrogen receptor assay; Estrogen Replacement in Atherosclerosis [study]; evoked response audiometry; extended relational algebra

ERA-ICA estradiol receptor assay immuno-cytochemical analysis

ERAS electronic residency application service

ERASME Efficacy of Renal Artery Stent Multicentre Evaluation

ERAV equine rhinitis A virus

ERBAC Excimer Laser, Rotablator, and Balloon Angioplasty Comparison [study]

ERBF effective renal blood flow

ERBV equine rhinitis B virus

ERC endoscopic retrograde cholangiography; enteric cytopathic human orphan-rhino-coryza [virus]; erythropoietin-responsive cell; ethical review committee; European Resuscitation Council

Erc erythrocyte

ER cap endoscopic resection cap

ERCC excision repair cross complementing

ERCoh event-related coherence

ERCP endoscopic retrograde cholangiopancreatography

Ercs erythrocytes

ERD erosive reflux disease; event-related desynchronization; evoked response detector

ERDA Energy Research and Development Administration

ERDIP electronic records development and implementation

ERE estrogen response element; external rotation in extension

EREP event-related evoked potential

ERF edge response function; Education and Research Foundation; end response function; esophagorespiratory fistula; external rotation in flexion; Eye Research Foundation

eRF eukaryotic release factor

E-RFC E-rosette forming cell

ERFS electrophysiologic ring-finger splinting

ERG electron radiography; electroretinogram, electroretinography; emergency response guidebook

ERGIC endoplasmic reticulum–Golgi intermediate compartment

ErgTX ergotoxin

ERHD exposure-related hypothermic death

ErHV erinaceid herpesvirus

ERI elective replacement indicator [pacemaker]; environmental response inventory; E-rosette inhibitor; erythrocyte rosette inhibitor

ERIA electroradioimmunoassay

ERIC Education Resources Information Center; Educational Resource Information Clearinghouse

ERICA European Risk and Incidence: A Coordinated Analysis

ERISA Employee Retirement Income Security Act

ERL extraneous residue limit

ERK extracellular signal-regulated kinase

ErLV *Erysimum* latent virus

ERM electrochemical relaxation method; extended radical mastectomy; ezrin, radixin, and moesin

ERMSa embryonal rhabdomyosarcoma

ERNA early return to normal activities [after acute myocardial infarction]; efferent renal nerve activity; equilibrium radionuclide angiocardiography

ERNST European Resuscitation Nimodipine Study

ERO effective regurgitant orifice [tricuspid regurgitation]; Eugenics Record Office

ERO$_2$ oxygen extraction ratio

EROD 7-ethoxyresorufin-*O*-deethylase

EROI epiphyseal region of interest

EROS elaboration of reactions for organic synthesis

ERP early receptor potential; effective refractory period; elodoisin-related peptide; emergency response team; endoscopic retrograde pancreatography; enzyme-releasing peptide; equine rhinopneumonitis; estrogen receptor protein; event-related potential

Er-PBMC E-rosette-negative peripheral blood mononuclear cell

ERPC evacuation of retained products of conception

ERPF effective renal plasma flow

ERPG emergency response planning guidelines

ERPLV effective refractory period of left ventricle

ERR excess relative risk

ERS enamel-renal syndrome; endoscopic retrograde sphincterectomy

E$_{rs}$ respiratory system elastance

ERSP event-related slow potential

ERSPC European Randomized Study of Screening for Prostatic Cancer

ERT emergency room thoracotomy, emergent resuscitative thoracotomy; enzyme replacement therapy; esophageal radionuclide transit;

estrogen replacement therapy; examination room terminal; external radiation therapy

ERTAS extended reticulothalamic activating system

ERTOCS, ERTOS European Randomised Trial of Ovarian Cancer Screening

ERU endorectal ultrasound

ERV Embu virus; enterolike virus; equine rhinopneumonitis virus; Estero Real virus; etched ringspot virus; expiratory reserve volume

ERVEV Erve virus

ERVSP estimated right ventricular systolic pressure

ERY erysipelas

Ery *Erysipelothrix*

ES ejection sound; elastic stocking; elastic support; electrical stimulus, electrical stimulation; electroshock; electrospray; electrotherapy system; Elejalde syndrome; embryonic stem; emergency service; emission spectrometry; end of systole; endometritis-salpingitis; endoscopic sclerosis; endoscopic sclerotherapy; endoscopic sphincterotomy; end stage [disease]; end systole; end to side; English speaking; enzyme substrate; epileptic seizures; epileptic syndrome; erythromycin stearate; esophageal; esophageal scintigraphy; esophagus; esterase; evoking strength; Ewing sarcoma; exfoliation syndrome; expectation score; experimental study; expert system; exterior surface; extra stimulus; extrasystole

Es einsteinium

E$_s$ secondary etiology; shear energy

ESA Electrolysis Society of America; electronic signature authentication; endocardial surface area; epidermal surface antigen; epididymal sperm aneuploidy; esterase; esterase A

ESAC extrastructurally abnormal chromosome

ESADDI estimated safe and adequate daily dietary intake

ESAS semiautomated instrument system

ESAT early screening of autistic traits; esterase activator

ESAW European statistics on accidents at work

ESB electrical stimulation of the brain; enhanced skill building; environmental specimen banking; esterase B

ESBL extended spectrum beta-lactamase

ESBY Electrical Stimulation vs. Coronary Artery Bypass [study]

ESC electromechanical slope computer; embryonic stem cell; endosystolic count; environmental stress cracking; epidural spinal cord; erythropoietin-sensitive stem cell; esterase C

ESCA electron spectroscopy for chemical analysis

ESCALAT, ESCALATE Efegatran and Streptokinase to Canalize Arteries Like Accelerated Tissue Plasminogen Activator [study]

ESCAPE Evaluation Study of Congestive Heart Failure and Pulmonary Artery Catheterization Effectiveness

ESCAT Early Self-Controlled Anticoagulation Trial

ESCC epidural spinal cord compression; esophageal squamous cell carcinoma

ESCH European Study Group on Cytogenetic Biomarkers and Health

Esch *Escherichia*

ESCN electrolyte and steroid cardiopathy with necrosis

ESCOBAR Emergency Stenting Compared to Conventional Balloon Angioplasty Randomized Trial

ESCODD European Standards Committee on Oxidative DNA Damage

EsCPS *Euxoa scandens* cypovirus

ESCS epidural spinal cord stimulation

ESD electronic submission document; electronic summation device; electrostatic discharge; emission spectrometric device; endoscopic submucosal dissection; end-systolic dimension; esterase-D; exoskeletal device

ESDI enhanced small device interface

ESDM early start Denver model

ESDN European Skeletal Dysplasia Network

ESE electrostatic unit [Ger. *electrostatische Einheit*]; evolutionary stable energy; exercise stress echocardiography

ESEM endoscopically suspected esophageal metaplasia; European Society for Engineering and Medicine

ESETCID European Study of Epidemiology and Treatment of Cardiac Inflammatory Diseases

ESF edge spread function; electron scatter function; electrosurgical filter; erythropoietic stimulating factor

ESFH European Society for Hemapheresis; Interdisciplinary European Society for Haemapheresis and Haemotherapy

ESFL end-systolic force-length relationship

ESG electrospinogram; endovascular stent graft; estrogen; exfoliation syndrome glaucoma

ESGE European Society of Gastrointestinal Endoscopy

ESHEL Association for the Planning and Development of Services for the Aged in Israel

ESHF end-stage heart failure

ESHG European Society of Human Genetics

ESHL early-stage Hodgkin lymphoma

ESHR elder spontaneously hypertensive rat

EsHV esocid herpesvirus

ESI elastase-specific inhibitor; electrospray ionization; emergency safety information; emergency severity index; enzyme substrate inhibitor; epidural steroid injection

ESIC electrical stimulation−induced contractions

ESIC-LCE electric stimulation−induced contractions, leg cycle ergometry

ESI-MS electrospray ionization mass spectrometry

ESIMV expiratory synchronized intermittent mandatory ventilation

ESIN elastic stable intramedullary nailing

ESIPT excited state intermolecular proton transfer

ESKAPE *Enterococcus faecium, Staphylococcus aureus, Klebsiella pneumoniae, Acinetobacter baumannii, Pseudomonas aeruginosa,* and *Enterobacter* species

ESL end-systolic length; E-selectin ligand; extracorporeal shockwave lithotripsy

ESLD end-stage liver disease

ESLF end-stage liver failure

ESLV elderberry symptomless virus

ESM ejection systolic murmur; endolymphatic stromal myosis; endoscopic specular microscope; ethosuximide

ESMC entropy sampling Monte Carlo

ESMIR Echocardiographic Selection of Patients for Mitral Regurgitation [study]

ESMIS Emergency Medical Services Management Information System

ESMS electrospray mass spectrometry

ESN educationally subnormal; estrogen-stimulated neurophysin; exposed seronegative

ESnet Energy Sciences Network

ESN(M) educationally subnormal-moderate

ESN(S) educationally subnormal-severe

ESO electrospinal orthosis; embolic signal onset

eso esophagoscopy; esophagus

ESOCAP European Study of Community Acquired Pneumonia

ESP early systolic paradox; echo spacing; effective sensory projection; effective systolic pressure; embryo storage problems; endometritis-salpingitis-peritonitis; end-systolic pressure; eosinophil stimulation promoter; epidermal soluble protein; especially; evoked synaptic potential; extrasensory perception

ESPA electrical stimulation−produced analgesia; extended sibling pair analysis

ESPAC European Study Group of Pancreatic Cancer

ESPC enhanced spectral pathology component

ESPEN European Society for Parenteral and Enteral Nutrition

EsPeR personalized risk estimation

ESPRIM European Study Prevention Research of Infarct With Molsidomine

ESPRIT Efficacy Safety Prospective Randomized Ibopamine Trial; European and Australian Stroke Prevention in Reversible Ischemia Trial; European Study of the Prevention of Reocclusion After Initial Thrombolysis; European Study Programme the Relevance of Immunology in Liver Transplantation; Evaluation of Subcutaneous Proleukin in a Randomized International Trial

ESPS European Secondary Prevention Study; European Stroke Prevention Study

ESPVR end-systolic pressure-volume relationship

ESQ early signs questionnaire

ESR Einstein stroke radius; electric skin resistance; electron spin resonance; emotional stress release; equipment service report; erythrocyte sedimentation rate; estrogen receptor; European Society of Radiology; extracytoplasmic stress response

ESRD End Stage Renal Disease [Program]; end-stage renal disease

ESRF end-stage renal failure; European Synchrotron Radiation Facility

ESRI Environmental Systems Research Institute

ESS earliest starting shift; earth and space sciences; elementary sulcal surface; empty sella syndrome; endostreptosin; Epworth sleepiness scale; erythrocyte-sensitizing substance; euthyroid sick syndrome; excited skin syndrome; exonic splicing silencer/suppressor; squamous self-healing epithelioma

ess essential

ESSENCE Efficacy Safety Subcutaneous Enoxaparin in Non-Q-Wave Coronary Events [study]; Electronic Surveillance System for Early Notification of Community-Based Epidemics

ESSEX European Scimed Stent Experience

ESSF external spinal skeletal fixation

ESSV Essaouira virus

EST Early Stroke Trial; electric shock threshold; electroshock therapy; endodermal sinus tumor; endometrial sinus tumor; endoscopic sphincterectomy; esterase; exercise stress test; expressed sequence tag

Est estradiol

est ester; estimation, estimated

ESTEEM European Standardised Telematic Tool to Evaluate EMG

esth esthetic, esthetics

Est,l elastance, lung

E-STP experimental short-term psychotherapy

Est,rs elastance, respiratory system

Est,w elastance, chest wall

ESU electrostatic unit; electrosurgical unit

E-sub excitor substance

ESUE emergency screening ultrasound examination

ESV end-systolic volume; esophageal valve

ESVEM Electrophysiologic Study vs. Electrocardiographic Monitoring

ESVH endoscopic saphenous vein harvesting

ESVI end-systolic volume index

ESVS endoscopic vascular surgery; epiurethral suprapubic vaginal suspension

ESWL extracorporeal shock wave litho-tripsy

ESWS end-systolic wall stress

E$_{syn}$ reversal potential

ET educational therapy; effective temperature; ejection time; embryo transfer; endothelin; endotoxin; endotracheal; endotracheal tube; end tidal; endurance time; enterostomal therapist; enterotoxin; epidermolytic toxin; epithelial tumor; esophageal temperature; esotropia; essential thrombocythemia; essential tremor; ethanol; etiocholanolone test; etiology; eustachian tube; examination terminal; exchange transfusion; exercise test; exercise treadmill; exfoliative toxin; expiration time; exploratory thoracoscopy

E:T, E/T effect/target ratio

ET-1 endothelin-1

ET$_3$ erythrocyte triiodothyronine

ET$_4$ effective thyroxine [test]

Et ethyl; etiology

et and [L. *et*]; end tidal

ETA electron transfer agent; elongation of tendon Achilles; endotracheal airways; endotracheal aspiration; ethionamide; exfoliative toxin A

ET-A, ET$_A$ endothelin A

ETAB extrathoracic assisted breathing

ETAC early treatment of atopic child

ETAF epidermal thrombocyte activating factor; epithelial thymus-activating factor

ETAG end-tidal anesthetic gas

et al and others [L. *et alii*]

ETAR equivalent tissue air ratio

ET-B, ET$_B$ endothelin B

ETBA endoscopic transaxillary breast augmentation

ETC electron transport chain; emergency trauma care; enterotoxigenic *Escherichia coli*; esophageal tracheal Combitube; estimated time of conception

ET$_c$ corrected ejection time

ETCC emergency team coordination course

ETCO$_2$, $_{et}$CO$_2$ end-tidal carbon dioxide

ETD eustachian tube dysfunction

ETDRS Early Treatment Diabetic Retinopathy Study

ETD(V) extrapolated tolerance dose (volume)

ETE end to end

ETEC enterotoxic/enterotoxigenic *Escherichia coli*

ETF electron-transferring flavoprotein; embryo toxic factor; eustachian tube function; extension teardrop fracture

ETFB electron transfer flavoprotein beta polypeptide

ETFDH electron-transferring flavoprotein dehydrogenase

ETG episode treatment group

ETH elixir terpin hydrate; ethanol; ethmoid

ETh excitability threshold

eth ether

ETHC elixir terpin hydrate with codeine

ETHR education, training, and human resources

ETI endotracheal intubation

ETIC Environmental Teratology Information Center

ETICBACK Environmental Teratology Information Center Backfile

ETIO etiocholanolone

etiol etiology

EtIV *Eriborus terebrans* ichnovirus

ETK erythrocyte transketolase

ETKTM every test known to man

ETL echo train length; expiratory threshold load

ETM erythromycin

ETNet Educational Technology Network

EtNP ethanolamine phosphate

EtNU ethyl nitrosourea

ETO estimated time of ovulation; ethylene oxide

Eto ethylene oxide

E-TOF electron time of flight

ETOH, EtOH ethanol

ETOX ethylene oxide

ETP electron transport particle; entire treatment period; ephedrine, theophylline, phenobarbital; eustachian tube pressure

ETPCO₂ end-tidal partial carbon dioxide

ETR effective thyroxine ratio; endothelin receptor

ETS educational testing service; electrical transcranial stimulation; electron transport system; electronic transimpedance scanning; electrosleep therapy; endoscopic transthoracic sympathectomy; environmental tobacco smoke; erythromycin topical solution; event timing system; expiration time signal; extracellular transport system

ET-ST endotracheal tube-stylet unit

ETT endotracheal tube; epinephrine tolerance test; exercise tolerance test; exercise treadmill test; extrathyroidal thyroxine

ET-TL endotracheal tube Trachlight unit

ETTP enhanced trusted third party

ETU emergency and trauma unit; emergency treatment unit; ethylene thiourea

ETV extravascular thermal volume

ETX etiology

EU Ehrlich unit; elementary unit; emergency unit; endotoxin unit; entropy unit; enzyme unit; esterase unit; etiology unknown; excretory urography; expected utility

Eu europium; euryon

EUA emergency use authorization; examination under anesthesia

EUBV Eubenangee virus

EUCAST European Committee on Antimicrobial Susceptibility Testing

EUCLID European Diabetes Controlled Trial of Lisinopril in Insulin-Dependent Diabetes Mellitus

EUCROMIC European Collaborative Research on Mosaicism in Chorionic Virus Sample

EUDB end-user database

EUFOS European Federation of Oto-Rhino-Laryngological Societies

EUHID encrypted universal health care identifier

EUL expected upper limit

EULAR European League Against Rheumatism

EUM external urethral meatus

EUP extrauterine pregnancy

EURAGE European Community Concerted Action on Aging

EURALIM European Alimentation Study

EURAMIC European Community Multicenter Study on Antioxidants, Myocardial Infarction, and Breast Cancer

EUREKA Unconventional Research Enabling Knowledge Acceleration

EURID European Registry for Implantable Cardioverter Defibrillators

EURO-ART European Angiojet Rapid Thrombectomy [study]

EUROASPIRE European Action on Secondary Prevention by Intervention to Reduce Events

EUROCARDI European Concerted Action for the Rapid Diagnosis of Myocardial Infarction

EUROCARE European Carvedilol Restenosis Trial

EURO-CAT European Cancer After Transplant [project]; European Register of Congenital Anomalies and Twins

EURODIAB ACE European Diabetes: Aetiology of Childhood Diabetes on an Epidemiological Basis

EURODIAB IDDM European Diabetes Centers Study of Complications in Patients with Insulin-Dependent Diabetes Mellitus

EURODIAB TIGER European Diabetes: Type I Genetic Epidemiology Resources

EURO-DIRECT European Direct Myocardial Revascularization in Regeneration of Endomyocardial Channels Trial

EUROHAZCON Congenital Anomalies Near Hazardous Waste Landfill Sites in Europe [study]

EURO-ISDN European Integrated Services Digital Network

EURONET European On-Line Network

EUROPA European Trial of Reduction of Cardiac Events with Perindopril in Stable Coronary Artery Disease

EuroQol European quality of life [scale]

EUROSCOP European Registry Society Study of Chronic Obstructive Pulmonary Diseases

EUROSTROKE European Collaborative Study of Incidence and Risk Factors for Ischemic and Hemorrhagic Stroke

EUROTOX European Committee on Chronic Toxicity Hazards

EUROWINTER European Study on Cold Exposure and Winter Mortality From Ischemic Heart Disease

EUS endorectal ultrasonography/ultrasound; endoscopic ultrasonography/ultrasound; external urethral sphincter

EUS-CPN endosonography-guided celiac plexus neurolysis

EUS-FNA endoscopic ultrasound fine-needle aspiration

Eust eustachian

EUS-TNB endoscopic ultrasound TruCut needle biopsy

EUV extreme ultraviolet laser

EV Ebola virus; eczema vaccinatum; ejected volume; electric vehicle; electronic patient record [EPR] value; emergency vehicle; encephalitis/encephalomyelitis virus; enteritis virus; enterovirus; entomopoxvirus; epidermodysplasia verruciformis; estradiol valerate; eustachian valve; evoked potential; excessive ventilation; expected value; extravascular

Ev, ev eversion

eV, ev electron volt

EV-69, 70, 71 human enteroviruses 69, 70, 71

EVA Epidemiological Study on Vascular and Cognitive Aging; ethyl violet azide; ethylene vinyl acetate; European Vascular Agency [study]

evac evacuate, evacuated, evacuation

EVADE Experience With Left Ventricular Assist Device With Exercise [trial]

eval evaluate, evaluated, evaluation

eval stud evaluation study

evap evaporated, evaporation

EVAR endovascular aneurysm repair

EVB electronic view box; esophageal variceal bleeding

EVC, EvC Ellis–van Creveld [syndrome]

EVCI expected value of clinical information

EVD external ventricular drain; extracardiac vascular disease; extravascular [lung] density

ever eversion, everted

EVF ethanol volume fraction

EVFMG exchange visitor foreign medical graduate

EVG electroventriculography

EVGLI European Working Group on *Legionella* Surveillance Centre

EVIL exposure to selected viruses in research laboratories

EVL electronic visualization laboratory

EVLT endovascular laser therapy; endovenous laser treatment

EVLW extravascular lung water

EVM electronic voltmeter; extravascular mass

EVNT event

EVOC emergency vehicle operator course

EVP episcleral venous pressure; evoked visual potential

EVPI expected value of perfect information

EVR evoked visual response; exudative vitreoretinopathy

EVRS early ventricular repolarization syndrome

EVS eligibility verification system; endovaginal sonography

EVSG endovascular stent grafting

EVT endovascular technology

EVTV extravascular thermal volume

EVV Everglades virus

EVRX exudative vitreoretinopathy, X-linked

EW emergency ward; estrogen withdrawal

E-W Edinger-Westphal [nucleus]

EWA exponentially weighted average

EWAs erythrocytes without antigens

EWB estrogen withdrawal bleeding

EWCM egg-white cervical mucus

EWGCP European Working Group on Cardiac Pacing

EWGLP European Workshop for Computer-Based Support for Clinical Guidelines and Protocols

EWHO elbow-wrist-hand orthosis

EWKY elder Wistar-Kyoto rat

EWL egg-white lysozyme; evaporation water loss; excess weight loss

EWPHE European Working Party on Hypertension in the Elderly

EWR European Wallstent Registry

EWS Ewing sarcoma

EWSR Ewing sarcoma breakpoint region

EX exfoliation; exsmoker

E(X) expected value of the random variable X

ex exacerbation; examination, examined, examiner; example; excision; exercise; exophthalmos; exposure; extraction

EXA electronic x-ray archives

exac exacerbation

EXACT Extended Release Adalat Canadian Trial

EXACTO Excimer Laser Angioplasty in Coronary Total Occlusion

EXAFS extended x-ray absorption fine structure

exam examination, examine, examined

EXBF exercise hyperemia blood flow

ExBRT external beam radiation therapy

exc excision

EXCEED Excellence Center for Eliminating ethnic/Racial Disparities

EXCEL Expanded Clinical Evaluation of Lovastatin [trial]

exch exchange

EXCITE Evaluation of Oral Xemilofiban in Controlling Thrombotic Events

excr excretion

EXE exemestane

ExEF ejection fraction during exercise

EXELFS extended electron loss fine structure

exer exercise

EXERT Exercise Rehabilitation Trial

exg exogenous

EXIT ex utero intrapartum therapy

EXO exonuclease; exophoria

exog exogenous

exoph exophthalmia

EXoS exoenzyme S

exos exostosis
EXP expiration
exp expansion; expectorant; experiment, experimental; expiration, expired; exponential function; exposure
exp lap exploratory laparotomy
EXPAPS Exeter Primary Angioplasty Pilot Study
expect expectorant
exper experiment, experimental
ExPGN extracapillary proliferative glomerulonephritis
expir expiration, expiratory, expired
expl exploratory
Expl Lap exploratory laparotomy
ExpNET Expert Network
exptl experimental
EXREM external radiation-emission [dose in] man
EXS external support

EXT exercise testing
Ext extraction, extract
ext extension; extensive; extensor; exterior; external; extract; extreme, extremity
extr extract
EXTRA Evaluation of XT Stent for Restenosis of Native Arteries
extrav extravasation
ext rot external rotation
extub extubation
EXU excretory urogram
exud exudate, exudation
EY egg yolk; epidemiologic year
EYA egg yolk agar
EYAV Eyach virus
EYAV-FR578 Eyach virus—France 578
EYAV-GER Eyach virus—Germany
EZ epileptogenic zone
Ez eczema
EZE ezetimibe

F

F bioavailability; a cell that donates F factor in bacterial conjugation; coefficient of inbreeding; a conjugative plasmid in F^+ bacterial cells; degree of fineness of abrasive particles; facies; factor; Fahrenheit; failure; false; family; farad; Faraday constant; fascia; fasting; fat; father; feces; fellow; female; fermentation; fertility; fetal; fibroblast; fibrous; field of vision; filament; *Filaria*; fine; finger; flexion; flow; fluorine; flux; focal [spot]; focus; foil; fontanel; foramen; force; form, forma; formula; fornix; fossa; fraction, fractional; fracture; fragment; free; French [catheter]; frequency; frontal; frontal electrode placement; function; fundus; *Fusiformis*; fusion; *Fusobacterium*; gilbert; Helmholz free energy; hydrocortisone; inbreeding coefficient; left foot electrode [vectorcardiography]; let there be made [L. *fiat*]; phenylalanine; variance ratio

°F degree Fahrenheit

F′ hybrid F plasmid

F⁻ bacterial cell lacking an F plasmid

F⁺ bacterial cell having an F plasmid

F₀, F₁ coupling factor

F₁, F₂, etc. first, second, etc., filial generation; years of fellowship study

FI, FII, etc. coagulation factors I, II, etc.

F344 Fischer 344 [rat]

f atomic orbital with angular momentum quantum number 3; farad; fasting; father; female; femto-; fiber, fibrous; fingerbreadth; fission; flexion; fluid; focal; foot; form, forma; formula; fostered; fraction; fracture; fragment; frequency; frontal; function; fundus; numerical expression of the relative aperture of a camera lens

f- femto- [10^{-15}]

FA factor analysis; false aneurysm; Families Anonymous; Fanconi anemia; far advanced; fatty acid; febrile antigen; femoral artery; fetal age; fibrinolytic activity; fibroadenoma; fibrosing alveolitis; field ambulance; field assessment; filterable agent; filtered air; first aid; flip angle; fluorescent antibody; fluorescent assay; fluoroalanine; folic acid; follicular area; food allergy; forearm; fortified aqueous [solution]; fractional anisotropy; free acid; Freund adjuvant; Friedreich ataxia; functional activity; functional administration

F/A fetus active

fa fatty [rat]

FAA folic acid antagonist; formaldehyde, acetic acid, alcohol; fumarylacetoacetic acid

FA-A Fanconi anemia A

FAAB female assigned at birth

FAAH fatty acid amide hydrolase

FAAN Fellow of the American Academy of Nursing

FAANP Fellow of American Academy of Nurse Practitioners

FAAPM Fellow of American Academy of Pain Management

FAB fast atom bombardment; formalin ammonium bromide; fragment, antigen binding; French-American-British [leukemia staging]; functional arm brace

FA-B Fanconi anemia B

Fab fragment, antigen binding

F(ab′)₂ fragment, antigen binding

Fabc fragment, antigen, and complement binding

FABER flexion in abduction and external rotation

FABF femoral artery blood flow

FAB-MS fast atom bombardment mass spectrometry

FABP fatty acid–binding protein; folate-binding protein

FAC familial adenomatosis coli; femoral arterial cannulation; ferric ammonium citrate; fetal abdominal circumference; fluorescent aromatic compound; 5-fluorouracil, Adriamycin, and cyclophosphamide; foamy alveolar cast; fractional area changes; free available chlorine; functional aerobic capacity

FA-C Fanconi anemia C

Fac factor

fac facility; to make [L. *facere*]

FACA Fanconi anemia complementation group A; Fellow of the American College of Anesthetists; Fellow of the American College of Angiology; Fellow of the American College of Apothecaries

FACAI Fellow of the American College of Allergy and Immunology

FACAS Fellow of the American College of Abdominal Surgeons

FACB Fanconi anemia complementation group B

Facb fragment, antigen, and complement binding

FACC Fanconi anemia complementation group C; Fellow of the American College of Cardiologists

FACCT Foundation for Accountability

FACD Fanconi anemia complementation group D; Fellow of the American College of Dentists

FACE Fellow of the American College of Endocrinology; fluorophore-assisted carbohydrate electrophoresis

FACEP Fellow of the American College of Emergency Physicians

FACES Family Adaptability and Cohesion Evaluation Scale; unique facies, anorexia, cachexia, and eye and skin lesions [syndrome]

FACET Flosequinan Angiotensin Converting Enzyme-Inhibitor Trial; Fosinopril Amlodipine Cardiovascular Events Trial

FACFP Fellow of the American College of Family Physicians

FACFS Fellow of the American College of Foot Surgeons

FACG Fellow of the American College of Gastroenterology

FACH forceps to aftercoming head

FACHA Fellow of the American College of Health Administrators; Fellow of the American College of Hospital Administrators

FACHE Fellow of the American College of Healthcare Executives

FACIT fibril-associated collagen with interrupted triple helixes

FACL fatty acid coenzyme ligase

FACLM Fellow of the American College of Legal Medicine

FACMTA Federal Advisory Council on Medical Training Aids

FACN Fellow of the American College of Nutrition

FACNHA Foundation of the American College of Nursing Home Administrators

FACNM Fellow of the American College of Nuclear Medicine

FACNP Fellow of the American College of Nuclear Physicians

FACO Fellow of the American College of Otolaryngology

FACOG Fellow of the American College of Obstetricians and Gynecologists

FACOS Fellow of the American College of Orthopaedic Surgeons

FACOSH Federal Advisory Council on Occupational Safety and Health

FACP Fellow of the American College of Physicians

FACPE Fellow of the American College of Physician Executives

FACPM Fellow of the American College of Preventive Medicine

FACR Fellow of the American College of Radiology

FACS Fellow of the American College of Surgeons; fluorescence-activated cell sorter

FACScan fluorescence-associated cell sorter scan

FACSM Fellow of the American College of Sports Medicine

FACT Flanagan Aptitude Classification Test; focused appendix computed tomography; functional assessment of cancer therapy

FAct fibrinolytic activity

FACT-B Functional Assessment of Cancer Therapy-Breast

FACT-G Functional Assessment of Cancer Therapy-General

FACTS Functional Angiometric Correlation with Thallium Scintigraphy [trial]

FACTT Fluorescent Amplification Catalyzed by T7-Polymerase Technique

FACWA familial amyotrophic chorea with acanthocytosis

FAD familial Alzheimer dementia; familial autonomic dysfunction; fetal activity acceleration determination; flash-induced afterdischarge; flavin adenine dinucleotide; flea allergy dermatitis [veterinary medicine]

FA-D Fanconi anemia D

FADF fluorescent antibody dark field

FADH$_2$ reduced form of flavin adenine dinucleotide

FADIR flexion in adduction and internal rotation

FADN flavin adenine dinucleotide

FADS fetal akinesia deformation sequence

FAdV fowl adenovirus

FAE fetal alcohol effect; follicle-associated epithelium

FA-E Fanconi anemia E

FAED food-avoidance emotional disorder

FAEE fatty acid ethyl ester

FAEES fatty acid ethyl ester synthase

FAEN Fellow of the Academy of Emergency Nursing

FAERS Food and Drug Administration Adverse Event Reporting System

FAES Foundation for Advanced Education in the Sciences

FAF fatty acid free; fibroblast-activating factor

FAH Federation of American Hospitals

FAHA Fellow of the American Heart Association

FAHIS Florida Abuse Hotline Information System

Fahr Fahrenheit

FaHV falconid herpesvirus

FAI first-aid instruction; free androgen index; functional aerobic impairment; functional assessment inventory

FAJ fused apophyseal joint

FAK focal adhesion kinase

FALCPA Food Allergen Labeling and Consumer Protection Act

FALG fowl antimouse lymphocyte globulin

FALP fluoro-assisted lumbar puncture

FALS familial amyotrophic lateral sclerosis; forward angle light scatter

FAM 5-fluorouracil, Adriamycin, and mitomycin C; fuzzy associative memory

Fam, fam familal, family

FAMA Fellow of the American Medical Association; fluorescence-assisted mismatch analysis; fluorescent antibody to membrane antigen

FAM-A functional area model of activity

FAM-D functional area model of data

FAME fatty acid methyl ester

FAMG family group

fam hist family history

FAMIS Fosinopril in Acute Myocardial Infarction Study

FAMMM familial atypical multiple-mole melanoma [syndrome]

FAMOUS Fragmin Advanced Malignancy Outcome Study

FAMP fludarabine

FAN femoral antegrade; fuchsin, amido black, and naphthol yellow

FANA fluorescent antinuclear antibody

F and R force and rhythm

FANEL Federation for Accessible Nursing Education and Licensure

FANPT Freeman Anxiety Neurosis and Psychosomatic Test

FANTASTIC Full Anticoagulation vs. Aspirin Ticlopidine After Stent Implantation [study]

FAO Food and Agriculture Organization

FAO$_2$ fractional alveolar oxygen

FAOF family assessment of occupational functioning

FAP familial adenomatous polyposis; familial amyloid polyneuropathy; fatty acid polyunsaturated; fatty acid poor; femoral artery pressure; fibrillating action potential; Fibrinolytics vs. Primary Angioplasty [trial]; fixed action potential; frozen animal procedure; functional ambulation profile

FAPA Fellow of the American Psychiatric Association; Fellow of the American Psychoanalytical Association

FAPHA Fellow of the American Public Health Association

FAPIS Flecainide and Propafenone Italian Study

FAPS Felodipine Atherosclerosis Prevention Study; French Aortic Plaque Study

FAPY formamidopyrimidine

FAQ frequently asked questions; functional assessment questionnaire

FAR fatal accident rate; federal acquisitions regulation; fractional albumin rate

far faradic

FARE Federation of Alcoholic Rehabilitation Establishments

FARS Fatality Analysis Reporting System

FARV Farallon virus

FAS Family Attitude Scale; fatty acid synthetase; Federation of American Scientists; fetal akinesia sequence; fetal alcohol syndrome

FASA Federated Ambulatory Surgery Association

FASB Financial Accounting Standards Board

FASC free-standing ambulatory surgical center

fasc fascicular, fasciculus

FASEB Federation of American Societies for Experimental Biology

FASHP Federation of Associations of Schools of the Health Professions

FAST ferment active solution therapy; Fitness, Arthritis, and Seniors Trial; flow-assisted, short-term [catheter]; fluorescent antibody staining technique; fluoro-allergosorbent test; focused abdominal sonography for trauma; focused assessment with sonography in trauma; Fourier acquired steady state; Frenchay Aphasia Screening Test; functional assessment stages

FASTEST Femoral Artery Stent Study

FAST-MI Field Ambulance Study of Thrombolysis in Myocardial Infarction

FAstV feline astrovirus

FAT family attitudes test; fluorescent antibody technique; fluorescent antibody test

FAT$_{DPA}$ fat dual-photon absorptiometry

FATIMA Fraxiparin Anticoagulant Therapy in Myocardial Infarction Study in Amsterdam

Fat$_{IVNA}$ fat in vitro neutron activation analysis

FATS face and thigh squeeze [position]; Familial Atherosclerosis Treatment Study; fast adiabatic trajectory in steady state

FatSat fat saturation

FAT$_{UWW}$ fat underwater weighing

FAV fascio-auriculovertebral [sequence]; feline ataxia virus; floppy aortic valve; fowl adenovirus

FAVS fascio-auriculo-vertebral spectrum

F$_{AW}$ airway flow

FAX, fax facsimile

FAZ Fanconi-Albertini-Zellweger [syndrome]; foveal avascular zone; fragmented atrial activity zone

FB factor B; fascicular block; fasting blood [test]; feedback; fiberoptic bronchoscopy; fingerbreadth; flexible bronchoscope, flexible bronchoscopy; foreign body; *Fusobacterium*

FBA fecal bile acid

FBAO foreign-body airway obstruction

F-BAR forward and backward autoregression

FBC full blood count

FBCOD foreign body of the cornea, oculus dexter (right eye)

FBCOS foreign body of the cornea, oculus sinister (left eye)

FBCP familial benign chronic pemphigus

FBD failed biopsy detection; forward/backward bending; functional bowel disorder

fBDE fractional balanced differential expression

FBDO foodborne disease outbreak

FbDP fibrin degradation products

FBDSS Foodborne Disease Surveillance System

FBE full blood examination

FBEC fetal bovine endothelial cell

FBF forearm blood flow; full breastfeeding

FBG fasting blood glucose; fibrinogen; foreign body granulomatosis

fbg fibrinogen

FBH familial benign hypercalcemia

FBHH familial benign hypocalciuric hypercalcemia

FBI flossing, brushing, and irrigation

FBID found in bed dead

FBJMSV Finkel-Biskis-Jinkins murine sarcoma virus

FBL follicular basal lamina

FBLN fibulin

FBM felbamate; fetal breathing movements; fractional/fractal brownian motion

FBN Federal Bureau of Narcotics; fibribillin

FBP femoral blood pressure; fibrin breakdown product; filtered backprojection; folate-binding protein; fructose-1, 6-biphosphatase

FBPM forward-backward Prony method

FBPsS Fellow of the British Psychological Society

FBR fetal breathing rate

FBS fasting blood sugar; feedback system; fetal bovine serum; film-based system

FBSC Frederick Biomedical Supercomputing Center

FBSS failed back surgery syndrome; field-based similarity searching

FC family coping; fasciculus cuneatus; fast component; febrile convulsions; feline conjunctivitis; ferric chloride; ferric citrate; fibrocyte; finger clubbing; finger counting; flow compensation; fluorescein conjugated; fluorocarbon; fluorocytosine; fold change; Foley catheter; follicle culture; foster care; fowl cholera; free cholesterol; frontal cortex; functional castration

5-FC flucytosine; 5-fluorocytosine

F+C flare and cells

Fc centroid frequency; fraction/centrifuge; fragment, crystallizable

Fc' fragment of immunoglobulin molecule produced by papain digestion

fc cutoff frequency; foot candles

FCA ferritin-conjugated antibodies; Freund's complete adjuvant; functional capacity assessment

FCAH familial cytomegaly adrenocortical hypoplasia [syndrome]

FCAP Fellow of the College of American Pathologists

FCAS familial cold autoinflammatory syndrome

FCAT Federative Committee on Anatomical Terminology

F cath Foley catheter

FCC Federal Communications Commission; follicular center cells; Food Chemicals Codex

fcc face-centered-cubic

f/cc fibers per cubic centimeter of air

FCCA familial congenital cardiac abnormality

FCCH family child care home

FCCL follicular center cell lymphoma

FCCP Fellow of the American College of Chest Physicians

FCCSET Federal Coordinating Committee for Science, Engineering, and Technology

FCD feces collection device; fibrocystic disease; fibrocystic dysplasia; focal cytoplasmic degradation

FCE fibrocartilaginous embolism

FceR fragment receptor for immunoglobulin E

FCF fetal cardiac frequency; fibroblast chemotactic factor

FCFC fibroblast colony-forming cell

FcγR fragment receptor for immunoglobulin G

FCH faculty contact hour; family care home; fetal cystic hygroma

FCHL familial combined hyperlipidemia

FChS Fellow of the Society of Chiropodists

FCHSP Flight Crew Health Stabilization Program

FCI fixed-cell immunofluorescence; folded cell index; food chemical intolerance; free fasciocutaneous flap

FCIM Federated Council for Internal Medicine

fCJD familial Creutzfeldt-Jakob disease

FCL fibroblast cell line

fcly face lying

FCM flow cytometry; fuzzy cognitive map [algorithm]

FCMC familial chronic mucocutaneous candidiasis; family-centered maternity care

FCMD Fukuyama congenital muscular dystrophy

FCMS Fellow of the College of Medicine and Surgery; Foix-Chavany-Marie syndrome

FCMW Foundation for Child Mental Welfare

FCN food contact notification

FCO Fellow of the College of Osteopathy

FCoV feline coronavirus

FCP F-cell production; femoral hole coronal positioning; final common pathway; Functional Communication Profile

FCPN fuzzy colored Petri net

FCPR fatigue crack propagation rate

FCPS Fellow of the College of Physicians and Surgeons

FCR flexor carpi radialis; fractional catabolic rate; Fuji computed radiography

FcR fragment receptor

FCRA fecal collection receptacle assembly; Fellow of the College of Radiologists of Australasia

FCRC Frederick Cancer Research Center

FcRγ fragment receptor gamma chain

FCS fasciocutaneoskeletal syndrome; fecal containment system; feedback control system; fetal calf serum; food contact substances; foot compartment syndrome

FCSP Fellow of the Chartered Society of Physiotherapy

FCST Fellow of the College of Speech Therapists

FCSW female commercial sex worker

FCT food composition table; fucosyl transferase

FCU familial cold urticaria; flexor carpi ulnaris

FCV feline calicivirus; fowl calicivirus

FCx frontal cortex

FCXM flow cytometric cross matching

FCZ fluconazole

FD familial dysautonomia; family doctor; fan douche; fatal dose; fetal danger; fibrin derivative; fibrous dysplasia; floppy disk; focal distance; Folin-Denis [assay]; follicular diameter; foot drop; forceps delivery; Fourier descriptor; fractal dimension; fracture-dislocation; freeze drying; functional days

FD1 from day 1

FD2 from day 2

FD$_{50}$ median fatal dose

Fd amino-terminal portion of the heavy chain of an immunoglobulin molecule; ferredoxin

fd fundus

FDA Fisher discriminant analysis; fluorescein diacetate; Food and Drug Administration; right frontoanterior [position]

FDA-CBER Food and Drug Administration Center for Biologics Evaluation and Research

FDAM fuzzy logic–based decision analysis module

FDAMA Food and Drug Administration Modernization Act

FDAW film digitizer acquisition workstation

FDB familial defective apolipoprotein B; First Databank

FDBL fecal daily blood loss

FDC factor-dependent cell; follicular dendritic cell

FD&C Food, Drug, and Cosmetic Act; food, drugs, and cosmetics

FDCA Food, Drug, and Cosmetic Act

FDCM familial dilated cardiomyopathy

FDCPA Food, Drug, and Consumer Product Agency

FDD fluorescent differential display; Food and Drugs Directorate; frequency division duplex

FDDC ferric dimethyldithiocarbonate

FDDI fiber distributed data interface; film distribution data interface

FDDS Family Drawing Depression Scale

FDE female day-equivalent; final drug evaluation

FDECU field-employable environmental control unit

FDF fast death factor; fractional dimension filtering

FDFQ Food/Drink Frequency Questionnaire

FDFT farnesyldiphosphate farnesyltransferase

FDG features of differential diagnosis; fluorine 18-labeled deoxyglucose; fluorodeoxyglucose

fdg feeding

FDGF fibroblast-derived growth factor

FDG-PET fluorodeoxyglucose positron emission tomography

FDH familial dysalbuminemic hyperthyroxinemia; focal dermal hypoplasia; formaldehyde dehydrogenase

FDI facial disability index; fibrillation detection interval; first dorsal interosseous [muscle]; frequency domain imaging; functional disability index; International Dental Federation [Fr. *Fédération Dentaire Internationale*]

FDIU fetal death in utero

FDK Feldkamp [algorithm]

FDL flexor digitorum longus

FDLMP first day of last menstrual period

FDLO fluorescent dye-labeled oligonucleotide

FDLV fer-de-lance virus

FDM fetus of diabetic mother; fibrous dysplasia of the mandible; finite differentiation method; fluorodeoxymannose

FDMP fluid depth at Morison's pouch

FDNB fluorodinitrobenzene

FDO fleet dental officer

FDOPA fluorodihydroxyphenylalanine

FDP family doctor practice; fibrin degradation product; fibrinogen degradation product; flexor digitorum profundus; fructose-1,6-diphosphate; left frontoposterior [position]

FDPase fructose-1,6-diphosphatase

FDPM frequency domain photon migration

FDPS farnesyl diphosphate synthetase

FDPSL farnesyl diphosphate synthetase-like

FDQB flexor digiti quinti brevis

FDR first-degree relative; fractional disappearance rate

FDS Fellow in Dental Surgery; fiber duodenoscope; flexor digitorum superficialis

FDSRCSEng Fellow in Dental Surgery of the Royal College of Surgeons of England

FDT frequency doubling technique; right frontotransverse [position]

FDTD finite difference time domain

FdUrd fluorodeoxyuridine

(F)dUTP fluorescent deoxyuridine triphosphate

FDV Fiji disease virus; foliar decay virus; Friend disease virus

FDWT fast dyadic wavelet transform

FDXD flat dynamic x-ray image detector

FDZ fetal danger zone

FE fatty ester; fecal emesis; fetal erythroblastosis; fetal erythrocyte; figure eight; finite element; fluid extract; fluorescent erythrocyte; forced expiration; formaldehyde-ethanol; frequency-encoded; frozen embryo

Fe female; ferret

F$_e$ fraction excreted

fe female

FEA finite element analysis

feb fever [L. *febris*]

FEBP fetal estrogen-binding protein

FEBS Federation of European Biochemical Societies

FEB SZ febrile seizures

FEC fixed excitation codebook; forced expiratory capacity; free erythrocyte coproporphyrin; free-standing emergency center; Friend erythroleukemia cell

FECG fetal electrocardiogram

FECH ferrochelatase

F$_{ECO_2}$ fractional concentration of carbon dioxide in expired gas

FECP free erythrocyte coproporphyrin

FECSR flexion-extension cervical spine radiography

FECT fibroelastic connective tissue

FECU factor VIII correctional unit

FECV feline enteric coronavirus

FECVC functional extracellular fluid volume

FED field emission display; figure-eight distribution; fish eye disease; functional esophageal disorder

FeD iron deficiency

Fed federal

FedNets Federal agency networks

FEDRIP Federal Research in Progress

FedStats federal statistics

FEE forced equilibrating expiration

FEEG fetal electroencephalography

FEER field echo with even echo rephasing

FEESST flexible endoscopic evaluation of swallowing with sensory testing

FEF forced expiratory flow

FEF$_{25-75}$ forced expiratory flow at 25% to 75% of forced vital capacity

FEF$_{50}$ forced expiratory flow at 50% of forced vital capacity

FEF$_{50}$/FIF$_{50}$ ratio of expiratory flow to inspiratory flow at 50% of forced vital capacity

FEFO first expired first out

FEFV forced expiratory flow volume

fEGG fast electrogastrogram

FEH focal epithelial hyperplasia

FEHBARS Federal Employee Health Benefit Acquisition Regulations

FEHBP Federal Employee Health Benefits Program

FEHBP-MSA Federal Employees Health Benefits Program-Medical Savings Account

Fe^{+2}Hgb ferromethemoglobin

Fe^{+3}Hgb ferrimethemoglobin

FeHV felid herpesvirus

FEIBA factor VIII bypassing activity

FEKG fetal electrocardiogram

FEL familial erythrophagocytic lymphohistiocytosis; free electron laser

Fel feline [veterinary medicine]

FELASA Federation of European Laboratory Animal Science Associations

FELC Friend erythroleukemia cell

FeLV, Felv feline leukemia virus [veterinary medicine]

FEM female; femoral, femur; finite element method; finite element model; finite element modeling techniques; fixed-effect model

fem female; femoral, femur

FEMA Federal Emergency Management Agency

FEMINA Felodipine ER and Metoprolol in the Treatment of Angina Pectoris

fem intern at inner side of the thighs [L. *femoribus internus*]

FEN flap endonuclease; fluids, electrolytes, nutrition

Fen fenfluramine

FENa, FE$_{Na}$ fractional excretion of sodium

FEO familial expansile osteolysis

FE$_{O_2}$, F$_{EO_2}$ fractional concentration of oxygen in expired gas

FEOBV fluoroethoxybenzylvesamicol

FEP fluorinated ethylene-propylene; free erythrocyte protoporphyrin; front-end processing; front-end processor

FEPB functional electronic peroneal brace

FEPP free erythrocyte protoporphyrin

FER flexion, extension, rotation; fractional esterification rate; functional entity relationship

fert fertility, fertilized

FES family environment scale; fat emboli syndrome, fat embolism syndrome; flame emission spectroscopy; forced expiratory spirogram; functional electrical stimulation

Fe/S iron/sulfur

FESO$_4$ ferrous sulfate

FESS functional endoscopic sinus surgery

FEST Fosinopril Efficacy/Safety Trial; Fosinopril on Exercise Tolerance [study]; Framework for European Services in Telemedicine

FeSV feline sarcoma virus

FET field-effect transistor; forced expiratory time; frozen embryo transfer

FETE Far Eastern tick-borne encephalitis

FETs forced expiratory time in seconds

FEUO for external use only

FEV familial exudative vitreoretinopathy; forced expiratory volume

FEV1, FEV$_1$ forced expiratory volume in one second

FEV$_{1\%}$ ratio of forced expiratory volume in 1 second to forced vital capacity

fev fever

FEVB frequency ectopic ventricular beat

fEVP flash-evoked visual potential

FEVR familial exudative vitreoretinopathy

FF degree of fineness of abrasive particles; fat free; father factor; fecal frequency; fertility

factor; field of Forel; filtration fraction; fine fiber; fine focus; finger flexion; finger to finger; fixation fluid; flat feet; flip-flop; fluorescent focus; follicular fluid; force fluids; forearm factor; forearm flow; forward flexion; foster father; free fluids; free fraction; fresh frozen; fundus firm

F-F femoro-femoral

F2F face-to-face

ff$^+$ fertility inhibition positive

ff$^-$ fertility inhibition negative

FFA Fellow of the Faculty of Anaesthetists; free fatty acid; fundus fluorescein angiography

FFAP free fatty acid phase

FFARCS Fellow of the Faculty of Anaesthetists of the Royal College of Surgeons

FFAST formal FAST computed tomography

FFB fat-free body; flexible fiberoptic bronchoscopy

FFC fixed flexion contracture; fluorescence flow cytometry; free from chlorine

FFCM Fellow of the Faculty of Community Medicine

FFD Fellow in the Faculty of Dentistry; finger-to-floor distance; focus-film distance; free-form deformations

FFDCA Federal Food, Drug, and Cosmetic Act

FFDD focal facial dermal dysplasia

FFDM full-field digital mammography

FFDSRCS Fellow of the Faculty of Dental Surgery of the Royal College of Surgeons

FFDW fat-free dry weight

FFE fast field echo; fecal fat excretion

FFF degree of fineness of abrasive particles; field-flow fractionation; flicker fusion frequency

FFG free fat graft

FFGA Fonseca and Flaming algorithm

FFHC federally funded health center

FFHom Fellow of the Faculty of Homeopathy

FFI family function index; fatal familial insomnia; foot function index; free from infection; fundamental frequency indicator

FFIT fluorescent focus inhibition test

FFL flexible fiberoptic laryngoscopy

FFM fat-free mass; friction force microscopy; fundus flavimaculatus

FFMDXA fat-free mass dual-energy x-ray absorptiometry

FFMHYD fat-free mass hydrodensitometry

FFNS fluticasone furoate nasal spray

FFOM Fellow of the Faculty of Occupational Medicine

FFP freedom from progression; fresh frozen plasma

FFQ food frequency questionnaire

FFR Fellow of the Faculty of Radiologists; filtering facepiece respirator [includes N95 masks]

FFROM full and free range of motion

FFS failure-free survival; fat-free solids; fee for service; femoro-facial syndrome

FFT fast Fourier transform; finite Fourier transform; flicker fusion test; flicker fusion threshold

FFTF freedom from treatment failure

FFU femur-fibula-ulna [syndrome]; focal forming unit

FFV feline foamy virus; fruit fly virus

FFW fat-free weight

FFWB foot flat, weight bearing

FFWC fractional free water clearance

FFWW fat-free wet weight

FG fasciculus gracilis; fast glycolytic [fiber]; Feeley-Gorman [agar]; fibrin glue; fibrinogen; Flemish giant [rabbit]

fg femtogram; flammable gas detector

FGA fibrinogen alpha; first-generation antipsychotic

FGB fibrinogen beta

FGC fibrinogen gel chromatography

FGD fatal granulomatous disease

FgDP fibrinogen degradation products

FGDS fibrogastroduodenoscopy

FGDY faciogenital dysplasia

FGF father's grandfather; fibroblast growth factor; fresh gas flow

FGF1 fibroblast growth factor 1

FGF2 fibroblast growth factor 2

FGFA fibroblast growth factor, acidic

FGFB fibroblast growth factor, basic

FGFR fibroblast growth factor receptor

FGG fibrinogen gamma; focal global glomerulosclerosis; fowl gammaglobulin

FGGM finite generalized gaussian mixture

FGH formylglutathione hydrolase

FGID functional gastrointestinal disorder

FGL fasting gastrin level; fasting glucose level

FGM father's grandmother; female genital mutilation

FGN fibrinogen; focal glomerulonephritis; fractional gaussian noise

FGP fundic gland polyp

FGR familial glucocorticoid resistance; finite time growth

FGS fibrogastroscopy; focal glomerular sclerosis; formal genesis syndrome

FGT fluorescent gonorrhea test

FH facial hemihyperplasia; familial hypercholesterolemia; familial hypertension; family history; fasting hyperbilirubinemia;

favorable histology; femoral hernia; femoral hypoplasia; femur head; fetal head; fetal heart; fibromuscular hyperplasia; field hospital; flat hyperplasia; follicular hyperplasia; Frankfort horizontal [plane]; fumarate hydratase

FH⁺ family history positive

FH⁻ family history negative

FH₄ tetrahydrofolic acid

fh fostered by hand

FHA familial hypoplastic anemia; Fellow of the Institute of Hospital Administrators; filamentous hemagglutinin

FHAB freshwater harmful algal blooms

FHADES Farm Hazard and Demographic Enumeration Survey

FHB flexor hallucis brevis

FH/BC frontal horn/bicaudate ratio

FHC familial hypercholesterolemia; familial hypertrophic cardiomyopathy; family health center; Ficoll-Hypaque centrifugation; Fuchs heterochromic cyclitis

FHD familial histiocytic dermatoarthritis; family history of diabetes; femoral head diameter; fetal heart disease

FHF fetal heart frequency; fulminant hepatic failure

fHg free hemoglobin

FHH familial hypocalciuric hypercalcemia; fawn-hooded hypertensive [rat]; fetal heart heard

FHI Family Health International; Fuchs' heterochromic iridocyclitis

FHIP family health insurance plan

FHIS Farm Health Interview Survey

FHIT fragile histidine triad

FHL flexor hallucis longus; Food Hygiene Laboratory; functional health literacy; functional hearing loss

FHM familial hemiplegic migraine; fathead minnow [cells]

FHN family history negative

FHNH fetal heart not heard

FHP family history positive; functional health pattern

FHPMHP family history of physical and mental health problems

FHPSAT Functional Health Pattern Screening Assessment Tool

FHR familial hypophosphatemic rickets; fetal heart rate

fH-R factor H receptor

FHRDC family history research diagnostic criteria

FHRH femoral head resurfacing hemiarthroplasty

FHRNST fetal heart rate nonstress test

FHRS Familial Hypercholesterolemia Regression Study

FHS Family Heart Study; fetal heart sound; fetal hydantoin syndrome; Floating Harbor syndrome; Framingham Heart Study

FH-S soluble fumarate hydratase

FHSA Family Health Service Authority

FHSD family history of sudden death

FHS-SCAN Family Heart Study Subclinical Atherosclerosis Network

FHT fast Hartley transform; fetal heart; fetal heart tone

FHTG familial hypertriglyceridemia

FH-UFS femoral hypoplasia-unusual facies syndrome

FHV falcon herpesvirus; flock house virus

FHVP free hepatic vein pressure

FHx family history

FI factor 1; fasciculus intrafascicularis; fever caused by infection; fibrinogen; fixed interval; flame ionization; follicular involution; food insecurity; food intolerance; forced inspiration; frontoiliac; full scan with interpolation

FIA feline infectious anemia [veterinary medicine]; fistula in ano; fluorescent immunoassay; focal immunoassay; Freund incomplete adjuvant

FIAC 2'-fluoro-5-iodo-aracytosine

FIB Fellow of the Institute of Biology; fibrin; fibrinogen; fibrositis; fibula

fib fiber; fibrillation; fibrin; fibrinogen; fibula

FIC finite-sample information criterion; Fogarty International Center; fractional inhibitory concentration

FICA faith and belief, importance, community, address/action; Federal Insurance Contributions Act; fluoroimmunocytoadherence

FICD Fellow of the Institute of Canadian Dentists; Fellow of the International College of Dentists

FiCO$_2$, FI$_{CO_2}$ fractional concentration of carbon dioxide in inspired gas

FICS Fellow of the International College of Surgeons

FICSIT Frailty and Injuries: Cooperative Studies of Intervention Techniques

FICU fetal intensive care unit

FID flame ionization detector; free induction decay; fungal immunodiffusion

FIDD fetal iodine deficiency disorder

FIELD Fenofibrate Intervention and Event Lowering in Diabetes [trial]

FIF feedback inhibition factor; fibroblast interferon; forced inspiratory flow; formaldehyde-induced fluorescence

FIF$_{50}$ forced inspiratory flow at 50% of forced vital capacity

FIFO first in, first out

FIFR fasting intestinal flow rate

FIFRA Federal Insecticide, Fungicide, and Rodenticide Act

FIG Flosequinan Investigator Group

FIGD familial idiopathic gonadotropin deficiency

FIGE field inversion gel electrophoresis

FIGLU, FIGlu formiminoglutamate, formiminoglutamic acid

FIGLU-uria formiminoglutaminaciduria

FIGO International Federation of Gynecology and Obstetrics [Fr. *Fédération Internationale de Gynécologie et d'Obstetrique*]

FIH familial isolated hypoparathyroidism; fat-induced hyperglycemia

fil filament; filial

filt filter, filtration

FIM familial infantile myasthenia; field ion microscopy; fimbria; fluorescence-imaged microdeformation; functional independence measure

FIMG familial infantile myasthenia gravis

FIMLT Fellow of the Institute of Medical Laboratory Technology

FIMS Interational Federation of Sports Medicine [Fr. *Fédération Internationale de Médecine du Sport*]

FIN fine intestinal needle

FINCC familial idiopathic nonarteriosclerotic cerebral calcification

FIND finding

FINESS First International New Intravascular Rigid-Flex Endovascular Stent Study

FINMONICA Finnish Monitoring Trends and Determinants in Cardiovascular Diseases

FINRISK Finland Cardiovascular Risk Study

FINV Fin V 707 virus

FIO$_2$, FiO$_2$ fractional concentration of oxygen in inspired gas

FI$_{O_2}$ forced inspiratory oxygen; fractional concentration of oxygen in inspired gas

FIP feline infectious peritonitis [veterinary medicine]; International Pharmaceutical Federation [Fédération Internationale Pharmaceutique]

FIPA familial intestinal polyatresia [syndrome]

FIPS Federal information processing standards; Frankfurt Isoptin Progression Study

FIPV feline infectious peritonitis virus

FIQ full-scale intelligence quotient

FIR far infrared; finite impulse response; fold increase in resistance; fractional intramural retention

FIRDA frontal, intermittent rhythmic delta activity

FIRM formal inference-based recursive modeling

FIRST Flolan International Randomized Survival Trial

FIS fatigue interview schedule; forced inspiratory spirogram; free induction signal

fis fission

FISAC Federal Information Services and Application Council

FISH Finnish Isradipine Study in Hypertension; fluorescence in situ hybridization

FISP fast imaging with steady state precision

FISS Fraxiparine in Stroke Study

fist fistula

FIT fluorescein isothiocyanate; Fracture Intervention Trial; fusion inferred threshold

FITC fluorescein isothiocyanate

FIUO for internal use only

FIV feline immunodeficiency virus [veterinary medicine]; forced inspiratory volume

FIV₁ forced inspiratory volume in one second

FIVC forced inspiratory vital capacity

FIVE familial isolated vitamin E [deficiency]

FIV-O feline immunodeficiency virus Oma [veterinary medicine]

FIV-P feline immunodeficiency virus Petaluma [veterinary medicine]

FIXAg factor IX antigen

FJN familial juvenile nephrophthisis

FJRM full joint range of movement

FJS finger joint size

FK feline kidney

FK506 tacrolimus

FKBP FK506 binding protein

FK-NN fuzzy K−nearest neighbor

FKT Fukunaga-Koontz transform

FL false lumen; fatty liver; feline leukemia; femur length; fibers of Luschka; fibroblast-like; filtration leukapheresis; focal length; follicular lymphoma; Friend leukemia; frontal lobe; full liquid; functional length; fuzzy logic

FL-2 feline lung [cells]

Fl fluid; fluorescence

fL femtoliter

fl femtoliter, filtered load; flexible, flexion; flow; fluid; fluorescent; flutter; foot-lambert

FLA fluorescent-labeled antibody; left frontoanterior

FLAC, FL/AC femur length/abdominal circumference ratio

flac flaccid, flaccidity

FLAIR fluid-attenuated inversion recovery

FLAIR-FLASH fluid-attenuated inversion recovery, fast low-angle shot

FLAK flow artifact killer

FLAP 5-lipooxygenase activating protein

FLARE Fluvastatin Angioplasty Restenosis [trial]

FLASH fast low-angle shot

FLAV Flanders virus

FLC family life cycle; fatty liver cell; fetal liver cell; Fourier linear combiner; free light chain; Friend leukemia cell

FLCL follicular large cell lymphoma

FlCV flame chlorosis virus

FLD fibrotic lung disease; field hospital; Fisher's linear discriminate [classification]; frontal lobe degeneration

fld fluid

fl dr fluid dram

FLDV flounder lymphocystis disease

FLE fiducial localization error

FLEQUIN Flecainide Compared to Oral Quinidine [study]

FLEV Flexal virus

FLEX Federation Licensing Examination

flex flexion, flexor

FLEXOR Focused Lesion Expansion Optimizes Result [trial]

FLG filaggrin

FLIC functional living index, cancer

FLICC Federal Library and Information Center Committee

FLK funny-looking kid

FLKS fatty liver and kidney syndrome

FLM fasciculus longitudinalis medialis; fraction of labeled mitosis

FLO Fourier linear combiner

floc flocculation

Flops floating point operations per second

fl oz fluid ounce

FLP fixed linear paralleling; functional limitations profile; left frontoposterior

FLR fluorescent-labeled reference; funny-looking rash

FLS fatty liver syndrome; Fellow of the Linnean Society; fibrous long-spacing [collagen]; filmless system; fixed least squares [algorithm]; flow-limiting segment

FLSP fluorescein-labeled serum protein

FLT left frontotransverse

FLU fluconazole; flumazenil; flunitrazepam; 5-fluorouracil; fluoxetine; fluphenazine; flutamide

flu influenza

FLUAV Influenza A virus

FLUBV Influenza B virus

FLUCV Influenza C virus

FLUENT Fluvastatin Long-Term Extension Trial

fluor fluorescence; fluorescent; fluorometry; fluoroscopy

fluoro fluoroscope, fluoroscopy

FLV feline leukemia virus [veterinary medicine]; Friend leukemia virus; fuzzy linguistic value

FM face mask; facilities management; family medicine; fat mass; feedback mechanism; fetal movement; fibrin monomer; fibromuscular; fibromyalgia; Fielding-Magliato [classification]; filtered mass; flavin mononucleotide; flowmeter; fluid movement; fluorescent microscopy; foramen magnum; forensic medicine; foster mother; frequency modulation; functional movement

FM2 flunitrazepam

Fm fermium

fM full mutation

f-M free metanephrine

fm femtometer; femtomole

FMA Frankfort mandibular angle; free of microcalcifications; full matrix analysis; functional motor activity

FMAP feeding mean arterial pressure

FMAT fetal movement acceleration test

f_{max} maximum frequency

FMC family medicine center; field medical card; flight medicine clinic; focal macular choroidopathy; foundation for medical care

FMCG fetal magnetocardiography

FMCL follicular mixed-cell lymphoma

FMD facility medical director; family medical doctor; fibromuscular dysplasia; flow-mediated dilation; foot and mouth disease; frontometaphyseal dysplasia

FMDI frequency modulation detection interference

FMDV foot and mouth disease virus

FME full mouth extraction

FMEA failure modes and effects analysis

Fmed median frequency

FMEG fetal magnetoencephalography

FMEL Friend murine erythroleukemia

FMEN familial multiple endocrine neoplasia

F-met, fMet formyl methionine

FMF familial Mediterranean fever; fetal movement felt; flow microfluorometry; forced midexpiratory flow

FMFD V familial multiple coagulation factor deficiency V

FMFM full mutation/full methylation

FMG five-mesh gauze; foreign medical graduate

FMGEMS Foreign Medical Graduate Examination in Medical Sciences

FMH family medical history; fat-mobilizing hormone; fetomaternal hemorrhage; fibromuscular hyperplasia; first metatarsal head

FMI fat mass index; Foods and Moods Inventory

FMIBMA fiber movement−induced biologic movement artifacts

FML flail mitral leaflet; fluorometholone

FMLA Family and Medical Leave Act

FMLP formylpeptide; *N*-formyl-methionyl-leucyl-phenylalanine

f-MLP *N*-formyl-methionyl-leucyl-phenylalanine

FMN first malignant neoplasm; flavin mononucleotide; frontomaxillonasal

FMNH, FMNH₂ reduced form of flavin mononucleotide

FMO flavin monooxygenase; fleet medical officer; flight medical officer

fmol femtomole

FMP faculty mentorship program; first menstrual period; fructose monophosphate

FMPIR fast multiplanar inversion recovery

FMPM full mutation/partial methylation

FMPP familial male precocious puberty

FMPSPGR fast multiplanar spoiled gradient recalled

FMR fragile site mental retardation (intellectual disability) [syndrome]; Friend-Moloney-Rauscher [antigen]

fMRA functional magnetic resonance angiography

F MRI fluorine magnetic resonance imaging

fMRI functional magnetic resonance imaging

FMRP fragile site mental retardation (intellectual disability) [syndrome] protein

FMS fat-mobilizing substance; fatty meal sonogram; Fellow of the Medical Society; fibromyalgia syndrome; Finnish Multicenter Study; Fragmin Multicenter Study; full mouth series

FMT fecal microbiota transplantation; Fragmin Multicenter Trial; frequency modulation detection threshold

FMTC familial medullary thyroid cancer

fMTT first-moment mean transit time

FMU first morning urine

F-MuLV Friend murine leukemia virus

FMX full mouth x-ray

FMZ flumazenil

FN false negative; fecal nitrogen; fibronectin; FitzHugh-Nagumo [model]; fluoride number

F-N finger to nose

fn function

FNA fine-needle aspiration

FNAB fine-needle aspiration biopsy

FNAC fine-needle aspiration cytology

fNaDC flounder sodium dicarboxylate

FNB fine-needle biopsy; food and nutrition board

FNBMD femoral neck bone mineral density

FnBPA fibronectin-binding protein A

FnBPB fibronectin-binding protein B

FNC Family Nurse Clinician; fatty nutritional cirrhosis; full nursing care

FNCJ fine-needle catheter jejunostomy

FND febrile neutrophilic dermatosis; frontonasal dysplasia; functional neck dissection

f-NE free norepinephrine

Fneg false negative

FNF false-negative fraction; femoral neck fracture

FNFMG foreign national foreign medical school graduate

FNH focal nodular hyperplasia

FNHR febrile nonhemolytic reaction

FNHTR febrile nonhemolytic transfusion reaction

FNIC Food and Nutrition Information Center

FNL fibronectin-like

FNLA Fellow of the National Lipid Association

f-NM free normetanephrine

FNN false nearest neighbor

FNP family nurse practitioner

FNR false-negative rate; fibronectin receptor

FNRA fibronectin receptor alpha

FNRB fibronectin receptor beta

FNRBL fibronectin receptor beta−like

FNS frontier nursing service; functional neuromuscular stimulation

FNT false neurochemical transmitter; farnesyltransferase

FNTA farnesyltransferase alpha

FNTB farnesyltransferase beta

FNTC fine-needle transhepatic cholangiography

FNZ flunarizine

FO fiberoptic; fish oil; foot arthrosis; foramen ovale; forced oscillation; fronto-occipital

Fo fomentation, fomenting

FOA Federation of Orthodontic Associations

FOAR facio-oculo-acoustico-renal [syndrome]

FOAVF failure of all vital forces

FOB father of baby; fecal occult blood; feet out of bed; fiberoptic bronchoscopy; foot of bed; functional observational battery

FOBT fecal occult blood test

FOC fronto-occipital circumference

FOCAL formula calculation

FOD figure of demerit [radiotherapy]; focus-to-object distance; free of disease

F-ODN fluorescein-labeled oligodeoxyribonucleotide

FOF found on floor

FOG fast oxidative glycolytic [fiber]

FOL folate

FOLR folate receptor

FOM figure of merit

FOMi 5-fluorouracil, vincristine, and mitomycin C

F-OMP fluorescein-labeled oligonucleoside methylphosphonate

FOOB fell out of bed

FOOD Feed or Ordinary Diet [trial]

FOOSH fell onto outstretched hand

FOP fibrodysplasia ossificans progressiva; forensic pathology

FOPR full outpatient rate

F-OPT fluorescein-labeled oligonucleoside phosphorothioate

For foramen; forensic

for foreign; formula

FORECAST Fractional Flow Reserve or Relative Fractional Velocity Reserve Evaluation of Coronary Artery Stenosis vs. Thallium

FORIMG foreign national international medical school graduate

form formula

FORT Fish Oil Restenosis Trial

FORTRAN formula translation

FORV Forecariah virus

FOS fast orthogonal search; fiberoptic sigmoidoscopy; fixation-off sensitivity; fractional osteoid surface; Framingham Offspring Study

FOSIT Fosamax International Trial

Fos-R foscarnet-resistant

Fos-R HIV foscarnet-resistant human immunodeficiency virus

FOSS Framingham Offspring Spouse Study

FOUV Foula virus

FOV field of view

FOX ferrous xylenol orange

FP false positive; familial porencephaly; family physician; family planning; family practice; family practitioner; Fanconi pancytopenia; fast pathway; femoropopliteal; fetoprotein; fibrinolytic potential; fibrinopeptide; fibrous proliferation; field pronouncement; filling pressure; filter paper; finite particle; fixation protein; flank pain; flash point; flavin phosphate; flavoprotein; flexor profundus; flow probe; fluid percussion; fluid pressure; fluorescence polarization; fluorescent probe; fluticazone propionate; follicular phase; food poisoning; food processing; forearm pronated; freezing point; frontoparietal; frontopolar; frozen plasma; full period; fusion peptide; fusion point

F-P frontopopliteal

F:P, F/P fluorescence/protein ratio

F1P, F-1-P fructose-1-phosphate

F6P, F-6-P fructose-6-phosphate

Fp fibrinopeptide; frontal polar electrode placement

fp flexor pollicis; foot-pound; forearm pronated; freezing point

FPA Family Planning Association; Federal Privacy Act; fibrinopeptide A/alpha; filter paper activity; fluorophenylalanine; foot progression angle

FpA fibrinopeptide A/alpha

FPB femoral popliteal bypass; fibrino-peptide B/beta; flexor pollicis brevis

FpB fibrinopeptide B/beta

FPBA fluorescence photobleaching analysis

FPBC false-positive blood culture

FPC familial polyposis coli; family planning clinic; fish protein concentrate

FPCA family practice comfort assessment

FpCA 1-fluoromethyl-2-*p*-chlorophenyl-ethylamine

FPD familial platelet disorder; fetopelvic disproportion; flame photometric detector; flat panel detector

FPDM fibrocalculous pancreatic diabetes mellitus

FPE fatal pulmonary embolism; field placement error; final prediction error

F-18-PET fluoride ion-positron emission tomography

FPF false-positive fraction; fibroblast pneumocyte factor

FPG fasting plasma glucose; fluorescence plus Giemsa; focal proliferative glomerulonephritis

FPGA field programmable gate array; field programmable generic array

FPGS folylpolyglutamate synthetase

FPH₂ reduced form of flavin phosphate

FPHE formaldehyde-treated pyruvaldehyde-stabilized human erythrocytes

FPHT fosphenytoin

FPI femoral pulsatility index; flat panel imager; fluid percussion injury; formula protein intolerance; Freiburg Personality Identification Questionnaire

FPIA fluorescence polarization immunoassay

FPK fructose phosphokinase

FPL familial partial lipodystrophy; fasting plasma lipids; flexor pollicis longus

FPLC fast protein liquid chromatography

FPLV feline panleukemia virus

FPM filter paper microscopic [test]; fine particle mass; full passive movements

fpm feet per minute

FPN ferric chloride, perchloric acid, nitric acid [solution]; fuzzy Petri net

FPNP Family Planning Nurse Practitioner

FPO faciopalatoosseous [syndrome]; Federation of Prosthodontic Organizations; freezing point osmometer

FPP faculty practice plan; free portal pressure

FPPG finger photoplethysmography

FPPH familial primary pulmonary hypertension

FPR false-positive rate; finger peripheral resistance; fluorescence photobleaching recovery; fractional proximal resorption; *N*-formylpeptide receptor

FPRA first-pass radionuclide angiogram

FPRH *N*-formylpeptide receptor homolog

FPRP false-positive report probability

FPS farnesylpyrophosphate synthetase; Fellow of the Pathological Society; Fellow of the Pharmaceutical Society; fetal PCB (polychlorinated biphenyl) syndrome; footpad swelling; frames per second

fps feet per second; frames per second

FPSA fractional positive surface area

FPSL farnesylpyrophosphate synthetase−like

FPS-R Faces Pain Scale-Revised

FPSTS false-positive serologic test for syphilis

FPT farnesyl protein transferase; femoropopliteal tibial

FPTase farnesyl-protein transferase

FPV Facey's Paddock virus; feline parvovirus; feline pseudoleukemia virus; feline pseudoleukopenia virus; femoral-popliteal vein; fosamprenavir; fowl plague virus; fowlpox virus; Fraser point virus

FPVB femoral popliteal vein bypass

FQHC federally qualified health center

FQPA Food Quality Protection Act

fQSR filtered QSR [ECG]

FR faculty rater; failure rate; fasciculus retroflexus; febrile reaction; feedback regulation; film-screen radiograph; Fischer-Race [notation]; fixed ratio; flocculation reaction; flow rate; fluid restriction; fluid resuscitation; fluid retention; framework region; free radical; frequency of respiration; frequent relapses

F2R factor II receptor

F&R force and rhythm

Fr fracture; francium; franklin [unit charge]; French; frequency or frequent

f_R respiratory frequency

Fr1 first fraction

FRA fibrinogen-related antigen; fluorescent rabies antibody

fra fragile

FRAC Food Research and Action Center

frac, fract fracture

FrAdV frog adenovirus

F( )R:Ag factor ( ) related antigen

FRAME Fund for the Replacement of Animals in Medical Experiments

FRAMI Fragmin in Acute Myocardial Infarction [study]

FRAP fluorescence recovery after photobleaching

FRAT free radical assay technique

FRAX fragile X [chromosome]

fra(X) chromosome X fragility; fragile X chromosome, fragile X syndrome

FRAXA fragile X syndrome A

FRAXE fragile X syndrome E

FRAXIDIS Fraxiparine in Post-Hospital Discharge [study]

FRAXIS Fraxiparine in Ischemic Syndromes [study]

FRAX-MR fragile X mental retardation (intellectual disability) [syndrome]

FRAXODI Fraxiparine Once Daily Injection [study]

Fr BB fracture of both bones

FRC Federal Radiation Council; fiber-reinforced composite; frozen red cells; functional reserve capacity; functional residual capacity

F( )R:C factor ( ) related cofactor activity

FRCD Fellow of the Royal College of Dentists; fixed-ratio combination drug

FRCGP Fellow of the Royal College of General Practitioners

FRCN Fellow of the Royal College of Nursing

FRCNA Fellow of the Royal College of Nursing, Australia

FRCOG Fellow of the Royal College of Obstetricians and Gynaecologists

FRCP Fellow of the Royal College of Physicians

FRCPA Fellow of the Royal College of Pathologists of Australia

FRCPath Fellow of the Royal College of Pathologists

FRCP(C) Fellow of the Royal College of Physicians of Canada

FRCPE Fellow of the Royal College of Physicians of Edinburgh

FRCPI Fellow of the Royal College of Physicians of Ireland

FRCPsych Fellow of the Royal College of Psychiatrists

FRCS Fellow of the Royal College of Surgeons

FRCS(C) Fellow of the Royal College of Surgeons of Canada

FRCSEd Fellow of the Royal College of Surgeons of Edinburgh

FRCSEng Fellow of the Royal College of Surgeons of England

FRCSI Fellow of the Royal College of Surgeons of Ireland

FRCVS Fellow of the Royal College of Veterinary Surgeons

FRD fumarate dehydrogenase

frd fumarate dehydrogenase

FRDA Friedreich ataxia

FRD A fumarate dehydrogenase A

FRDA-Acad Acadian Friedreich ataxia

FRD B fumarate dehydrogenase B

FRD C fumarate dehydrogenase C

FRD D fumarate dehydrogenase D

FRE Fischer rat embryo; flow-related enhancement

FREFLEX force reflecting exoskeleton

FREIR Federal Research on Biological and Health Effects of Ionizing Radiation

frem fremitus

freq frequency

FRES Fellow of the Royal Entomological Society

FRESCO Florence Randomized Elective Stenting in Acute Coronary Occlusion [study]

FRESH Food Reeducation for Elementary School Health

FRET fluorescence resonance energy transfer

FRF Fertility Research Foundation; follicle-stimulating hormone releasing factor

FRFC functional renal failure of cirrhosis

FRFSE fast relaxation fast spin echo

FRH follicle-stimulating hormone releasing hormone

FRh fetal rhesus monkey [kidney cell]

FRhK fetal rhesus monkey kidney [cell]

FRHS fast-repeating high sequence

FRIC Fragmin in Unstable Coronary Artery Disease [trial]

frict friction

FRIPHH Fellow of the Royal Institute of Public Health and Hygiene

FRISC Fragmin During Instability in Coronary Artery Disease [trial]

FRISC-II Fragmin and/or Revascularization during Instability in Coronary Artery Disease [trial]

FRIV frijoles virus

FRJM full range joint movement

FRMedSoc Fellow of the Royal Medical Society

FrMLV Friend murine leukemia virus

FRMS Fellow of the Royal Microscopical Society

FrMV Frangipani mosaic virus

FRNN fuzzy rough nearest neighbor [algorithm]

FRNS Fryns syndrome

FRO floor reaction orthosis

fROAT flounder renal organic anion transporter

FROC free receiver operating characteristic

FROG French Rotablator Group [study]

FROM full range of motion; full range of movements

FROST French Optimal Stenting Trial

FRP follicle-stimulating hormone releasing protein; functional refractory period

FRS Fellow of the Royal Society; ferredoxin-reducing substance; first rank symptom; fragment separator; furosemide

FRSH Fellow of the Royal Society of Health

FRT Family Relations Test; full recovery time

Fru fructose

FRV full-length retroviral [sequence]; functional residual volume

Frx fracture

Frzbs frizzled related protein

FS factor of safety; Fanconi syndrome; feasibility study; febrile seizure; Felty syndrome; fetoscopy; fibrin sealant; fibromyalgia syndrome; fibrosarcoma; field stimulation; file server; fine structure; Fisher syndrome; flexible sigmoidoscope; fluorescence spectrometry; food security; food service; forearm supination; fractional shortening; fracture site; fragile site; frequency-shifted [imaging]; Friesinger score; frozen section; full scale; full sensitivity; full soft [diet]; full strength; functional shortening; function study; functional system; human foreskin [cells]; simple fracture

%FS percent fractional shortening

F/S female, spayed [veterinary medicine]; frozen section

FSA fast simulated annealing; flexible spending account

FSB fetal scalp blood

FSBA fluorosulfonylbenzoyladenosine

FSBP finger systolic blood pressure

FSBS finger-stick blood sugar

FSBT Fowler single breath test

FSC finite sample criterion; Food Standards Committee; forward scatter

FSCCL follicular small cleaved cell lymphoma

FSCR flexible surface coil-type resonator

FSD focus-skin distance

FSE fast spin echo; febrile status epilepticus; feline spongiform encephalopathy; fetal scalp electrode; filtered smoke exposure

FSE-IR fast spin echo inversion recovery

FSEV *Figulus subleavis* entomopoxvirus

FSF fibrin stabilizing factor; final sperm fraction; front surface fluorescence

FSG fasting serum glucose; focal segmental sclerosis

FSGHS focal segmental glomerular hyalinosis and sclerosis

FSGN focal sclerosing glomerulonephritis

FSGS focal segmental glomerulosclerosis

FSH fascioscapulohumeral; focal and segmental hyalinosis; follicle-stimulating hormone

FSHB follicle-stimulating hormone, beta chain

FSHD facioscapulohumeral muscular dystrophy

FSH/LR-RH follicle-stimulating hormone and luteinizing hormone releasing hormone

FSHR follicle-stimulating hormone receptor

FSH-RF follicle-stimulating hormone releasing factor

FSH-RH follicle-stimulating hormone releasing hormone

FSHSMA fascioscapulohumeral spinal muscular atrophy

FSI foam stability index; Food Sanitation Institute; functional status index

FSIQ full-scale intelligence quotient

FSIS Food Safety and Inspection Service

FSL fasting serum level

FSM finite state machine

FSMA Food Safety Modernization Act

FSMB Federation of State Medical Boards

FSMC forward support medical company

FSN functional stimulation, neuromuscular

FSOP free-standing surgical outpatient facility

FSP familial spastic paraplegia; femoral hole sagittal positioning; fibrinogen split products; fibrin split products; fine suspended particles

F-SP special form [L. *forma specialis*]

FSPB finite-size pencil beam

FSPGR fast spoiled gradient-recalled acquisition in steady state

FSQ Functional Status Questionnaire

FSR Fellow of the Society of Radiographers; film screen radiography; force sensing resistor; force sensing retractor; forward stepping regression; fragmented sarcoplasmic reticulum; full scale range; fusiform skin revision

FSRS functional status rating system

FSS focal segmental sclerosis; Freeman-Sheldon syndrome; functional system scale; French steel sound; fuzzy shell segmentation [algorithm]

FST foam stability test

FSU family service unit; functional spine unit; functional subunit

FSUM focused segmented ultrasound machine

FSV feline fibrosarcoma virus [veterinary medicine]; Fort Sherman virus; forward stroke volume

FSVP Foreign Supplier Verification Program

FSW female sex worker; field service worker

FT Fallot tetralogy; false transmitter; family therapy; farnesyl transferase; fast twitch; fatigue trial; femorotibial; fibrous tissue; fingertip; follow through; force target; Fourier transform; free testosterone; free thyroxine; full term; function test

FT₃ free triiodothyronine

FT₄ free thyroxine

Ft ferritin

fT free testosterone

ft foot, feet

FTA femorotibial angle; fibrin tissue adhesive; fluorescent titer antibody; fluorescent treponemal antibody

FTA-ABS, FTA-Abs fluorescent treponemal antibody, absorbed [test]

FTAG, F-TAG fast-binding target-attaching globulin

FTAS familial testicular agenesis syndrome

FTase farnesyl transferase

FTAT fluorescent treponemal antibody test

FTB front to back

FTBD fit to be detained; full-term born dead

FTBE focal tick-borne encephalitis

FTBI fractionated total body irradiation

FTBS Family Therapist Behavioral Scale

FTC Federal Trade Commission; Fibrinolysis Trialists Collaboration; fibulotalocalcaneal; follicular thyroid carcinoma; frequency threshold curve; frequency tuning curve

ftc foot candle

FTD femoral total density; frontotemporal dementia

FTDS familial testicular dysgenesis syndrome

FTE full-time equivalent

FTEE full-time employee equivalent

FTF finger to finger

FTFT fast time frequency transform

FTG full-thickness graft

FTH ferritin heavy chain; fracture threshold

FTI farnesyl transferase inhibitor; free thyroxine index

FT₃I free triiodothyronine index

FT₄I free thyroxine index

FTIR Fourier transform infrared; functional terminal innervation ratio

FTKA failed to keep appointment

FTL ferritin light chain

ftL foot lambert

FTLB full-term live birth

ft lb foot pound

FTLD frontotemporal lobar degeneration

FTLV feline T-lymphotropic lentivirus

FTM fluid thioglycolate medium; fractional test meal

FTMS Fourier transform mass spectrometry

FTN finger to nose

FTNB full-term newborn

FTND full-term normal delivery

FTO fructose-terminated oligosaccharide

FTP file transfer protocol [sending and receiving files from remote computers on the Internet]

FTQ Fagerström Tolerance Questionnaire

FTR fractional tubular reabsorption

FTS family tracking system; feminizing testis syndrome; fetal tobacco syndrome; fissured tongue syndrome; flexor tenosynovitis; thymulin [Fr. *facteur thymique sérique*]

FTSG full-thickness skin graft

FTT failure to thrive; fat tolerance test; Fibrinolytic Therapy Trialists

FTTA fertile thoughts to all

FTU fluorescence thiourea

FTVD full-term vaginal delivery

FU fecal urobilinogen; fetal urobilinogen; fluorouracil; flux unit; follow-up; fractional urinalysis; fundus

F/U follow-up, fundus of umbilicus

F&U flanks and upper quadrants

5-FU 5-fluorouracil

Fu Finsen unit

FUB functional uterine bleeding

FUC fucosidase

Fuc fucose

FUCA fucosidase alpha

FUCA1 alpha-L-fucosidase

FUDR, FUdR fluorodeoxyuridine

FUE follicular unit extraction

FUF functional unification formalism

FUFA free volatile fatty acid

FUKAV Fukuoka virus

FULL fully formed anatomical structure

FUM 5-fluorouracil and methotrexate; fumarate; fumigation

FUMIR 5-fluorouracil, mitomycin C, radiation

FUMP fluorouridine monophosphate

FUN follow-up note

FUNC functional concept

funct function, functional

FUO fever of unknown origin

FUOV follow-up office visit

FUR 5-fluorouracil and radiation; fluorouracil riboside; fluorouridine; follow-up report; furin membrane-associated receptor

FUS feline urologic syndrome; first-use syndrome; focused ultrasound surgery; fusion

FuSV Fujinami sarcoma virus

FUT fibrinogen uptake test; follicular unit transplantation; fucosyl transferase

FUTP fluoridine triphosphate

FV femoral vein; fetal vaccinia; fever virus; fibroma virus; filiform virus; flow velocity; fluid volume; foamy virus; Fomede virus; Friend virus; Frog virus

Fv variable region antibody fragment

F(v) velocity distribution function

FVA Friend virus anemia

FVB Friend virus B-type

FVC false vocal cord; femoral vein cannulation; forced vital capacity

FVCC First Virtual Congress of Cardiology

FVD fluid volume deficit

FVE forced volume expiration

FVI flow velocity interval

FVL factor V Leiden mutation; femoral vein ligation; flow volume loop; force, velocity, length

FVOP finger venous opening pressure

FVP flexible video pericardioscopy; Friend virus polycythemia

FVPC follicular variant of papillary carcinoma

FVPF Family Violence Prevention Fund

FVR feline viral rhinotracheitis; forearm vascular resistance

FVRS Fellow in Vitreoretinal Surgery

FVS fetal valproate syndrome

FVT follicular-variant-translocation

f/V$_T$ frequency/tidal volume ratio

FW Felix-Weil [reaction]; Folin-Wu [reaction]; fragment wound

Fw F wave

fw fresh water

FWA Family Welfare Association

FWB full weight bearing

FWD forward; full ward diet

FWHM full width at half maximum

FWPCA Federal Water Pollution Control Administration

FWPV fowlpox virus

FWR Felix-Weil reaction; Folin-Wu reaction

FWTM full-width tenth maximum

FX factor X; fluoroscopy; fornix; fracture; frozen section

Fx fracture

fx fracture; friction

FXa factor Xa

FXD fexofenadine

Fx-dis fracture-dislocation

FXN function

FXS fragile X syndrome

fx/V$_T$ frequency/tidal volume ratio

FY fiscal year; full year

FYI for your information

FYMS fourth-year medical student

FZ focal zone; furazolidone

Fz frontal midline placement of electrodes

FZS Fellow of the Zoological Society

G

G acceleration; conductance; free energy; gallop; ganglion; gap; gas; gastrin; gauge; gauss; genome, genomic; geometric efficiency; giga; gingiva, gingival; glabella; globular; globulin; glucose; glycine; glycogen; goat; gold inlay; gonidial; good; goose; grade; Grafenberg spot; gram; gravida; gravitation constant; Greek; green; guanidine; guanine; guanosine; gynecology; unit of force of acceleration

G- giga- $[10^9]$

G° standard free energy

G₀ quiescent phase of cells leaving the mitotic cycle

1G first generation

G1 well-differentiated tumor

G₁ presynthetic gap

2G second generation

G2 moderately differentiated tumor

G₂ postsynthetic gap

G3 poorly differentiated tumor

G4 undifferentiated tumor

g force [gravity]; gap; gauge; gender; grain; gram; gravity; group; ratio of magnetic moment of a particle to the Bohr magneton; unit of standard acceleration due to gravity

γ lowercase Greek letter gamma; carbon separated from the carboxyl group by two other carbon atoms; constituent of the gamma protein plasma fraction; heavy chain of immunogammaglobulin; monomer in fetal hemoglobin; photon

ᵍ relative centrifugal force

GA Gamblers Anonymous; gastric analysis; gastric antrum; general anesthesia; general angiography; general appearance; generalized anxiety; genetic algorithm; gentisic acid; germ cell antigen; gestational age; gibberellic acid; gingivoaxial; glucoamylase; glucose; glucose/acetone; glucuronic acid; Golgi apparatus; gramicidin A; granulocyte adherence; granuloma annulare; guessed average; gut associated; gyrate atrophy

G/A globulin/albumin ratio

GA1 genetic algorithm 1

GA2 genetic algorithm 2

Ga gallium; granulocyte agglutination

Gα G protein subunit alpha complex

ga gauge

GAA gossypol acetic acid

GAAS Goldberg Anorectic Attitude Scale

GABA, gaba gamma-aminobutyric acid

GABA_A gamma-aminobutyric acid ionotropic receptor family A

GABA_B gamma aminobutyric acid ionotropic receptor family B

GABA_C gamma aminobutyric acid ionotropic receptor family C

GABAT, GABA-T gamma-aminobutyric acid transaminase

GABHS group A beta-hemolytic *Streptococcus*

GABI German Angioplasty Bypass Intervention [trial]; German Angioplasty Bypass Surgery Investigation

GABOA gamma-amino-beta-hydroxybutyric acid

GABRA gamma-aminobutyric acid alpha receptor

GAC general ambulatory care

GACELISA immunoglobulin G capture enzyme-linked immunosorbent assay

GACT government activity

GAD generalized anxiety disorder; glutamic acid decarboxylase

GADFLI general absorbed dose and fluence investigation

GADH gastric alcohol dehydrogenase

GADS gonococcal arthritis/dermatitis syndrome

GAdV goat adenovirus

GAEIB Group of Advisors on the Ethical Implications of Biotechnology

GAERS genetic absence epilepsy rats from Strasbourg

GAF global assessment of functioning

GAFeSV Gardner-Arnstein feline sarcoma virus

GAFG goal attainment follow-up guide

GAG glycosaminoglycan; group-specific antigen

GAH glyceraldehyde

GAHM genioglossus advancement and hyoid myotomy

GAHS galactorrhea, amenorrhea, hyperprolactinemia syndrome

GaHV gallid herpesvirus

GAIN Genetic Association Information Network; Glycine Antagonist GV150526 in Acute Stroke [trial]

GaIN Georgia Interactive Network for Medical Information

GAIP human $G_α$ interacting protein

GAIPAS General Audit Inpatient Psychiatric Assessment Scale

GAIT-ER-AID Gait Explanation and Reasoning Aid

GAL galactose; galactosyl; glucuronic acid lactone

Gal galactose

gal galactose; gallon

GALBP galactose-binding protein

GALC, GalC galactocerebroside

GALE galactose epimerase

GALK galactokinase

GalN galactosamine

GalNAc *N*-acetylgalactosamine

GALNS galactosamine-4-sulfatase

Gal-1-P galactose-1-phosphate

GalR galanin receptor

GALT galactose-1-*p*-uridyltransferase; gut-associated lymphoid tissue

GALV gibbon ape leukemia virus

Galv, galv galvanic

GAM geographical analysis machine

GAME immunoglobulins G, A, M, and E

GAMIS German-Austrian Myocardial Infarction Study

GAMM generalized abstract medical model

GAMP German-Austrian Multicenter Project

GAMS German-Austrian Multicenter Study

GAMV Gamboa virus

GAN giant axon neuropathy

G and D growth and development

gang, gangl ganglion, ganglionic

GANS granulomatous angiitis of the nervous system

GAO general accounting office

GAP D-glyceraldehyde-3-phosphate; Global AIDS Program; glottal area patency; growth-associated protein; guanosine triphosphatase activating protein

GAPD, GAPDH glyceraldehyde-3-phosphate dehydrogenase

GAPDP glyceraldehyde-3-phosphate dehydrogenase pseudogene

GAPNA Gerontological Advanced Practice Nurses Association

GAPO growth retardation, alopecia, pseudoanodontia, and optic atrophy [syndrome]

GAPs geriatric assessment programs

GAPST global average peristimulus time

GARS German-Austrian Reinfarction Study; glycine amide phosphoribosyl synthetase

GART genotype antiretroviral resistance test

GARV Garba virus

GAS galactorrhea-amenorrhea syndrome; gastric acid secretion; gastrin; gastroenterology; general adaptation syndrome; General Anxiety Scale; generalized arteriosclerosis; global anxiety score; global assessment scale; goal attainment scale; group A *Streptococcus*; growth arrest–specific

GASA growth-adjusted sonographic age

GASCIS German-Austrian Space-Occupying Cerebellar Infarction Study

GASP Group Against Smoking Pollution

gastroc gastrocnemius

GAT gamma-aminobutyric acid transporter; gelatin agglutination test; geriatric assessment team; Gerontological Apperception Test; group adjustment therapy

GATB Global Alliance for Tuberculosis Drug Development

GATR group attribute

GAUS German Activator Urokinase Study

GAVI Global Alliance for Vaccines and Immunization

GAWTS genomic amplification with transcript sequencing

GAXS German and Austrian Xamoterol Study

GB gallbladder; gigabyte; glial bundle; goofballs; Guillain-Barré [syndrome]

Gβ G protein subunit beta complex

Gb gigabit; gilbert

gB glycoprotein B

GBA ganglionic blocking agent; gender-based analysis; gingivobuccoaxial

GBAP glucocerebrosidase pseudogene

GBCA gadolinium-based contrast agent

GBD gallbladder disease; gender behavior disorder; glass blower's disease; Global Burden of Disease [study]; granulomatous bowel disease

GBF/DIME Geographic Base File Dual Independent Map Encoding

GBG glycine-rich beta-glycoprotein; gonadal steroid-binding globulin

GBH gamma-benzene hexachloride; graphite benzalkonium-heparin

GBHA glyoxal-bis-(2-hydroxyanil)

GBI globulin-binding insulin

GBIA Guthrie bacterial inhibition assay

GBL glomerular basal lamina

GBLC geometric broken line closure

GBM glioblastoma multiforme; glomerular basement membrane

GBP gabapentin; galactose-binding protein; gastric bypass; gated blood pool

GBpd gigabits per day

Gbps gigabits per second

Gbq gigabequerel

GBR guided bone regeneration

GBS gallbladder series; gastric bypass surgery; general biopsychosocial screening; glycerine-buffered saline; group B *Streptococcus*, group B streptococci; Guillain-Barré syndrome

GBSS Gey's balanced saline solution; Guillain-Barré-Strohl syndrome

GC ganglion cell; gas chromatography; general circulation; general closure; general condition; generalizability coefficient; generalized coherence; genetic counseling; geriatric care; germinal center; giant cell; glucocerebrosidase; glucocorticoid; goblet cell; Golgi cell; *Gonococcus;* gonorrhea; granular casts; granulomatous colitis; granulosa cell; group-specific component; guanine cytosine; guanylate cyclase; guanylyl cyclase

Gc galactocerebroside; gigacycle; *Gonococcus;* group-specific component

gC glycoprotein C

GCA gastric cancer area; giant cell arteritis

g-cal gram calorie

GCAP germ-cell alkaline phosphatase

GCAT Guideline Compliance Assessment Tool

GCB gonococcal base

GC-B guanylate cyclase B

gCBF global cerebral blood flow

GCBM glomerular capillary basement membrane

GCD graft coronary disease

GCDFP gross cystic disease fluid protein

GCF growth-rate−controlling factor

GCFT gonococcal/gonorrhea complement fixation test

GCG galactosyl ceramide beta-galactosidase; Genetics Computer Group; glucagon

GCGR glucagon receptor; glucocorticoid receptor

GCH granular clinical history

GCI General Cognitive Index; glottal closure instant

GCIIS glucose controlled insulin infusion system

GCK glomerulocystic kidney; glucokinase

GCL giant cell lesion; globoid cell leukodystrophy

GCLO gastric *Campylobacter*-like organism

GCM Gorlin-Chaudhry-Moss [syndrome]

g-cm gram-centimeter

gCMRO₂ global cerebral oxygen uptake

GC-MS, GC/MS gas chromatography/mass spectrometry

GCN geometric constraint network; giant cerebral neuron

GCNA Genetic Confidentiality and Nondiscrimination Act

GCNF glial cell−derived neurotrophic factor

g-coef generalizability coefficient

GCOP glucocorticoid-induced osteoporosis

GCP geriatric cancer population; German Cardiovascular Prevention [study]; good clinical practices; granulocyte chemotactic protein

GCPS Greig cephalopolysyndactyly syndrome

GCQ general community quarantine

GCR glucocorticoid receptor; Group Conformity Rating

GCRC General Clinical Research Center

GCRG giant cell reparative granuloma

GCRS gynecologic chylous reflux syndrome

GCS general clinical services; Gianotti-Crosti syndrome; Glasgow Coma Scale; global coordinate system; glucocorticosteroid; glutamylcysteine synthetase; glycine cleavage system

GCSA Gross cell surface antigen

GCSE generalized convulsive status epilepticus

G-CSF granulocyte colony-stimulating factor

GCSFR granulocyte colony-stimulating factor receptor

GCSP glycine cleavage system protein

GCT general care and treatment; germ cell tumor; giant cell thyroiditis; giant cell tumor

GC(T)A giant cell (temporal) arteritis

GC-TEA gas chromatography thermal energy analyzer

GCTTS giant cell tumor of tendon sheath

GCU gonococcal urethritis

GCV ganciclovir; great cardiac vein

GCVF great cardiac vein flow

GCV-TP ganciclovir triphosphate

GCW glomerular capillary wall

GCWM General Conference on Weights and Measures

GCY gastroscopy

GD gadolinium; gastroduodenal; Gaucher disease; gender dysphoria; general diagnostics; general dispensary; gestational day; Gianotti disease; gonadal dysgenesis; Graves disease; growth and development; growth delay

G&D growth and development

Gd gadolinium

gD glycoprotein D

gD2 glycoprotein D2

GDA gastroduodenal artery; general daily activity; germine diacetate; Graves disease autoantigen

GDAC Generic Drugs Advisory Committee

GDB gas density balance; Genome Database; guide dogs for the blind

GDC General Dental Council; giant dopamine-containing cell; Guglielmi detachable coil

Gd-CDTA gadolinium-cyclohexane-diamine-tetraacetic acid

GDCMS German Dilated Cardiomyopathy Study

Gd-DOTA gadolinium-tetra-azacyclododecatetraacetic acid

Gd-DTPA gadolinium-diethylene-triamine-pentaacetic acid

GDE Genetic Data Environment

Gd-EDTA gadolinium ethylene-diamine-tetraacetic acid

GDEP general dielectrophoretic [force]

GDF gel diffusion precipitin; growth differentiation factor

GDH glucose dehydrogenase; glutamate dehydrogenase; glycerophosphate dehydrogenase; glycol dehydrogenase; gonadotropin hormone; growth and differentiation hormone

GDI common gateway interface; guanidine nucleotide dissociation inhibitor

GDID genetically determined immunodeficiency disease

GDIR glucose-dependent insulinotropic receptor

g/dL grams per deciliter

GDM gestational diabetes mellitus

GDMO general duties medical officer

GdMP gadolinium mesoporphyrin

GDMS glow discharge mass spectrometry

gDNA genomic deoxyribonucleic acid

GDNF glial cell line—derived neutrophilic factor

GDP gel diffusion precipitin; gross domestic product; guanosine diphosphate

GDPR General Data Protection Regulation

GDS General Dental Service; geriatric depression scale; Global Deterioration Scale; Gordon Diagnostic System; gradual dosage schedule; guanosine diphosphate dissociation stimulator

GDT geometrically deformable template

GDU gastroduodenal ulcer

GDUFA Generic Drug User Fee Amendment

GDW glass distilled water

GDXY XY gonadal dysgenesis

GE gastric emptying; gastroemotional; gastroenteritis; gastroenterology; gastroenterostomy; gastroesophageal; gastrointestinal endoscopy; gel electrophoresis; generalized epilepsy; generator of excitation; genetic enhancement; genome equivalent; gentamicin; glandular epithelium; grade of evidence; gradient echo; guanidoethyl

G-E gradient echo

G/E granulocyte/erythroid ratio

Ge germanium

gE glycoprotein E

GEA gastric electrical activity; gastro-epiploid artery

GEART Gemfibrozil Atherosclerosis Regression Trial

GEB gum elastic bougie

GEC galactose elimination capacity; glomerular epithelial cell

GECC Government Employees' Clinic Center

GEE generalized estimating equation

GEF gastroesophageal fundoplication; glossoepiglottic fold; gonadotropin enhancing factor; guanosine nucleotide exchange factor

GEFS+ generalized epilepsy with febrile seizures plus

Ge^{-G} Gerbich negative

GEH glycerol ester hydrolase

GEHR Good European Health Record

GEI Genes and Environment Initiative

GEJ gastroesophageal junction

gel gelatin

GELIA German Experience with Low-Intensity Anticoagulation

GEM geriatric evaluation and management; guidelines element model

GEMISCH Generalized Medical Information System for Community Health

GEM-Q guidelines element model-quality

GE-MRI gradient echo magnetic resonance imaging

GEMS gel electrophoresis mass spectrometry; generic error-modeling system

GEMS/Food Global Environment Monitoring System/Food Contamination Monitoring and Assessment Programme

GEMSS glaucoma, lens ectopia, microspherophakia, stiffness, shortness [syndrome]

GEMT German Eminase Multicenter Trial

GEN gender; generation

Gen genetic, genetics; genus

gen general; genital

GeneCIS Genetic Clinical Information System

GENESIS General Ethnography and Needs Evaluations; Genes in Stroke [study]

genet genetic, genetics

GENE-TOX Genetic Toxicology [database]

genit genitalia, genital

GENNET Genetic Network

GENOA Genetics of Atherosclerosis [study]

GENOVA generalized analysis of variance

GENPS genital neoplasm-papilloma syndrome

GenRF gene reference into function

GENT gentamicin

GEO Gene Expression Omnibus; genetically enhanced organism

GEOSS Global Earth Observation System of Systems

GEP gastroenteropancreatic; gene expression profiling; gustatory evoked potential

GEPG gastroesophageal pressure gradient

GEPIC granulocyte elastase alpha-1 proteinase inhibitor complex

GEP-NET gastroenteropancreatic neuroendocrine tumor

GER gas exchange region; gastroesophageal reflux; geriatrics; granular endoplasmic reticulum

Ger geriatric, geriatrics; German

GERD gastroesophageal reflux disease

geriat geriatric, geriatrics

GeriROS geriatric review of systems

GERL Golgi-associated endoplasmic reticulum lysosome

GEROD Generator of Body Data

Geront gerontologic, gerontologist, gerontology

GERRI geriatric evaluation by relative rating instrument

GERV Germiston virus

GES gastroesophageal sphincter; glucose-electrolyte solution

GEST, gest gestation, gestational

GET gastric emptying time; general endotracheal [anesthesia]; graded treadmill exercise test

GETT general by endotracheal tube

GETV Getah virus

GEU geriatric evaluation unit

Gev giga electron volt

GEWS Gianturco expandable wire stent

GEX gas exchange

G$_{exg}$ exogenous glucose

GF gastric fistula; gastric fluid; germ free; glass factor; glomerular filtration; gluten free; grandfather; growth factor; growth failure

Gf gastric fluid

gf gram-force

GFA genetic function approximation; glial fibrillary acidic [protein]

GF-AAS graphite furnace atomic absorption spectroscopy

GFAP glial fibrillary acidic protein

GFAT glutamine:fructose-6-phosphate amidotransferase

GFATM Global Fund to Fight AIDS, Tuberculosis, and Malaria

GFCI ground-fault circuit interrupter

GFD gingival fibromatosis-progressive deafness [syndrome]; gluten-free diet

GFFS glycogen and fat-free solid

GFH glucose-free Hanks [solution]

GFI glucagon-free insulin; goodness-of-fit index; ground-fault interrupter

GfIV *Glypta fumiferanae* ichnovirus

GFL giant follicular lymphoma

Gflops gigaflops [billions of floating point operations per second]

G-FOBT guaiac-based fecal occult blood test

GFP gamma-fetoprotein; gel-filtered platelet; glomerular filtered phosphate; green fluorescent protein

GFR glomerular filtration rate

GFRP growth factor response protein

GFS global focal sclerosis; guafenesin

GFV Gabek Forest virus

GG gamma globulin; genioglossus; glycylglycine

Gγ G protein subunit gamma complex

γG immunoglobulin G

gG glycoprotein G

gg gynogenetic

GGA general gonadotropic activity

GGC gamma-glutamyl carboxylase

GGCS, g-GCS gamma-glutamyl cysteine synthetase

GGE generalized glandular enlargement; gradient gel electrophoresis

GGED Graphical Gene Expression Database

GGF geniculate ganglion fossa

GGFC gammaglobulin-free calf [serum]

GGG glycine-rich gamma-glycoprotein

GGH glycine-glycine-histidine

GGI Gillette Gait Index

GGM glucose-galactose malabsorption

GGMRF generalized gaussian Markov random field

GGO ground glass opacification

GG or S glands, goiter, or stiffness

GGPNA gamma-glutamyl-*p*-nitroanilide

GGR global genomic repair

GGT gamma-glutamyl transferase; gamma-glutamyl transpeptidase; geranylgeranyltransferase

GGTB glycoprotein 4-beta-galactosyl transferase

GGTP gamma-glutamyl transpeptidase

GGV *Gaeumannomyces graminis* virus; Gan Gan virus; generalized gross validation

GgV *Gaeumannomyces graminis* virus

GGVB gelatin, glucose, and veronal buffer

GGYV Gadgets Gully virus

GH general health; general hospital; genetic hemochromatosis; genetic hypertension; genetically hypertensive [rat]; geniohyoid; growth hormone

GHA generalized harmonic analysis; glucoheptanoic acid; Group Health Association

GHAA Group Health Association of America

GHAP Global Healthcare Application Project

GHAT German Hip Arthroplasty Trial**

GHB gamma hydroxybutyrate
GHb glycated hemoglobin
GHBA gamma-hydroxybutyric acid
GHBMO general hazardous materials behavior model
GHBP growth hormone binding protein
GHC group health cooperative
GHCH giant hepatic cavernous hemangioma
GHD growth hormone deficiency
GHDD Ghosal hematodiaphyseal dysplasia
GHDNet Global Health Disaster Network
GHEI Global Health Equity Initiative
GHEV *Goeldichironomus holoprasinus* entomopoxvirus
GHF growth hormone factor
GHHOS Glasgow Homeopathic Hospital Outcome Scale
GHL growth hormone−like
GHMM Generalized Hidden Markov Model
GHNet Global Health Network
GHP group health plan; growth hormone promotor
GHPM general health policy model
GHPQ General Health Perception Questionnaire
GHPS Global Health Professionals Survey
GHQ General Health Questionnaire
GHR granulomatous hypersensitivity reaction; growth hormone receptor
GHRA geriatric health risk appraisal
GHRF growth hormone−releasing factor
GHRFR growth hormone−releasing releasing factor
GH-RH growth hormone−releasing hormone
GHRHR growth hormone−releasing hormone receptor
GHRI general health rating index
GH-RIF growth hormone release inhibiting factor
GH-RIH growth hormone release inhibiting hormone
GHRP growth hormone−releasing peptide
GHSAG Global Health Security Action Group
GHSG German Hodgkin Study Group
GHT generalized Hough transform; Glaucoma Hemifield Test
GHV goose hepatitis virus; growth hormone variant
GHWs general hospital wards
GHz gigahertz
GI galvanic isolation; gastrointestinal; gelatin infusion [medium]; giant interneuron; gingival index; globin insulin; glomerular index; glucose intolerance; granuloma inguinale; growth inhibition; primigravida

GI$_{50}$ concentration required to inhibit cell growth by 50%
G$_i$ inhibitory guanyl-nucleotide−binding protein
gi gill
GIA gastrointestinal anastomosis
GIB gastrointestinal bleeding
GIBF gastrointestinal bacterial flora
GIBS generalized iterative bayesian simulation
GICA gastrointestinal cancer
GID gender identity disorder
GIF gastric intrinsic factor; gonadotropin-inhibiting factor; graphic interchange format; growth hormone−inhibiting factor
GIFB growth hormone inhibitory factor, brain
GIFIC graphical interface for intensive care
GIFT gamete intrafallopian transfer; granulocyte immunofluorescence test
GIGO garbage in, garbage out
GIH gastrointestinal hemorrhage; growth-inhibiting hormone
GIHINA Genetic Information Health Insurance Nondiscrimination Act
GII gastrointestinal infection; secundigravida
GIII tertigravida
GIK Glucose-Insulin-Kalium [pilot trial]; glucose-insulin-potassium
GIM general internal medicine; gonadotropin-inhibiting material
GIMC general internal medicine clinic
GIN Grosse Isle Anthrax Project
GINA Genetic Information Nondiscrimination Act; Global Initiative for Asthma
Ging, ging gingiva, gingival
g-ion gram-ion
GIP gastric inhibitory polypeptide; gastric inlet patch; giant cell interstitial pneumonia; glucose-dependent insulinotropic peptide; gonorrheal invasive peritonitis
GIPR gastric inhibitory polypeptide receptor
GIPSI Gradual Inflation at Optimum Pressure vs. Stent Implantation [study]
GIQLI Gastrointestinal Quality of Life Index
GIR global improvement rating; Grosse Isle Rinderpest Project
GIS gas in stomach; gastrointestinal series; geographic information system; guaranteed income supplement
GISAID Global Initiative on Sharing all Influenza Data
GISRS Global Influenza Surveillance and Response System
GISSI Grupo Italiano per lo Studio della Streptochinasi nell'Infarto Miocardico

GIST gastrointestinal stromal tumor

GIT gastrointestinal tract

GITS gastrointestinal therapeutic system

GITSG Gastrointestinal Tumor Study Group

GITT gastrointestinal transit time; glucose insulin tolerance test

GIV Great Island virus

GJ gap junction; gastric juice; gastrojejunostomy

gJ glycoprotein J

GJA-S gastric juice aspiration syndrome

GK galactokinase; glomerulocystic kidney; glucokinase; glycerol kinase

GKD glycerol kinase deficiency

GKI glucose potassium insulin

GKRS gamma knife radiosurgery

GL gland; glomerular layer; glomerulus; glycolipid; glycosphingolipid; glycyrrhizin; graphics library; greatest length; gustatory lacrimation

GL-4 glycophospholipid

Gl glabella

gL glycoprotein L

gl gill; gland, glandular

g/L, g/l grams per liter

GLA galactosidase A; gamma-linolenic acid; gingivolinguoaxial

glac glacial

GLAD glenolabral articular disruption; gold-labeled antigen detection

gland glandular

GLAP D-glyceraldehyde-3-phosphate

GLAT galactose + activator

GLB galactosidase beta

GLC gas-liquid chromatography

Glc glucose

glc glaucoma

GlcA gluconic acid

GLCB beta-glucuronidase

GLCLC glutamylcysteine synthase

GLC-MS gas-liquid chromatography mass spectrometry

GlcN glucosamine

GlcNAc N-acetylglucosamine

GlcUA D-glucuronic acid

GLD globoid cell leukodystrophy; glutamate dehydrogenase

GLDH glutamic dehydrogenase

GLH germinal layer hemorrhage; giant lymph node hyperplasia; gray level histogram

GLI glicentin; glioblastoma; glucagon-like immunoreactivity; guideline interchange format

GLIF guided lumbar interbody fusion; guideline interchange format

GLIIRA green light–induced infrared absorption

GLIM generalized linear interactive model

GLM general linear model

GLN glutamine

Gln glucagon; glutamine

gln glutamine

GLNH giant lymph node hyperplasia

GLNN galanin

GlnRS glutaminyl transfer ribonucleic acid synthase

GLO glyoxylase

GLO1 glyoxylase 1

glob globular; globulin

G-LOC G-induced loss of consciousness

GLOM glenoid labrum ovoid mass

GLP glucagon-like peptide; glucose-L-phosphate; glycolipoprotein; good laboratory practice; group living program

GLPC gas liquid phase chromatography

GLPR glucagon-like peptide receptor

GLR generalized likelihood ratio; graphic level recorder

GLRA glycine receptor alpha

GLRB glycine receptor beta

GLS generalized least square [estimator]; generalized lymphadenopathy syndrome

GLTN glomerulotubulonephritis

GLTT glucose-lactate tolerance test

GLU glucose; glucuronidase; glutamate; glutamic acid

GLU-5 five-hour glucose tolerance test

Glu glucuronidase; glutamic acid; glutamine

Glu2 glucose transporter 2

glu glucose; glutamic acid

Glu-A glutathione-agarose

GLUC glucosidase

gluc glucose

GLUD glutamate dehydrogenase

GLUDP glutamate dehydrogenase pseudogene

GLUL glutamate (ammonia) ligase

GluproRS glupropyl transfer ribonucleic acid synthase

GLUR, GluR glutamate receptor

GLUS granulomatous lesion of unknown significance

GLUT glucose transporter

GLV *Giardia lamblia* virus; gibbon ape leukemia virus; Gross leukemia virus

GLVR gibbon ape leukemia virus receptor

Glx glucose; glutamic acid

GLY, Gly, gly glycine

glyc glyceride

GlySH glyphosphate-surfactant herbicide

GlyCAM glycosylation-dependent cell adhesion molecule

GM gastric mucosa; gastrocnemius; Geiger-Müller [counter]; general medicine; genetic manipulation; geometric mean; giant melanosome; glyceryl methacrylate; gram; grand mal [seizure]; grand multiparity; grandmother; granulocyte-macrophage; graph-based model; Grateful Med; gray matter; growth medium

G-M Geiger-Müller [counter]

G/M granulocyte/macrophage

GM⁺ gram positive

GM⁻ gram negative

Gm an allotype marker on the heavy chains of immunoglobins

gM glycoprotein M

gm gram

g-m gram-meter

GMA glyceral methacrylate

GMB gastric mucosal barrier; granulomembranous body

GMBF gastric mucosa blood flow

GMC general medical clinic; General Medical Council [UK]; giant migratory contraction; grivet monkey cell

gm cal gram calorie

gm/cc grams per cubic centimeter

GMCD grand mal convulsive disorder

GM-CFC granulocyte-macrophage colony forming cell

GM-CFU granulocyte-macrophage colony forming unit

GM-CSA granulocyte-macrophage colony-stimulating activity

GM-CSF, (GM)-CSF granulocyte-macrophage colony-stimulating factor

GMD general message description; geometric mean diameter; glycopeptide moiety modified derivative

GME graduate medical education; granulomatous meningoencephalomyelitis

GMENAC Graduate Medical Education National Advisory Committee

G-MEPP giant miniature end plate potential

GMF gastric magnetic field; glial maturation factor

GMH germinal matrix hemorrhage

GMHA glycidyl methacrylate modified hyaluronic acid

GMK green monkey kidney [cells]

GMKV Gomoka virus

GML gut mucosa lymphocyte

g/mL, g/ml grams per milliliter

gm/L, gm/l grams per liter

gm-m gram-meter

GMN gradient moment nulling; moment reduction gradient

GMO genetically modified organism

g-mol gram-molecule

GMoV glycine mottle virus

GMP genetically modified product; glucose monophosphate; good manufacturing practice; Good Manufacturing Process standards; granule membrane protein; guanosine monophosphate

3′,5′-GMP guanosine 3′,5′-cyclic phosphate

GMPR guanine monophosphate reductase

GMPS guanosine 5′-monophosphate synthetase

GMR gallops, murmurs, rubs; gradient moment reduction; gradient motion rephasing

GMRH germinal matrix related hemorrhage

GMRI gated magnetic resonance imaging

GMS General Medical Service; geriatric mental state; Gilbert-Meulengracht syndrome; glyceryl monostearate; Gomori methenamine silver [stain]; goniodysgenesis, mental retardation (intellectual disability), short stature [syndrome]

GM&S general medicine and surgery

GMSC General Medical Services Committee

GMSP Galen Model for Surgical Procedures

GMT geometric mean titer; gingival margin trimmer; Göteborg Metoprolol Trial

GMV glycine mosaic virus; golden mosaic virus; gram molecular volume; green mottle virus

GMW gram molecular weight

GN gaze nystagmus; glomerulonephritis; glucose nitrogen [ratio]; gnotobiote; graduate nurse; gram negative; guanine nucleotide

G/N glucose/nitrogen ratio

Gn gnathion; gonadotropin

GNA general nursing assistance

GNAT guanine nucleotide binding protein, alpha transducing

GNAZ guanosine nucleotide binding alpha Z polypeptide

GNB ganglioneuroblastoma; gram-negative bacillus; guanine nucleotide binding [protein]

GNBM gram-negative bacillary meningitis

GNBT guanine nucleotide binding protein, beta transducing

GNC gender nonconforming; general nursing care; General Nursing Council [UK]; geriatric nurse clinician

GND gram-negative diplococci

GNDF giant cell−derived neurotropic factor

GNDFR giant cell−derived neurotropic factor−responsive

GNG gluconeogenesis

GNID gram-negative intracellular diplococci

GNN genetic neural network

GNP geriatric nurse practitioner; gerontologic nurse practitioner

GNR gram-negative rods

GnRF gonadotropin-releasing factor

GnRH gonadotropin-releasing hormone

GnRHa gonadotropin-releasing hormone agonist

GnRHR gonadotropin-releasing hormone receptor

GNRP guanine nucleotide−releasing protein

GNS German Nutrition Study

G/NS glucose in normal saline [solution]

GnSAF/GnSIF gonadotropin surge attenuating/inhibitory factor hormone

GNSWA Genetic Nurses and Social Worker's Association

GNTP Graduate Nurse Transition Program

GNUDI gerontological nursing U-diagnose instrument

GO gastro[o]esophageal; geroderma osteodysplastica; glucose oxidase; glutamic oxylacetic [acid]; gonorrhea

GΩ gigaohm [one billion ohms]

G&O gas and oxygen

Go gonion

GOA generalized osteoarthritis

GoAdV goose adenovirus

GOARN Global Outbreak Alert and Response Network

GOAT Galveston Orientation and Amnesia Test

GOBAB gamma-hydroxy-beta-aminobutyric acid

GOBI Growth and Development Charting the Road to Health, Oral Rehydration Therapy, Breast Feeding, Immunization

GOC granulose cell oocyte

GOE gas, oxygen, and ether

GOES Groningen orthopedic exit strategy

GOG Gynecologic Oncology Group

GOH geroderma osteodysplastica hereditaria

GOLD Global Initiative on Obstructive Lung Disease

GOMBO growth retardation, ocular abnormalities, microcephaly, brachycephaly, oligophrenia [syndrome]

GON gonococcal ophthalmia neonatorum; greater occipital nerve

GOND glaucomatous optic nerve damage

GOQ glucose oxidation quotient

GOR general operating room

GORAI Geriatric Oral Rehabilitation Assessment Index

GOS Glasgow outcome score; gum optical shield

GOSIP Government Open Systems Intercommunications Profile

GOT glucose oxidase test; glutamate oxaloacetate transaminase; goal of treatment

GOTM glutamic-oxaloacetic transaminase, mitochondrial

GOTS geriatric outpatient telephone screening

GOx glucose oxidase

GP gangliocytic paraganglioma; ganglionic plexi, plexus; gastroplasty; general paralysis, general paresis, general practice, general practitioner; genetic prediabetes; genetic programming; geometric progression; globus pallidus; glucose phosphate; glutamic pyruvic [acid]; glutathione peroxidase; glycerophosphate; glycopeptide; glycophorin; glycoprotein; Goodpasture syndrome; gram positive; grass pollen; guinea pig; gutta percha

G-P Grassbeger-Procaccia [algorithm]

G/P gravida/para

G-1-P glucose-1-phosphate

GP1 genetic programming 1

GPI glycoprotein I

GP2 genetic programming 2

G3P, G-3-P glyceraldehyde-3-phosphate; glycerol-3-phosphate

G6P, G-6-P glucose-6-phosphate

Gp glycoprotein

G$_p$ guanine nucleotide-binding protein

gp gene product; glycoprotein; group

GPA glenopolar angle; Global Program on AIDS; glycophorin A; Goodpasture antigen; grade point average; granulomatosis with polyangiitis; Group Practice Association; guinea pig albumin

GpA glycophorin A

GPAIS guinea pig anti-insulin serum

G6Pase, G-6-Pase glucose-6-phosphatase

GPASS General Practice Administration System for Scotland

GPB glossopharyngeal breathing; glycophorin B

GPC gastric parietal cell; gel permeation chromatography; General Practitioners Committee; giant papillary conjunctivitis; glycerolphosphorylcholine; glycophorin C; granular progenitor cell; guinea pig complement

GPCA gastrin-producing cell antibody

GPCI geographic practice cost index

GPCOV guinea pig type C oncovirus

GPCR G protein−coupled receptor

GPD glucose-6-phosphate dehydrogenase; glycerol-phosphate dehydrogenase

G3PD glucose-3-phosphate dehydrogenase

G6PD, G-6-PD glucose-6-phosphate dehydrogenase

G-6-PDA glucose-6-phosphate dehydrogenase enzyme variant A

G6PDH, G-6-PDH glucose-6-phosphate dehydrogenase reduced

G6PDL glucose-6-phosphate dehydrogenase-like

GPE globus pallidus externus; granulocyte colony stimulating factor promoter element; guinea pig embryo

GPEBP granulocyte colony stimulating factor promoter element binding protein

GPEP General Professional Education of the Physician

GP/ES gait pathology expert system

GPET graphic plan evaluation tool

GPF glomerular plasma flow; granulocytosis-promoting factor; greater palatine foramen

GPGG guinea pig gammaglobulin

GPh Graduate in Pharmacy

GPhC General Pharmaceutical Council [UK]

GPHIN Global Public Health Intelligence Network

GPHN giant pigmented hairy nevus

GP-HPLC gel permeation high-performance liquid chromatography

GPHV guinea pig herpesvirus

GPI general paralysis of the insane; globus pallidus internus; glucose phosphate isomerase; glycoprotein I; glycosylphosphatidylinositol; guinea pig ileum

G6PI glucose-6-phosphate isomerase

GP-IB general purpose interface bus

GPIbα glycoprotein Ib alpha

GpIbβ glycoprotein Ib beta

GPII General Practice Immunisation Incentives

GPIMH guinea pig intestinal mucosal homogenate

GPIPID guinea pig intraperitoneal infectious dose

GPK guinea pig kidney [antigen]

GPKA guinea pig kidney absorption [test]

GPLN Global Polio Laboratory Network

GPLV guinea pig leukemia virus

Gply gingivoplasty

GPM general preventive medicine; giant pigmented melanosome

GPm medial globus pallidus

GPMAL gravida, para, multiple births, abortions, and live births

GPN glossopharyngeal nerve; graduate practical nurse

GPNA Genetic Privacy Nondiscrimination Act

GPOA primary open-angle glaucoma

GPP generalist physician program; gross primary production

GPPQ General Purpose Psychiatric Questionnaire

GPPT Göteborg Primary Prevention Trial

GPRBC guinea pig red blood cell

GPS global positioning system; Goodpasture syndrome; gray platelet syndrome; guinea pig serum; guinea pig spleen

GPSYCH geriatric psychiatry

GPT General Population Trial; glutamate-pyruvate transaminase; glutamic-pyruvic transaminase

GpTh group therapy

GPU guinea pig unit

GPUT galactose phosphate uridyl transferase

GPV Global Programme for Vaccines and Immunization; goose parvovirus

GPVI glycoprotein VI

GPWW group practice without walls

GPX, GPx glutathione peroxidase

GQAP general question-asking program

GQAQ guidelines quality assessment questionnaire

GR gamma rays; gastric resection; general relief; general research; generalized rash; glucocorticoid receptor; glutathione reductase; good recovery; graded response; gravid; gravity resistance; growth rate

gr grade; graft; grain; gram; gravity; gray; gross

gr⁺ gram positive

gr⁻ gram negative

GRA gated radionuclide angiography; glucocorticoid-remedial aldosteronism; gonadotropin-releasing agent

GRABS group A beta-hemolytic streptococcal pharyngitis

GRACE Gianturco Roubin Stent in Acute Closure Evaluation

grad gradient; gradually; graduate

GRADE Grading of Recommendations Assessment, Development and Evaluation

GRAE generally regarded as effective

GRAIL Gene Recognition and Analysis Internet Link

GRAMI Gianturco Roubin Second Generation Coronary Stent in Acute Coronary Infarction

gran granule, granulated

GRAND Glaxo Receptor Antagonist Against Nottingham Deep Vein Thrombosis Study

GRANDDAD growth delay, aged facies, normal development, deficiency of subcutaneous fat [syndrome]

GRAPE Glycoprotein Receptor Antagonist Potency Evaluation [study]

GRAPPA Generalized Autocalibrating Partially Parallel Acquisition

GRAS generally recognized as safe

GRASP Glaxo Restenosis and Symptoms Project

GRASS gradient recalled acquisition in a steady state

GRASSIC Grampian Asthma Study of Integrated Care

grav gravid

grav 1, grav I pregnancy one, primigravida

grav 2, grav II pregnancy two, secundagravida

GRB growth factor receptor binding protein

GRC growth factor regulated [ion] channel

GRD gastroesophageal reflux disease; gender role definition

grd ground

GRE global relative entropy; glucocorticoid response element; gradient-recalled echo; gradient-refocused echo; Graduate Record Examination

GREAT Genome Recognition and Exon Assembly Tool; Grampian Region Early Antistreplase Trial

GRECC Geriatric Research, Education, and Clinical Center

GRECO German Recanalization of Coronary Occlusion [trial]; German Recombinant Plasminogen Activator [study]

GREP get regular expression and print

GRF gastrin-releasing factor; gelatin-resorcinol-formalin; genetically related macrophage factor; Gibbs random field; glutamyl transpeptidase—releasing factor; gonadotropin-releasing factor; ground reaction force; growth hormone—releasing factor

GRG glucocorticoid receptor gene; glycine-rich glycoprotein; guidelines review group

GRH growth hormone—releasing hormone

GRHR gonadotropic-releasing hormone receptor

GrHV gruid herpesvirus

GRIA glutamate receptor, ionotropic, ampa

GRIF growth hormone release inhibiting factor

GRIFFIN Graphics Investigation of Familial Information

GR II Gianturco Roubin Second Generation Coronary Stent Trial

GRIK glutamate receptor, ionotropic, kainate

GRINA glutamate receptor, ionotropic, *N*-methyl-D-aspartate A

GRINB glutamate receptor, ionotropic, *N*-methyl-D-aspartate B

GRIPS Göttingen Risk, Incidence, and Prevalence Study

GRL glass reflection light

GRMP granulocyte membrane protein

GRN graduate registered nurse; granules; granulin

GrN gram negative

Grn green

gRNA genomic ribonucleic acid; guide ribonucleic acid

GRO growth-regulated oncogene; growth-related [protein]

GROB growth-related protein beta

GROD granular osmophilic deposit

GROG growth-related protein gamma

GROU group

GRP gastrin-releasing peptide; glucose-regulated protein

GrP gram positive

$Gr_1P_0AB_1$ one pregnancy, no births, one abortion

GRPR gastrin-releasing peptide receptor

GRPS glucose-Ringer-phosphate solution

GRS gastrin receptor scintigraphy; Golabi-Rosen syndrome

GRV ground reaction vector

GRW giant ragweed [test]

gr wt gross weight

GS gallstone; Gardner syndrome; gas spectrometry; gastric shield; gastrocnemius; general surgery; gestational score; Gilbert syndrome; Gitelman syndrome; glomerular sclerosis; glucagon secretion; glucosamine; glucosamine sulfate; glutamine synthetase; gluteal set; glycogen synthase; goat serum; Goldenhar syndrome; Goodpasture syndrome; graft survival; granulocytic sarcoma; grip strength; Griselli syndrome; group section; group specific

G/S glucose and saline

G6S glucosamine-6-sulfatase

G_s stimulatory G protein

gs group specific

g/s gallons per second

GSA generalized simulated annealing; general somatic afferent; Gerontological Society of America; Gross virus antigen; group-specific antigen; guanidinosuccinic acid

Gsa G protein stimulatory alpha subunit

GSBG gonadal steroid-binding globulin

G-SBS guanosine substrate-binding strand

GSC gas-solid chromatography; germline stem cell; gravity settling culture

GSCN giant serotonin-containing neuron

GSD genetically significant dose; Gerstmann-Sträussler disease; gestational sac diameter; glutathione synthetase deficiency; glycogen storage disease

GSD-0 glycogen storage disease zero

GSE General Self-Efficacy [scale]; general somatic efferent; gluten-sensitive enter-opathy

GSEV *Geotrupes sylvaticus* entomopox-virus

GSF galactosemic fibroblast; generalized structure function; genital skin fibroblast

GSFR granulocyte colony stimulating factor receptor

GSH glomerulus stimulating hormone; golden Syrian hamster; L-alpha-glutamyl-L-cysteinyl-glycine; reduced glutathione

GSH-EE glutathione ethyl ester

GSH-Px glutathione peroxidase

GSHV ground squirrel hepatitis B virus

GSI global severity index

GSIV Great Saltee Island virus

GSM generic semantic [data] modeling; global system for mobile communication; group sequential method

GS-MS gas spectrography/mass spectrophotometry

GSN gelsonin; giant serotonin-containing neuron

GSoA Gerontological Society of America

GSP galvanic skin potential

GSPECT, gSPECT gated single photon emission computed tomography

GsplV *Glypta* sp. ichnovirus

GSPS Global School Personnel Survey

GSR galvanic skin response; generalized Shwartzman reaction; glutathione reductase

GSRS Gastrointestinal Symptom Rating Scale

GSS gamete-shedding substance; General Social Survey; genome survey sequence; Gerstmann-Sträussler-Scheinker [disease]; glutathione synthetase; granulomatous slack skin

GSSD Gerstmann-Sträussler-Scheinker disease

GSSG oxidized glutathione

GSSG-R glutathione reductase

GSSI general solvent-solute interaction

GSSR generalized Sanarelli-Shwartzman reaction

GST glutathione-*S*-transferase; gold salt therapy; gold sodium thiomalate; graphic stress telethermometry; group striction

GSTA glutathione-*S*-transferase alpha

GST1L glutathione-*S*-transferase-1−like

GSTM glutathione-*S*-transferase mu

GSTP glutathione-*S*-transferase pi

GSTT glutathione-*S*-transferase theta

GSV gestational sac volume; greater saphenous vein

GSVD general singular value decomposition

GSVT greater saphenous vein thrombophlebitis

GSW gunshot wound

GSWA gunshot wound, abdominal

GSWH gunshot wound to head

GSYY Grimsey virus

GT gait training; galactosyl transferase; gastrostomy; generation time; genetic therapy; gingiva treatment; Glanzmann thrombasthenia; glucose therapy; glucose tolerance; glucose transport; glucuronyl transferase; glutamyl transpeptidase; glycityrosine; granulation tissue; great toe; greater trochanter; group tensions; group therapy

G&T gowns and towels

GT1 to GT10 glycogen storage disease, types 1 to 10

gt drop [L. *gutta*]

g/t granulation time; granulation tissue

GTA gene transfer agent; Glanzmann thrombasthenia; glycerol teichoic acid

GTB gastrointestinal tract bleeding

GTCS generalized tonic-clonic seizures

GTD gestational trophoblastic disease

GTDS Giesen Tumor Documentation System

GTE green tea extract

GTEM gigahertz transverse electromagnetic [cell]

GTF general transcription factor; glucose tolerance factor; glucosyl-transferase

GTH gonadotropic hormone

GTHR generalized thyroid hormone resistance

GTI grid tiler

GTM generalized tendomyopathy

GTN gestational trophoblastic neoplasia; glomerulotubulonephritis; glyceryl trinitrate

GTO Golgi tendon organ

GTP glutamyl transpeptidase; guanosine triphosphate

GTPase guanosine triphosphatase

gt-PET ground truth positron emission tomography

GTPV goatpox virus

GTR galvanic tetanus ratio; granulocyte turnover rate; guided tissue regeneration

GTS Gilles de la Tourette syndrome; glucose transport system

GTSS Global Tobacco Surveillance System

GTT gelatin-tellurite-taurocholate; glucose tolerance test

gtt. drops [L. *guttae*]

G tube gastric tube

GTV gross tumor volume

GTX *Goniopora* toxin; gonyautoxin

GTX$_2$ gonyautoxin II

GTX$_3$ gonyautoxin III

GU gastric ulcer; genitourinary; glucose uptake; glycogenic unit; gonococcal urethritis; gravitational ulcer; guanethidine

GUA group of units of analysis

Gua guanine

GUARANTEE Global Unstable Angina Registry and Treatment Evaluation

GUCA guanylate cyclase activator

GUD genitourinary dysplasia

GUI graphic user interface

GUIDE Guidance by Ultrasound Imaging for Decision Endpoints [trial]

GUIDE II Guidance by Ultrasound for Interventional Decision Endpoints II [trial]

GUK guanylate kinase

GULHEMP general physique, upper extremity, lower extremity, hearing, eyesight, mentality, and personality [scale]

GUM genitourinary medicine

GUNM Georgetown University Nursing Model

Guo guanosine

GURV Gurupi virus

GUS genitourinary sphincter; genitourinary system

GUSTO Globus Ubiquitous Supercomputing Testbed Organization

GUSTO-I Global Utilization of Streptokinase and Tissue Plasminogen Activator for Occluded Coronary Arteries [trial]

GUSTO-IIa Global Use of Strategies to Open Occluded Arteries [trial]

GUSTO-IIb Global Use of Strategies to Open Occluded Arteries in Acute Coronary Syndromes [trial]

GUSTO-III Global Use of Strategies to Open Occluded Coronary Arteries [trial]

GUSTO-IV Global Use of Streptokinase and Tissue Plasminogen Activator for Occluded Arteries [trial]

Guttat. drop by drop [L. *guttatim*]

GV gas ventilation; gastric volume; generalized vaccinia; gentian violet; germinal vesicle; granulosis virus; griseoviridan; Gross virus

GVA general visceral afferent [nerve]

GVB gelatin-Veronal buffer

GVBD germinal vesicle breakdown

GVE general visceral efferent [nerve]

GVF good visual fields; gradient vector flow

GVG gamma-vinyl-gamma-aminobutyric acid

GVH, GvH graft versus host

GVHD, GvHD graft-versus-host disease

GVHR, GvHR graft-versus-host reaction

GVL graft versus leukemia

G vs HD graft-versus-host disease

GVTY gingivectomy

GW germ warfare; gigawatt; glycerin in water; gradual withdrawal; group work; guidewire

G/W glucose in water

GWAFD Genée-Wiedemann acrofacial dysostosis

GWAS genome-wide association studies

GWB general well-being

GWDT gray-weighted distance transformation [imaging]

GWE glycerol and water enema

GWG generalized Wegener granulomatosis

GWN gaussian white noise

GWTG Get with the Guidelines

GWUHP George Washington University Health Plan

GX glycinexylidide; histopathologic grade of tumor cannot be assessed

Gx gastroschisis

GXD Gene-Expression Database

GXT graded exercise test

Gy gray

GY-1 graduate year one

GYN, Gyn, gyn gynecologic, gynecologist, gynecology

GypV gypsy virus

GYTS Global Youth Tobacco Survey

GZ Guilford-Zimmerman [test]

H

H bacterial antigen in serologic classification of bacteria [Ger. *Hauch*, breath]; deflection in the His bundle [ECG]; dose equivalent; draft [L. *haustus*]; electrically induced spinal reflex; enthalpy; fucosal transferase-producing gene; heart; heavy; height; hemagglutination; hemisphere; hemolysis; henry; heparin; heroin; high; hippocampus; histidine; *Histoplasma*; histoplasmosis; Holzknecht unit; homosexual; horizontal; hormone; horse; hospital; Hounsfield unit; hour; human; hydrogen; hydrolysis; hygiene; hyoscine; hypermetropia; hyperopia; hypodermic; hypothalamus; magnetic field strength; magnetization; mustard gas; oersted

H⁺ hydrogen ion
[H⁺] hydrogen ion concentration
H₀ null hypothesis
H1/2 half-value layer
H1, ¹H, H¹ alternate hypothesis; first [heart] sound; halistatin; protium
H2, ²H, H² deuterium; second [heart] sound
H3, ³H, H³ third [heart] sound; tritium
4H hypothalamic hamartoblastoma, hyperphalangeal hypoendocrine, hypoplastic anus [syndrome]
h hand rearing; heat transfer coefficient; hecto; height; henry; hour; human; hundred; hypodermic; negatively staining region of a chromosome; Planck constant; secondary constriction; specific enthalpy
h- hecto- [10²]
HA H antigen; Hakim-Adams [syndrome]; halothane anesthesia; Hartley [guinea pig]; headache; health affairs; health alliance; health authority; hearing aid; height age; hemadsorption; hemagglutinating antibody; hemagglutination; hemagglutinin; hemolytic anemia; hemophiliac with adenopathy; hepatic adenoma; hepatic artery; hepatitis A; hepatitis-associated; heteroduplex analysis; heterophil antibody; Heyden antibiotic; high anxiety; hippocampal asymmetry; hippuric acid; histamine; histocompatibility antigen; Horton arteritis; hospital administration; hospital admission; hospital apprentice; Hounsfield unit; human albumin; hyaluronic acid; hydroxyapatite; hydroxylamine; hyperactive; hyperalimentation; hyperandrogenism; hypersensitivity alveolitis; hypothalamic amenorrhea
H/A head to abdomen; headache

1HA hydroxyapatite; hydroxylamine
HA2 hemadsorption virus 2
Ha absolution hypermetropia; hamster; Hartmann number
ha hectare
HAA hearing aid amplifier; hemolytic anemia antigen; hepatitis-associated antigen; hepatitis-associated aplastic anemia; hospital activity analysis
HA Ag hepatitis A antigen
HAART highly active antiretroviral therapy
HAAS Honolulu-Asia Aging Study
hAAT human α₁-antitrypsin
HAB harmful algal bloom; histoacryl blue
HABA 2(4'-hydroxyazobenzene) benzoic acid
HABF hepatic artery blood flow
HABP hospital-acquired bacterial pneumonia
HA-BP high-affinity binding protein
HABP/VABP hospital-acquired bacterial pneumonia/ventilator-associated bacterial pneumonia
HACCP hazard analysis and critical control point system
HACE high-altitude cerebral edema
HACEK *Haemophilus, Actinobacillus, Cardiobacterium, Eikenella, Kingella*
HACER hypothalamic area controlling emotional response
HAChT high-affinity choline transport
HACR hereditary adenomatosis of the colon and rectum
HACS Hazard-Assessment Computer System; hyperactive child syndrome
hACSP human adenylate cyclase–stimulating protein
HACT health care activity
HAD health care alternatives development; hemadsorption; HIV-associated dementia; hospital administration, hospital administrator; hospital anxiety and depression [scale]; human immunodeficiency virus–associated dementia
HAd hemadsorption; hospital administrator
HADD hydroxyapatite deposition disease
HADH hydroxyacyl CoA dehydrogenase
HAd-I hemadsorption-inhibition
HADS hospital anxiety and depression scale
HAdV 1 to 51 human adenoviruses 1 to 51
HAdV-A to F human adenoviruses A to F
HAE health appraisal examination; hearing aid evaluation; hepatic artery embolism; hereditary angioneurotic edema
Hae *Haemophilus influenzae aegyptius*
HAEC Hirschsprung-associated enterocolitis; human aortic endothelial cell

HAF hepatocellular altered focus; hyperalimentation fluid

HaF Hageman factor

HAFP human alpha-fetoprotein

HAG heat-aggregated globulin

HAGG hyperimmune antivariola gamma-globulin

HAGH hydroxyacyl-glutathione hydrolase

HAGL humeral avulsion of glenohumeral ligament

HAH halogenated aromatic compound

HAHS Harvard Alumni Health Study

HAHTG horse antihuman thymus globulin

HAI health care–associated infection; hemagglutination inhibition; hepatic arterial infusion; hospital-acquired infection

H&A Ins health and accident insurance

HAIR-AN hyperandrogenism, insulin resistance, and acanthosis nigricans [syndrome]

HaK hamster kidney

HAL hand-assisted laparoscopy; Heart Attacks in London [study]; hemorrhoidal artery ligation; hepatic artery ligation; hybrid artificial liver; hypoplastic acute leukemia

hal halogen; halothane

HALC high affinity, low capacity

HALF high amplitude, low frequency; Homocysteine, Atherosclerosis, Lipid and Familial Hypercholesterolemia [study]

HALFD hypertonic albumin-containing fluid demand

halluc hallucinations

HALO Halotestin

HALP hand-assisted laparoscopic proctocolectomy; hyperalphalipoproteinemia

HALT Hypertension and Lipid Trial

HALT MI Hu23F2G Anti-Adhesion to Limit Cytotoxic Injury Following Acute Myocardial Infarction [study]

HALV human acquired immunodeficiency syndrome lymphotropic virus

HaLV hamster leukemia virus

HAM hearing aid microphone; helical axis in motion; hemolymph anticoagulation medium; human albumin microsphere; human alveolar macrophage; human T-cell lymphotropic virus–associated myelopathy; hypoparathyroidism, Addison disease, and mucocutaneous candidiasis [syndrome]

HAM-1, -2 histocompatibility antigen modifier types 1 and 2

HAm human amnion

HAMA Hamilton anxiety [scale]; human antimurine antibody

HA-MA methacrylated hyaluronic acid

HAMD Hamilton depression [scale]

HAMDCT Hospital Authority Master Disease Code Table

HAMIT Heparin in Acute Myocardial Infarction Trial

HaMSV, Ha-MSV Harvey murine sarcoma virus

HAN heroin-associated nephropathy; hyperplastic alveolar nodule

HANA hemagglutinin neuraminidase

H and E hematoxylin and eosin

HANDI Hemophilia and AIDS/HIV Network for the Dissemination of Information

Handicp handicapped

HaNDL headache and neurologic deficits with cerebrospinal fluid lymphocytosis

HANE hereditary angioneurotic edema; Hydrochlorothiazide, Atenolol, Nitrendipine, Enalapril [study]

HANES Health and Nutrition Examination Survey

hANF human atrial natriuretic factor

h ANP human atrial natriuretic peptide

HANSA Healthcare Advanced Networked System Architecture

HAODM hypoplasia anguli oris depressor muscle

HAP Handicapped Aid Program; Hazardous Air Pollutants [list]; hazardous air pollution; health alliance plan; hepatic arterial phase; heredopathia atactica polyneuritiformis; high-altitude peristalsis; histamine acid phosphate; hospital-acquired pneumonia; hospital admissions program; Human Activity Profile; humoral antibody production; hydrolyzed animal protein; hydroxyapatite; hypoxic abdominal perfusion

HAp hydroxyapatite

HAPA hemagglutinating anti-penicillin antibody

HAPC high-amplitude peristaltic contraction; hospital-acquired penetration contact

HAPE high-altitude pulmonary edema

HAPI Heparin as an Alternative to Promote Patency in Acute Myocardial Infarction [study]

HAPORT Heart Attack Patient Outcome Research Team [study]

HAPPHY Heart Attack Primary Prevention in Hypertension

HAPS hepatic arterial perfusion scintigraphy

HAPSA Home Assessment Program for Successful Aging

HaPV hamster polyomavirus

HAPVC hemianomalous pulmonary venous connection

HAPVD hemianomalous pulmonary venous drainage

HAPVR hemianomalous pulmonary venous return

HaPyV hamster polyomavirus

HAQ health assessment questionnaire

HAQDI Heath Assessment Questionnaire Disability Index

HAR head airway region; high-altitude retinopathy

HARD hydrocephalus, agyria, retinal dysplasia [syndrome]

HARD ± E hydrocephalus, agyria, retinal dysplasia with or without encephalocele [syndrome]

HAREM heparin assay rapid easy method

HARH high-altitude retinal hemorrhage

HARK humiliation, afraid, rape, kick [violence screening tool]

HARM harmonics from the injected signal; heparin assay rapid method

HAROLD Hypertension and Ambulatory Recording in the Old

HARP harmonic phase; Harvard Atherosclerosis Reversibility Project; homeless and at-risk population; hospital admission risk profile

HARS histidyl-RNA synthetase; human AIDS reporting system

HART Heparin-Aspirin Reperfusion Trial; hyperfractionated accelerated radiation therapy; Hypertension Audit of Risk Factor Therapy [study]

HART II Heparin and Reperfusion Therapies [study]

HARTS Hoechst Adverse Reaction Terminology System

HAS Hamilton Anxiety Scale; health advisory service; health assessment system; Helsinki Aging Study; Hemostatic System Activation Substudy; highest asymptomatic; Hirulog Angioplasty Study; hospital administrative service; hospital advisory service; human albumin solution; hydrocephalus due to stenosis of the aqueduct of Sylvius; hyperalimentation solution; hypertensive arteriosclerotic

HASCVD hypertensive arteriosclerotic cardiovascular disease

HASHD hypertensive arteriosclerotic heart disease

HASI Hirulog Angioplasty Study Investigators

HASM human airway smooth muscle

HASMC human aortic smooth muscle cell

HASP Hospital Admissions and Surveillance Program

HASS highest anxiety subscale score

HASTE half-Fourier acquisition single-shot turbo spin echo

HAstV 1 to 8 human astroviruses 1 to 8

HAT hair apposition technique; Halsted Aphasia Test; head, arm, trunk; Health Attribution Test; heparin-associated thrombocytopenia; heterophil antibody titer; histone acetyltransferase; home asthma telemonitoring; hospital arrival time; human African trypanosomiasis; hypoxanthine, aminopterin, and thymidine; hypoxanthine, azaserine, and thymidine

3-HAT 3-hydroxyanthranilic acid

HATG horse antihuman thymocyte globulin

HATH Heterosexual Attitudes Toward Homosexuality [scale]

HATT heparin-associated thrombocytopenia and thrombosis

HATTS hemagglutination treponemal test for syphilis

HaTx hanatoxin

HAU hemagglutinating unit

HAV hemadsorption virus; hepatitis A virus

HAVOC Hematoma and Vascular Outcome Complications [study]

HAVS hand-arm vibration syndrome

HAWIC Hamburg-Wechsler Intelligence Test for Children

HAZ height-for-age Z-score

HAZMAT, HazMat, hazmat hazardous material

HAZOP hazard and operability

HAZR hazardous substance

HAZUS Hazard US [method]

HAZWOPER hazardous waste operations and emergency response

HB health board; heart block; heel to buttock; held back; hemoglobin; hepatitis B; His bundle; hold breakfast; housebound; hybridoma bank; hyoid body

Hb hemoglobin

HBA bundle of His electrogram; heated blood agar [test]

HbA hemoglobin A, adult hemoglobin

HBA$_1$ glycosylated hemoglobin

HBAb hepatitis B antibody

HBABA hydroxybenzeneazobenzoic acid

HbA1c, HbA$_{1c}$ glycosylated hemoglobin

HBAg hepatitis B antigen

HBB hemoglobin beta chain; hospital blood bank; hydroxybenzyl benzimidazole

HbBC hemoglobin binding capacity

HBBW hold breakfast blood work

HBC hereditary breast cancer; hit by car [veterinary medicine]

HB$_c$, HBC, HBc hepatitis B core [antigen]

HbC hemoglobin C

HBCAB, HBcAb hepatitis B core antibody

HBCAG, HBcAg, HB$_c$Ag hepatitis B core antigen

HBCG heat-aggregated Calmette-Guérin bacillus

HbCO carboxyhemoglobin

Hb CS hemoglobin Constant Spring

HBCT helical biphasic contrast-enhanced computed tomography

HbCV *Haemophilus influenzae* conjugate vaccine

HBD has been drinking; homozygous by descent; hydroxybutyric dehydrogenase; hypophosphatemic bone disease

HbD hemoglobin D

hBD human beta-defensin

HBDH hydroxybutyrate dehydrogenase

hBDNF human brain-derived neurotrophic factor

HBDT human basophil degranulation test

HBE His bundle electrogram

HbE hemoglobin E

HB$_e$ hepatitis B early antigen

HBeAb/Ag hepatitis B e-antibody/antigen

HBEAG, HB$_e$Ag, HBeAg hepatitis B early antigen

HBEC human brain endothelial cell

HB-EGF heparin-binding epidermal growth factor

HBF hand blood flow; hemispheric blood flow; hemoglobinuric bilious fever; hepatic blood flow; hypothalamic blood flow

HbF fetal hemoglobin; hemoglobin F

Hbg hemoglobin

HBGA histo–blood group antigen

HBGF heparin-binding growth factor

HBGM home blood glucose monitoring

HBGR hemoglobin-gamma regulator

HbH hemoglobin H

HBHC hospital-based home care

HBHCT hospital-based home care team

Hb-Hp hemoglobin-haptoglobin

HBI hemibody irradiation; high serum-bound iron

HBIG, HBIg hepatitis B immunoglobulin

HBL hepatoblastoma

HBLA human B-cell lymphocyte antigen

H$_2$ blockers histamine blockers

HBLV human B-cell lymphotropic virus

HBM health belief model; hypertonic buffered medium

HbM hemoglobin Milwaukee

HBMEC human brain microvascular endothelial cell

HbMet methemoglobin

HBMP Human Brain Map Project

hBNP human brain natriuretic peptide

HBO hyperbaric oxygen, hyperbaric oxygenation

HbO, HbO$_2$ oxyhemoglobin

HBOC hereditary breast-ovarian cancer

HBOT hyperbaric oxygen therapy

HBoV human bocavirus

HBP heartbeat period; hepatic binding protein; high blood pressure; hospital-based practice

HbP primitive hemoglobin

HBPV HB virus

HBr hydrobromic acid

HbR reduced hemoglobin

HBS hepatitis B surface [antigen]; hyperkinetic behavior syndrome

HB$_s$ hepatitis B surface [antigen]

HbS hemoglobin S; sickle cell hemoglobin

HBsAb hepatitis B surface antibody

HBsAb/Ag hepatitis B surface antibody/antigen

HBSAG, HBsAg, HB$_s$AG, HB$_s$Ag hepatitis B surface antigen

HBsAg/adr hepatitis B surface antigen manifesting group-specific determinant *a* and subtype-specific determinants *d* and *r*

HBSC hematopoietic blood stem cell

HBSS Hank's balanced salt solution

HbSS hemoglobin SS

HBT brevetoxin; human brain thromboplastin; human breast tumor

HBT-B brevetoxin B

Hb$_{tot}$ total hemoglobin

HBV hepatitis B vaccine; hepatitis B virus; high biologic value

HBV-MN membranous nephropathy associated with hepatitis B virus

HBVS hepatitis B virus integration site

HBW Healthbeat Wales [study]; high birth weight

HbZ hemoglobin Z, hemoglobin Zürich

HC hair cell; hairy cell; Hajdu-Cheney [disease]; handicapped; head circumference; head compression; Health Canada; health care; health checkup; healthy control; heart catheterization; heart cycle; heat conservation; heavy chain; hematochromatosis; hemicholinium; hemoglobin concentration; hemorrhagic colitis; heparin cofactor; hepatic catalase; hepatitis C; hepatocellular; hepatocellular cancer; hereditary coproporphyria; hexachloroethane; Hickman catheter; high calorie; hip circumference; hippocampus; histamine challenge; histochemistry; home care; homocysteinuria; Hospital Corps; house call; Huntington chorea; hyaline casts; hybrid capture [assay]; hydraulic concussion; hydrocarbon; hydrocortisone; hydroxycorticoid; hyoid cornu; hypercholesterolemia; hypertrophic cardiomyopathy

H&C hot and cold

4HC 4-hydroperoxy-cyclophosphamide

Hc hexachloroethane; *Histoplasma capsulatum*; hybrid capture [assay]; hydrocolloid

HCA health care associate; heart cell aggregate; hepatocellular adenoma; hierarchical clustering analysis; home care aide; Hospital Corporation of America; hybrid capture assay; hydrocortisone acetate; hypothermic circulatory arrest

HCa high calcium

HC/AC head circumference/abdominal circumference ratio

hCaCC human calcium-sensitive chloride channel

HCAEC human coronary artery endothelial cell

HCAP handicapped

HCATT hyperbaric care air transport team

HCA/W home care aide/worker

HCB hexachlorobenzene

HCC health call center; health care–related common component; hepatitis contagiosa canis; hepatocellular carcinoma; history of chief complaint; hospital computer center; hydroxycholecalciferol

25-HCC 25-hydroxycholecalciferol

HCCA health care commuting area; hepatocellular carcinoma; hereditary cortical cerebellar atrophy; hilar cholangiocarcinoma 4-hydroxycinnamic acid

HCCAA hereditary cysteine C amyloid angiopathy

HCCH hexachlorocyclohexane

HCCS hereditary cancer consulting service

HCD health care delivery; heavy-chain disease; high-calorie diet; high-carbohydrate diet; homologous canine distemper; human Chagas disease

HCE health care establishment; health care expertise; hypoglossal carotid entrapment

HCEA Health Care Education Association

HC-EAS hybrid capture expansion analysis system

HCF [fetal] head-to-cervix force; healthy control female; heparin cofactor; hereditary capillary fragility; highest common factor; hypocaloric carbohydrate feeding

HCFA Health Care Financing Administration

hCFSH human chorionic follicle-stimulating hormone

HCG, HcG, hCG human chorionic gonadotropin

HCH Health Care for the Homeless; hemochromatosis; hexachlorocyclohexane; hygroscopic condenser humidifier

HCHB hemichorea-hemiballismus

HCHP Harvard Community Health Plan

HCHWA hereditary cerebral hemorrhage with amyloidosis

HCHWA-D hereditary cerebral hemorrhage with amyloidosis, Dutch type

HCI Health Commons Institute; human collagenase inhibitor; human-computer interface

HcImp hydrocolloid impression

HCIN high-grade cervical intraepithelial neoplasia

HCIS Health Care Information System

HCK hematopoietic cell kinase

HCL hairy cell leukemia; human cultured lymphoblasts

HCl hydrogen chloride

HCLF high carbohydrate, low fiber

HCLU health care libraries unit

HCM health care management; hospital communication module; hypertrophic cardiomyopathy

HCMM hereditary cutaneous malignant melanoma

HCMV human cytomegalovirus

HCN health communication network; hereditary chronic nephritis

HCO health care organization

HCO$_3^-$ bicarbonate

HCOP health center opportunity program

HCoV human coronavirus

HCP handicapped; health care personnel; health care professional; health care provider; hematopoietic cell phosphatase; hepatocatalase peroxidase; hereditary coproporphyria; hexachlorophene; high cell passage; home care platform; hydrophobic class pair; hyperplasia with chronic pancreatitis

H&CP hospital and community psychiatry

HCPCS Healthcare Common Procedure Coding System

HCPH hematopoietic cell phosphatase

HCPOTP health care professionals other than physicians

HCPP health care prepayment plan

HCPS hantavirus cardiopulmonary syndrome

HCQ hydroxychloroquine

HCQI health care quality improvement

HCQIA Health Care Quality Improvement Act

HCR heme-controlled repressor; host cell reactivation; hysterical conversion reaction

HCRE Homeopathic Council for Research and Education

hCRH human corticotropin-releasing hormone

Hcrit hematocrit

H-CRT high-resolution cathode ray tube

HCS Hajdu-Cheney syndrome; Hazard Communication Standard; health care support; hemocystic spot; high confidence [information] system; hourglass contraction of the stomach; human chorionic somatotropin; human cord serum

17-HCS 17-hydroxycorticosteroid

hCS human chorionic somatomammotropin

HCSD Health Care Studies Division

hCSM human chorionic somatomammotropin

HCSS hypersensitive carotid sinus syndrome

HCSUS HIV Cost and Services Utilization Study

HCT health check test; helical computed tomography; hematocrit; hematopoietic cell transplantation; historic control trial; homocytotrophic; human calcitonin; hydrochlorothiazide; hydrophobic class torsion; hydroxycortisone

Hct hematocrit

hCT human calcitonin; human chorionic thyrotropin

HCTA health care technology assessment; helical compound tomographic angiography

HCTC Health Care Technology Center

HCTD hepatic computed tomography density

HCTS high cholesterol and tocopherol supplement

HCTU home cervical traction unit

HCTZ hydrochlorothiazide

HCU hand-carried ultrasound; health care unit; homocystinuria; hyperplasia cystica uteri

HCUP Healthcare Cost and Utilization Project

HCUPnet Healthcare Cost and Utilization Project Network

HCV hepatitis C virus; hog cholera virus

HCVD hemorrhagic cerebrovascular disease; hypertensive cardiovascular disease; hypoxic coronary vasodilatation

HCVE human cardiac valve endothelium

HCVS human coronavirus sensitivity

HCW health care worker

Hcy homocysteine

HD distilled mustard [gas]; Haab-Dimmer [syndrome]; Hajna-Damon [broth]; Hansen disease; hard disk; hearing distance; heart disease; helix destabilizing [protein]; hemidesmosome; hemidiaphragm; hemodialysis; hemolytic disease; hemolyzing dose; hemorrhagic dengue; herniated disk; high density; high dose; hip disarticulation; Hirschsprung disease; histopathologic damage; Hodgkin disease; homeodomain; hormone dependent; house dust; human defensin; human diploid

[cells]; Huntington disease; hydatid disease; hydrodensitometry; hydroxydopamine

H&D Hunter and Driffield [curve]

HD₅₀ 50% hemolyzing dose of complement

HDA heteroduplex analysis; high disease activity; Huntington's Disease Association; hydroxydopamine

HDAC histone deacetylase

HDACI histone deacetylase inhibitors

HDAd helper-dependent adenovirus

HD-AF hemidesmosome-anchoring filament

HDAg hepatitis delta antigen

HDARAC high-dose cytarabine

HDBH hydroxybutyric dehydrogenase

HDC hand drive control; Health Care Financing Administration Data Center; high-dose chemotherapy; histidine decarboxylase; hospital dialysis center; human diploid cell; hypodermoclysis

HDCS human diploid cell strain

HDCT high-dose chemotherapy

HDCV human diploid cell rabies vaccine

HDD hard disk device; high-dosage depth; Higher Dental Diploma

HDDRISC Heart Disease and Diabetes Risk Indicators in a Screened Cohort [study]

HDE high-dose epinephrine; humanitarian device exemption

HDES Heidelberg Diet and Exercise Study

HDF hemodiafiltration; host defense factor; human diploid fibroblast

HDFP Hypertension Detection and Follow-up Program

3H-DFP tritiated diisopropyl-fluorophosphonate

HDG high-dose group

HDH heart disease history

Hdh huntingtin; Huntington disease homolog

3H-DHE tritiated dihydroergocryptine

HDI Hamilton depression inventory; hemorrhagic disease of infants; hexamethylene diisocyanate; high-definition imaging; hospital discharge index

HDIC hepatodiaphragmatic interposition of colon

HDIR high-dose ionizing radiation; high isodose range

HDIVIG high-dose intravenous immunoglobulin

HDL hardware description language; high-density lipoprotein

HDLBP high-density lipoprotein binding protein

HDL-C high-density lipoprotein−cholesterol complex

HDL-c high-density lipoprotein cell surface

HDLP high-density lipoprotein

HDLS hereditary diffuse leukoencephalopathy with spheroids

HDLW distance from which a watch ticking is heard by the left ear

HDM house dust mite

HDMA Healthcare Distribution Management Association

HDMP high-dose methylprednisolone

HDMTX high-dose methotrexate

HDMTX-CF high-dose methotrexate citrovorum factor

HDMTX-LV high-dose methotrexate leucovorin

HDN health data network; hemolytic disease of the newborn

hDNA heteroduplex deoxyribonucleic acid; hybrid deoxyribonucleic acid

HDP heart disease program; hexose diphosphate; high-density polyethylene; hydrogen diphosphonate; hydroxydimethylpyrimidine

HDPAA heparin-dependent platelet-associated antibody

HDPE high-density polyethylene

HDPs homeopathic drug provings

HDR high-dose radiation; high dose rate

HDRA histoculture drug response assay

HDRBC head-damaged red blood cells

HDRF Heart Disease Research Foundation

HDRS Hamilton Depression Rating Scale

HDRV human diploid rabies vaccine

HDRW distance from which a watch ticking is heard by the right ear

HDS Hamilton Depression Scale; Health Data Services; health delivery system; Healthcare Data Systems; herbal and dietary supplement; herniated disk syndrome; Hospital Discharge Survey; Hypertension in Diabetes Study

HDSA Huntington's Disease Society of America

HDSCR health deviation self-care requisites

HDT high-dose treatment

HDU hemodialysis unit; high-dependency unit

HDV hemorrhagic disease virus; hepatitis D virus, hepatitis delta virus

HDZ hydralazine

HE half-scan with extrapolation; hard exudate; hektoen enteric [agar]; hemagglutinating encephalomyelitis; hematoxylin-eosin [stain]; hemoglobin electrophoresis; hepatic encephalopathy; hereditary elliptocytosis; high exposure; hollow enzyme; human enteric; hydroxyethyl; hyperextension; hypertensive encephalopathy; hypogonadotropic eunuchoidism

H&E hematoxylin and eosin; hemorrhage and exudate; heredity and environment

H/E hematoxylin/eosin

He heart

HEA hexone-extracted acetone; human erythrocyte antigen

HEADDFIRST Hemicraniectomy and Durotomy from Massive Hemispheric Infarctions: A Proposed Multicenter, Prospective Randomized Study

HEADLAMP Health and Environment Analysis for Decision Making: Linkage and Monitoring Project

HEAL health education assistance loan; Hospital and Emergency Ambulance Link

HealSB Health Standards Board

HEALTH ABC Dynamics of Health, Aging and Body Composition [study]

HealthSTAR Health Services, Technology, Administration, and Research

HEAP heparin and early patency

HEART Healing and Early Afterload Reducing Therapy [study]; Health Education and Research Trial; Hyperlipidemia, Epidemiology, Atherosclerosis Risk-Factor Trial; Hypertension and Ambulatory Recording Venetia Study

HEAT human erythrocyte agglutination test

HEB hematoencephalic barrier

HEBSWEB Health Education Board for Scotland's Website

HEC hamster embryo cell; Health Education Council; human endothelial cell; hydroxyergocalciferol; hydroxyethyl cellulose

HECC high-end computing and computation

HECCWG High End Computing and Computation Working Group

HED hereditary ectodermal dysplasia; hydrotropic electron donor; hydroxyephedrine; hypohidrotic ectodermal dysplasia; unit skin dose [radiation; Ger. *Haut-Einheits-Dosis*]

HEDH hypohidrotic ectodermal dysplasia—hypothyroidism [syndrome]

HEDIS Health Employer Data and Information Set

HEENT head, ears, eyes, nose, and throat

HEEP health effects of environmental pollutants

HEF hamster embryo fibroblast; human embryo fibroblast

HeFT heart failure trial

HEG hemorrhagic erosive gastritis; hexaethylene glycol

HEHR highest equivalent heart rate

HEI Health Effects Institute; high-energy intermediate; highly exposed individual; homogeneous enzyme immunoassay; human embryonic intestine [cells]

HEI-AR Health Effects Institute-Asbestos Research

HEIR health effects of ionizing radiation; high-energy ionizing radiation

HEIS high-energy ion scattering

HEK human embryo kinase; human embryonic kidney

HEL hen egg white lysozyme; human embryonic lung; human erythroleukemia

HeLa Henrietta Lacks [cells]

Heliox helium and oxygen

HELF human embryo lung fibroblast

HELLIS Health, Literature, Library, and Information Services

HELLP hemolysis, elevated liver enzymes, and low platelet count [syndrome]

HELP Hawaii early learning profile; Health Education Library Program; Health Emergency Loan Program; Health Evaluation and Learning Program; Health Evaluation Through Logical Processing; Heart European Leaders Panel [study]; heat escape lessening posture; heparin-induced extracorporeal low-density lipoprotein precipitation; Heroin Emergency Life Project; Hospital Equipment Loan Project; Hospitalized Elderly Longitudinal Project

HELP NSAID *Helicobacter* Eradication for Lesion Prevention with Nonsteroidal Anti-inflammatory Drugs [study]

HELPS Hypertension, Exercise, and Lifestyle Programs for Seniors [study]

HELVETICA Hirudin in European Restenosis Prevention Trial vs. Heparin Treatment in Percutaneous Transluminal Coronary Angioplasty

HEM hematologist, hematology; hematuric; hemophilia; hemorrhage; hemorrhoids; high-electrolyte meal

HEMA health data manager application; Health Education Media Association 2-hydroxyethyl methacrylate

hemat hematologist, hematology

HEMB hemophilia B

hemi hemiparalysis, hemiparesis; hemiplegia

HEMO, hemo hemodialysis

HEMOA Hemophilia A Mutation Database

HEMOSTAT Hemostasis with ProstarXL vs. Angioseal After Coronary Intervention Trial

HEMPAS hereditary erythrocytic multi-nuclearity with positive acidified serum

HEMRI hereditary multifocal relapsing inflammation

HEMS Helicopter Emergency Medical Service [UK]; hospital engineering management system

HEN home enteral nutrition

hENaC human epithelial sodium channel

HeNe helium neon

HEP hemolysis end point; hepatic; hepatoerythropoietic porphyria; high egg passage [virus]; high-energy phosphate; home exercise program; human epithelial cell; Hypertension in Elderly Persons [trial]

HEp-1 human cervical carcinoma cells

HEp-2 human laryngeal tumor cells

Hep hepatic; hepatitis

hEP human endorphin

HEPA high-efficiency particulate air [filter respirator]

HEP A, HepA hepatitis A

HEP B, HepB hepatitis B

HepBsAg hepatitis B surface antigen

HEP C hepatitis C

HEP D hepatitis D

HEPES N-2-hydroxyethylpiperazine-N-2-ethanesulfonic [acid]

HEPM human embryonic palatal mesenchymal [cell]

HEPOD hereditary expansile polyostotic dysplasia

HEPT 1-[(2-hydroxyethoxy)methyl]-6-(phenylthio)thymine

HER hemorrhagic encephalopathy of rats; hernia; human epidermal growth factor receptor

HER2, Her-2 human epidermal growth factor receptor 2

hered hereditary, heredity

HERN Human T-cell Leukemia Virus European Research Network

hern hernia, herniated

HERO Hirulog Early Reperfusion/Occlusion [study]

HEROICS How Effective Are Revascularization Options in Cardiogenic Shock? [trial]

HERS Health Evaluation and Referral Service; Heart and Estrogen-Progestin Re-placement Study; hemorrhagic fever with renal syndrome; HIV Research Study; Hysterectomy Educational Resources and Services

HERT hospital emergency response team

HES health examination survey; hematoxylin-eosin stain; human embryonic skin; human embryonic spleen; hydroxyethyl starch; hypereosinophilic syndrome; hyperprostaglandin E syndrome

HeSCA Health Sciences Communications Association

HESI Health and Environmental Sciences Institute
HET Health Education Telecommunications; helium equilibration time
Het heterophil
het heterozygous
HETA health evaluation and technical assistance
HETE hydroxyeicosatetraenoic [acid]
HETP height equivalent to a theoretic plate; hexaethyltetraphosphate
HEV health and environment; hemagglutinating encephalomyelitis virus; hemorrhagic enteritis virus; hepatitis E virus; hepato-encephalomyelitis virus; high endothelial venule; high endothelial vessel; human enterovirus
HeV hepatitis viruses
HEV-A, B, C, D human enteroviruses A, B, C, and D
HEW [Department of] Health, Education, and Welfare
HEX hexaminidase; hexosaminidase
Hex hexamethylmelamine
HEXA Hexosaminidase A Locus Database
HEX A, hex A hexosaminidase A
HEX B, hex B hexosaminidase B
HEX C, hex C hexosaminidase C
HF Hageman factor; half-Fourier; haplotype frequency; hard filled; hay fever; head forward; head of fetus; heart failure; helper factor; hemofiltration; hemorrhagic factor; hemorrhagic fever; Hertz frequency; high fat; high flow; high frequency; hippocampal formation; human factor; human fibroblast; humidifier fever; hydrogen fluoride; hyper-flexion
Hf hafnium; hippocampal formation
hF half-Fourier
hf half; high frequency
HFA Health for All; height for age; high-functioning autism
HFAK hollow-fiber artificial kidney
HFB human fetal brain
HFBA heptafluorobutyric acid
HFC hard filled capsule; high-frequency component; high-frequency current; histamine-forming capacity; hydrofluorocarbon
HFD hemorrhagic fever of deer; high-fiber diet; high-flux dialysis; high forceps delivery; high-frequency Doppler; hospital field director; human factors design
HFDA high film density area
HFDK human fetal diploid kidney
HFDL human fetal diploid lung
HFE, HFe hemochromatosis
HFEC human foreskin epithelial cell
HFECG high-frequency electrocardiography
HFF human foreskin fibroblast

HFG hand-foot-genital [syndrome]
HFGC human fetal glial cell
HFH hemifacial hyperplasia
HFHV high frequency, high volume
HFI hereditary fructose intolerance; high-Fourier imaging; high-frequency information; human fibroblast interferon
HFIF human fibroblast interferon
HFIFPPV high-frequency interrupted flow positive pressure ventilation
HFIS high-frequency insertion system
HFJV high-frequency jet ventilation
HFK human foreskin keratinocyte
HFL human fetal lung
HFM hand, foot, and mouth [disease]; hemifacial microsomia
HFMA Healthcare Financial Management Association
HFO high field open; high-frequency oscillation/oscillator
HFO-A high-frequency oscillatory [ventilation] action
HFOV high-frequency oscillatory ventilation
HFP hexafluoropropylene; high-frequency pulsation; hypofibrinogenic plasma
HFPEF heart failure with preserved ejection fraction
HFPPV high-frequency positive pressure ventilation
HFPV high-frequency percussive ventilation
HFR high-frequency recombination
Hfr heart frequency; high frequency
HFREF heart failure with reduced ejection fraction
HFRND high frequency and responsibility nursing diagnosis
HFRS hemorrhagic fever with renal syndrome
HFS hemifacial spasm; Hospital Financial Support
hfs hyperfine structure
hFSH, HFSH human follicle-stimulating hormone
HFSP Hanukah factor serine protease
HFST hearing for speech test
HFT high-frequency transduction; high-frequency transfer
Hft high-frequency transfer
HFTT high-frequency induced thermotherapy
HFU hand-foot-uterus [syndrome]
HFV high-frequency ventilation; human foamy virus
HG hand grip; herpes gestationis; Heschl's gyrus; high glucose; human gonadotropin; human growth; hypoglycemia
hg hectogram; hemoglobin
HGA homogentisic acid; human granulocytic anaplasmosis

HGAC high gain adaptive control
hGalR human galanin receptor
Hgb hemoglobin
HGD high-grade dysplasia
HGDB Human Genome Database
Hge hemorrhage
HGF hematopoietic growth factor; hepatocyte growth factor; human gingival fibroblast; hyperglycemic-glucogenolytic factor
Hg-F fetal hemoglobin
HGFL hepatocyte growth factor−like [protein]
HGF-R hepatocyte growth factor receptor
HGF/SF hepatocyte growth factor/scatter factor
HGG herpetic geniculate ganglionitis; human gammaglobulin; hypogammaglobulinemia
HGH, HgH, hGH human growth hormone
HGHRF human growth hormone−releasing factor
HGI Human Gene Index
HGIN high-grade intraepithelial neoplasia
HGL heregulin
HGM heterotropic gastric mucosa; hog gastric mucosa; human gene mapping; human glucose monitoring
HGMCR human genetic mutant cell repository
HGMD, HGMDB Human Gene Mutation Database
HGMP Human Genome Mapping Project
HGMP RC Human Genome Mapping Project Resource Centre
HGO hepatic glucose output; human glucose output
HGP hepatic glucose production; Human Genome Project; hyperglobulinemic purpura
HGPRT hypoxanthine guanine phosphoribosyl transferase
HGPS hereditary giant platelet syndrome; Hutchinson-Gilford progeria syndrome
HGPT hypoxanthine-guanosine phosphoribosyl transferase
hGR human glucocorticoid receptor
hGRH human growth hormone−releasing hormone
HGS hand grip strength
HGTS Human Gene Therapy Subcommittee
HGV hepatitis G virus
HH halothane hepatitis; handheld; hard of hearing; healthy hemophiliac; healthy human; Henderson-Hasselbalch equation; hiatal hernia; Hodgkin-Huxley [model]; holistic health; home help; hydralazine acid hydrazone; hydroxyhexamide; hypergastrinemic hyperchlorhydria; hyperhidrosis; hypogonadotropic hypogonadism; hyporeninemic hypoaldosteronism

H&H hematocrit and hemoglobin
Hh hedgehog
HHA health hazard appraisal; hereditary hemolytic anemia; home health agency; home health aid; hypothalamo-hypophyseoadrenal [system]
HH handheld assist
HHANES Hispanic Health and Nutrition Examination Survey
HHAV human hepatitis A virus
HHb hypohemoglobinemia; un-ionized hemoglobin
HHC heart healthy controls; home health care; household contact; hypocalciuric hypercalcemia
HHCC home health care classification
HHCS high-altitude hypertrophic cardiomyopathy syndrome
HHD high heparin dose; home hemodialysis; hypertensive heart disease
HHE health hazard evaluation; hemiconvulsion, hemiplegia, epilepsy [syndrome]; hypotonic hyporesponsive episode
HHEs hypotonic-hyporesponsive episodes
HHFAST handheld focused assessment with sonography for trauma
HHG hypertrophic hypersecretory gastropathy; hypogonadotropic hypogonadism
HHH hyperornithinemia, hyperammonemia, homocitrillinuria [syndrome]
HHHH hereditary hemihypotrophy, hemiparesis, hemiathetosis [syndrome]
HHHO hypotonia, hypomentia, hypogonadism, obesity [syndrome]
HHI hereditary hearing impairment
HHIE Hearing Handicap Inventory for the Elderly
HHIE-S Hearing Handicap Inventory for the Elderly-Screening Version
HHIS hospital in home information system
HHM high humidity mask; Hodgkin-Huxley equation for muscles; humoral hypercalcemia of malignancy
H + Hm compound hypermetropic astigmatism
HHMI Howard Hughes Medical Institutes
HHMMTV human homologue of mouse mammary tumor virus
HHN handheld nebulizer
HHNA Home Healthcare Nurses Association
HHNC hyperosmolar nonketotic diabetic coma
HHNK hyperglycemic hyperosmolar nonketotic [coma]
HHNS hyperosmolar hyperglycemic nonketotic syndrome
HHP Honolulu Heart Program
HHPA hexahydrophthalic anhydride

HHR hydralazine, hydrochlorothiazide, and reserpine

HHRG home health resource group

HHRH hereditary hypophosphatemic rickets with hypercalciuria; hypothalamic hypophysiotropic releasing hormone

HHS [Department of] Health and Human Services; Hearing Handicap Scale; Helsinki Heart Study; hereditary hemolytic syndrome; Honolulu Heart Study; human hypopituitary serum; hyperglycemic hyperosmolar syndrome; hyperkinetic heart syndrome

HHSSA Home Health Services and Staffing Association

HHT head halter traction; hereditary hemorrhagic telangiectasia; heterotopic heart transplantation; homoharringtonine; hydroxyheptadecatrienoic acid

HHV human herpesvirus

HHV 1 to 8 human herpesviruses 1 to 8

HI half-scan with interpolation; hazard index; head injury; health informatics; health insurance; hearing impaired; heart infusion; hemagglutination inhibition; hepatobiliary imaging; high impulsiveness; histidine; hormone independent; hormone insensitivity; hospital insurance; humoral immunity; hydroxyindole; hyperglycemic index; hypomelanosis of Ito; hypothermic ischemia

H-I hemagglutination-inhibition

Hi histamine; histidine

HIA Hearing Industries Association; heat infusion agar; hemagglutination inhibition antibody or assay

HIAA Health Insurance Association of America

5-HIAA 5-hydroxyindoleacetic acid

HIB heart infusion broth; hemolytic immune body; *Haemophilus influenzae* type B [vaccine]

Hib *Haemophilus influenzae* type B [vaccine]

HIBAC Health Insurance Benefits Advisory Council

HIBC health industry bar code

HIBCC Health Industry Business Communications Council

HIC handling-induced convulsions; health insurance claim; Heart Information Center; hydrophobic-interaction chromatography

HICA hydroxyisocaproic acid

HIC-CPR high-impulse compression cardiopulmonary resuscitation

HICH hypertensive intracranial hemorrhage

HiCn cyanmethemoglobin

HICPAC Healthcare Infection Control Practices Advisory Committee

HI-CPR high-impulse cardiopulmonary resuscitation

HID headache, insomnia, depression [syndrome]; herniated intervertebral disk; human infectious dose; hyperkinetic impulse disorder; hypertension in diabetes

HIDA Health Industry Distributors Association; hepato-iminodiacetic acid

HIDAC high-density avalanche chamber

HIDDEL health information disclosure, description, and evaluation language

HIE human intestinal epithelium; hyperimmunoglobulin E; hypoxic-ischemic encephalopathy

HIES hyper-immunoglobulin E syndrome

HIF higher integrative functions; hypoxia-inducible factor

HIFBS heat-inactivated fetal bovine serum

HIFC hog instrinsic factor concentrate

HIFCS heat-inactivated fetal calf serum

HiFOS High-Frequency Oscillation Study

HIFU high-intensity focused ultrasound

HIG, hIG human immunoglobulin

HIg hyperimmunoglobulin

HIGS Hemophilia Inhibitor Genetics Study

HIH hypertensive intracerebral hemorrhage

HIHA high impulsiveness, high anxiety

HiHb hemiglobin (methemoglobin)

HII Health Industries Institute; health information infrastructure; Health Insurance Institute; hemagglutination inhibitor immunoassay

HIL health information locator

HILA high impulsiveness, low anxiety

HILDA human interleukin in DA [cells]

HILI herbal and dietary supplement–induced liver injury

HIM health information management; hepatitis–infectious mononucleosis; hexosephosphate isomerase; hyperimmunoglobulin M

HIMA Health Industry Manufacturers Association

HIMAC heavy ion medical accelerator in Chiba

HIMC hepatic intramitochondrial crystalloid

HIMEC human intestinal microvascular endothelial cells

HIMO Healthcare Information Management Officer

HIMP high-dose intravenous methylprednisolone

HIMS health care information management system

HIMSS Healthcare Information Management and Support System; Healthcare Information and Management Systems Society

HIMT hemagglutination inhibition morphine test

HIN health information network; Hemophilia in the Netherlands [study]

HI:NC health information: nursing component
h-index Hirsch Index
HINF health information science
HINT health care information networks and technologies; hierarchical interpolation; Holland Interuniversity Nifedipine/Metoprolol Trial
Hint Hinton [test]
HIO health insuring organization; hypoiodism
HIOMT hydroxyindole-*O*-methyl transferase
HIOS high index of suspicion
HIP health illness profile; health insurance plan/program; help for incontinent people; heparan sulfate/heparin interacting protein; homograft incus prosthesis; hospital insurance program; hydrostatic indifference point
HIPA heparin-induced platelet activation
HIPAA Health Insurance Portability and Accountability Act
HIPC Health Information Policy Council; health insurance purchasing collective; health insurance purchasing cooperative
HIPDM *N*-trimethyl-*n*-(2-hydroxyl-3-methyl-5-iodobenzyl)-1,3-propendiamine
HIPE Hospital Inpatient Enquiry
HIPEC hyperthermic intraperitoneal chemotherapy
HiPIP high-potential iron protein
HIPO hemihypertrophy, intestinal web, preauricular skin tag, and congenital corneal opacity [syndrome]; Hospital Indicator for Physicians Orders
HIPOS Hypertension in Pregnancy: Offspring Study
HiPPI high-performance parallel interface
HiPRF high pulse-repetition frequency
HIPS health information processing system; Heparin Delivery with Infusasleeve Catheter Prior to Stent Implantation [study]; Heparin Infusion Prior to Stenting [study]
HIR head injury routine; health care information repository; homogeneity isodose range
HIRL₁ homogeneity isodose range limited to the inferior
HIRMIT High-Risk Myocardial Ischemia Trial
HIRS health care-specific incident reporting scheme
HIS health information system; Health Interview Survey; Hemodilution in Stroke [study]; histatin; histidine; Hormones in Stroke [study]; hospital information system; Hungarian Isradipine Study; hyperimmune serum
His, his histidine
HISA health care information system architecture

HISAAP Hunter Illawarra Study of Airways and Air Pollution
HISB Health Insurance Standards Board
HISCC Healthcare Information Standards Coordinating Committee
HISKEW Health Information Skeletonized Eligibility Write-off
HISP Health Information System Programme
HIS-PACS hospital information system picture archiving and communication system
HISPP Healthcare Informatics Standards Planning Panel
HISSG Healthcare Information System Sharing Group; Hospital Information Systems Sharing Group
HIST hospital in-service training
hist histamine; history
HISTLINE History of Medicine Online
Histo histoplasmin skin test
histol histologic, histologist, histology
HIT health information technology; health integration team; hemagglutination inhibition test; heparin-induced thrombocytopenia; High-Density Lipoprotein Cholesterol Intervention Trial; Hirudin for the Improvement of Thrombolysis [study]; histamine inhalation test; hypertrophic infiltrative tendinitis
HITB, HiTB *Haemophilus influenzae* type B
HITF Health Insurance Trust Fund
HITS high-intensity transient signal; HIV Testing Survey; hurt, insult, threaten, scream
HIT-SK Hirudin for the Improvement of Thrombolysis with Streptokinase
HITT heparin-induced thrombocytopenia and thrombosis
HITTS heparin-induced thrombosis-thrombocytopenia syndrome
HIU hyperplasia interstitialis uteri
HIV human immunodeficiency virus
HIV Ag human immunodeficiency virus antigen
HIV/AIDS human immunodeficiency virus/acquired immunodeficiency syndrome
HIVAN human immunodeficiency virus–associated nephropathy
HIV-D human immunodeficiency virus dementia
HIV-G human immunodeficiency virus–associated gingivitis
HIVRAD HIV Vaccine Research and Design
HIVRT human immunodeficiency virus reverse transcriptase
HIZ high-intensity zone
HJ Henderson-Jones [disease]; Highlands J [virus]; Howell-Jolly [bodies]
HJB high jugular bulb
HJR hepatojugular reflex

HJV Highlands J virus
HK hand to knee; heat killed; heel to knee; hexokinase; human kidney
H-K hand to knee
hK2 human glandular kallikrein 2
HKA hip-knee-ankle
HKAFO hip-knee-ankle-foot orthosis
HKAO hip-knee-ankle orthosis
HKB hybrid knowledge base
HKC human kidney cell
HKLM heat-killed *Listeria monocytogenes*
HKS hyperkinesis syndrome
HL hairline; hairpin loop; hairy leukoplakia; half-life; hallux limitus; health level; hearing level; hearing loss; heparin lock; hepatic lipase; histiocytic lymphoma; histocompatibility locus; Hodgkin lymphoma; human leukocyte; hydrolethalus [syndrome]; hyperlipidemia; hypermetropia, latent; hypertrichosis lanuginosa
H&L heart and lung
H/L hydrophil/lipophil ratio
Hl hypermetropia, latent
hl, hL hectoliter
HL7 health level 7
HLA histocompatibility leukocyte antigen; histocompatibility locus antigen; homologous leukocyte antibody; horizontal long axis; human leukocyte antigen; human lymphocyte antigen
HL-A human leukocyte antigen
HLAA Hearing Loss Association of America; human leukocyte antigen A
HLAB human leukocyte antigen B
HLAC human leukocyte antigen C
HLAD human leukocyte antigen D
HLA-DP human leukocyte antigen, DP subregion
HLA-DQ human leukocyte antigen, DQ subregion
HLA-DR human leukocyte antigen, DR subregion
HLA-LD human lymphocyte antigen–lymphocyte defined
HLA-SD human lymphocyte antigen–serologically defined
HLB hydrophilic-lipophilic balance; hypotonic lysis buffer
HLBI human lymphoblastoid interferon
HLC heat loss center
HLCL human lymphoblastoid cell line
HLD hepatolenticular degeneration; herniated lumbar disk; [von] Hippel–Lindau disease; hypersensitivity lung disease
HLDH heat-stable lactic dehydrogenase
HLDM high-level data model

HLEG hydrolysate lactalbumin Earle glucose
HLF heat-labile factor; hepatic leukemia factor; high-level fluoroscopy
HLGT high-level group term
HLH helix-loop-helix; hemophagocytic lymphohistiocytosis
hLH human luteinizing hormone
HLHS hypoplastic left heart syndrome
HLI human leukocyte interferon
H-L-K heart, liver, and kidneys
HLL hypoplastic left lung
HLLAPI high-level language application programming interface
HLM heart-lung machine; hypermobile lateral meniscus
HLN hilar lymph node; hyperplastic liver nodules
HLP hepatic lipoperoxidation; hind leg paralysis; holoprosencephaly; hyperkeratosis lenticularis perstans; hyperlipoproteinemia
HLQ high-level question
HLR heart-lung resuscitation; heart/lung ratio; high-level resistance
HLS Health Learning System; high-level segmentation; [von] Hippel–Lindau syndrome
HLT heart-lung transplantation; high l-leucine transport; high-level term; human lipotropin; human lymphocyte transformation
HLTx heart-lung transplant
HLV hamster leukemia virus; herpeslike virus; hypoplastic left ventricle
HLVS hypoplastic left ventricle syndrome
HM hand movements; health maintenance; heart murmur; Heller myotomy; hemifacial microsomia; hemodynamic monitoring; hemosiderin-laden macrophages; Holter monitoring; home management; homosexual male; hospital management; human milk; hydatidiform mole; hyperbaric medicine; hyperimmune mouse
Hm manifest hypermetropia
hm hectometer
HMA health care management alternatives; heteroduplex mobility assay; human monocyte antigen; hydroxymethionine analogue
HMAB human monocyte antigen B
HMAC Health Manpower Advisory Council
HMAS hyperimmune mouse ascites
HMB homatropine methobromide; human milk bank; hydroxymethylbilane
HMBA hexamethylene bisacetamide
7-HMBA 7-hydroxymethyl-7-methyl-benz-[α] anthracene
HMBANA Human Milk Banking Association of North America
HMBS hydroxymethylbilane synthetase

HMC hand-mirror cell; health maintenance cooperative; heroin, morphine, and cocaine; hospital management committee; human mesothelial cell; hypertelorism, microtia, clefting [syndrome]

HMCA hydroxymethyl-cyclophenyl adenine

HMCCMP human mammary carcinoma cell membrane proteinase

HMD head-mounted display [computer graphics]; hyaline membrane disease

HMDC health maintenance and diagnostic center

HMDP hydroxymethylenediphosphonate

HME Health Media Education; heat and moisture exchanger; heat, massage, and exercise; hemimegalencephaly

HMEC human mammary epithelial cell

HMEF heat and moisture exchanger filter

HMF hydroxymethylfurfural

HMFG human milk fat globulin

HMG high-mobility group; human menopausal gonadotropin; 3-hydroxy-3-methyl-glutaryl

hMG human menopausal gonadotropin

HMG CoA 3-hydroxy-3-methylglutaryl coenzyme A

HMH health level message handling

HMI healed myocardial infarct; health and medical informatics; human-machine interface; hypomelanosis of Ito

HMIC Health Management Information Consortium

HMIG hazardous materials identification guide

HMIS hazardous materials identification system; hazardous materials information system; hospital management information system

HMK high-molecular-weight kininogen

HML human milk lysosome

HMM heavy meromyosin; hexamethyl-melamine; hidden Markov model

HMMA 4-hydroxy-3-methoxymandelic acid

HMMER hidden Markov marker and profiles

HMMF human monocyte-derived macrophage

HMN hereditary motor neuropathy

H-MNPM [Department of] Health Education and Welfare Medicus Nursing Process Methodology

HMO health maintenance organization; heart minute output

HMOX heme oxygenase

HMP hexose monophosphate pathway; hot moist packs

HMPA hexamethylphosphoramide

HMPAO, HM-PAO hexamethyl-propyleneamine oxime

HMPG hydroxymethoxyphenylglycol

HMPS hexose monophosphate shunt

HMPT hexamethylphosphorotriamide

HMPV human metapneumovirus

HMQC heteronuclear multiple-quantum correlation

HMR health maintenance recommendations; health maintenance record; health management resources; histiocytic medullary reticulosis

HMRI Hospital Medical Records Institute

H-mRNA H-chain messenger ribonucleic acid

HMRT hazardous materials response team

HMRTE human milk reverse transcriptase enzyme

HMRU hazardous materials response unit

HMS hexose monophosphate shunt; Household Multipurpose Survey; hypermobility syndrome

HMSA health manpower shortage area; hydroxymethane sulfonate

HMSAS hypertrophic muscular subaortic stenosis

hMSH human Mut S homologue

HMSN hereditary motor and sensory neuropathy

HMSS Hospital Management Systems Society

HMT hematocrit; histamine-*N*-methyltransferase; hospital management team

HMTA hexamethylenetetramine

HMU hydroxymethyl-uracil

5-HMU 5-hydroxymethyl uridine

HMVEC human microvascular endothelial cell

HMW high molecular weight

HMW-AGT high-molecular-weight AGT forms

HMW-BCGF high-molecular-weight B-cell growth factor

HMWC high-molecular-weight component

HMWGP high-molecular-weight glycoprotein

HMWK high-molecular-weight kininogen

HMX heat, massage, and exercise

HN head and neck; head nurse; hemagglutinin neuraminidase; hematemesis neonatorum; hemorrhage of newborn; hereditary nephritis; high necrosis; hilar node; histamine-containing neuron; home nursing; human nutrition; hypertrophic neuropathy

H&N head and neck

HNA health care network architecture; heparin neutralizing activity

HNAD hyperosmolar nonacidotic diabetes

HNB human neuroblastoma

HNBD has not been drinking
HNC Holistic Nurse, Certified; hypernephroma cell; hyperosmolar nonketotic coma; hypothalamoneurohypophyseal complex
HNF hepatocyte nuclear factor
HNF1A hepatocyte nuclear factor-1-alpha
HNKC hyperosmolar nonketotic coma
HNKDS hyperosmolar nonketotic diabetic state
HNL histiocytic necrotizing lymphadenitis
HNMT histamine *N*-methyltransferase
HNN hierarchical neural network
HNP hereditary nephritic protein; herniated nucleus pulposus; human neurophysin; human neutrophil protein
HNPCC hereditary nonpolyposis colorectal cancer; Hereditary Non-Polyposis Colorectal Cancer [Database]; human nonpolyposis colorectal cancer
HNPP hereditary neuropathy with liability to pressure palsies
HNR harmonic/noise ratio
hnRNA heterogeneous nuclear ribonucleic acid
hnRNP, HNRP heterogeneous nuclear ribonucleoprotein
HNRPG heterogeneous nuclear ribonucleoprotein peptide G
HNS head and neck surgery; home nursing supervisor
HNSCC head and neck squamous cell carcinoma
HNSHA hereditary nonspherocytic hemolytic anemia
HNTD highest nontoxic dose
HNV has not voided; health network venture
HO hand orthosis; heterotopic ossification; high oxygen; hip orthosis; history of; Holt-Oram [syndrome]; house officer; hyperbaric oxygen
H/O, h/o history of
Ho horse; [Cook-Medley] hostility scale
HOA hip osteoarthritis; hypertrophic osteoarthropathy
HoaRhLG horse anti-rhesus lymphocyte globulin
HoaTTG horse antitetanus toxoid globulin
HOB head of bed
HOC human ovarian cancer; hydroxycorticoid; hypertrophic obstructive cardiomyopathy
HOCA high-osmolar contrast agent
HOCAP Hypertrophic Obstructive Cardiomyopathy Ablation Pacing [study]
HOCM high-osmolar contrast medium; hypertrophic obstructive cardiomyopathy
HOD hyperbaric oxygen drenching

HOF hepatic outflow
HoFF height of fundus
HoFH homozygous familial hypercholesterolemia
HOGA hyperornithinemia with gyrate atrophy
HOH hard of hearing
HOI hospital onset of infection
HoIg horse immunoglobulin
HOKPP hypokalemic periodic paralysis
HoLAP holmium laser ablation of the prostate
HOLON health object library online
HOM high-osmolar medium
HOMA homeostasis model assessment
HOME Home Observations for Measurement of the Environment
Homeop homeopathy
HOMER-D home rehabilitation-dialysis
HOMO highest occupied molecular orbital
HOMSTRAD Homologous Structure Alignment Database
HON Health on the Net
HONC hyperosmolar nonketotic coma
HONK hyperosmolar nonketosis
HoNOS Health of the Nation Outcome Scale
HOOD hereditary onycho-osteodysplasia
HOODS hereditary onycho-osteodysplasia syndrome
HOOE heredopathia ophthalmo-otoencephalica
HOOP Health Online Outreach Project
HOP high oxygen pressure; holoprosencephaly-polydactyly [syndrome]
HOPE Health Outcomes Prevention Evaluation; Healthcare Options Plan Entitlement; health-oriented physical education; holistic orthogonal parameter estimation; Hospital Outcomes Project for the Elderly; Hypertensive Old People in Edinburgh [study]
HOPG highly oriented pyrolytic graphite
HOPI history of present illness
HOPP hepatic occluded portal pressure
HOPWA housing opportunities for people with AIDS
hor horizontal
HORG health care organization
HOS health opinion survey; high-order spectrum; Holt-Oram syndrome; human osteosarcoma; hypo-osmotic swelling
HoS horse serum
HOSA Health Occupations Students of America
HOSE Hierarchically Ordered Spherical Description of Environment
Hosp, hosp hospital

HOST health care open systems and trials; hybrid open-system technology; hypo-osmotic shock treatment

HOT health-oriented telecommunication; Hormones Opposed by Tamoxifen [trial]; human old tuberculin; hyperbaric oxygen therapy; Hypertension Optimal Treatment [study]

HOT MI Hyperbaric Oxygen and Thrombolysis in Myocardial Infarction [study]

HOTS hypercalcemia, osteolysis, T-cell syndrome

HOVERGEN Homologous Vertebrate Genes [database]

HOX, Hox homeobox [protein]

HOWARD Hand-Wrist Assisting Robotic Device

Ho:YAG holmium:yttrium-aluminum-garnet [laser]

HP halogen phosphorus; handicapped person; haptoglobin; hard palate; Harvard pump; health profession(al); health profile; health promotion; heater probe; heat production; heel to patella; *Helicobacter pylori*; hemiparkinsonism; hemipelvectomy; hemiplegia; hemoperfusion; *Haemophilus pleuropneumoniae*; heparin; hepatic porphyria; high permeability; high potency; high power; high pressure; high protein; highly purified; horizontal plane; horsepower; hospital participation; hot pack; house physician; human pituitary; hydrophilic petrolatum; hydrostatic pressure; hydroxypyruvate; hyperparathyroidism; hypersensitivity pneumonitis; hypophoria

H&P history and physical examination

Hp haptoglobin; hematoporphyrin; hemiplegia

HPA Health Care Practice Act; Health Policy Agenda for the American People; health promotion advocates; *Helix pomatia* agglutinin; hemagglutinating penicillin antibody; *Histoplasma capsulatum* polysaccharide antigen; human platelet alloantigen; human platelet antigen; humeroscapular periarthritis; hybridization protection assay; hypertrophic pulmonary arthropathy; hypophyseal-adrenal axis; hypothalamic-pituitary-adrenal [axis]; hypothalamo-pituitary-adrenocortical [system]; hypothalamopituitary axis

HPAA hydroperoxyarachidonic acid; hydroxyphenylacetic acid; hypothalamo-pituitary-adrenal axis

HPAC high-performance affinity chromatography; hypothalamo-pituitary-adrenocortical

HPAE, HPAEC high-performance anion exchange

HPAEC-PAD high-performance anion exchange chromatography with pulsed amperometric detection

HPAFT hereditary persistence of alfa-fetoprotein

H-PAGE horizontal polyacrylamide gel

HPAH hydralazine pyruvic acid hydrazone

HPAI highly pathogenic avian influenza

HPASE high-performance application for science and engineering

HPB hepatobiliary

HPBC hyperpolarizing bipolar cell

HPBF hepatotrophic portal blood factor

HPBL human peripheral blood leukocyte

HPC health professional card; hemangiopericytoma; high-performance computing; hippocampal pyramidal cell; history of present complaint; holoprosencephaly; hydroxypropylcellulose

HPCA human progenitor cell antigen

HPCC high-performance computing and communications

HPCE high-performance capillary electrophoresis

HPCHA high−red cell phosphatidylcholine hemolytic anemia

HPD hearing protective device; hereditary progressive dystonia; high-protein diet; home peritoneal dialysis

HPDR hypophosphatemic D-resistant rickets

HPE hepatic portoenterostomy; high-permeability edema; history and physical examination; holoprosencephaly; hydrostatic permeability edema

HPETE hydroxyperoxy-eicosatetranoic [acid]

HPeV human parechovirus

HPF heparin-precipitable fraction; hepatic plasma flow; high-pass filter; high-power field; hypocaloric protein feeding

hpf high-power field; hours postfertilization

HPFH hereditary persistence of fetal hemoglobin

hPFSH, HPFSH human pituitary follicle-stimulating hormone

HPG high-purity germanium; hypothalamic-pituitary-gonadal [axis]

hPG, HPG human pituitary gonadotropin

HpGe hyperpure germanium

HPGL Hewlett Packard graphic language

HPH *Helix pomatia* hemocyanin; hygromycin B phosphotransferase

Hp-HB haptoglobulin-hemoglobin complex

HPI hepatic perfusion index; high pathogenicity island; history of present illness

HPIEC high-performance ion-exchange chromatography

HPIV 1 to 4 human parainfluenza viruses 1 to 4

HPL human parotid lysozyme; human peripheral lymphocyte; human placental lactogen

hPL human placental lactogen; human platelet lactogen

HPLA hydroxyphenyl lactic acid

HPLAC high-pressure liquid-affinity chromatography

HPLC high-performance liquid chromatography; high-power liquid chromatography; high-pressure liquid chromatography

HPLC-MS high-performance liquid chromatography mass spectrometry

HPLE hereditary polymorphic light eruption

HPLH hypoplastic left heart

HPM high-performance membrane

HPMC human peripheral mononuclear cell; hydroxypropylmethylcellulose

hPMS human postmeiotic segregation

HPN Health Provider Network; hepsin; home parenteral nutrition; hypertension

hpn hypertension

HPNA Hospice and Palliative Nurses Association

HPNAT high-performance networking application team

HPNS high-pressure neurologic syndrome

HPNSP high-performance network service provider

HPO high-pressure oxygen; hydroperoxide; hydrophilic ointment; hypertrophic pulmonary osteoarthropathy

HPOA hypertrophic pulmonary osteoarthropathy

HPP hereditary pyropoikilocytosis; history of presenting problems

HPP, hPP human pancreatic polypeptide; hydroxyphenylpyruvate; hydroxypyrozolopyrimidine

HPPA hydroxyphenylpyruvic acid

HPPC health plan purchasing cooperative

HPP-CFC high proliferative potential colony-forming cell

HPPD hours per patient day; hydroxyphenylpyruvate dioxygenase

hppd hours per patient-day

HPPH 5-(4-hydroxyphenyl)-5-phenyl-hydantoin

HPPK 6-hydroxymethyl-7,8-dihydropterin pyrophosphokinase

HPPO high partial pressure of oxygen; hydroxyphenyl pyruvate oxidase

HPQ Health Perceptions Questionnaire

HPR haptoglobin-related gene; health practices research

HPr human prolactin

hPRL human prolactin

HPRP human platelet-rich plasma

HPRT hypoxanthine phosphoribosyltransferase

HpRz hairpin ribozyme

HPS Hantavirus pulmonary syndrome; Health Protection Scotland; [Simvastatin] Heart Protection Study; Helsinki Policemen Study; hematoxylin, phloxin, and saffron; Hermansky-Pudlak syndrome; high pain sensitivity; high-protein supplement; His-Purkinje system; Hopkins Precursors Study; human platelet suspension; hypertrophic pyloric stenosis; hypothalamic pubertal syndrome

HPSA health professional shortage area

HPSL health professions student loan

HPSS high-performance storage system

HPT histamine provocation test; human placental thyrotropin; hyperparathyroidism; Hypertension Prevention Trial; hypothalamo-pituitary-thyroid [system]

1°HPT primary hyperparathyroidism

2°HPT secondary hyperparathyroidism

HPTH hyperparathyroid hormone

HPTIN human pancreatic trypsin inhibitor

HPTLC high-performance thin-layer chromatography

HPTN HIV Prevention Trials Network

HPU heater probe unit

HPV *Hemophilus pertussis* vaccine; hepatic portal vein; human papillomavirus; human parvovirus; hypoxic pulmonary vasoconstriction

HPVD hypertensive pulmonary vascular disease

HPV-DE high-passage virus-duck embryo

HPV-DK high-passage virus-dog kidney

HPVG hepatic portal venous gas

HPVM high-performance virtual machine

HPW hypergammaglobulinemic purpura of Waldenström

HP/W health promotion/wellness

HPX high peroxidase; hypophysectomized

Hpx hemopexin

HPZ high pressure zone

[3H] QNB (−)-[3H] quinuclidinyl benzilate

HQSAR hologram quantitative structure-activity relationship

HR hairpin ribozyme; hallux rigidus; handwriting recognition; hazard ratio; heart rate; hematopoietic reconstitution; hematopoietic resistance; hemorrhagic retinopathy; hepatorenal; higher rate; high resolution; high risk; histamine receptor; histamine release; hormonal response; hormone receptor; hospital record; hospital report; hospitalization rate; human resources; hydroxyethylrutoside; hyperimmune reaction; hypersensitive response; hypertensive rat; hypophosphatemic rickets; hypoxic reaction

H&R hysterectomy and radiation

hr hairless [mouse]; homologous repeat; host-range [mutant]; hour

HRA health record analyst; health risk appraisal; heart rate audiometry; heart-reactive antibody; hereditary renal adysplasia; high right atrium; histamine release activity; Human Resources Administration

H2RA histamine₂-receptor antagonist; H₂-receptor antagonist

HRAE high right atrium electrogram

HRBC horse red blood cell

HRC health reference center; hereditary renal cancer; high-resolution chromatography; horse red cell; human rights committee

h/rCRF human recombinant corticotropin-releasing factor

HRCT, HR-CT high-resolution computed tomography

HRE hepatic reticuloendothelial [cell]; high-resolution electrocardiography; hormone receptor enzyme; hormone response element

HR-EEG high-resolution electroencephalography

HREH high-renin essential hypertension

HREM high-resolution electron microscopy

HRF health-related facility; heart rate fluctuations; histamine-releasing factor; homologous restriction factor; human readable format

HRG, HRGP histidine-rich glycoprotein

HRH2 histamine receptor H2

HR-HPV high-risk human papillomavirus

HrHRF human recombinant histamine-releasing factor

HRI high-resolution imaging

HRIG, HRIg human rabies immunoglobulin

HRL head rotation to the left

HRLA human reovirus−like agent

HRM health risk management; Heidelberg Retracing Model

HRmax maximal heart rate

HRMS health records management system; high-resolution multisweep [imaging]

hRNA heterogeneous ribonucleic acid

HRNB Halstead-Reitan Neuropsychological Battery

hROAT human renal organic anion transporter

HRP harm-reduction program; high-risk patient; high-risk pregnancy; histidine-rich protein; horseradish peroxidase

HRPC hormone-refractory prostate cancer; hormone-resistant prostatic cancer

HRPD Hamburg Rating Scale for Psychiatric Disorders

hr-PET high-resolution positron emission tomography

HRPT hyperparathyroidism

HRQL, HRQOL health-related quality of life

HRR Hardy-Rand-Rittler [color vision test]; head rotation to the right; heart rate range

HRRI heart rate retardation index

HRS Hamilton Rating Scale; Hamman-Rich syndrome; Haw River syndrome; health and rehabilitative services; Health and Retirement Study; Heart Rhythm Society; hepatorenal syndrome; high rate of stimulation; hormone receptor site; humeroradial synostosis

HRSA Health Resources and Services Administration

HRSD Hamilton Rating Scale for Depression; Hirschsprung disease

HRSP high-resolution storage phosphor

HRSUB submaximal heart rate

HRT heart rate; Heidelberg retinal tomography; hormone replacement therapy; Hormone Replacement Trial

HRTE human reverse transcriptase enzyme

HRTEM high-resolution transmission electron microscopy

HRUS high-resolution ultrasound

HRV heart rate variability; human reovirus; human rhinovirus; human rotavirus

HRV-A, -B human rhinoviruses A and B

HS Haber syndrome; habitual snoring; half scan; half strength; Hallopeau-Siemens [syndrome]; hamstring; hand surgery; harmonic scalpel; Hartmann solution; head sling; health services; health statistics; healthy subject; heart sounds; heat stable; heavy smoker; heel slide; Hegglin syndrome; heme synthetase; hemorrhagic septicemia; hemorrhagic shock; Henoch-Schönlein [purpura]; heparan sulfate; hereditary spherocytosis; herpes simplex; hidradenitis suppurativa; hippocampal system; home surgeon; homologous serum; horizontally selective; Horner syndrome; horse serum; hospital ship; hospital staff; hospital stay; hours of sleep; house surgeon; human serum; Hurler syndrome; hybrid sign; hypercoagulable state; hypereosinophilic syndrome; hypersensitive site; hypersensitivity; hypertonic saline; hypothalamic syndrome

H/S helper/suppressor ratio; hysterosalpingography

H&S hemorrhage and shock; hysterectomy and sterilization

hs history; hospitalization

h.s. at bedtime [L. *hora somni*]

HSA Hazardous Substances Act; health savings account; Health Services Administration; Health Services Australia; health systems agency; hereditary sideroblastic anemia; horse serum albumin; human serum albumin; hypersomnia—sleep apnea

HSAG N-2-hydroxyethylpiperazine-N-2-ethanesulfonate-saline-albumin-gelatin

HSAM highly selective affinity modification

HSAN hereditary sensory and autonomic neuropathy

HSAP heat-stable alkaline phosphatase

HSAS hydrocephalus due to stenosis of aqueduct of Sylvius; hypertrophic subaortic stenosis

HSC Hand-Schüller-Christian [syndrome]; Health and Safety Commission; health sciences center; health screening center; hematopoietic stem cell; hepatic stellate cell; human skin collagenase

HSCD Hand-Schüller-Christian disease

HSCL Hopkins Symptom Check List

HS-CoA reduced coenzyme A

HSCR Hirschsprung disease

hs-CRP, hsCRP high-sensitivity C-reactive protein

HSCS health state classification system; Hypertension-Stroke Cooperative Study

HSCSG Hypertension-Stroke Cooperative Study Group [trial]

HSCT hematopoietic stem cell transplantation

HSD Hallervorden-Spatz disease; highly sulfated domain; high-speed data; honestly significant difference; hydroxysteroid dehydrogenase; hypertonic saline and dextran

H(SD) Holtzman Sprague-Dawley [rat]

HSDB Hazardous Substances Data Bank

HSDD hypoactive sexual desire disorder

HSDO health services delivery organization

HSE health, safety, and environment; heat stress element; hemorrhagic shock and encephalopathy; herpes simplex encephalitis; high salt extract; human serum esterase

hSEAP human secreted alkaline phosphatase

HSEES Hazardous Substances Emergency Events Surveillance [system]

HSEP heart synchronized evoked potential

HSES hemorrhagic shock—encephalopathy syndrome

HSF heat shock factor; hepatocyte stimulatory factor; histamine sensitizing factor; hypothalamic secretory factor

HSG Health Service Guideline; herpes simplex genitalis; human salivary gland; hysterosalpingogram, hysterosalpingography

hSGF human skeletal growth factor

HSGP human sialoglycoprotein

HSH Health Smart Home [database]; hypomagnesemia with secondary hypocalcemia

HSHC hydrocortisone hemisuccinate

HSI health service indicator; health supervision index; heat stress index; hue saturation intensity; human seminal plasma inhibitor

HSIL high-grade squamous intraepithelial lesion

HSIL/CA high-grade squamous intraepithelial lesion/cancer

HSIS Health Services Information System

HSK herpes simplex keratitis

HSL hormone-sensitive lipase

HSLC high-speed liquid chromatography

HSM health system model; heparin surface modified; hepatosplenomegaly; hierarchical storage management; holosystolic murmur

HSMHA Health Services and Mental Health Administration

HSN hereditary sensory neuropathy; hospital satellite network

HSNU atrophic humeral shaft nonunion

HSO health service organization

hSOD human superoxide dismutase

HSP health care security policy; Health Systems Plan; heat shock protein; Hemorrhagic Stroke Project; hemostatic screening profile; Henoch-Schönlein purpura; hereditary spastic paraparesis; high-scoring segment pair; Hospital Service Plan; human serum prealbumin; human serum protein

hsp heat shock protein

HS PACS high-speed picture archive and communication system

HSPG, HS-PG heparan sulfate-proteoglycan

HSPM hippocampal synaptic plasma membrane

HSPN Henoch-Schönlein purpura nephritis

HSP$_p$ heat shock protein promoter

HSQ health status questionnaire; home screening questionnaire

HSQB Health Standards and Quality Bureau

HSQC heteronuclear single-quantum correlation

HSR Harleco synthetic resin; health services research; heated serum reagin; homogeneously staining region; hypersensitivity reaction

HSRC Health Services Research Center; Human Subjects Review Committee

HSRCCT high spatial resolution cine computed tomography

HSRD hypertension secondary to renal disease

HSR&D health services research and development

HS-RDEB recessively inherited dystrophic epidermolysis bullosa of Hallopeau and Siemens

HSRI Health Systems Research Institute
HSRPROJ Health Services Research Project in Progress
HSRS Health-Sickness Rating Scale
HSRV human spuma retrovirus
HSS Hallermann-Streiff syndrome; Hallervorden-Spatz syndrome; health services support; Henoch-Schönlein syndrome; highspeed supernatant; hyperstimulation syndrome; hypertonic saline solution; hypertrophic subaortic stenosis
HSSCC hereditary site-specific colon cancer
HSSD hospital sterile supply department
HSSU hospital sterile supply unit
HST health sciences and technology
HSTAR health services and technology assessment research
HSTAT Health Science/Technology Assessment Text
HSTF heat shock transcription factor; heat stress transferring factor; human serum thymus factor
HSTM health state transition matrix
HSUS Health Services Utilization Study
HSV herpes simplex virus; high selective vagotomy; hyperviscosity syndrome
HSV-1 herpes simplex virus type 1
HSV-2 herpes simplex virus type 2
HSVE herpes simplex virus encephalitis
HSVT high-speed valve tester
HSVTK, HSVtk herpes simplex virus thymidine kinase
HSyn heme synthase
HT Hashimoto thyroiditis; head trauma; hearing test; hearing threshold; heart; heart transplant, heart transplantation; hemagglutination titer; hereditary tyrosinemia; hierarchical term; high-frequency transduction; high temperature; high tension; high threshold; histologic technician; home treatment; hospital treatment; Hough transform; Hubbard tank; human thrombin; hydrocortisone test; hydrotherapy; hydroxytryptamine; hypermetropia, total; hypertension, hypertensive; hypertext; hyperthyroidism; hypertransfusion; hypodermic tablet; hypothalamus; hypothyroidism
H&T hospitalization and treatment
³HT tritiated thymidine
5-HT 5-hydroxytryptamine
Ht height of heart; heterozygote; hyperopia, total; hypothalamus
H$_t$ dose equivalent to individual tissues
hT human telomerase
ht heart; heart tones; height; high tension
HTA health technology assessment; heterophil transplantation antigen; human thymocyte

antigen; hydroxytryptamine; hypophysiotropic area
HTACS human thyroid adenyl-cyclase stimulator
ht aer heated aerosol
HT(ASCP) Histologic Technician certified by the American Society of Clinical Pathologists
HTB house tube feeding; human tumor bank
HTC hepatoma cell; hepatoma tissue culture; home telecare; homozygous typing cell
Htc hematocrit
HTCMS home telecare management system
HTCVD hypertensive cardiovascular disease
HTD human therapeutic dose
HTDW heterosexual development of women
hTERT human telomerase reverse transcriptase
HTF heterothyrotropic factor; house tube feeding; HpaII tiny fragment; human tubal fluid
HTG hypertriglyceridemia
HTGL hepatic triglyceride lipase
HTGS high-throughput genomic sequence
HTH helix-turn-helix; high-test hypochlorite; homeostatic thymus hormone; hypothalamus
Hth hypothermic
HTHD hard thoracic herniated disk; hypertensive heart disease
HTIG human tetanus immune globulin
HTK heel to knee
HTL hamster tumor line; hearing threshold level; histotechnologist; human T-cell leukemia; human thymic leukemia
HTLA high titer, low avidity; human T-lymphocyte antigen
HTL(ASCP) Histotechnologist certified by the American Society of Clinical Pathologists
HTLF human T-cell leukemia virus enhancer factor
HTLV human T-lymphotropic virus
HTLV 1, 2 human T-lymphotropic viruses 1 and 2
HTLV-III human T-cell lymphotrophic virus type III
HTLV-MA cell membrane antigen associated with human T-lymphotropic virus
HTLVR human T-lymphotropic virus receptor
HTMT hybrid technology multi threaded technology
HTN Hantaan [-like virus]; histatin; hypertension; hypertensive nephropathy
HTO high tibial osteotomy; high turnover osteoporosis; hospital transfer order
HTOF healthy tissue overdose factor

HTOR 5-hydroxytryptamine oxygenase regulator

HTP House-Tree-Person [test]; hydroxytryptophan; hypothromboplastinemia

5-HTP 5-hydroxy-l-tryptophan

HtPA hexahydrophthalic anhydride

HTPN home total parenteral nutrition

HTR hemolytic transfusion reaction; histidine transport regulator; 5-hydroxytryptamine receptor

hTR human telomerase RNA; human thyroid receptor

HTRAK health maintenance tracking system

hTRb human thyroid receptor beta

HTRCCT high temporal resolution cine computed tomography

HTS Hamilton Twin Study; head trauma syndrome; HeLa tumor suppression; high-throughput screening; high-titer screening; Home Telecare System; human thyroid-stimulating hormone, human thyroid stimulator; hypertonic saline

hTS human thymidylate synthase

HTSAB human thyroid-stimulating antibody

HTSC home telecare service center

hTSC human thiazide-sensitive sodium-chloride cotransporter

HTSH, hTSH human thyroid-stimulating hormone

HTST high temperature, short time

HTT 5-hydroxytryptamine transformer

HTTP hypertext transfer protocol

HTTPD hypertext transfer protocol daemon

HTTPS secure hypertext transfer protocol; support hypertext transfer protocol

HTV herpes-type virus

HTVD hypertensive vascular disease

HTX heterotaxy, X-linked; histrionicotoxin

HTx heart transplantation

HU heat unit; hemagglutinating unit; hemolytic unit; Hounsfield unit; human urine, human urinary; hydroxyurea; hyperemia unit

Hu human

HUAA home uterine activity assessment

HUB HELIOS unification bus

HUBNET Hospital and University of Buffalo Library Resource Network

HUC human uroepithelial cell; hypouricemia

HUCBC human umbilical cord blood cells

HuCS human-centered system

HuEPO human erythropoietin

HU-FSH human urinary follicle-stimulating hormone

HUGO Human Genome Organization

HUGV Hughes virus

HUI headache unit index; Health Utilities Index

HUIFM human leukocyte interferon milieu

HuIFN human interferon

HUK human urinary kallikrein

HUM Hilbert uniqueness method

Hum humerus

HUMAN hyper utilities mechatronic assistant

HUMANE human-oriented universal medical assessment system under network environment

HUP Hospital Utilization Project

HUR hydroxyurea

HURA health in underserved rural areas

HURT hospital utilization review team

HUS heel ultrasonography; hemolytic uremic syndrome; hyaluronidase unit for semen

HuSA human serum albumin

HuSMC human smooth muscle cell

HUT head-up tilt

hut histidine utilization

HUTHAS human thymus antiserum

HuTV human torovirus

HUV human umbilical vein

HUVEC human umbilical vein endothelial cell

HUVS hypocomplementemic urticarial vasculitis syndrome

HV hallux valgus; Hantaan virus; has voided; heart volume; hepatic vein; hepatitis viruses; herpesvirus; high voltage; high volume; histologically verified; His ventricle; hospital visit; hyperventilation; hypervolemia; hypovirus

H&V hemigastrectomy and vagotomy

H$_v$ heat of evaporation

hv hypervariable region

HVA hallux valgus angle; hazard vulnerability analysis; homovanillic acid

HVAC heating, ventilating, and air conditioning

HVC Health Visitor's Certificate

HVCT helical volume scan computed tomography

HVD Hantavirus disease; hypertensive vascular disease

HVDRR hypocalcemic vitamin D−resistant rickets

HVE hepatic venous effluence; high-voltage electrophoresis

HVEM herpesvirus entry mediator

HVG host versus graft [disease]

HVGS high-voltage galvanic stimulation

HVJ hemagglutinating virus of Japan

HVL half-value layer; high viral load

hvl half-value layer

HVLP high volume, low pressure

HVM high-velocity missile

HVOO hepatic venous outflow obstruction

HVPC high-voltage pulsed current

HVPE high-voltage paper electrophoresis
HVPG hepatic venous pressure gradient
HVPGS high-voltage pulsed galvanic stimulation
HVR hepatic vascular resistance; hypervariable region; hypoxic ventilation response
HVS herpesvirus of Saimiri; herpesvirus sensitivity; high vaginal swab; high-voltage spike and wave [discharge]; high-voltage stimulation; high-volume screening; hyperventilation syndrome; hyperviscosity syndrome
HVSD hydrogen-detected ventricular septal defect
HVT half-value thickness; herpesvirus of turkeys
HVTEM high-voltage transmission electron microscopy
HVTN HIV Vaccine Trials Network
HVUS hypocomplementemic vasculitis urticaria syndrome
HVWP hepatic vein wedge pressure
HW half-width; healing well; heart weight; heartworm [veterinary medicine]; hypertriglyceridemic waist
HWB hot water bottle
HWBW heart weight/body weight [ratio]
HWC Health and Welfare, Canada
HWCD Hans-Weber-Christian disease
HWD heartworm disease
HWE Hardy-Weinberg equilibrium; healthy worker effect; hot water extract
HWP hepatic wedge pressure; hot wet pack
HWS hot water soluble
HX histiocytosis X; hydrogen exchange; hypophysectomized; hypoxanthine
Hx hallux; hemopexin; history; hypoxanthine
hx hospitalization
HXB hexabrachion
HXIS hard x-ray imaging spectrometry
HXM hexamethylmelamine
HXR hypoxanthine riboside
Hy hypermetropia; hyperopia; hypophysis; hypothenar; hysteria
HYC hycanthone methylsulfonate
Hy-C Hydralazine vs. Captopril [trial]

HYCAT Hytrin Community Assessment Trial
HYCONES Hybrid Connectionist Expert System
HYCX hydrocephalus due to congenital stenosis of aqueduct of Sylvius
HYD hydralazine; hydrated, hydration; hydrocortisone; hydrodensitometry; hydroxyurea
hydr hydraulic
hydro hydrotherapy
HYE healthy years equivalent
hyg hygiene, hygienic, hygienist
HYL, Hyl hydroxylysine
HYNON Hypertension Non-Drug Treatment [cooperative study]
HYP hydroxyproline; hypnosis
Hyp hydroxyproline; hyperresonance; hypertrophy; hypothalamus
hyp hypophysectomy, hypophysis
HyperGEN Hypertension Genetic Epidemiology Network
hyper-IgE hyperimmunoglobulinemia E
hypn hypertension
hypno hypnosis
Hypo hypodermic, hypodermic injection
hypox hypophysectomized
HYPP hyperkalemic periodic paralysis
HYPPOS Hypertensive Population Survey
HYPREN Hypertension Under Prazosin and Enalapril [study]
HypRF hypothalamic releasing factor
HYPRO, HyPro hydroxyproline
hys, hyst hysterectomy; hysteria, hysterical
HYSTENOX Enoxaparin Following Hysterectomy [study]
HyTk hybromycin-thymidine kinase
HYVET Hypertension in the Very Elderly Trial
HZ herpes zoster
Hz hertz
HZFesV Hardy-Zuckerman feline sarcoma virus
Hz/G hertz/gauss
HZO herpes zoster ophthalmicus
HZV herpes zoster virus

I

I carcinoma of the vaginal wall; electric current; endometrial carcinoma in situ confined to the corpus uteri; immediate; implantation; impression; inactive; incisor [permanent]; increase; independent; index; indicated; indirect; induction; inertia; inhalation; inhibited [pacemaker]; inhibition, inhibitor; inosine; insoluble; inspiration, inspired; insulin; intake; intensity; intermediate; intermittent; internal; internal medicine; intervention; intestine; involvement of a single lymph node; iodine; ionic current; ionic strength; iris; ischemia; isochromosome; isoleucine; isotope; isotropic; nuclear spin quantum number

I2 intervention implementation

I-131 iodine-131

i electric current; incisor [deciduous]; insoluble; isochromosome; optically inactive

ι lowercase Greek letter iota

IA ibotenic acid; image analysis; immediately available; immune adherence; immunoadsorbent; immunobiologic activity; impedance angle; indolaminergic accumulation; indole acetic acid; indolic acid; indulin agar; infantile autism; infected area; inferior angle; information assurance; inhibitory antigen; inpatient admission; intelligent agent; internal auditory; intraalveolar; intraamniotic; intraaortic; intraarterial; intraarticular; intraatrial; intraauricular; intracellular anchor; intrinsic activity; invasive aspergillosis; irradiation area; isopropyl alcohol

I&A identification and authentication; irrigation and aspiration

Ia endometrial carcinoma in situ, length of uterine cavity less than 8 cm; immune response gene-associated antigen

IAA imidazoleacetic acid; indoleacetic acid; infectious agent, arthritis; insulin autoantibody; International Antituberculosis Association; interruption of the aortic arch; iodoacetic acid

IAAA inflammatory abdominal aortic aneurysm

IAAR imidazoleacetic acid ribonucleotide

IAB Industrial Accident Board; initial intentional bias; intraabdominal; intraaortic balloon

IABA intraaortic balloon assistance

IABC, IABCP intraaortic balloon counterpulsation

IABM idiopathic aplastic bone marrow

IABP intraaortic balloon pump

IABS International Association for Biological Standards

IAC image analysis cytometry; immuno-affinity chromatography; ineffective airway clearance; internal auditory canal; interposed abdominal compression; intraarterial catheter; intraarterial chemotherapy

IAC CPR interposed abdominal compression cardiopulmonary resuscitation

IACD implantable automatic cardioverter-defibrillator; intraarterial conduction defect

IACFP International Association for Correctional and Forensic Psychology

IACI idiopathic arterial calcification of infancy

IACOV Iaco virus

IACP intraaortic counterpulsation

IACS International Academy of Cosmetic Surgery

IACUC institutional animal care and utilization committee

IACV International Association of Cancer Victors and Friends

IAD inactivating dose; instructional advance directive; internal absorbed dose; internal age distribution; intraset distance

IADH inappropriate antidiuretic hormone

IADHS inappropriate antidiuretic hormone syndrome

IADL instrumental or intermediate activities of daily living

IADR International Association for Dental Research

IAds immunoadsorption

IADSA, IA-DSA intraarterial digital subtraction angiography

IAEA International Atomic Energy Agency

IAET International Association for Enterostomal Therapy

IAF idiopathic alveolar fibrosis; 5-iodoacetamidofluorescein

IAFC International Association of Fire Chiefs

IAFF International Association of Fire Fighters

IAFI infantile amaurotic familial idiocy

IAFN International Association of Forensic Nurses

IAG International Association of Gerontology and Geriatrics; International Academy of Gnathology

IAGP International Association of Geographic Pathology

IAGUS International Association of Genito-Urinary Surgeons

IAH idiopathic adrenal hyperplasia; implantable artificial heart; intraabdominal hypertension

IAHA idiopathic autoimmune hemolytic anemia; immune adherence hemagglutination

IAH/ACS intraabdominal hypertension/abdominal compartment syndrome

IAHC International Association for Human Caring

IAHD idiopathic acquired hemolytic disorder

IAHS infection-associated hemophagocytic syndrome

IAHSS International Association for Healthcare Security & Safety

IAI integral access interface; intraabdominal infection; intraabdominal injury

IAIHG International Autoimmune Hepatitis Group

IAIMS Integrated Academic Information Management System; Integrated Advanced Information Management System

IAIS insulin autoimmune syndrome

IAM immune adhesion molecule; Institute of Aviation Medicine; internal auditory meatus

i am intraamniotic

IAMA Infection in Atherosclerosis and Use of Macrolide Antibiotics [study]

IAMM International Association of Medical Museums

IAMS International Association of Microbiological Societies

IAN idiopathic aseptic necrosis; indole acetonitrile

iANP immunoreactive atrial natriuretic peptide

IANPHI International Association of National Public Health Institutes

IAO immediately after onset; intermittent aortic occlusion; International Association for Orthodontics; International Association of Orthodontists

IA OCA oculocutaneous albinism type IA

IAOM International Association of Orofacial Myology

IAP idiopathic acute pancreatitis; immunosuppressive acidic protein; incident action plan; inosinic acid pyrophosphorylase; Institute of Animal Physiology; integrin-associated protein; intermittent acute porphyria; International Academy of Pathology; International Academy of Proctology; International Atherosclerosis Project; intraabdominal pressure; intraarterial pressure; intracellular action potential; intracisternal A-type particle; islet-activating protein

IAPAC International Association of Physicians in AIDS Care

IAPB International Agency for the Prevention of Blindness

IAPG interatrial pressure gradient

IAPM International Academy for Preventive Medicine

IAPP International Association for Preventive Pediatrics; islet amyloid polypeptide

IAPSRS International Association of Psychosocial Rehabilitation Services

IAPV intermittent abdominal pressure ventilation

IAQ indoor air quality

IAR immediate asthma reaction; inhibitory anal reflex; iodine-azide reaction

IARC International Agency for Research on Cancer

IARF ischemic acute renal failure

IARG International Anticoagulant Review Group [study]

IARS image archival and retrieval system

IARSA idiopathic acquired refractory sideroblastic anemia

IART intraoperative avidination radionuclide therapy

IAS immunosuppressive acidic substance; infant apnea syndrome; insulin autoimmune syndrome; interatrial septum; interatrial shunting; internal anal sphincter; International Acquired Immune Deficiency Syndrome Society; International AIDS Society; intraamniotic saline

IASA interatrial septal aneurysm

IASD iatrogenic atrial septal defect; interatrial septal defect; interauricular septal defect

IASH isolated asymmetric septal hypertrophy

IASHS Institute for Advanced Study of Human Sexuality

IASL International Association for the Study of the Liver

IASLC International Association for the Study of Lung Cancer

IASP International Association for the Study of Pain

IASSH Italian Acute Stroke Study with Hemodilution

IAT instillation abortion time; intrinsic accuracy test; invasive activity test; iodine azide test

IATI, IaTI inter-alpha-trypsin inhibitor

IATIL inter-alpha-trypsin inhibitor, light chain

IAV intermittent assisted ventilation; intra-arterial vasopressin

IAVB incomplete atrioventricular block

IAVI International AIDS Vaccine Initiative

IAVM intramedullary arteriovenous malformation

IB idiopathic blepharospasm; immune body; inclusion body; index of body build; infectious bronchitis; instantaneous boundary; Institute of Biology; interface bus; ipratropium bromide

Ib endometrial carcinoma in situ, length of uterine cavity more than 8 cm tumor

I_b background sodium current

ib in the same place [L. *ibidem*]

IBAT intravascular bronchoalveolar tumor

IBAV Ibaraki virus

IBB intestinal brush border

IBBB intra−blood-brain barrier

IBBBB incomplete bilateral bundle branch block

IBC inflammatory breast cancer; inflammatory breast carcinoma; Institutional Biosafety Committee; iodine-binding capacity; iron-binding capacity; isobutyl cyanoacrylate

IBCA isobutyl-2-cyanoacrylate

IBCLC International Board-Certified Lactation Consultant

IBC-R Injury Behavior Checklist-Revised

IBD identical by descent; inflammatory bowel disease; integrated balloon display; irritable bowel disease

IBDlist Inflammatory Bowel Disease List

IBDQ Inflammatory Bowel Disease Questionnaire

IBDU unclassified inflammatory bowel disease

IBDV infectious bursal disease virus

IBE immunoreactive beta-endomorphin; International Bureau for Epilepsy

IBED Inter-African Bureau for Epizootic Diseases

IBEN individual behavior

IBF immature brown fat; immunoglobulin-binding factor; Insall-Burstein-Freeman [instrumentation]; intestinal blood flow

IBG insoluble bone gelatin

IBI interbeat interval; intermittent bladder irrigation; ischemic brain infarction

ibid in the same place [L. *ibidem*]

IBIDS ichthyosis, brittle hair, impaired intelligence, decreased fertility, short stature [syndrome]; International Bibliographic Information on Dietary Supplements

IBIS Invasive Bacterial Infection Surveillance [study]

IBK infectious bovine keratoconjunctivitis

IBM inclusion body myositis; intact bridge mastoidectomy

IBMIR instant blood-mediated inflammatory reaction

IBMP International Board of Medicine and Psychology

IBMTR International Bone Marrow Transplantation Registry

IBMX 3-isobutyl-1-methylxanthine

IBNR incurred but not reported

IBO information-bearing object

IB OCA oculocutaneous albinism type IB

IBP insulin-like growth factor binding protein; International Biological Program; intra-aortic balloon pumping; iron-binding protein

IBPMS indirect blood pressure measuring system

IBQ Illness Behavior Questionnaire

IBR infectious bovine rhinotracheitis

IBRO International Brain Research Organization

IBRV infectious bovine rhinotracheitis virus

IBS identical by state; imidazole buffered saline; immunoblastic sarcoma; integrated backscatter; Iowa Breakfast Study; irritable bowel syndrome; isobaric solution

IBSA iodinated bovine serum albumin

IBS-C irritable bowel syndrome with constipation

IBS-D irritable bowel syndrome with diarrhea

IBSN infantile bilateral striated necrosis

IBSP integrin-binding sialoprotein

IBSS International Bibliography of the Social Sciences

IBT immunobead binding test; ink blot test

IBTR ipsilateral breast tumor recurrence

IbTX iberiotoxin

IBU ibuprofen; international benzoate unit

i-Bu isobutyl

IBV infectious bronchitis vaccine; infectious bronchitis virus; Ivorian bacilliform virus

IBW ideal body weight

IBX Independence Blue Cross

IC icteric, icterus; immune complex; immunocompetent; immunoconjugate; immunocytochemistry; immunocytotoxicity; impedance cardiogram; imprinting center; indirect calorimetry; individual counseling; infection control; inferior colliculus; information and communication; informed consent; inner canthal; inorganic carbon; inspiratory capacity; inspiratory center; institutional care; integrated circuit; integrated concentration; intensive care; intercostal; intermediate care; intermittent catheterization; intermittent claudication; internal capsule; internal carotid; internal conjugate; interstitial cell; interstitial cystitis; intracapsular; intracardiac; intracarotid; intracavitary; intracellular; intracerebral; intracisternal; intracranial; intracutaneous; intraoperative cholangiography; invasive candidiasis; irritable colon; ischemic colitis; islet cells; isovolumic contraction

IC 1/2/3 intermediate care 1/2/3

IC$_{50}$ inhibitory concentration of 50%

ICA immunocytochemical analysis; independent component analysis; internal carotid artery; intracranial aneurysm; islet cell antibody

ICAA International Council on Alcohol and Addictions; Invalid Children's Aid Association

ICAAC Interscience Conference on Antimicrobial Agents and Chemotherapy

ICAb islet cell antibody

IC-AFM intermittent-contact mode atomic force microscopy

ICAI intelligent computer-aided instruction

ICAM improved chemical agent monitor; induced endothelial cell adhesion molecule; integrated computer-aided manufacturing

ICAM-1, -2, -3 intracellular adhesion molecules 1, 2, 3

ICAMI International Committee Against Mental Illness

ICAO internal carotid artery occlusion

ICARIS Intervention Cardiology Risk Stratification [study]

ICARUS Islet Cell Antibody Register User Study

ICASO International Committee of Acquired Immunodeficiency Syndrome Service Organisations

ICAT International Comprehensive Anatomical Terminology

ICBDMS International Clearinghouse for Birth Defects Monitoring Systems

ICBF inner cortical blood flow

ICBG idiopathic calcification of basal ganglia

ICBM International Consortium for Brain Mapping

ICBN intercostobrachial nerve

ICBP intracellular binding protein

ICBPG improved chemical and biological protective glove

ICBR increased chromosomal breakage rate

ICC immunocompetent cells; immunocytochemistry; Indian childhood cirrhosis; induction compliance checklist; infection control committee; intensive coronary care; interchromosomal crossing over; interclass correlation coefficient; intercluster constraint; internal conversion coefficient; International Certification Commission; interventional cardiac center; intraclass correlation coefficient; intracranial cavity; invasive cervical cancer; Italian Cancer Classification

ICCE intracapsular cataract extraction

iCCK immunoreactive cholecystokinin

ICCM idiopathic congestive cardiomyopathy

ICCR International Committee for Contraception Research

ICCS International Classification of Clinical Services

ICCs interstitial cells of Cajal

ICCU intensive coronary care unit; intermediate coronary care unit

ICD I-cell disease; immune complex disease; impedance cardiogram; implantable cardioverter-defibrillator; impulse-control disorder; induced circular dichroism; initial cardioverter-defibrillator; initial claudication distance; Institute for Crippled and Disabled; intercanthal distance; International Center for the Disabled; International Classification of Diseases, Injuries, and Causes of Death; International Common Denomination; International Statistical Classification of Diseases and Health-Related Problems; intracardiac defibrillator; intracervical device; intrauterine contraceptive device; ischemic coronary disease; isocitrate dehydrogenase; isolated conduction defect

ICD-10 International Statistical Classification of Diseases and Health-Related Problems, 10th Revision

ICDA International Classification of Diseases, Adapted

ICD/BPA International Classification of Diseases as adapted by the British Paediatric Association

ICDC implantable cardioverter-defibrillator catheter

ICD-9-CM International Classification of Diseases, 9th Revision, Clinical Modification

ICDH isocitrate dehydrogenase

ICD/IPD inner canthal distance/interpupillary distance

ICD-O International Classification of Diseases-Oncology

ICDRC International Contact Dermatitis Research Center

ICDREC International Computer Database for Radiation Accident Case Histories

ICDS Integrated Child Development Scheme; International Cardiac Doppler Society

ICE ice, compression, elevation; ichthyosis-cheek-eyebrow [syndrome]; ifosfamide, carboplatin, etoposide; immunochemical evaluation; in case of emergency; integrated clinical encounter; integration, codification and evaluation; interleukin converting enzyme; intracardiac echocardiography; iridocorneal endothelial [syndrome]

ICECA International Committee for Electronic Communication on Acquired Immunodeficiency Syndrome

ICECG intracardiac electrocardiography

ICED Index of Co-existent Diseases

ICEEG intracranial electroencephalography

ICE-GTC intractable childhood epilepsy with generalized tonic clonic seizures

ICER incremental cost-effectiveness ratio; inducible cyclic adenosine monophosphate early repressor

ICES information collection and evaluation system

ICET induced current electrical impedance tomography

ICEUS intracaval endovascular ultrasound

ICF immunodeficiency, centromeric instability, facial anomalies [syndrome]; indirect centrifugal flotation; informed consent form; intensive care facility; intercellular fluorescence; interciliary fluid; intermediate-care facility; International Cardiology Foundation; intracellular fluid; intravascular coagulation and fibrinolysis

ICFA incomplete Freund adjuvant; induced complement-fixing antigen

ICFF important clinical field finding

ICF(M)A International Cystic Fibrosis (Mucoviscidosis) Association

ICF-MR intermediate-care facility for the mentally retarded (intellectual disability)

ICF/MR intensive care facilities for mental retardation (intellectual disability)

ICG impedance cardiogram; impedance cardiography; indocyanine green; isotope cisternography

ICGC indocyanine green clearance; International Cancer Genome Consortium

ICGN immune-complex glomerulonephritis

ICH idiopathic cortical hyperostosis; immunocompromised host; infectious canine hepatitis; Institute of Child Health; International Conference on Harmonisation; intracerebral hematoma; intracranial hemorrhage; intracranial hypertension

ICHD Inter-Society Commission for Heart Disease Resources

ICHPER·SD International Council for Health, Physical Education, Recreation, Sport, and Dance

ICHPPC International Classification of Health Problems in Primary Care

IcHV Ictalurid herpesvirus

ICI intracardiac infection

ICi intracisternal

ICIC International Classification of Primary Care

ICIDH International Classification of Impairments, Disabilities, and Handicaps

ICIN Intracoronary Streptokinase Trial of the Interuniversity Cardiology Institute of the Netherlands

ICIS imaging center information system

iCJD iatrogenic Creutzfeldt-Jakob disease

ICJR International Congress for Joint Reconstruction

ICL idiopathic CD4 T-cell lymphocytopenia; implantable collamer lens; implantable contact lens; intracranial lesion; iris-clip lens; isocitrate lyase

I$_{Cl}$ chloride ionic current

ICLA International Committee on Laboratory Animals

ICLAS International Council for Laboratory Animal Science

ICLH Imperial College, London Hospital

ICLP isolated cleft lip or palate

ICM inner cell mass; integrated conditional model; intelligent cardiovascular monitor; intercostal margin; International Confederation of Midwives; intersecting core model; intracellular multiplication; intracytoplasmic membrane; introduction to clinical medicine; ion conductance modulator; isolated cardiovascular malformation

icm intracellular multiplication

ICMA immunochemiluminometric assay

ICMF intercostal muscle flap

ICMI Inventory of Childhood Memories and Imaginings

ICML International Congress on Medical Librarianship

ICMP Internet control message protocol

ICMSF International Commission on Microbiological Specifications for Foods

ICN intensive care nursery; International Council of Nurses

ICNα intracellular concentration of sodium

ICNB International Committee on Nomenclature of Bacteria

ICNC intracerebral nuclear cell

ICNIRP International Commission on Non-Ionizing Radiation Protection

ICNND Interdepartmental Committee on Nutrition in National Defense

ICNP International Classification of Nursing Practice

ICNV International Committee on Nomenclature of Viruses

ICO idiopathic cyclic oedema; impedance cardiac output; infection control officer; intermittent cardiac output

ICOHCS Ishi Town Preschool Children Oral Health Care Study

ICOMS input, constraints, output, and mechanisms

ICOPER International Cooperative Pulmonary Embolism Registry

ICP incident command post; incubation period; indwelling catheter program; infantile cerebral palsy; infection-control practitioner; infectious cell protein; inflammatory cloacogenic polyp; insecticidal crystal protein; integrated care pathway/planning; interactive closest point; interdisciplinary care plan; intermittent catheterization protocol; intracranial pressure; intracytoplasmic; intrahepatic cholestasis of pregnancy; iterative closest point

ICPA International Commission for the Prevention of Alcoholism

ICPB International Collection of Phytopathogenic Bacteria

IC/PBS interstitial cystitis and painful bladder syndrome

ICPC International Classification of Primary Care

ICPC-PLUS International Classification of Primary Care, with extension and electronic version

ICPEMC International Commission for Protection Against Environmental Mutagens and Carcinogens

ICPI Intersociety Council on Pathology Information

ICP-MS inductively coupled plasma mass spectrometer; inductively coupled plasma mass spectrometry

ICPR International Commission on Stage Grouping and Presentation of Results

ICR [distance between] iliac crests; Institute for Cancer Research; intermittent catheter routine; International Congress of Radiology; international consensus report; intracardiac catheter recording; intracavitary radium; intracorneal ring; intracranial reinforcement; ion cyclotron resonance

ICRAC calcium release—activated calcium current

ICRC infant care review committee; International Committee of the Red Cross; Islet Cell Resource Center

ICRD Index of Codes for Research Drugs

ICRE International Commission on Radiological Education

ICRETT International Cancer Research Technology Transfer

ICREW International Cancer Research Workshop

ICRF Imperial Cancer Research Fund

I-CRF immunoreactive corticotropin-releasing factor

ICRF-159 razoxane

ICRP International Commission on Radiological Protection; International Committee on Radiation Protection

ICRS Index Chemicus Registry System

ICRT intracoronary radiation therapy

ICRU International Commission on Radiation Units and Measurements

ICS ileocecal sphincter; image criteria score; immotile cilia syndrome; immunocytochemical staining; impulse-conducting system; incident command system; information and communication system; inhaled corticosteroids; integrated case study; intensive care, surgical; intercellular space; intercostal space; intercuspidation splint; International College of Surgeons; International Cytokine Society; intracellular segment; intracranial stimulation; Iohexol Cooperative Study; irritable colon syndrome

I&CS information and communication system

ICSA islet cell surface antibody

ICSB International Committee on Systematic Bacteriology

ICSC idiopathic central serous choroidopathy

ICS$_f$ final intercuspidation splint

ICSG International Cooperative Study Group

ICSH International Committee for Standardization in Hematology; interstitial cell-stimulating hormone

ICS-HSH Information and Communication System Health Smart Home

ICSI Institute for Clinical Systems Integration; intracytoplasmic sperm injection

ICSK intracoronary streptokinase

ICSO intermittent coronary sinus occlusion

ICSP Interagency Council on Statistical Policy; International Council of Societies of Pathology

ICSS intracranial self-stimulation

I/CSS informed consent support system

ICSTI International Council for Scientific and Technical Information

ICSU International Council of Scientific Unions

ICT icteric, icterus; indirect Coombs test; induction chemotherapy; inflammation of connective tissue; information and communications technology; insulin coma therapy; intensive conventional therapy; intermittent cervical traction; interstitial cell tumor; intracardiac thrombus; intracranial tumor; isovolumic contraction time

Ict icterus

iCT immunoreactive calcitonin

ICTDR International Centers for Tropical Disease Research

ICTMM International Congress on Tropical Medicine and Malaria

ICTS idiopathic carpal tunnel syndrome

ICTV International Committee for the Taxonomy of Viruses

ICTVdB International Committee on Taxonomy of Viruses Database

ICTX intermittent cervical traction

ICU immunologic contact urticaria; infant care unit; intensive care unit; intermediate care unit

ICUS intracoronary ultrasound

ICV internal cerebral vein; intracellular volume; intracerebroventricular

icv intracerebroventricular

ICVA intracranial vertebral artery

ICVS International Cardiovascular Society

ICW intensive care ward; intermediate care ward; intracellular water

ICWS integrated clinical workstation

ICx immune complex; inter-cartridge exchange

ICZN International Code of Zoological Nomenclature

ID identification; identifier; idiotype; iditol dehydrogenase; immunodeficiency; immunodiffusion; immunoglobulin deficiency; inappropriate disability; incapacitating dose; incision and drainage; inclusion disease; index of discrimination; individual dose; infant death; infectious disease; infective dose; inhibitory dose; initial diagnosis; initial dose; initial dyskinesia; injected dose; inside diameter; interdigitating; interhemispheric disconnection; internal diameter; interstitial disease; intradermal; intraduodenal

I-D intensity-duration

I&D incision and drainage

ID$_{50}$ median incapacitating dose; median infective dose

Id infradentale; interdentale; the same [L. *idem*]

id the same [L. *idem*]

IDA idamycin; iduronidase; image display and analysis; iminodiacetic acid; insulin-degrading activity; intelligent data analysis; iron deficiency anemia

IDAMAP intelligent data analysis in medicine and pharmacology

IDAV immunodeficiency-associated virus

IDB image database

IDBS infantile diffuse brain sclerosis

IDC idiopathic dilated cardiomyopathy; infiltrating ductal carcinoma; interdigitating cell

iDC immature dendritic cell

IDCI intradiplochromatid interchange

IDCOP idealized design of clinical office practice

IDCS Idiopathic Dilated Cardiomyopathy Study

IDCT inverse discrete cosine transform

IDD idealized dose distribution; insulin-dependent diabetes; intellectual and developmental disability; intraluminal duodenal diverticulum; Inventory to Diagnose Depression

IDDF investigational drug data form

IDDM insulin-dependent diabetes mellitus

IDDM-MED insulin-dependent diabetes mellitus multiple epiphyseal dysplasia [syndrome]

IDDP immediate drug development project

IDDT immune double-diffusion test

IDE insulin-degrading enzyme; integrated development environment; intelligent drive electronics; investigational device exemption

IDEA Individuals with Disabilities Education Act; Internet Database of Evidence-based Abstracts and Articles

IDEF Integrated [Computer-Aided Manufacturing] Definition

i-DENT Internet Dental Epidemiology System Produced by Tokushima University

iDEP insulator-based dielectrophoretic device

IDET intradiskal electrothermal annuloplasty; intradiskal electrothermal therapy

IDF International Diabetes Federation; inverse document frequency

IDFT inverse discrete Fourier transform

IDG intermediate dose group

IDH intraductal hyperplasia; isocitrate dehydrogenase

IDHS Indian Diet Heart Study

IDI immunologically detectable insulin; induction-delivery interval; integrated discrimination improvements; interdentale inferius

I-5DI type I 5′deiodinase

IDIC Internal Dose Information Center

idic isodicentric

IDIS International Drug Information Service; intraoperative digital substraction angiography

IDISA intraoperative digital subtraction angiography

IDK internal derangement of knee

IDL Index to Dental Literature; interface definition language; intermediate density lipoprotein; intermediate differentiation of lymphocytic lymphoma; isodose line

IDL-C, IDL-c intermediate-density lipoprotein–cholesterol complex

IDLH immediate danger to life and health

IDM idiopathic disease of myocardium; immune defense mechanism; indirect method;

infant of diabetic mother; intermediate-dose methotrexate; inverse different moment

IDMC independent data monitoring committee

ID-MS isotope dilution mass spectrometry

IDN integrated delivery network

iDNA intercalary deoxyribonucleic acid

IDP imidodiphosphonate; immunodiffusion procedure; inflammatory demyelinating neuropathy; initial dose period; inosine diphosphate

IDPH idiopathic pulmonary hemosiderosis

IDPN iminodipropionitrile; inflammatory demyelinating polyneuropathy

IDQ Individualized Dementia Questionnaire

IDR intradermal reaction; item discrimination ratio

IDS iduronate sulfatase; immune deficiency state; infectious diseases service; inhibitor of DNA synthesis; integrated delivery system; International Documentation System; intraduodenal stimulation; Inventory for Depressive Symptomatology; investigational drug service

IdS interdentale superius

IDSA Infectious Diseases Society of America; intraoperative digital subtraction angiography

IDSAN International Drug Safety Advisory Network

IDS-CRC International Documentation System-Colorectal Cancer

IDSRN Integrated Delivery System Research Network

IDS-SR Inventory for Depressive Symptomatology Systems Review

IDT immune diffusion test; instillation delivery time; interdisciplinary team; intradermal typhoid [vaccine]

IDU idoxuridine; injection drug use; injection drug user; intravenous drug user; iododeoxyuridine

IDUA iduronidase

IdUA iduronic acid

IDUR idoxuridine

IdUrd idoxuridine

IDUS injecting drug user

IDV indinavir; intermittent demand ventilation

IDVC indwelling venous catheter

IDW initial deflection width

IDWT inverse discrete wavelet transform

IDX 4'-iodo-4'-deoxyoxorubicin

Idx cross-reactive idiotype

IE imaging equipment; immediate early; immunizing unit [Ger. *Immunitäts Einheit*]; immunoelectrophoresis; infective endocarditis; information economics; information engineering; inner ear; inspiratory exerciser; intake energy; internal elastica; intraepithelial

I/E inspiratory/expiratory ratio; internal/external

I$_E$ involvement of a single extrahepatic organ or site

I:E inspiratory/expiratory ratio

ie, i.e. that is [L. *id est*]

IEA immediate early antigen; immunoelectroadsorption; immunoelectrophoretic analysis; infectious equine anemia; inferior epigastric artery; International Epidemiological Association; intravascular erythrocyte aggregation

IEBC International Entomopathogenic Bacillus Center

IEC independent ethics committee; information, education, communication; injection electrode catheter; inpatient exercise center; International Electrotechnical Commission; intestinal epithelial cell; intraepithelial carcinoma; ion-exchange chromatography

IECa intraepithelial carcinoma

IECG intracardiac electrocardiography

IED improvised explosive device; inflammatory eye disease; inherited epidermal dysplasia; intermittent explosive disorder

IEE inner enamel epithelium

IEED involuntary emotional expression disorder

IEEE Institute of Electrical and Electronics Engineers

IEEG intracranial electroencephalography

IEF International Eye Foundation; isoelectric focusing

IEG immediate early gene

IEGM intracardiac electrogram

I-EHR integrated electronic health record

IEI isoelectric interval

IEL internal elastic lamina; intraepithelial lymphocyte

IEM immuno-electron microscopy; inborn error of metabolism

IEMA immunoenzymatic assay

IEMCT individualized epidural morphine conversion tool

IEMG integrated electromyogram; integrated electromyography

IEOP immunoelectro-osmophoresis

IEP immunoelectrophoresis; individualized education program; isoelectric point

IEPR International EECP Patient Registry

IERIV Ieri virus

IES impact of events scale; inferior esophageal sphincter

IESS Intergroup Ewing Sarcoma Study

IET intrauterine exchange transfusion

IETF Internet Engineering Task Force

IETT immediate exercise treadmill testing

IF idiopathic fibroplasia; idiopathic flushing; immersion foot; immunofluorescence; impact factor; indirect fluorescence; infrared; inhibiting factor; initiation factor; instantaneous flow; instantaneous frequency; insufficiency fracture; integrate and fire; intensifying factor; interbody fusion; interferon; interior facet; intermediate filament; intermediate frequency; internal fixation; interstitial fibrosis; interstitial fluid; interventional fluoroscopy; intrinsic factor; involved field

IF1, IF2, IF3 interferons 1, 2, 3

I$_f$ hyperpolarization-activated current

IFA idiopathic fibrosing alveolitis; immunofluorescence assay; immunofluorescent antibody; incomplete Freund's adjuvant; indirect fluorescent antibody; indirect fluorescent assay; International Fertility Association; International Filariasis Association

IFAA International Federation of Associations of Anatomists

IFABP intestinal fatty acid binding protein

IFAP ichthyosis follicularis, atrichia, photophobia [syndrome]

IFAT indirect fluorescent antibody test

IFBC International Food Biotechnology Council

IFC intermittent flow centrifugation; intrinsic factor concentrate

IFCC International Federation of Clinical Chemistry and Laboratory Medicine

IFCR International Foundation for Cancer Research

IFCS inactivated fetal calf serum

IFDS isolated follicle-stimulating hormone deficiency syndrome

IFE immunofixation electrophoresis; interfollicular epidermis

IFEV Ife virus

IFF inner fracture face

IFFH International Foundation for Family Health

IFFS International Federation of Fertility Societies

IFG impaired fasting glucose; inferior frontal gyrus; interferon gamma

IFGO International Federation of Gynecology and Obstetrics

IFGS interstitial fluid and ground substance

IFGT irradiation and fusion gene transfer

IFHGS International Federation of Human Genetics Societies

IFHNOS International Federation of Head and Neck Oncologic Societies

IFHP International Federation of Health Professionals

IFHPMSM International Federation for Hygiene, Preventive Medicine, and Social Medicine

IFHRO International Federation of Health Records

IFI immune interferon; intensified follow-up indicator; invasive fungal infection

IFIP International Federation for Information Processing

IFL immunofluorescence

IFLrA recombinant human leukocyte interferon A

IFM internal fetal monitor; isoleucine, phenylalanine, and methionine

IFMBE International Federation for Medical and Biological Engineering

IFME International Federation for Medical Electronics

IFMP International Federation for Medical Psychotherapy

IFMSA International Federation of Medical Student Associations

IFMSS International Federation of Multiple Sclerosis Societies

IFN interferon

IFNA interferon alpha

IFN α, β, γ interferon alpha, beta, and gamma

If nec if necessary

IFNG interferon gamma

IFNGT interferon gamma transducer

I-FOBT immunochemical fecal occult blood test

IFOS International Federation of Oto-Rhino-Laryngological Societies

IFP inflammatory fibroid polyp; insulin, compound F [hydrocortisone], prolactin; interactive filtered projection; intermediate filament protein; International Federation for Psychotherapy; intimal fibrous proliferation; intrapatellar fat pad

IFPM International Federation of Physical Medicine

IFPMA International Federation of Pharmaceutical Manufacturers & Associations

IFR infrared; inspiratory flow rate

IFRA indirect fluorescent rabies antibody [test]

IFRP International Fertility Research Program

IFRT involved field radiotherapy

IFS interstitial fluid space

IFSE International Federation of Science Editors

IFSM information system; International Federation of Sports Medicine

IFSP individualized family service plan

IFSSH International Federation of Societies for Surgery of the Hand; International Forum for Social Science and Health

IFT immunofluorescence test; inverse Fourier transform

IF/TA interstitial fibrosis/tubular atrophy

IFU interferon unit

IFV interstitial fluid volume; intracellular fluid volume

IFX infliximab

IG immature granule; immunoglobulin; insulin and glucose; intergenic; interstitial glucose; intragastric; irritable gut

Ig immunoglobulin

IGA infantile genetic agranulocytosis

IgA immunoglobulin A

IgA1, IgA2 subclasses of immunoglobulin A

IgAGN immunoglobulin A glomerulonephritis

IgAN immunoglobulin A nephropathy

IGBP iatrogenic gallbladder perforation

IGC immature germ cell; intragastric cannula

IG-CAM immunoglobulin of cell adhesion molecule

IGCP intraglomerular capillary pressure

IGD idiopathic growth hormone deficiency; Integrated Genome Database; interglobal distance; isolated gonadotropin deficiency

IgD immunoglobulin D

IgD1, IgD2 subclasses of immunoglobulin D

IGDM infant of mother with gestational diabetes mellitus

IGE idiopathic generalized epilepsy; impaired gas exchange

IgE immunoglobulin E

IgE1 subclass of immunoglobulin E

IGF insulin-like growth factor

IGF-1 insulin-like growth factor 1

IGFBP insulin-like growth factor binding protein

IGF-1-BP insulin-like growth factor 1 binding protein

IGFBP-3 IGF-binding protein 3

IGFET insulated gate field effect transistor

IGF-1-KIRA insulin-like growth factor 1 kinase receptor activation

IGFL integral green fluorescence

IGFR insulin-like growth factor receptor

IGF1R insulin-like growth factor receptor type 1

IgG immunoglobulin G

IgG1, IgG2, IgG3, IgG4 subclasses of immunoglobulin G

IgG-SC immunoglobulin G–secreting cells

IGH immunoreactive growth hormone

IgH immunoglobulin heavy chain

IgHC immunoglobulin heavy chain constant region

IGHD immunoglobin delta heavy chain; isolated growth hormone deficiency

IGHE immunoglobulin epsilon heavy chain

IGHL inferior glenohumeral ligament

IGHV immunoglobulin heavy chain variable region

IGI intelligent graphic interface; Internet Healthcare Coalition

IGIF interferon-gamma-inducing factor

IGIV intravenous immune globulin

IGKDEL immunoglobulin kappa deleting element

IGL immunoglobulin lambda; immunoglobulin light chain

IGLJ immunoglobulin lambda light chain J

IGLL immunoglobulin lambda–like

IGLLC inferior glenohumeral ligament labral complex

iGluR ionotropic glutamate receptor

IGM Internet Grateful Med

IgM immunoglobulin M

IgM1 subclass of immunoglobulin M

IgMN immunoglobulin M nephropathy

IGNS image-guided neurosurgery

IGO1 immunoglobulin kappa orphan 1

IGOS Image-Guided Orthopaedic Surgery [project]

IGP intestinal glycoprotein

IGR immediate generalized reaction; integrated gastrin response

IGRA interferon-gamma release assay

iGrid international grid

IGS image-guided surgery; implantable gastric stimulation; inappropriate gonadotropin secretion; internal guide sequence

Igs immunoglobulins

IgSC immunoglobulin-secreting cell

IGSF immunoglobulin superfamily

IGSS immunogold silver staining

IGT impaired glucose tolerance

IGTT intravenous glucose tolerance test

IGUV Iguape virus

IGV intrathoracic gas volume

IH idiopathic hirsutism; idiopathic hypercalciuria; idiopathic hypersomnia; immediate hypersensitivity; incompletely healed; indirect hemagglutination; industrial hygiene; infantile hydrocephalus; infectious hepatitis; inguinal hernia; inhibiting hormone; in hospital; inner half; inpatient hospital; intermittent heparinization; intimal hyperplasia; intracranial hematoma; iron hematoxylin

IHA idiopathic hyperaldosteronism; indirect hemagglutination; indirect hemagglutination antibody; intrahepatic atresia

IHAC Industrial Health and Advisory Committee

IHAPS interactive health appraisal system

IHBT incompatible hemolytic blood transfusion

IHC idiopathic hemochromatosis; idiopathic hypercalciuria; immunohistochemical [staining]; immunohistochemistry; inner hair cell; interactive health communication system; Internet Healthcare Coalition; intrahepatic cholestasis

IHCA individual health care account; isocapnic hyperventilation with cold air

IHCM ichthyosis hystrix, Curth-Macklin [type]

IHCP Institute of Hospital and Community Psychiatry

IHD in-center hemodialysis; intermittent hemodialysis; ischemic heart disease

IHDI ischemic heart disease index

IHDP Infant Health and Development Program

IHDPORT Ischemic Heart Disease Patient Outcomes Research Team

IHD SDP Ischemic Heart Disease Shared Decision-Making Program

IHES idiopathic hypereosinophilic syndrome

IHF Industrial Health Foundation; integration host factor; interhemispheric fissure; International Hospital Foundation

IHGD isolateral human growth deficiency

IHH idiopathic hypogonadotropic hypogonadism; idiopathic hypothalamic hypogonadism; infectious human hepatitis

IHHS idiopathic hyperkinetic heart syndrome

IHI Institute for Healthcare Improvement

IHIS integrated hospital information system

IHL International Homeopathic League

IHM in-hospital malnutrition

IHN integrated health care network

IHO idiopathic hypertrophic osteoarthropathy

IHOU in-hospital observation unit

IHP idiopathic hypoparathyroidism; idiopathic hypopituitarism; individualized health plan; inositol hexaphosphate; interhospitalization period; inverted hand position

IHPC intrahepatic cholestasis; intraperitoneal hyperthermic chemotherapy

IHPH intrahepatic portal hypertension

IHPP Intergovernmental Health Project Policy

IHQL index of health-related quality of life

IHR International Health Regulations; intrahepatic resistance; intrinsic heart rate

IHRA isocapnic hyperventilation with room air

IHRB Industrial Health Research Board

IHS idiopathic hypereosinophilic syndrome; inactivated horse serum; Indian Health Service; innovative health care system; integrated health system; International Headache Society; International Health Society; intracranial hypotension syndrome

IHSA iodinated human serum albumin

IHSC immunoreactive human skin collagenase

IHSS idiopathic hypertrophic subaortic stenosis

IHT insulin hypoglycemia test; intravenous histamine test; ipsilateral head turning

I5HT intraplatelet serotonin

IHW International Histocompatibility Workshop

II carcinoma of the subvaginal tissue without involving the pelvic wall; endometrial carcinoma involving the corpus and cervix but no other tissues; icterus index; image intensification/intensifier; involvement or two or more lymph nodes on the same side of the diaphragm

I&I illness and injuries

Ii incision inferius

IIA internal iliac artery

IIC ineffective individual coping; intraoperative imprint cytology

IICP increased intracranial pressure

IID independent identically distributed [nucleotides]; insulin-independent diabetes

IIDM insulin-independent diabetes mellitus

IIE idiopathic ineffective erythropoiesis; implantable insulin pump

II$_E$ localized involvement of an extrahepatic organ or site

IIEF International Index of Erectile Function

i-IEL intestinal intraepithelial lymphocyte

IIF immune interferon; indirect immunofluorescence; intracellular ice formation; isolated intraperitoneal fluid

IIFT intraoperative intraarterial fibrinolytic therapy

IIG imagineering interest group; interactive image-guided [surgery]

IIGR ipsilateral instinctive grasp reaction

IIH idiopathic infantile hypercalcemia

IIHD Israeli Ischemic Heart Disease [study]

III endometrial carcinoma extending outside the uterus but not outside the true pelvis; involvement of two or more lymph node regions on both sides of the diaphragm [staging system for Hodgkin disease]; vaginal carcinoma extending to pelvic wall

III$_E$ localized involvement of an extrahepatic organ or site [staging system for Hodgkin disease]

III-para tertipara

III$_S$ localized involvement of the spleen

III$_{SE}$ localized involvement of an extrahepatic organ and spleen

IIME Institute for International Medical Education

IIMS Interest in Internal Medicine Scale

IINB intrapleural intercostal nerve block

IIP idiopathic interstitial pneumonia; idiopathic intestinal pseudoobstruction; increased intracranial pressure

II-para secundipara

I-123 IPPA I-123 Iodo-Phenylpentadecanoic Acid [Viability Multicenter Study]

IIR infinite impulse response

IIS intensive immunosuppression; International Institute of Stress

IIT induction of immune tolerance; ineffective iron turnover; intensive insulin therapy; interactive image tool; isolated islet transplantation

IITF Information Infrastructure Task Force

IIUK Intraoperative Intra-Arterial Urokinase [study]

IIVS Institute for In Vitro Sciences

IJ ileojejunal; internal jugular; intrajejunal; intrajugular

IJCAI International Joint Conferences on Artificial Intelligence

IJD inflammatory joint disease

IJP inhibitory junction potential; internal jugular pressure

IJV internal jugular vein

IK immobilized knee; immune body [Ger. *Immunekörper*]; *Infusoria* killing [unit]; interstitial keratitis

I-K immunoconglutinin

I$_K$ potassium current

I$_k$ delayed rectifier current

I$_{K(AC, Adoi)}$ acetylcholine and adenosensitive potassium current

I$_{K-Ach}$ acetylcholine-induced potassium current

I$_{KAdo}$ outward inwardly rectifying potassium current

I$_{K(ATP)}$, I$_{K-ATP}$ ATP-sensitive potassium current

IKDC International Knee Documentation Committee

IKE Internet key exchange protocol; ion kinetic energy

I$_{KI}$ inward rectifier current

I$_{Kp}$ plateau potassium current

I$_{Kr}$ rectified potassium current

IKU *Infusoria* killing unit

IL ileum; iliolumbar; immature lung; incisolingual; independent laboratory; inguinal ligament; inspiratory load; instant library; intensity load; interleukin; internal loop; intestinal lymphocyte; intracellular loop; intralumbar; intraocular lens

IL-1 to 15 interleukins 1 to 15

ILA insulin-like activity; International Leprosy Association

ILa incisolabial

ILAE International League Against Epilepsy

ILAR Institute for Laboratory Animal Research

ILB infant, low birth [weight]; initial lung burden

ILBBB incomplete left bundle branch block

ILBW infant, low birth weight

ILC ichthyosis linearis circumflex; incipient lethal concentration; interstitial laser coagulation

ILD interstitial lung disease; intraoperative localization device; ischemic leg disease; ischemic limb disease; isolated lactase deficiency

ILDBP interleukin-dependent deoxyribonucleic acid–binding protein

ILE information-laden event; isoleucine

ILe, Ile isoleucine

ILED infrared light emission diode

IleRS isoleucyl RNA synthetase

ILEV Ilesha virus

ILRFA inline radiofrequency ablation

ILGA International Lesbian and Gay Association

ILGF insulin-like growth factor

ILH immunoreactive luteinizing hormone

ILHV Ilheus virus

ILI influenzalike illness

ILIS intelligent laboratory information system

ILL interlibrary loan; intermediate lymphocytic lymphoma

ILLE inverted with lower limbs extended

ILLP indeterminate lobular lymphocytic panniculitis

ILM insulin-like material; internal limiting membrane

ILMA, I-LMA intubating laryngeal mask airway

ILMS Israel Longitudinal Mortality Study

ILNR intralobar nephrogenic rest

ILo iodine lotion

ILP inadequate luteal phase; insufficiency of luteal phase; insulin-loaded polymer; interstitial laser photocoagulation; interstitial lymphocytic pneumonia; isolated limb perfusion

ILR interleukin receptor; irreversible loss rate

IL-1R to 15R interleukin 1 to 15 receptors

ILRA interleukin receptor alpha

IL1-RA interleukin-1 receptor antagonist

ILRB interleukin receptor beta

ILRCFS Iowa Lipid Research Clinics Family Study

ILS idiopathic leucine sensitivity; idiopathic lymphadenopathy syndrome; increase in life span; infrared liver scanner; integrated library system; intermittent light stimulation; intralobal sequestration

ILSA Italian Longitudinal Study on Aging

ILSI International Life Sciences Institute

ILSS integrated life support system; intraluminal somatostatin

ILT iliotibial tract

ILTV infectious laryngotracheitis virus

ILUS intraluminal ultrasound

ILV independent lung ventilation; instantaneous lung volume [recording]

ILVEN inflamed linear verrucous epidermal nevus

ILY intermedilysin

IM idiopathic myelofibrosis; immuno-suppressive method; implementation monitoring; Index Medicus; indomethacin; industrial medicine; infection medium; infectious mononucleosis; information management; inner membrane; innocent murmur; inspiratory muscles; intensity modulated; intermediate; intermediate megaloblast; intermediate metabolizer; internal malleolus; internal mammary [artery]; internal margin; internal medicine; internal monitor; intramedullary; intrametatarsal; intramuscular; invasive mole; isolated microcalcification

I-M incudomalleolar

2IM 2-ipomeanol

Im imidazole

im intramuscular

IMA immunometric assay; Industrial Medical Association; inferior mesenteric artery; installation medical authority; Interchurch Medical Assistance; intermetatarsal angle; internal mammary artery; internal maxillary artery; Irish Medical Association

IMAA iodinated macroaggregated albumin

IMAB internal mammary artery bypass

IMAC image management archiving and communications; immobilized metal affinity capture; information management, archiving, and communication; Intervention in Myocarditis and Acute Cardiomyopathy [study]

IMACS image archiving and communication system; image management and communication system

IMAGE integrated molecular analysis of gene expression; International Metoprolol/Nifedipine Angina Exercise Trial; International Multicenter Angina Exercise [study]; International Multicenter Aprotinin Graft Patency Experience [trial]

IMAGES Intravenous Magnesium Efficacy in Stroke [trial]

IMAI internal mammary artery implant

I$_{max}$ maximum [drug-induced] inhibition

IMB intensity-modulated beam [radiotherapy]; intermenstrual bleeding

IMBC indirect maximum breathing capacity

IMBI Institute of Medical and Biological Illustrators

IMC indigent medical care; information-memory-concentration [test]; intelligent monitoring and control; interdigestive migrating contractions; internal mammary chain; internal medicine clinic; internal model control; International Medical Corps; intestinal mast cell

IMCD inner medullary collecting duct

IMCI Integrated Management of Childhood Illness

IMC-N inframammary crease-to-nipple distance

IMCT Information-Memory-Concentration Test; International Multicentre Trial

IMCU intermediate medical care unit

IMD immunodeficiency; immunologically mediated disease; information management department; institution for mentally disabled; intratumoral microvessel density

ImD$_{50}$ median immunizing dose

IMDC intramedullary metatarsal decompression

IMDD idiopathic midline destructive disease

IMDDI individual molecular dataset diversity index

IMDG International Maritime Dangerous Goods [code]

IMDM Iscove's modified Dulbecco's medium

IMDP imidocarb dipropionate

IMDRF International Medical Device Regulators Forum

IME independent medical examination; indirect medical education

IMEG innovations in medical education grant

IMEL International Medical Electronic Link

IMEM improved minimum essential medium

IMEP Investigation in Menopausal Women of the Effect of Estradiol and Progesterone on Cardiovascular Risk Factors

IMET isometric endurance test

IMEX image segmentation

IMF idiopathic myelofibrosis; immunofluorescence; inframammary fold; installation medical facility; intermaxillary fixation;

intermediate filament; International Myeloma Foundation; intramaxillary fixation; Irish Medicines Formulary

IMG industry-made graft; inferior mesenteric ganglion; internal medicine group; international medical graduate

IMGG intramuscular gammaglobulin

IMGT International Immuno-Genetics Database

IMH idiopathic myocardial hypertrophy; indirect microhemagglutination [test]

IMHP 1-(iodomercuri)-2-hydroxypropane

IMHS intramedullary hip screw

IMHT indirect microhemagglutination test

IMI immunologically measurable insulin; impending myocardial infarction; Imperial Mycological Institute; inferior myocardial infarction; intelligent medical implant; intermeal interval; internal motility index; intramuscular injection

Imi imipramine

IMIA International Medical Informatics Association

IMIA-NI International Medical Informatics Association-Nursing Informatics

IMIA-NI/SIG International Medical Informatics Association-Nursing Informatics, Special Internet Group

IMIC International Medical Information Center

IMIMC interdigestive migrating myoelectric complex

IMIS Integrative Molecular Information System

IML intermediolateral

IMLA intramural left anterior [artery]

IMLAD intramural left anterior descending [artery]

IMLNS idiopathic minimal lesion nephrotic syndrome

ImLy immune lysis

IMM immunization [database]; inhibitor-containing minimal medium; inner mitochondrial membrane; internal medial malleolus

immat immature, immaturity

IMMC interdigestive migrating motor complex

immun immune, immunity, immunization

IMN internal mammary node

IMO idiopathic multicentric osteolysis; Irish Medical Organisation

imoa instantaneous maximum over the array

immobil immobilization, immobilize

IMP idiopathic myeloid proliferation; impression; incomplete male pseudohermaphroditism; individual Medicaid practitioner; inosine 5'-monophosphate; intramembranous particle;

intramuscular compartment pressure; *N*-iso-propyl-*p*-iodoamphetamine

Imp impression

imp impacted, impaction; impaired

IMPA incisal mandibular plane angle

IMPAC Information for Management, Planning, Analysis, and Coordination

IMPACT Immunisation Monitoring Programme Active; Initiatives to Mobilize for the Prevention and Control of Tobacco Use; Integrilin to Minimize Platelet Aggregation and Prevent Coronary Thrombosis [trial]; Interdisciplinary Maternal Perinatal Australasian Clinical Trials; International Mexiletine and Placebo Antiarrhythmia Coronary Trial

IMPACT-II Integrilin to Minimize Platelet Aggregation and Coronary Thrombosis [trial]

IMPACT-AMI Integrilin to Minimize Platelet Aggregation and Prevent Coronary Thrombosis-Acute Myocardial Infarction [trial]

IMPACT-Stent Integrilin to Minimize Platelet Aggregation and Coronary Thrombosis in Stenting [trial]

IMPATH interactive microcomputer patient assessment tool for health

IMPC International Myopia Prevention Center

IMPD inosine-5'-monophosphate dehydrogenase

IMPDH inosine-5'-monophosphate dehydrogenase

IMPDHL inosine-5'-monophosphate dehydrogenase-like

IMPG interphotoreceptor matrix proteoglycan

IMPR integrated microscopy resource

IMPRESS Intramural Low Molecular Weight Heparin for Prevention of Restenosis Study

IMPROVED Influence of Introduction of Mycophenolate Mofetil and Reduction of Cyclosporine on Renal Dysfunction After Cardiac Transplantation [study]

IMPS Inpatient Multidimensional Psychiatric Scale; intact months of patient survival

Impx impacted

IMR individual medical record; infant mortality rate; infant mortality risk; Institute for Medical Research; integrated microscopy resource; intelligent medical record

IMRI intraoperative magnetic resonance imaging

IMRT intensity modulated radiotherapy

IMS image management system; immunomagnetic separation; incurred in military service; Indian Medical Service; industrial methylated spirit; information management system; integrated medical services; international metric system; Internet map server; ion mobility spectrometry

IMSI international mobile subscriber identity

IMSN International Medication Safety Network

iMSP ideal midsagittal plane

IMSS in-flight medical support system

IMT immunomodulatory therapy; indomethacin; induced muscular tension; inflammatory myofibroblastic tumor; inspiratory muscle training; intimal mean thickness

IM&T information management and technology

IMU Index of Medical Underservice

IMV inferior mesenteric vein; informative morphogenetic variant; intelligent magic view [imaging]; intermittent mandatory ventilation; intermittent mechanical ventilation; intracellular mature virion; isophosphamide, methotrexate, and vincristine

IMViC, imvic indole, methyl red, Voges-Proskauer, citrate [test]

IMVP idiopathic mitral valve prolapse

IMVS Institute of Medical and Veterinary Science

IN icterus neonatorum; impetigo neonatorum; incidence; incompatibility number; infundibular nucleus; insulin; integrase; interneuron; interstitial nephritis; intranasal; irritation of nociceptors

In index; indium; inion; insulin; inulin

in inch

in^2 square inch

in^3 cubic inch

INA infectious nucleic acid; inferior nasal artery; instrumentation amplifier; International Neurological Association

I$_{Na}$ sodium current

INAA instrumental neutron activation analysis

INABIS First Internet World Congress for Biomedical Sciences

INAD infantile neuroaxonal dystrophy

INAH isonicotinic acid hydrazide

INANE International Academy of Nursing Editors

INB internuclear bridging; ischemic necrosis of bone

inbr inbreeding

INC inside needle catheter; intensive neonatal care; internodular cortex

inc incision; inclusion; incompatibility; incontinent; increase, increased; increment; incurred

INCB International Narcotics Control Board

INCD infantile nuclear cerebral degeneration

IN-CHF Italian Network Congestive Heart Failure

INCL infantile neuronal ceroid lipofuscinosis

incl inclusion or include

INCLEN International Clinical Epidemiology Network

incr increase, increased; increment

incur incurable

IND indomethacin; industrial medicine; investigational new drug

ind indirect; induction

INDANA Individual Data Analysis of Antihypertensive Intervention Trials

indep independent

indic indicated, indication

indig indigestion

indiv individual

INDO indoleamine-2,3-dioxygenase; indomethacin

INDOR internuclear double resonance

indust industrial

INE infantile necrotizing encephalomyelopathy

INEPT insensitive nuclei enhanced by polarization transfer

INET image network

INF infant, infantile; infected, infection, infective; inferior; infirmary; infundibulum; infusion; interferon; intravenous nutritional fluid

Inf influenza

inf infant, infantile; inferior

INF APC inferoapical

infect infected, infection, infective

INFH ischemic necrosis of femur head

Inflamm inflammation, inflammatory

inf mono infectious mononucleosis

InfoMAP information management and assessment process

INFORMM Information Network for On-line Retrieval and Medical Management

INFSEC information security

INFV Inner Farne virus

ING isotope nephrogram

ing inguinal

InGP indolglycerophosphate

INH Indian hedgehog homolog; inhalation; inhibitor; isoniazid; isonicotinic acid hydrazide

INHA inhibin alpha

inhal inhalation

INHB inhibin beta

INHBA inhibitin beta A

INHBB inhibitin beta B

INHBC inhibitin beta C

inhib inhibiting, inhibition

INH-PT isonicotinic acid hydrazide preventive therapy
INI intranuclear inclusion
INIRC International Non-Ionizing Radiation Committee
inj injection; injured, injurious, injury
INJECT International Joint Efficacy Comparison of Thrombolytics [trial]; International Joint Evaluation of Coronary Thrombolysis [trial]
inject injection
INJR injury or poisoning
INK injury not known
INKV Inkoo virus
INL International Nursing Library
INLINIS Ireland-Netherlands Lisinopril-Nifedipine Study
INLSD ichthyosis and neutral lipid storage disease
i-NMDS international nursing minimum dataset
INN in-network; International Nonproprietary Name; intestinal noise
innerv innervated, innervation
innom innominate
INNOVO Inhaled Nitric Oxide Compared to Ventilatory Support Without Inhaled Nitric Oxide [trial]
INO inosine; internuclear ophthalmoplegia
Ino inosine
INOC isonicotinoyloxycarbonyl
inoc inoculated, inoculation
inorg inorganic
iNOS inducible macrophage-type nitric oxide synthase
Inox inosine, oxidized
INP idiopathic neutropenia
INPAV intermittent negative-pressure assisted ventilation
INPC isopropyl *N*-phenyl carbamate
INPEA isopropyl nitrophenylethanolamine
INPH iproniazid phosphate
INPHO Information Network for Public Health Officials; Integrated Network for Public Health Officials
INPP1 inositol polyphosphate 1-phosphatase
INPV intermittent negative-pressure ventilation
INQ interior nasal quadrant
InQ inquiry mode questionnaire
InQ(R) inquiry mode questionnaire, reliability assessment
INR international normalized ratio
INREM internal roentgen-equivalent, man
INRIA Institut National de Recherche en Informatique et en Automatique [National Institute for Research in Computer Science and Control]

INROAD In-Stent Restenosis Optimal Angioplasty Device [trial]
INRT involved node radation therapy
INS idiopathic nephrotic syndrome; implantable neurostimulator; information networking system; Infusion Nurses Society; insulin; insurance
Ins insulin; insurance, insured
ins insertion; insulin; insurance, insured
INSECT intensity normalized stereotaxic environment for classification of tissues
insem insemination
INSIGHT International Nifedipine Study Intervention as a Goal in Hypertension Treatment
insol insoluble
INSP, Insp inspiration
INSPIRE Increasing Participation in Cardiac Rehabilitation [study]; Intravascular Ultrasound Study Predictor of Restenosis [trial]
INSR insulin receptor
INSRR insulin receptor–related receptor
INSS international neuroblastoma staging system
Inst institute
instab instability
instill instillation
insuf insufflation
insuff insufficiency, insufficient; insufflation
INT interference; intermediate; intermittent; intern, internal; internship; interval; intestinal; intima; *p*-iodonitrotetrazolium
Int international; intestinal
int internal
INTACT International Nifedipine Trial on Antiatherosclerotic Therapy
INTEG integument
INTEL-SAT international communication satellite
INTERCEPT Incomplete Infarction Trial of European Research Collaborators Evaluating Prognosis Post-Thrombolysis
INTERHEALTH Integrated Programme for Community Health and Noncommunicable Diseases
InterLymph International Lymphoma Epidemiology Consortium
INTERMAP International Study of Macronutrients and Blood Pressure
intern internal
Internat international
INTERSALT International Study of Salt and Blood Pressure
INTERSEPT International Sepsis Trial
intes intestine
Intest intestine, intestinal
Int/Ext internal/external

INTH intrathecal
INTIMA Infusion of Tissue Plasminogen-Activator in Myocardial Infarction at the Acute Phase [study]
in-TIME Intravenous Lanoteplase for Treating Infarcting Myocardium Early [trial]
Intmd intermediate
Int Med internal medicine
INTOX, Intox intoxication
INTR intermittent
INTRO-AMI Integrilin and Reduced Dose of Thrombolysis in Acute Myocardial Infarction
Int Rot internal rotation
INTRP Inventory of Negative Thoughts in Response to Pain
INTRUC Introducing Catheter [study]
Int trx intermittent traction
intub intubation
INV inferior nasal vein; Inini virus
Inv, inv inversion; involuntary
INVEST International Verapamil SR/Trandolapril [study]
invest investigation
Inv/Ev inversion/eversion
inv ins inverted insertion
INVM isolated noncompaction of left ventricular myocardium
invol involuntary
involv involved, involvement
inv(p+q−), inv(p−q+) pericentric inversion
IO incisal opening; inferior oblique; inferior olive; internal os; interorbital; intestinal obstruction; intraocular; intraoperative; intraosseous
I&O in and out; intake and output
I/O input/output; intake/output
Io ionium; onset of inspiration
IO$_2$ inspired oxygen
IOA inner optic anlage; International Osteopathic Association
IOC International Organizing Committee on Medical Librarianship; intern on call; intraoperative cholangiography
IOCG intraoperative cholangiogram
IOCM iso-osmolar contrast medium
IOD information object model; injured on duty; integrated optical density; interorbital distance
IOE intraoperative echocardiography
IOECS intraoperative electrocortical stimulation
IOERT intraoperative electron beam radiation therapy
IOFB intraocular foreign body
IOH idiopathic orthostatic hypotension
IOHDR intraoperative high dose rate
IOL induction of labor; intraocular lens

IOM inferior orbitomental; infraorbital margin; Institute of Medicine; Institute of Occupational Medicine; interosseous membrane; intraoperative monitoring
IOML infraorbitomeatal line
IOMP International Organization for Medical Physics
IOMSN International Organization of Multiple Sclerosis Nurses
ION ischemic optic neuropathy
IONDT Ischemic Optic Neuropathy Decompression Trial
IONM intraoperative neuromonitoring
IOP improving organizational performance; intensive outpatient; intraocular pressure
IOPR intraoperative patient representation
IOR index of refraction; index of response; interoperable object reference
IORT intraoperative radiotherapy
IOS infant observation scale; International Organization for Standardization; intraoperative sonography
IOS RF intact outlet strut resonance frequency
IOT intraocular tension; intraocular transfer; ipsilateral optic tectum
IOTA information overload testing aid
IOTEE intraoperative transesophageal echocardiography
IOTF International Obesity Task Force
IOU intensive care observation unit; international opacity unit
IOUS intraoperative ultrasound
IOV inside-out vesicle
IOVA intraocular vision aid
IP icterus praecox; imaging plate; immune precipitate; immunoblastic plasma; immunoperoxidase technique; inactivated pepsin; incisoproximal; incisopulpal; incontinentia pigmenti; incubation period; induced potential; induction period; infection prevention; inflation point; infundibular process; infusion pump; inhibition period; inorganic phosphate; inosine phosphorylase; inositol phosphate; inpatient; instantaneous pressure; intermediate purity; International Pharmacopoeia; Internet protocol; interpeduncular; interphalangeal; interpupillary; intestinal pseudoobstruction; intramuscular pressure; intraperitoneal; intrapulmonary; inverse planning; inverted papilloma; ionization potential; ischemic preconditioning; isoelectric point; isoproterenol; L'Institut Pasteur
IP1 incontinentia pigmenti 1
IP$_1$ inositol-1-phosphate
IP2 incontinentia pigmenti 2
IP$_3$ inositol triphosphate
IP$_4$ inositol 1,3,4,5-tetraphosphate

Ip peak of inspiratory effort
I_p ionic current pump
ip intraperitoneal
i/p inpatient
IPA idiopathic pulmonary arteriosclerosis; immunoperoxidase assay; incontinentia pigmenti achromians; independent physician association; independent practice association; individual practice association; infantile papular acrodermatitis; International Pediatric Association; International Pharmaceutical Association; International Psychoanalytical Association; International Psychogeriatric Association; intrapleural analgesia; isopropyl alcohol; marker for detecting ovarian cancer
I_pa pulse average intensity
IPAA ileal pouch−anal anastomosis; International Psychoanalytical Association
IPAB Independent Payment Advisory Board
IPAC Information Policy Advisory Committee
IPAG The Influenza and Pneumonia Action Group
IPAP inspiratory positive airway pressure
IPAQ International Physical Activity Questionnaire
I-para primipara
IPAT Institute of Personality and Ability Testing; Iowa Pressure Articulation Test
iPAT integrated Parallel Acquisition Techniques
IPB injury-prone behavior; integrated problem-based curriculum
IPBH intraparenchymal brain hemorrhage
IPC infection prevention and control [measures]; intermittent pneumatic compression; International Poliomyelitis Congress; interpeduncular cistern; interpersonal process of care; ion pair chromatography; ischemic preconditioning; isopropyl carbamate; isopropyl chlorophenyl
IPCD infantile polycystic disease
IPCFC intermittent pneumatic calf and foot compression
IPCL intrapapillary capillary loop
IPCP interdisciplinary patient care plan
IPCS International Program on Chemical Safety; intrauterine progesterone contraception system
IPD idiopathic Parkinson disease; idiopathic protracted diarrhea; immediate pigment darkening; impedance plethysmography; increase in pupillary diameter; incurable problem drinker; inflammatory pelvic disease; intermittent peritoneal dialysis; intermittent pigment darkening; International Pharmacopeal Database; interocular phase difference; interpupillary distance; Inventory of Psychosocial Development

IPE infectious porcine encephalomyelitis; interstitial pulmonary emphysema
IΦE International Partnership in Health Information Education
IPEH intravascular papillary endothelial hyperplasia
IPF idiopathic pulmonary fibrosis; infection-potentiating factor; insulin promoter factor; interstitial pulmonary fibrosis
IPFM integral pulse frequency modulation
IPFM/SDC integral pulse frequency modulation/Smith delay compensator
IPG impedance plethysmography; inspiration-phase gas
iPGE immunoreactive prostaglandin E
IPH idiopathic portal hypertension; idiopathic pulmonary hemosiderosis; idiopathic pulmonary hypertension; inflammatory papillary hyperplasia; International Partnership for Health; interphalangeal; intraparenchymal hemorrhage; intraperitoneal hemorrhage
IPHR inverted polypoid hamartoma of the rectum
IPI interpotential interval; interpulse interval
IPIA immunoperoxidase infectivity assay
IPITA International Pancreas and Islet Transplant Association
IPJ interphalangeal joint
IPK intractable plantar keratosis
IPKD infantile polycystic kidney disease
IPL inner plexiform layer; intense pulsed light; intrapleural
IPM impulses per minute; inches per minute; interphotoreceptor matrix
IPMA intraductal papillary mucinous adenoma
IPMB borderline intraductal papillary mucinous neoplasm
IPMC intraductal papillary mucinous carcinoma
IPMI information processing in medical imaging
IPMN intraductal papillary mucinous neoplasm
IPMS inhibited power motive syndrome
IPMT intraductal papillary mucinous tumor
IPN immunization program nurse; infantile polyarteritis nodosa; infectious pancreatic necrosis; interductal papillary neoplasm; intern progress note; interpeduncular nucleus; interstitial pneumonitis
IPNA isopropyl noradrenalin
IPNV infectious pancreatic necrosis virus
IPO improved pregnancy outcome
IPOF immediate postoperative fitting
IPOIC immediate postoperative instillation of intravesical chemotherapy

IPOP immediate postoperative prosthesis
IPP independent practice plan; individual patient profile; inflatable penile prosthesis; inorganic pyrophosphate; inspiratory plateau pressure; intermittent positive pressure; intracisternal A-particle–promoted polypeptide; intrahepatic partial pressure; intrapericardial pressure
Ipp interpulse potential
IPPA inspection, palpation, percussion, and auscultation; iodophenylpentadecanoic acid
IPPB intermittent positive-pressure breathing
IPPB-I intermittent positive-pressure breathing, inspiration
IPPHS International Primary Pulmonary Hypertension Study
IPPI interruption of pregnancy for psychiatric indication
IPPO intermittent positive-pressure inflation with oxygen
IPPPSH International Prospective Primary Prevention Study in Hypertension
IPPR integrated pancreatic polypeptide response; intermittent positive-pressure respiration
IPPV intermittent positive-pressure ventilation
IPPYV Ippy virus
IPQ intimacy potential quotient
IPR imidozaline-preferring receptor; immediate phase reaction; independent professional review; Institute for Process Control and Robotics; insulin production rate; interval patency rate; intraparenchymal resistance; ipratropium; iproniazid
IP₃R IP_3R inositol 1,4,5-triphosphate receptor
i-Pr isopropyl
IPRD intellectual product
IPRL isolated perfused rat liver/lung
iProClass integrated protein classification
IPRT interpersonal reaction test
IPS idiopathic pain syndrome; idiopathic postprandial syndrome; immersive projection system; inches per second; infundibular pulmonary stenosis; initial prognostic score; intensive care unit point system; intermittent photic stimulation; interpractice system; intrapartum stillbirth; intraperitoneal shock; ischiopubic synchondrosis
ips inches per second
IPSB index of proximity to stability boundary
IPSC inhibitory postsynaptic current
IPSC-E Inventory of Psychic and Somatic Complaints in the Elderly
IPSF immediate postsurgical fitting
IPSID immunoproliferative small intestine disease

IPSP inhibitory postsynaptic potential
IPSS inferior petrosal sinus sampling; International Prostate Symptom Score
IPT immunoperoxidase technique; immunoprecipitation; information processing theory; interpersonal psychotherapy; isoniazid preventive therapy; isoproterenol
IPTG isopropyl-β-thiogalactopyranoside; isopropyl thiogalactose
iPTH immunoassay for parathyroid hormone; immunoreactive parathyroid hormone
IPTT Initiative for Pharmaceutical Technology Transfer
IPTX intermittent pelvic traction
IpTX imperatoxin
IpTxa imperatoxin A
IpTxi imperatoxin I
IPU inpatient unit
IPV inactivated poliomyelitis vaccine/virus; infectious pustular vaginitis; infectious pustular vulvovaginitis; interpersonal violence, intimate partner violence; intrapulmonary vein
IPW interphalangeal width
IPZ insulin protamine zinc
IQ inhibitory quotient; institute of quality; intelligence quotient
IQAS internal quality assurance system
IQB individual quick blanch
IQCODE information questionnaire on cognitive decline in the elderly
IQOLA International Quality of Life Assessment
IQR interquartile range
IQ&S iron, quinine, and strychnine
IQW interactive query workstation
IR drop of voltage across a resistor produced by a current; ileal resection; immediate release; immune response; immunization rate; immunoreactive; immunoreagent; in room; impedance rheography; index of response; individual reaction; inferior rectus; inflow resistance; information retrieval; infrared; infrarenal; inside radius; insoluble residue; inspiratory reserve; inspiratory resistance; insulin resistance; intermediate representation; internal resistance; internal rotation; interventional radiology; intrarectal; intrarenal; inversion recovery; inverted repeat; irritant reaction; ischemia-reperfusion; isovolumic relaxation
I-R Ito-Reenstierna [reaction]
I/R ischemia/reperfusion
Ir immune response; iridium
ir immunoreactive; intrarectal; intrarenal
IRA ileorectal anastomosis; immunoradioassay; immunoregulatory alpha-globulin;

inactive renin activity; individual regression analysis; infarct-related artery; inwardly rectifying

IR-ACTH immunoreactive adrenocorticotropic hormone

IRAD International Registry of Acute Aortic Dissection

IrANP, ir-ANP immunoreactive atrial natriuretic peptide

IR-APAP immediate release acetaminophen

IRAR Immunization Registry Annual Report

IRAS Insulin Resistance Atherosclerosis Study

IR-AVP immunoreactive arginine-vasopressin

IRB immunoreactive bead; institutional review board

IRBBB incomplete right bundle branch block

IRBC immature red blood cell; infected red blood cell

ir-BNP immunoreactive brain natriuretic peptide

IRBP intestinal retinol-binding protein

IRC implant-related complications; inspiratory reserve capacity; instantaneous resonance curve; International Red Cross; International Research Communications System

IRCA intravascular red cell aggregation

IRCC International Red Cross Committee

IRCU intensive respiratory care unit

IRD infantile Refsum disease; isorhythmic dissociation

IrDA infrared data association

IRDM insulin-resistant diabetes mellitus

IRDP insulin-related DNA polymorphism

IRDS idiopathic respiratory distress syndrome; infant respiratory distress syndrome

IRE intelligent rules element; internal rotation in extension; iron regulatory element; iron-responsive element; irreversible electroporation; isolated rabbit eye

IREBP iron-responsive element binding protein

IRED infrared emission detection; infrared light-emitting diode

IREE infrared ray electronic endoscopy

IRES internal ribosome entry site; ischemia residua

IRF idiopathic retroperitoneal fibrosis; impulse response function; installation response force; interferon regulatory factor; internal rotation in flexion

IRFL integral red fluorescence

IRFPA infrared focal plan array

IRG immunoreactive gastrin; immunoreactive glucagon

IRGH immunoreactive growth hormone

IRGl immunoreactive glucagon

IRH Institute for Research in Hypnosis; Institute for Religion and Health; intrarenal hemorrhage

IRHCS immunoradio-assayable human chorionic somatomammotropin

IRhGH immunoreactive human growth hormone

IRhPL immunoreactive human placental lactogen

IRI immunoreactive insulin; [near]-infrared interreactance; insulin resistance index

IRIA indirect radioimmunoassay

IRIg insulin-reactive immunoglobulin

IRIS immune reconstitution inflammatory syndrome; Integrated Risk Information System; interleukin regulation of immune system; International Research Information Service; Isosents for Reperfusion Intervention Study

IRIV immuno-potentiating reconstituted influenza virosome; Irituia virus

IRK inwardly rectifying potassium [channel]

IRLED, IR-LED infrared light-emitting diode

IRM industry reference material; information resource management; innate releasing mechanism; insect resistance management; Institute of Rehabilitation Medicine

IRMA immunoradiometric assay; intraretinal microvascular abnormalities

iRNA immune ribonucleic acid; informational ribonucleic acid

ir-NP immunoreactive natriuretic peptide

IROS intelligent robots and systems; ipsilateral routing of signal

IROX iridium oxide

IRP immunoreactive plasma; immunoreactive proinsulin; incus replacement prosthesis; insulin-releasing polypeptide; interstitial radiation pneumonitis; intraocular retinal prosthesis

IRPA International Radiation Protection Association

IRPA/INIRC International Radiation Protection Association's International Non-Ionizing Radiation Committee

IRPTC International Registry of Potentially Toxic Chemicals

IRR incident/rate ratio; insulin receptor−related receptor; intrarenal reflux

Irr irradiation; irritation

IRRD Institute for Research in Rheumatic Diseases

irreg irregular, irregularity

irrig irrigate, irrigation

IRS immunoreactive secretion; incident reporting scheme; infrared sensor; infrared spectrophotometry; insulin receptor species; insulin receptor substrate; insulin-related substrate; Intergroup Rhabdomyosarcoma Study; internal resolution site; International Rhinologic Society; Invasive Reperfusion Study; ionizing radiation sensitivity

IRS-1, -2 insulin receptor substrates 1 and 2

IRSA idiopathic refractory sideroblastic anemia; iodinated rat serum albumin

IRSE inversion recovery spin-echo

IRT immunoreactive trypsin; interresponse time; interstitial radiotherapy; intestinal replacement therapy; item response theory

IRTIS Integrated Radiation Therapy Information System

IRTO immunoreactive trypsin output

IRTU integrating regulatory transcription unit

IRU industrial rehabilitation unit; interferon reference unit

IRV inferior radicular vein; inspiratory reserve volume; intelligent radiology workstation; inverse ratio ventilation

IrVd Iresine viroid

IRW intelligent radiology workstation

IRX Information Retrieval Experimental Workbench

IS ileal segment; iliosacral; immediate sensitivity; immune serum; immunostaining; immunosuppression; impingement syndrome; incentive spirometer; index of sexuality; infant size; infantile spasms; information services; information system; infundibular septum; insertion sequence; in situ; insulin secretion; interaction site; intercellular space; intercostal space; interictal spike; international standards; interstitial space; interventricular system; intracardiac shunt; intraspinal; intrasplenic; intrastriatal; intraventricular septum; invalided from service; inversion sequence; ischemic score; isoproterenol

I-S incudostapedial

Is incision superius

is in situ; island; islet; isolated

ISA ileosigmoid anastomosis; Information Science Abstracts; Instrument Society of America; Instrumentation, Systems, and Automation Society; intracarotid sodium amytal; intraoperative suture adjustment; intrinsic simulating activity; intrinsic stimulation activity; intrinsic sympathomimetic activity; iodinated serum albumin; irregular spiking activity

I$_{sa}$ spatial average intensity [pulse]

ISAAA International Service for the Acquisition of Agri-Biotech Applications

ISAAC International Study of Asthma and Allergies in Childhood

ISADH inappropriate secretion of antidiuretic hormone

ISAGA immunosorbent agglutination assay

ISAM indexed sequential access manager; interferometric synthetic aperture microscopy; Intravenous Streptokinase in Acute Myocardial Infarction [trial]

I$_{sapa}$ spatial average, pulse average intensity

ISAPS International Society of Aesthetic Plastic Surgery

ISAR individualizable drug-eluting stent system to abrogate restenosis; Intracoronary Stenting and Antithrombotic Regimen [trial]

I$_{sata}$ spatial average, temporal average intensity

ISB incentive spirometry breathing

ISBI International Society for Burn Injuries

ISBP International Society for Biochemical Pharmacology

ISBT International Society for Blood Transfusion

ISC immunoglobulin-secreting cells; information system center; innerstrand crosslink; insoluble collagen; intensive supportive care; International Society of Cardiology; International Society of Chemotherapy; intershift coordination; interstitial cell; irreversibly sickled cell

IS&C image save and carry

Isc short circuit current

ISCAB Israeli Coronary Artery Bypass [study]

ISCAS International Society for Computer-Aided Surgery

ISCB International Society for Computational Biology

ISCD International Society for Clinical Densitometry

ISCF interstitial cell fluid

ISCL integrated secure communication layer

ISCLT International Society for Clinical Laboratory Technology

ISCM International Society of Cybernetic Medicine

ISCN International System for Human Cytogenetic Nomenclature

ISCO immunostimulating complex [vaccine]; Information System for Clinical Oncology

ISCOAT Italian Study on Complications of Oral Anticoagulant Therapy

ISCOM immune stimulatory complexes in matrix

ISCP infection surveillance and control program; International Society of Comparative Pathology

ISCVS International Society for Cardiovascular Surgery

ISCW immunosuppression of streptococcal wall

ISD immunosuppressive drug; implant support device; Information Services Division; inhibited sexual desire; intermediate sulfate domain; International Society of Dermatology; interset distance; interstimulus distance; interventricular septal defect; isosorbide dinitrate

ISDB information source database

ISDN integrated services digital network; isosorbide dinitrate

iSDR inducible stable DNA replication

ISE inhibited sexual excitement; intelligent synthesis environment; International Society of Endocrinology; International Society of Endoscopy; inversion spin-echo pulse sequence; ion-selective electrode

ISEFT ion-sensitive field-effect transistor

ISEK International Society of Electrophysiology and Kinesiology

ISEM immunosorbent electron microscopy

ISF interstitial fluid

ISFC International Society and Federation of Cardiology

ISFV interstitial fluid volume; Isfahan virus

ISG Ibopamine Study Group [trial]; immune serum globulin

ISGE International Society of Gastroenterology

ISH in situ hybridization; icteric serum hepatitis; internal self helper; International Society of Hematology; International Society of Hypertension; isolated septal hypertrophy; isolated systolic hypertension

ISHAM International Society for Human and Animal Mycology

ISHT International Society for Heart Transplantation

ISHTAR Implementing Secure Healthcare Telematics Application

ISI infarct size index; information science innovations; initial slope index; injection scan interval; injury severity index; Institute for Scientific Information; insulin sensitivity index; International Sensitivity Index; International Standardized Index; interstimulus interval

ISIH interspike interval histogram

ISIS image-selected in vivo spectroscopy; imaging science and information system; Information Society Initiative for Standardization; information system—imaging system; integrated survey information system; intelligent selection and imaging studies; interactive

system for image selection; International Infarct Survival [Trial]; International Study of Infarct Survival

ISIS-2 Second International Infarct Survival [trial]

ISIT interactive simulation and identification tool

ISKDC International Study of Kidney Diseases in Childhood

ISKV Issyl-Kul virus

ISL inner scapular line; instrumental spatial linkage; International Society of Lymphology; interspinous ligament; isoleucine

ISLAND Infant Size Limitation: Acute N-Acetylcysteine Defense [trial]

ISLAV Isla Vista virus

ISM industrial-scientific-medical; Information Source Map; International Society of Microbiologists; intersegmental muscle

ISMB Intelligent System for Molecular Biology

ISMED International Society on Metabolic Eye Disease

ISMH International Society of Medical Hydrology and Climatology

ISMHO International Society for Mental Health Online

ISMN isosorbide mononitrate

ISMP Institute for Safe Medication Practices

ISN integrated service network; International Society of Nephrology; International Society of Neurochemistry

ISNCC International Society of Nurses in Cancer Care

ISO incident safety officer; International Organization for Standardization; isoprenaline

iso isoproterenol; isotropic

ISOBM International Society for Oncodevelopmental Biology and Medicine

isol isolated, isolation

isom isometric

ISP distance between iliac spines; international standardized profile; Internet service provider; interspace; interstitial pressure; intraspinal; isoproterenol

I$_{sp}$ spatial peak intensity [pulse]

ISPC intermittent sequential pneumatic compression

ISPCR in situ polymerase chain reaction

ISPI integrated services protocol instrument

ISPN International Society of Psychiatric-Mental Health Nurses

ISPO International Society for Prosthetics and Orthotics

ISPOCD International Study of Post-operative Cognitive Dysfunction

ISPOT International Study of Perioperative Transfusion

I_spta spatial peak, temporal average intensity

I_sppa spatial peak, pulse average intensity

ISPRM International Society of Physical and Rehabilitation Medicine

ISPS International Society of Pediatric Surgery

ISPT interspecies ovum penetration test

isq unchanged [L. *in status quo*]

ISR image service representative; information storage and retrieval; injection site reaction; Institute for Sex Research; Institute of Surgical Research; insulin secretion rate; intelligent stroke registry; International Sanitary Regulations

ISRE interferon-stimulated response element

ISRI Information Science Research Institute

ISRM International Society of Reproductive Medicine

ISRT involved site radiation therapy

ISS idiopathic short stature; immunostimulatory sequence; infantile sialic acid storage [disease]; inferior sagittal sinus; injury severity scale; injury severity score; instructional support services; International Society of Surgery; invasive surgical staging; ion-scattering spectroscopy; ion surface scattering; isotonic saline solution

ISSCBW Inter-Service Sub-Committee on Biological Warfare

ISSD infantile sialic acid storage disease

ISSHP International Society for the Study of Hypertension in Pregnancy

ISSI interspinous surgical staging; interview schedule for social interaction; Israeli Study of Surgical Infections

ISSIR International Society of Sexual and Impotence Research

ISSM International Society for Sexual Medicine

ISSN international standard serial number

ISSX International Society for the Study of Xenobiotics

IST inappropriate sinus tachycardia; insulin sensitivity test; insulin shock therapy; International Society on Toxicology; International Stroke Trial; isometric systolic tension

IS&T Society for Imaging Science and Technology

ISTAHC International Society of Technology Assessment in Healthcare

ISTC [Department of] Industry, Science, and Technology of Canada

ISTD International Society of Tropical Dermatology

ISTM International Society of Travel Medicine

ISTU isometric strength testing unit

ISU International Society of Urology

I-sub inhibitor substance

ISUP International Society of Urological Pathology

ISV integrated simulation and verification

ISVP infectious subviral particle; intermediate subviral particle

ISW interstitial water

ISWI incisional surgical wound infection

ISY intrasynovial

IT iliotibial; immunologic test; immunotherapy; immunotoxin; implantation test; individual therapy; inferior turbinate; information technology; inhalation test; inhalation therapy; injection time; insulin therapy; intensive therapy; intentional tremor; intermittent traction; internal telomere; interstitial tissue; intradermal test; intratesticular; intrathecal; intrathoracic; intratracheal; intratracheal tube; intratuberous; intratumoral; ischial tuberosity; isolation transformer; isomeric transition

I/T information technology; intensity/time

I&T intolerance and toxicity

I-T interrupter technique

IT² Internet technology for the twenty-first century

ITA inferior temporal artery; information transmission analysis; internal thoracic artery; International Tuberculosis Association

I_ta temporal average intensity

ITAM immunoreceptor tyrosine activation motif

ITAV Itaituba virus

ITB iliotibial band

ITBS iliotibial band syndrome

ITC imidazolyl-thioguanine chemotherapy; infant toddler checklist; inferior temporal cortex; information and communication technology; Interagency Testing Committee; in the canal [hearing aid]; intrathecal chemotherapy; intratubular fluid concentration; isothermal titration calorimetry; isothiocyanate

ITc International Table calorie

ITCM information technology for crises management teams

ITCP idiopathic thrombocytopenic purpura

ITCVD ischemic thrombotic cerebrovascular disease

ITD idiopathic torsion dystonia; intensely transfused dialysis; intratypic differentiation; iodothyronine deiodinase

ITE information technology equipment; insufficient therapeutic effect; in the ear [hearing aid]; in-training examination; intrapulmonary interstitial emphysema

ITEA intermittent thoracic epidural anesthesia

ITEM information and communication technology for medicine

IT-ESD insulation-tipped (diathermic knife) endoscopic submucosal dissection

ITET isotonic endurance test

ITF Interagency Tack Force; interferon; intestinal trefoil factor

ITFS iliotibial tract friction syndrome; incomplete testicular feminization syndrome

ITG integrin

ITGA integrin alpha

ITGB integrin beta

ITH interstitial hyperthermia

ITh, ith intrathecal

IThP intrathyroidal parathyroid

ITI immunotolerance induction; inter-alpha-trypsin inhibitor; International Trachoma Initiative; intertrial interval

ITIH2 inter-alpha-trypsin inhibitor, heavy chain 2

ITIL inter-alpha-trypsin inhibitor, light chain

ITIM immunoreceptor tyrosine-based inhibition motif

ITIV Itimirim virus

ITL information technology laboratory

ITLC instant thin-layer chromatography

ITM improved Thayer-Martin [medium]; intermediate transient memory; intrathecal methotrexate; Israel turkey meningoencephalitis

ITMTX intrathecal methotrexate

ITO indium tin oxide

I$_{(to)}$ transient outward current

ITOU intensive therapy observation unit

ITP idiopathic thrombocytopenic purpura; immune thrombocytopenia; immunogenic thrombocytopenic purpura; increased torque production; individualized treatment plan; inosine triphosphate; inositol 1,4,5-triphosphate; islet cell tumor of the pancreas; isotachophoresis

I$_{tp}$ temporal peak intensity

ITPA Illinois Test of Psycholinguistic Abilities; inosine triphosphatase

ITPASMT International Tissue Plasminogen Activator/Streptokinase Mortality Trial

ITPK inositol 1,4,5-triphosphate-3-kinase

ITPKA inositol 1,4,5-triphosphate-3-kinase A

ITPKB inositol 1,4,5-triphosphate-3-kinase B

ITPR inositol 1,4,5-triphosphate receptor

ITPV intratracheal pulmonary ventilation; Itaporanga virus

ITQ inferior temporal quadrant

ITQV Itaqui virus

ITR intraocular tension recorder; intratracheal; inverted terminal repeat; isotretinoin

ITRA itraconazole

ITRI Inhalation Toxicology Research Institute

ITS infective toxic shock; insulin-transferrin-selenium; intelligent tutoring system; International Twin Study; Israeli Thrombolytic Survey

ITSHD isolated thyroid-stimulating hormone deficiency

ITT insulin tolerance test; intent [or intention] to treat; internal tibial torsion

IT&T information technology and telematics

ITU intensive therapy unit; International Telecommunication Union; international toxic unit

ITUV Itupiranga virus

ITV inferior temporal vein

ITx intestinal transplantation

ITZ itraconazole

IU immunizing unit; infection unit; integral uniformity; international unit; intrauterine; in utero; 5-iodouracil

iu infectious unit

IUA intrauterine adhesions

IUAT International Union Against Tuberculosis

IUATLD International Union Against Tuberculosis and Lung Disease

IUB International Union of Biochemistry

IUBMB International Union of Biochemistry and Molecular Biology

IUBS International Union of Biological Sciences

IUC idiopathic ulcerative colitis; intrauterine catheter; inward unidirectional current

IUCD intrauterine contraceptive device

IUD intrauterine death; intrauterine device

IUDR, IUdR iodeoxyuridine

IUF isolated ultrafiltration

IUFB intrauterine foreign body

IUG infusion urogram; intrauterine gas; intrauterine growth

IUGR intrauterine growth rate; intrauterine growth retardation

IUHPE International Union for Health Promotion and Education

IUI intrauterine insemination

IUIS International Union of Immunological Societies

IU/L international units per liter

IUM internal urethral meatus; intrauterine [fetus], malnourished; intrauterine membrane

IU/min international units per minute

IUMS International Union of Microbiological Societies

IUP intrauterine pregnancy; intrauterine pressure

IUPAC International Union of Pure and Applied Chemistry

IUPAP International Union of Pure and Applied Physics

IUPAT intrauterine pregnancy at term

IUPD intrauterine pregnancy delivered

IUPESM International Union for Physical and Engineering Sciences in Medicine

IUPHAR International Union of Basic and Clinical Pharmacology

IUPS International Union of Physiological Sciences

IUPTB intrauterine pregnancy, term birth

IURES International Union of Reticuloendothelial Societies

IUT intrauterine transfusion

IUVDT International Union against Venereal Diseases and the Treponematoses

IV endometrial carcinoma extending outside the true pelvis or involving the bladder and rectum; ichnovirus; ichthyosis vulgaris; immunodeficiency virus; initial visit; interventricular; intervertebral; intravaginal; intravascular; intravenous; intraventricular; intravertebral; invasive; in vivo; in vitro; involvement of one or more extralymphatic organs [staging system for Hodgkin disease]; iodine value; iridescent virus; iridovirus; isometric virus; symbol for class 4 controlled substances

iv intravascular; intravenous

IVA interpretative value analysis; intraoperative vascular angiography; isovaleric acid

IVa endometrial carcinoma spreading to adjacent organs; vaginal carcinoma with metastases to adjacent organs

IVACG International Vitamin A Consultative Group

IVAP in vivo adhesive platelet

IVAS intracorporeal ventricular assist system

IVB intraventricular block

IVb endometrial carcinoma spreading to distant organs; vaginal carcinoma with metastases to distant organs

IVBAT intravascular bronchioalveolar tumor

IVBC intravascular blood coagulation

IVC inferior vena cava; inspiratory vital capacity; integrated vector control; intravaginal culture; intravascular coagulation; intravenous cholangiogram, intravenous cholangiography; intraventricular catheter

IVCC intravascular consumption coagulopathy

IVCD intraventricular conduction defect

IVCH intravenous cholangiography

IVC-LA inferior vena cava and left atrium

IVCP inferior vena cava pressure

IVCR inferior vena cava reconstruction

IVCT inferior vena cava thrombosis; intravenously enhanced computed tomography

IVCV inferior venacavography; Ivy vein clearing virus

IVD intervertebral disk; in vitro diagnostic device

IVDA/IVDU intravenous drug abuse/abuser—intravenous drug use/user

IVDMIA in vitro diagnostic multivariate index assay

iVDPV immunodeficiency-associated vaccine-derived poliovirus

IVDSA intravenous digital subtraction angiography

IVET in vivo expression technology

IVF interventricular foramen; intervertebral foramen; intravascular fluid; intravenous fluid; in vitro fertilization

IVFA intravenous fluorescein angiography

IVF-ET in vitro fertilization—embryo transfer

IVGG intravenous gammaglobulin

IVGTT intravenous glucose tolerance test

IVH intravenous hyperalimentation; intraventricular hemorrhage; in vitro hyperploidy

IVI intravenous infusion

IVIG, IVIg, ivIG intravenous immunoglobulin

IVISTAT Intravenous Immunoglobulin or Sulfamethoxazole/Trimethoprim as Additional Therapy for Systemic Vasculitis [study]

IVJC intervertebral joint complex

IVL intravascular lymphomatosis; involucrin

I-VLBW intubated very low birthweight

IVM intravascular mass; in vitro maturation

IVMG intravenous magnesium sulfate

IVMP intravenous methylprednisolone

IVN intravenous nutrition

IVNA in vivo neutron activation

IVNAA in vivo neutron activation analysis

IVNR interventional neuroradiology

IVOTTS Irvine viable organ—tissue transport system

IVOX intravascular oxygenator

IVP intravenous push; intravenous pyelogram, intravenous pyelography; intraventricular pressure; intravertebral vacuum phenomenon

IVPB intravenous piggyback

IVPF isovolume pressure flow curve

IVPSB International Veterinary Pathology Slide Bank

IVR idioventricular rhythm; interactive voice response; intravaginal ring; isolated volume responder

IVRA intravenous regional anesthesia

IVRS interactive voice response system
IVRT isovolumic relaxation time
IVS inappropriate vasopressin secretion; intervening sequence; interventricular septum; intervillous space
IVSA International Veterinary Students Association
IVSCT in vitro skin corrosivity test
IVSD interventricular septal defect; intraventricular septum in diastole
IVSR-UC intravenous steroids—ulcerative colitis
IVST intraventricular septal thickness
IVT index of vertical transmission; interventional video tomography; interventricular trigone; intrasound vibration test; intravenous transfusion; intraventricular; in vitro tetraploidy; isovolumetric time
IVTT in vitro transcription and translation
IVTTT intravenous tolbutamide tolerance test
IVU intravenous urography
IVUS intravascular ultrasound

IVUS/QCA Intravascular Ultrasound Quantitative Coronary Angiography [study]
IVV influenza virus vaccine; intravenous vasopressin
IVW image-viewing workstation
IW inner wall; inpatient ward; input word
IWB indeterminate Western blot [test]; index of well-being
IWGMT International Working Group on Mycobacterial Taxonomy
IWHRC Internet World Health Research Center
IWHS Iowa Women's Health Study
IWI inferior wall infarction; interwave interval
IWL insensible water loss; interwave latency
IWMI inferior wall myocardial infarct
IWPS info-window presentation system
IWRP Individualized Written Rehabilitation Program
IWS Index of Work Satisfaction
IXDB X Chromosome Integrated Database
IY$_W$ weighted incremental yield
IZ infarction zone

J dynamic movement of inertia; electric current density; flux density; joint; joule; journal; juvenile; juxtapulmonary-capillary receptor; magnetic polarization; polypeptide chain in polymeric immunoglobulins; reference point following the QRS complex, at the beginning of the ST segment [ECG]; sound intensity

J flux

j jaundice

JA jet area; judgment analysis; juvenile atrophy; juxtaarticular

JACADS Johnston Atoll chemical agent destruction system

JACV Jacareacanga virus

JAE juvenile absence epilepsy

JAHIS Japanese Association of Healthcare Information System

JAI juvenile amaurotic idiocy

JAK Janus kinase

JAK-STAT Janus kinase signal transducers and activators of transcription

JAM junction-associated membrane

JAMA *Journal of the American Medical Association*

JAMG juvenile autoimmune myasthenia gravis

JAMIA *Journal of the American Medical Informatics Association*

JaMSPUK Japanese Multicenter Study for Pro-Urokinase

JAMV Jamanxi virus

JAN Japanese accepted name

JANET Joint Academic Network

JAOA *Journal of the American Osteopathic Association*

JAPV Japanaut virus

JARIV Jari virus

JAS Jenkins Activity Survey; juvenile ankylosing spondylitis

JASTRO Japanese Society for Therapeutic Radiology and Oncology

jaund jaundice

JAV Johnston Atoll virus

JB jugular bulb

JBE Japanese B encephalitis

JBS Johanson-Blizzard syndrome

JC Jakob-Creutzfeldt [disease]; Joint Commission [formerly JCAHO]; joint contracture

J/C joules per coulomb

jc juice

JCA juvenile chronic arthritis

JCAAI Joint Council of Allergy, Asthma and Immunology

JCAE Joint Committee on Atomic Energy

JCAH Joint Commission on Accreditation of Hospitals

JCAHO Joint Commission on Accreditation of Healthcare Organizations [obsolete; now called the Joint Commission]

JCAI Joint Council of Allergy and Immunology

JCC Joint Committee on Contraception

JCD Jakob-Creutzfeldt disease

JcDNV *Junonia coenia* densovirus

JCF juvenile calcaneal fracture

JCM Japanese Collection of Microorganisms

JCML juvenile chronic myelogenous leukemia

JCN Jefferson Cancer Network

JCP juvenile chronic polyarthritis

JCPyV JC polyomavirus

JCQ job contentment questionnaire

JCRB Japanese Collection of Research Bioresources

jct junction

JCV Jakob-Creutzfeldt virus; Jamestown Canyon virus

JD jejunal diverticulitis; juvenile diabetes

JDF Juvenile Diabetes Foundation

JDM juvenile diabetes mellitus

JDMS juvenile dermatomyositis

JDRF Juvenile Diabetes Research Foundation International

JDV Juan Diaz virus

JE Japanese encephalitis; junctional escape

JEB junctional epidermolysis bullosa

JECFA Joint Expert Committee on Food Additives

JEE Japanese equine encephalitis

Jej, jej jejunum

JEMBEC agar plates for transporting cultures of gonococci

JER junctional escape rhythm

JES junkies, ex-users, substitute drug users

JET joint engineering team; junctional ectopic tachycardia

JEV Japanese encephalitis virus

JF joint fluid; jugular foramen; junctional fold

JFET junction field effect transistor

JFS jugular foramen syndrome

JG, jg juxtaglomerular

JGA juxtaglomerular apparatus

JGC juxtaglomerular cell

JGCT juvenile granulosa cell tumor; juxtaglomerular cell tumor

JGI jejunogastric intussusception; juxtaglomerular granulation index
JGP juvenile general paresis
JH jet height; juvenile hormone
J$_H$ heat transfer factor
JHA juvenile hormone analogue
JHITA Joint Healthcare Information Technology Association
JHMO junior hospital medical officer
JHPS Johns Hopkins Precursors Study
JHR Jarisch-Herxheimer reaction
JI jejunoileal; jejunoileitis; jejunoileostomy
JIA juvenile idiopathic arthritis
JIB jejunoileal bypass
JIC joint information center
JIFSAN Joint Institute for Food Safety and Applied Nutrition
JIH joint interval histogram
JIMI Japanese Intervention Trial in Myocardial Infarction
JIPID Japan International Protein Information Center
JIS Japanese industrial standard; juvenile idiopathic scoliosis
JISC Joint Information Systems Committee
JIT just-in-time
JJ jaw jerk; jejunojejunostomy
J/K joules per kelvin
J/kg joules per kilogram
JL jet length
J-LN Jervell and Lange-Nielsen [syndrome]
JLO judgment of line orientation
JLP juvenile laryngeal papilloma
JLRCPS Jerusalem Lipid Research Clinic Prevalence Study
JMD juvenile macular degeneration
JME juvenile myoclonic epilepsy; juvenile myoclonus epilepsy
JMHTS Japanese Society of Multiphasic Health Testing and Service
J-MIX Japanese medical record information exchange
JMS Juberg-Marsidi syndrome; junior medical student
JMWH *Journal of Midwifery and Women's Health*
JN Jamaican neuropathy
Jn junction
JNA Jena Nomina Anatomica
JNC Joint National Committee
JNC-V Fifth Report of the Joint National Committee on Detection, Evaluation, and Treatment of High Blood Pressure
JNC-VI Sixth Report of the Joint National Committee on Detection, Evaluation, and Treatment of High Blood Pressure
JND just noticeable difference

JNK Jun N-terminal kinase
JNP Jadassohn nevus phakomatosis
JNPA juvenile nasopharyngeal angiofibroma
JNPV juncopox virus
jnt joint
JOAG juvenile open-angle glaucoma
JOAV Joa virus
JOC joint operations center
JOD juvenile-onset diabetes
JODM juvenile-onset diabetes mellitus
JOIV Joinjakaka virus
JOR jaw opening response
JOS jaw osteosarcoma
jour journal
JP Jackson-Pratt [drain]; Japanese Pharmacopeia; joining peptide; juvenile periodontitis
JPA juvenile pilocytic astrocytoma
JPB junctional premature beat
JPC junctional premature contraction
JPD juvenile plantar dermatosis
JPEG Joint Photographic Experts Group
JPI Jackson Personality Inventory
JPN *Journal of Psychosocial Nursing*
JPS Japanese Pancreatic Society; joint position sense
JPSTH joint peristimulus histogram
JR Jolly reaction; junctional rhythm
JRA juvenile rheumatoid arthritis
JRC-CVT Joint Review Committee on Education in Cardiovascular Technology
JRC-DMS Joint Review Committee on Diagnostic Medical Sonography
JRC/EMT Joint Review Committee for Emergency Medical Technicians
JROM joint range of motion
JRT junctional recovery time
JS jejunal segment; Job syndrome; junctional slowing
J/s joules per second
JSAIR Japanese Society of Angiography and Interventional Radiology
JSATO$_2$ jugular vein oxygen saturation
JSDN Japan Standardized Disease Names
JSLIST joint service lightweight integrated suit technology
JSP Java server pages
JSRT Japanese Society of Radiologic Technology
JSRV Jaagsiekte sheep retrovirus
JSV Jerry-Slough virus
JT jejunostomy tube; junctional tachycardia
J/T joules per tesla
jt joint
JTPS juvenile tropical pancreatitis syndrome
Ju jugale
JUA Joint Underwriting Association

jug jugular
JUGV Jugra virus
junct junction
JUNV Junin virus
JURV Jurona virus
JUTV Jutiapa virus
juv juvenile
juxt near [L. *juxta*]
JV jugular vein; Junin virus
JVC jugular venous catheter

JVD jugular venous distension
JVP jugular vein pulse; jugular venous pressure; jugular venous pulsations
JVPT jugular venous pulse tracing
JWG joint working group
JWOCN Journal of Wound, Ostomy, and Continence Nursing
JWS Jackson-Weiss syndrome
Jx junction
JXG juvenile xanthogranuloma

K

K absolute zero; burst of diphasic slow waves in response to stimuli during sleep [EEG]; capsular antigen [Ger. *Kapsel*, capsule]; carrying capacity; cathode; coefficient; constant; constant improvement factor; electron capture; electrostatic capacity; equilibrium constant; ionization constant; kallikrein inhibiting unit; kanamycin; Kell factor; kelvin; kerma; kidney; Kilham [virus]; killer [cell]; kilo-; kilodalton; kinetic energy; *Klebsiella*; knee; lysine; modulus of compression; number 1024 in computer core memory; potassium [L. *kalium*]; uppercase Greek letter kappa; vitamin K

κ lowercase Greek letter kappa; magnetic susceptibility

K₁ phylloquinone

K₁, K₂ empirical Rohrer constants

K4 fourth Korotkoff sound

K5 fifth Korotkoff sound

K9 canine [veterinary medicine]

17-K 17-ketosteroid

k Boltzmann constant; constant; kilo; kilohm

KA alkaline phosphatase; kainic acid; keratoacanthoma; keto acid; ketoacidosis; King-Armstrong [unit]; knowledge acquisition; knowledge aggregate

K/A ketogenic/antiketogenic ratio

K_A association constant

Ka cathode

K_a absorption rate constant; acid ionization constant; affinity constant; association constant

kA kiloampere

ka cathode

KAAD kerosene, alcohol, acetic acid, and dioxane

KAAS Keele assessment of auditory style

KABC Kaufman Assessment Battery for Children

KADV Kadam virus

KAF conglutinogen-activating factor; killer-assisting factor; kinase activating factor

KAFO knee-ankle-foot orthosis

KAIV Kaikalur virus

KAL Kallmann [syndrome]

KAL1 Kallmann gene

KALP Kallmann pseudogene

KAMI Koch Acute Myocardial Infarction [study]

KAMIT Kentucky Acute Myocardial Infarction Trial

KAMV Kamese virus

kan kanamycin

KanR, kan^r kanamycin resistance

KANV Kannamangalam virus

KAO knee-ankle orthosis

KAP knowledge, attitudes, and practice

kappa a light chain of human immunoglobulins

KAPS Kuopio Atherosclerosis Prevention Study

KARV Karimabad virus

KAS Katz Adjustment Scales; Kennedy-Alter-Sung [syndrome]

KASV Kasba virus; Kasokero virus

KAT kanamycin acetyltransferase; knowledge acquisition tool; Kuopio Angioplasty Gene Transfer Trial

kat katal

kat/L, kat/l katals per liter

K_ATP adenosine triphosphate potassium channel

KAU King-Armstrong unit

KaV Kawino virus

KB human oral epidermoid carcinoma cells; Kashin-Bek [disease]; ketone body; kilobase; kilobyte; Kleihauer-Betke [test]; knee brace; knowledge base

K-B Kleihauer-Betke [test]; Kuo-Bean [model]

Kb kilobit

K_b base ionization constant; binding constant

kb kilobase; kilobyte

KBD knowledge base dictionary

KBG syndrome of multiple abnormalities [original patient's initials]

KBI knowledge-based information

KBM knowledge base manager

kbp kilobase pair

Kbps kilobits per second

kBq kilobecquerel

KBS Klüver-Bucy syndrome; knowledge-based system

KBTA knowledge-based temporal abstraction

KBV Kachemak Bay virus

KC cathodal closing; keratoconjunctivitis; keratoconus; knee-to-chest; Kupffer cell

kC kilocoulomb

kc kilocycle

K Cal, Kcal, kcal kilocalorie

KCC cathodal closing contraction; Kulchitzky cell carcinoma

KCCT kaolin-cephalin clotting time

KCD kinostatic change detector
K cell killer cell
KCF key clinical finding
KCG kinetocardiogram
kCi kilocurie
KCl potassium chloride
KCO transfer coefficient
KCP knowledge, concern, and first-aid practices
kcps kilocycles per second
KCS Kenny-Caffey syndrome; keratoconjunctivitis sicca
kc/s kilocycles per second
KCSS Keio Cooperative Stroke Study
KCT, KCTe cathodal closing tetanus; kaolin clotting time
KCTe cathodal closing tetanus
KCV Kern Canyon virus
KD cathodal duration; Kawasaki disease; Kennedy disease; killed; Krabbe disease
K$_D$ dissociation constant
K$_d$ degradation constant; dissociation constant; distribution coefficient; partition coefficient
kd, kDa kilodalton
KDA known drug allergies
KDAPPIMT Kawasaki Disease Aneurysm Prevention Protocol and Italian Multicenter Trial
KDB kinase insert domain; knowledge database
KDC kidney disease treatment center
KDD knowledge discovery in databases
KDD-R knowledge discovery in databases using rough sets
KDI knowledge and distributed intelligence
kdn kidney
KDNA kinetoblast deoxyribonucleic acid
KDO ketodeoxyoctonate
KDOQI Kidney Disease Outcomes Quality Initiative
KDS Kaufman Developmental Scale; King-Denborough syndrome; knowledge data system; Kocher-Debré-Semelaigne [syndrome]; Kupfer-Detre system
KDT cathodal duration tetanus
KDV Kadipiro virus
kdyn kilodyne
KE Kendall compound E; kethoxal; kinetic energy; Krining estimator
K$_e$ exchangeable body potassium
KED Kendrick extrication device
KEDS Kids Eating Disorder Survey
KEDV Kedougou virus
Kel elimination constant
K$_{em}$ elimination rate constant

KEMRI Kenyan Medical Research Institute
KEMV Kemerovo virus
KENV Kenai virus
Kera keratitis
KERMA kinetic energy released per unit mass
KERV Kentucky equine respiratory virus
KESS Knowles-Eccersley-Scott Symptom [questionnaire]
KETV Ketapang virus
KEUV Keuraliba virus
keV kiloelectron volt
KEYV Keystone virus
KF Kayser-Fleischer [rings]; Kenner fecal medium; kidney function; Klippel-Feil [syndrome]; knowledge finder
K-F Kayser-Fleischer [rings]
K$_f$ Klenow fragment
kf flocculation rate in antigen-antibody reaction; kilogram force
KFAB kidney-fixing antibody
KFAO knee-foot-ankle orthosis
KFC Ketanserin for Carcinoid [trial]; Ketanserin on Fibroblast Culture [study]
K$_{fc}$ filtration coefficient
KFD Kyasanur forest disease
KFDV Kyasanur Forest disease virus
KFR Kayser-Fleischer ring
KFS Klippel-Feil syndrome
KFSD keratosis follicularis spinulosa decalvans
KG ketoglutarate; knowledge graph
kG kilogauss
kg kilogram
KG-1 Koeffler Golde-1 [cell line]
kg-cal kilocalorie
kg/cm^2 kilogram per square centimeter
KGD ketoglutarate dehydrogenase
KGF keratocyte growth factor
kgf kilogram force
KGFR keratocyte growth factor receptor
kg/L kilograms per liter
KGM keratinocyte growth medium
kg-m kilogram-meter
kg/m kilograms per meter
kg-m/s^2 kilogram-meter per second squared
Kgn kininogen
kgps kilograms per second
17-KGS 17-ketogenic steroid
KGS ketogenic steroid
KH K-homologous; K-homology; Krebs-Henseleit [buffer]
K24H potassium, urinary 24-hour
KHAV Khabarovsk virus; Kharagysh virus; Khasan virus
KHB Krebs-Henseleit buffer

KHb potassium hemoglobinate
KHC kinetic hemolysis curve
KHD kinky hair disease
KHF Korean hemorrhagic fever
KHM keratoderma hereditaria mutilans
KHN Knoop hardness number
KHP King's Honorary Physician
KHS King's Honorary Surgeon; kinky hair syndrome; Krebs-Henseleit solution
kHz kilohertz
KI karyopyknotic index; Krönig's isthmus; potassium iodide
KIA Kligler iron agar
KIC ketoisocaproate; ketoisocaproic acid
KICB killed intracellular bacteria
KID keratitis, ichthyosis, and deafness [syndrome]; kinase insert domain
KIDI knowledge of infant development inventory
KIF knowledge information format; knowledge interchange format
KIHD Kuopio Ischemic Heart Disease Risk Factor Study
kilo kilogram
KIMSA Kirsten murine sarcoma
KIMSV, KiMSV Kirsten murine sarcoma virus
KIMV Kimberley virus
KIN keratinocytic intraepidermal neoplasia
KIND Kyushu University Hospital Information Network Database
KINDS Kinmen Neurologic Disorders Survey
KINV Kindia virus
KIP key intermediary protein
KiP kilopascal
KIPS key indicators, probes, and scoring method
KIR killer immunoglobulin receptor; killer-cell immunoglobulin-like receptor
Kir inward rectified potassium [channel]
KIRA kinase receptor activation
KISS keep it simple and safe; keep it simple, stupid; key integrative social system; Kobe Idiopathic Cardiomyopathy Survival Study; saturated solution of potassium iodide
KIST Korea Institute of Science and Technology
KISV Kismayo virus
KIT Kahn Intelligence Test
KIU kallikrein inactivation unit
KIVA keto isovaleric acid
KJ, kj knee jerk
kJ kilojoule
KK knee kick
kkat kilokatal
KKS kallikrein-kinin system
KKV Kaeng Khoi virus

KL Karhunen-Loéve [transform]; kidney lobe; Kit ligand; Klebs-Loeffler [bacillus]; Kleine-Levin [syndrome]
kl kiloliter
KLAV Klamath virus
KLC Karhunen-Loève coefficient
Klebs *Klebsiella*
KLH keyhole limpet hemocyanin
KLK kallikrein
KLKR kallikrein
KLM killed *Mycobacterium*
KLS kidneys, liver, and spleen; Kreuzbein lipomatous syndrome
KLT Karhunen-Loève transform
KLV Kalanchoe latent virus
KM kanamycin; knowledge management; knowledge map
K$_m$ Michaelis-Menten constant
km kilometer
k$_m$ metabolic constant
km^2 square kilometer
KMC K-means clustering analysis
kMc kilomegacycle
K-MCM potassium-containing minimum capacitation medium
kMc/s kilomegacycles per second
KMEF keratin, myosin, epidermin, and fibrin
kmps kilometers per second
KMPV Kammavanpettai virus
Km^R kanamycin residue
KMS kabuki make-up syndrome; knowledge management system; kwashiorkor-marasmus syndrome
K-MSV Kirsten murine sarcoma virus
KMV killed measles virus vaccine
KN knowledge networking
Kn kanamycin; knee; Knudsen number
kN kilonewton
kn knee
K nail Küntscher nail
KNG kininogen
KNN K-nearest neighbor; Kohonen neural network
k-NN K-nearest neighbor
KnoME knowledge management environment
KNRK Kirsten sarcoma virus in normal rat kidney
KNS kinesin
KNSL kinesin-like
KO keep on; keep open; killed organism; knee orthosis; knockout
kΩ kilohm
KOC cathodal opening contraction
KO-DMEM Knockout Dulbecco Modified Eagle Medium
k$_{off}$ off-rate constant
KOH potassium hydroxide

KOKV Kokobera virus
KOL key opinion leader
KOLV Kolongo virus
KOOLV Koolpinyah virus
KOOV Koongol virus
KOR keep-open rate
KOPS thousand operations per second
KOTV Kotonkan virus
KOUV Koutango virus
KOWV Kowanyama virus
KP Kaufmann-Peterson [base]; keratitic precipitate; keratitis punctata; kidney protein; killed parenteral [vaccine]; *Klebsiella pneumoniae*
K$_p$ partition coefficient
kPa kilopascal
kPa·s/l, kPa·s/L kilopascal seconds per liter
KPB ketophenylbutazone; potassium phosphate buffer
KPC keratoconus posticus circumscriptus
KPD kidney paired donation
KPE Kelman pharmacoemulsification
KPI kallikrein-protease inhibitor; karyopyknotic index
kpm kilopodometer
KPR key pulse rate
KPS Karnofsky Performance Status
KPT kidney punch test
KPTI Kunitz pancreatic trypsin inhibitor
KPTT kaolin partial thromboplastin time
KPV kangaroo poxvirus; key process variable; killed parenteral vaccine; killed polio vaccine
KPWIN KnowledgePro for Windows
KPyV Kilham polyomavirus
KQC key quality characteristics
KQML knowledge query and manipulation language
KR key ridge; knowledge representation; Kopper-Reppart [medium]
Kr krypton
kR kiloroentgen
KRAS, KRas V-Ki-ras2 Kirsten rat sarcoma
KRB Krebs-Ringer buffer
KRBG Krebs-Ringer bicarbonate buffer with glucose
KRBS Krebs-Ringer bicarbonate solution
KRDU Knowledge Resources Development Unit
KRIS Kaunas-Rotterdam Intervention Study
KRIV Kairi virus
KRP Kolmer test with Reiter protein [antigen]; Krebs-Ringer phosphate
KRR knowledge representation and reasoning
KRRS kinetic resonance Raman spectroscopy

KRS knowledge representation syntax
KRT keratin
KRV Kilham rat virus
KS Kabuki syndrome; Kallmann syndrome; Kaposi sarcoma; Kartagener syndrome; Kawasaki syndrome; keratan sulfate; ketosteroid; Klinefelter syndrome; Korsakoff syndrome; Kozhevnikov syndrome; Kveim-Siltzbach [test]
17-KS 17-ketosteroid
K-S Kearns-Sayre [syndrome]
ks kilosecond
KSC cathodal closing contraction
KSHV Kaposi sarcoma–associated herpesvirus
KSIV Karshi virus
KS/OI Kaposi sarcoma with opportunistic infection
KSOM Kohonen's self-organizing map
KSOV Kaisodi virus
KSP Karolinska Scales of Personality; kidney-specific protein; kinesin spindle protein
K$_{sp}$ solubility product
17-KSR 17-ketosteroid reductase
KSS Kearns-Sayre syndrome; Kearns-Sayre-Shy [syndrome]; Knee Society Score; knowledge source server
KSSO knowledge support system zero
KST cathodal closing tetanus; kallistatin
KSV Kao Shuan virus
KT kidney transplant, kidney transplantation; kinesiotherapist; kinesiotherapy
K$_t$ turnover rate constant
KTA kidney transplant alone
KTI kallikrein-trypsin inhibitor
KTM Kops-Tissot-Monro [mask]
KTRV Keterah virus
KTS Klippel-Trenaunay syndrome
KTSA Kahn test of symbol arrangement
KTU knowledge transfer and utilization
Kt/V dialyzer clearance of urea; dialysis time/volume of distribution of urea
KTW, KTWS Klippel-Trenaunay-Weber [syndrome]
KTX kaliotoxin
KTx kidney transplant
KU kallikrein unit; Karmen unit
Ku kurchatovium; Peltz factor
K$_u$ urinary rate coefficient
kU$_A$/L kilounits of antibody per liter
KUB kidneys and upper bladder; kidneys, ureters, and bladder
KUf ultrafiltration coefficient
KUMIS Kumamoto University Myocardial Infarction Study
KUN Kunjin [virus]
KUNV Kunjin virus

KUS kidney, ureter, spleen
KV kanamycin and vancomycin; kidney vacuolating virus; killed vaccine
K$_v$ voltage-gated potassium [channel]
kV, kv kilovolt
kVA kilovolt-ampere
kvar kilovar
KVBA kanamycin-vancomycin blood agar
kVcp, kvcp kilovolt constant potential
KVE Kaposi varicelliform eruption
KVLBA kanamycin-vancomycin laked blood agar
KVO keep vein open
kVp, kvp kilovolt peak
KW Keith-Wagener [finding]; Kimmelstiel-Wilson [syndrome]; Kugelberg-Welander [syndrome]
kW, kw kilowatt
Kw weighted kappa

K$_w$ dissociation constant of water
KWAV Kwatta virus
KWB Keith-Wagener-Barker [classification]
KWD Kimmelstiel-Wilson disease
KWE Kumar-Welti-Ernst [method]
kWh, kW-hr, kw-hr kilowatt-hour
KWIC key word in context
K wire Kirschner wire
KWord 32-bit word
KWS Kimmelstiel-Wilson syndrome; Kugelberg-Welander syndrome
K-XRF K x-ray fluorescence
KYCS Kiryat Yovel Community Study
KYN kynurenic acid
KYN-OH kynurenine-3-hydroxylase
KYSMI Kyoto Shiga Myocardial Infarction [study]
KZ ketoconazole

L

L angular momentum; Avogadro constant; boundary [L. *limes*]; coefficient of induction; diffusion length; inductance; *Lactobacillus*; lambda; lambert; latent heat; latex; Latin; leader sequence; left; *Legionella*; *Leishmania*; length; lente insulin; lethal; leucine; levo-; lewisite; lidocaine; ligament; light; light sense; lingual; *Listeria*; liter; liver; low; lower; lumbar; luminance; lymph; lymphocyte; outer membrane layer of cell wall of gram-negative bacteria; pound [L. *libra*]; radiance; self-inductance; syphilis [L. *lues*]; threshold [L. *limen*]

Λ uppercase Greek letter lambda

λ lowercase Greek letter lambda; craniometric point; decay constant; an immunoglobulin light chain; mean free path; microliter; thermal conductivity; wavelength

L₊ limes tod [the smallest amount of toxin which will produce a toxic reaction]

L0 no evidence of lymph node metastases

L₀ limes zero [limes nul, the largest amount of toxin that will not produce a toxic reaction]

L1 acute lymphoblastic leukemia with lymphoblasts, scanty cytoplasm, and inconspicuous nucleoli; lymph node metastases assessed

L1, L2, L3, L4, L5 first, second, third, fourth, and fifth lumbar vertebrae

L2 acute lymphoblastic leukemia with large pleomorphic blasts, abundant cytoplasm, and prominent nucleoli

L₂ area [length square]

L3 acute lymphoblastic leukemia having blast with basophilic vacuolated cytoplasm

L₃ volume [length cube]

L/3 lower third

l azimuthal quantum number; left; length; lethal; levorotatory; liter; long; longitudinal; specific latent heat

LA laboratory aide or assistant; lactic acid; lactic acidemia; large amount; laser angioplasty; late abortion; late antigen; latex agglutination; left angle; left arm; left atrium; left auricle; leucine aminopeptidase; leukemia antigen; leukoagglutination; leuprolide acetate; levator ani; Lightwood-Albright [syndrome]; linear addition; linguoaxial; linoleic acid; lobuloalveolar; local anesthesia; local anesthetic; long acting; long arm; long

axis; low anxiety; Ludwig angina; lupus anticoagulant; lymphocyte antibody

L&A light and accommodation; living and active

L/A liver/aorta

LA50 total body surface area of burn that will kill 50% of patients (lethal area)

La labial; lambda; lambert; lanthanum

LAA left atrial appendage; left atrial area; left auricular appendage; leukemia-associated antigen; leukocyte ascorbic acid

LAAM ʟ-alpha acetylmethadol; levo-alpha-acetylmethadol

LAAO ʟ-amino acid oxidase

LA/Ao left atrial/aortic ratio

LAB, lab laboratory

LABA long-acting beta agonist

LabBase laboratory database

LABBB left anterior bundle branch block

LABC locally advanced breast cancer

LABE labetalol

LABP laboratory procedure

LA-BP low-affinity binding protein

LABV left atrial ball valve

LabVISE Laboratory Reporting Scheme in Virology and Serology

LAC La Crosse [virus]; lactase; lansoprazole, amoxicillin, clarithromycin; large area coverage; lateral crural convexity; left atrial circumflex [artery]; left atrial contraction; linear attenuation coefficient; linguoaxiocervical; long-arm cast; low-amplitude contraction; lung adenocarcinoma cells; lupus anticoagulant

LaC labiocervical

Lac laceration; lactation

LACD left apex cardiogram, calibrated displacement

LACI lacidipine; lipoprotein-associated coagulation inhibitor

LACN local area communications network

LacR lactose repressor

Lacr lacrimal

LACS long-chain acyl-coenzyme A synthetase

Lact lactate, lactating, lactation; lactic

Lact hyd lactalbumin hydrolysate

LACV La Crosse virus

LAD lactic acid dehydrogenase; laser-assisted drug delivery; left anterior descending [coronary artery]; left atrial defect; left axis deviation; leukocyte adhesion deficiency; leukocyte antibody detection assay; ligament augmentation device; linoleic acid depression; lipoamide dehydrogenase; lymphocyte-activating determinant

LADA laboratory animal dander allergy; latent autoimmune diabetes in the adult, latent autoimmune diabetes of adults; left acromio-dorsoanterior [position]; left anterior descending artery

LADB left [coronary] descending branch

LADCA left anterior descending coronary artery

LADD lacrimal-auricular-dental-digital [syndrome]; left anterior descending diagonal [coronary artery]

LADH lactic acid dehydrogenase; liver alcohol dehydrogenase

LAD-MIN left axis deviation, minimal

LADP left acromio-dorso-posterior [position]; left anterior descending arterial pressure

LADS Lors American Data System

LAE left atrial enlargement

LAEDV left atrial volume in end diastole

LAEI left atrial emptying index

LAESV left atrial volume in end systole

LAF laminar air flow; Latin American female; left anterior fascicle; leukocyte-activating factor; lymphocyte-activating factor

LAFB left anterior fascicular block

LAFR laminar air flow room

LAFU laminar air flow unit

LAG labiogingival; laparoscopy-assisted gastrectomy; leukocyte antigen group; linguoaxiogingival; lymphangiogram; lymphocyte activation gene

LaG labiogingival

LAGB laparoscopic adjustable gastric band

LAH lactalbumin hydrolysate; left anterior hemiblock; left atrial hypertrophy; Licentiate of Apothecaries Hall; lithium aluminum hydride

LAHB left anterior hemiblock

LAHC low affinity, high capacity

LAHF low amplitude, high frequency

LAHT laser-assisted hair transplantation

LAHV leukocyte-associated herpesvirus

LAI latex particle agglutination inhibition; leukocyte adherence inhibition

LaI labioincisal

LAID left anterior internal diameter

LAIF leukocyte adherence inhibition factor

LAIT latex agglutination inhibition test

LAIV live attenuated influenza vaccine

LAK lymphokine-activated killer [cells]

LAL left axillary line; limulus amebocyte lysate; low air loss; lysosomal acid lipase

LaL labiolingual

LALB low air-loss bed

LALI lymphocyte antibody—lymphocytolytic interaction

LALL lymphomatous acute lymphoblastic leukemia

LALV Lucerne Australian latent virus

LAM laminectomy; laminin; lamivudine; late ambulatory monitoring; Latin American male; left anterior measurement; left atrial myxoma; linear associative memory; lipoarabinomannan; lymphangioleiomyomatosis; lymphocyte adhesion molecule

Lam laminectomy

LAMA laminin A

LAMB laminin B; lentigines, atrial myxoma, mucocutaneous myxomas, blue nevi [syndrome]

L-AmB liposomal AmBisome [amphotericin]

LAMBR laminin B receptor

LAMC laminin C

LAMMA laser microprobe mass analyzer

LAMP limbic system—associated membrane protein; loop-mediated isothermal amplification; lysosome-associated membrane protein

LAN local area network; long-acting neuroleptic

LANC long-arm navicular cast

LANE lidocaine, atropine, naloxone, epinephrine

LANSS Leeds Assessment of Neuropathic Symptoms and Signs

LANV Laguna Negra virus; left atrial neovascularization

LAO left anterior oblique; left atrial overload; Licentiate of the Art of Obstetrics

LAP laboratory accreditation program; laparoscopy; laparotomy; latency-active promoter; latency-associated protein; left arterial pressure; left atrial pressure; leucine aminopeptidase; leukemia-associated phenotype; leukemia-associated phosphoprotein; leukocyte alkaline phosphatase; liver-enriched transcriptional activator protein; low atmospheric pressure; lyophilized anterior pituitary

Lap laparoscopy; laparotomy

LapCAC laparoscopic compression anastomosis clip

Lap & dye laparoscopy and injection of dye

LAPIS Late Potentials in Myocardial Infarction Study

LAPSE long-term ambulatory physiologic surveillance

LAPSS Los Angeles Prehospital Stroke Screen

LAPW left atrial posterior wall

LAQ long-arc quad

LAR laryngology; late asthmatic response; late reaction; left arm recumbent; legally authorized representative; leukocyte antigen related; long-acting release; low anterior resection

Lar larynx; left arm reclining

LARA Low-Dose Aspirin Trial on Restenosis After Angioplasty

LARab laryngeal abductor

LARad laryngeal adductor

LARC leukocyte automatic recognition computer; long-acting reversible contraceptive

LARD lacrimo-auriculo-radio-dental [syndrome]

L-Arg L-arginine

LARIS laser atomization resonance ionization spectroscopy

LARS laparoscopic antireflux surgery; laser angioplasty in the treatment of restenosis developing within coronary stents; leucyltRNA synthetase

LARVH laparoscopically-assisted radical vaginal hysterectomy

Laryngol laryngology

LAS laboratory automation system; lateral amyotrophic sclerosis; laxative abuse syndrome; left anterior-superior; leucine acetylsalicylate; linear alkylsulfonate; local adaptation syndrome; long arm splint; lower abdominal surgery; lymphadenopathy syndrome; lymphangioscintigraphy

LASA linear-analogue self-assessment; lipid-associated phenotype

LASAF low quantities of acetylsalicylic acid in atrial fibrillation

LASA-P linear-analogue self-assessment-Pristman

LASAR Local Alcohol and Stent Against Restenosis [trial]

LASA-S linear-analogue self-assessment-Selby

LASE laser-assisted spinal endoscopy

LASEK laser-assisted subepithelial keratomileusis

LASER light amplification by stimulated emission of radiation

LASH left anterior superior hemiblock

LA SI linearly additive, spatially invariant

LASIK laser-assisted in situ keratomileusis

L-ASP L-asparaginase

LASS labile aggregation stimulating substance

LAST Left Anterior Small Thoracotomy [study]

LASTAC laser transluminal angioplasty catheter

LASTLHY Latin American Study of Lacidipine in Hypertension

LASV Lassa virus

LAT lactic acidosis threshold; latency-associated transcript; lateral; lateral atrial tunnel; latex agglutination test; latissimus dorsi; left anterior trigone; left atrial thrombus; less acute mode of transportation; limbal autograft transplantation; L-type amino acid transporter; lysolecithin acyltransferase

Lat latent; lateral; Latin

Lat bend lateral bending

LATC lateral talocalcaneal

LATCH literature attached to charts; Lower Anchorages and Tethers for Children [system]

LATE Late Assessment of Thrombolytic Efficacy [trial]

L·atm liter atmosphere

LATP left atrial transmural pressure

LATPT left atrial transesophageal pacing test

LATS long-acting thyroid stimulator

LATS-P long-acting thyroid stimulator-protector

LATu lobuloalveolar tumor

LAUP laser-assisted uvulopalatoplasty

LAV liquid-assisted ventilation; lymphadenopathy-associated virus

Lav lavatory

LAVA laser angioplasty versus angioplasty; Leiden Artificial Valves and Anticoagulation [study]

LAVH laparoscopy-assisted vaginal hysterectomy

LAW left atrial wall

LAX, LAx long axis

Lax laxative; laxity

LAX-DSS long axis discrete subaortic stenosis

Lax oc laxative of choice

LB lamellar body; large bowel; left breast; left bronchus; left bundle; left buttock; leiomyoblastoma; lipid body; live birth; liver biopsy; loose body; low back; lung biopsy; Luria-Bertani [medium]

L&B left and below

Lb *Leishmania brasiliensis*; pound [L. *libra*]; pound force

lb pound [L. *libra*]

LBA laser balloon angioplasty; left basal artery

LBB left bundle branch; low back bending

LBBB left bundle branch block

LBBsB left bundle branch system block

LBC lidocaine blood concentration; liquid-based cytology; lymphadenosis benigna cutis

LBCD left border of cardiac dullness

LBCF Laboratory Branch complement fixation [test]

LBD lamellar body density; large bile duct; left border of dullness; Lewy body dementia; ligand-binding domain; lower back disorder; lumbar body density

LBF *Lactobacillus bulgaricus* factor; limb blood flow; liver blood flow

Lbf pound force

Lbf-ft pound force foot

LBH length, breadth, height

LBI low back injury; low serum-bound iron

Lb/in² pounds per square inch

LBL labeled lymphoblast; lymphoblastic lymphoma

LbL layer by layer

LBM last bowel movement; lean body mass; loose bowel movement; lung basement membrane

L-BMAA L-beta-*N*-methylamino-L-alanine

LBMT lansoprazole, bismuth, metronidazole, tetracycline

LBNP lower body negative pressure

LBO large bowel obstruction

LBP lipopolysaccharide-binding protein; local binary pattern; low back pain; low blood pressure; lumbar back pain

LBPF long bone or pelvic fracture

LBPP lower body positive pressure

LBPQ Low Back Pain Questionnaire

LBQC large-base quad cane

LBRF louse-borne relapsing fever

LBS low back syndrome; Lübeck Blood [Pressure] Study; lumbar back strain; Lutheran Brotherhood Study; lysine-binding site

LBSA lipid-bound sialic acid

LBT low back tenderness/trouble

LBTI lima bean trypsin inhibitor

Lb tr pound troy

LBV Lagos bat virus; left brachial vein; lung blood volume

LB-V left bundle ventricle

LBW lean body weight; low birth weight

LBWI low-birth-weight infant

LBWR lung/body weight ratio

LC Laënnec cirrhosis; Langerhans cell; laparoscopic cholecystectomy; large chromophobe; late clamped; lateral canthotomy; lateral cortex; lecithin cholesterol acyltransferase; left circumflex [coronary artery]; lethal concentration; Library of Congress; life care; light chain; linguocervical; lipid cytosomes; liquid chromatography; liquid crystal; liver cirrhosis; living children; location component; locus ceruleus; long chain; low calorie; low contrast; lower calyceal; lung cancer; lung cell; lymphocyte count

LC₀ maximum sublethal concentration

LC₅₀ median lethal concentration

LCA Leber congenital amaurosis; left carotid artery; left circumflex artery; left coronary artery; leukocyte common antigen; lithocholic acid; liver cell adenoma; lymphocyte chemotactic activity

LCα low calcium

LCAH lipoid congenital adrenal hyperplasia

LCAL large cell anaplastic lymphoma

LCAM liver cell adhesion molecule

LCAO linear combination of atomic orbitals

L-CAPS Low-Density Lipoprotein Coronary Atherosclerosis Prospective Study

LCAR late cutaneous anaphylactic reaction

LCAS Lipoprotein and Coronary Atherosclerosis Study

LCAT lecithin cholesterol acyltransferase

LCATA lecithin cholesterol acetyltransferase alpha

LCB Laboratory of Cancer Biology; Leber congenital blindness; left costal border; lymphomatosis cutis benigna

LCBF local cerebral blood flow

LCBI laboratory-confirmed bloodstream infection

LCC lactose coliform count; left circumflex coronary [artery]; left common carotid [artery]; left coronary cusp; life cycle cost; lipid-containing cell; liver cell carcinoma; L-type calcium channel

LCCA late cortical cerebellar atrophy; leukoclastic angiitis

LCCE Lamaze Certified Childbirth Educator

LCCME Liaison Committee on Continuing Medical Education

LCCS lethal congenital contracture syndrome; lower cervical cesarean section

LCCSCT large cell calcifying Sertoli cell tumor

LCD lattice corneal dystrophy; liquid crystal diode; liquid crystal display; liquor carbonis detergens [coal tar solution]; localized collagen dystrophy; low-calcium diet

LC-DCP low-contact dynamic compression plate

LCDD light chain deposition disease

LCDV lymphocystis disease virus

LCE leg cycle ergometry

LCED liquid chromatography with electrochemical detection

LCF least common factor; left circumflex [coronary artery]; lymphocyte culture fluid

LCFA, L-cFA long-chain fatty acid

LCFU leukocyte colony-forming unit

LCG Langerhans cell granule; Langerhans cell granulomatosis; liquid crystal glasses

LCGL large cell granulocytic leukemia

LCGME Liaison Committee on Graduate Medical Education

LCGR lutropin-choriogonadotropin receptor

LCGU local cerebral glucose utilization

LCH Langerhans cell histiocytosis

LCh Licentiate in Surgery

L-CHAD long-chain 3-hydroxyacyl coenzyme A dehydrogenase

LCI length complexity index

LCIN low-grade cervical intraepithelial neoplasia

LCIS lobular carcinoma in situ

LCL lateral collateral ligament; left coronary leaflet; Levinthal-Coles-Lillie [body]; lower confidence limit; lower control limit; lymphoblastoid cell line; lymphocytic lymphosarcoma; lymphoid cell line

LCLC large cell lung carcinoma

LCLo lowest lethal concentration

LCM laser-capture microdissection; latent cardiomyopathy; left costal margin; leukocyte-conditioned medium; lowest common multiple; lymphatic choriomeningitis; lymphocytic choriomeningitis

LCME Liaison Committee on Medical Education

LCMG long-chain monoglyceride

L/cm H₂O liters per centimeter of water

LC-MS, LC/MS liquid chromatography-mass spectrometry

LCMV lymphocytic choriomeningitis virus

LCN lateral cervical nucleus; left caudate nucleus; line correlated noise; lipocalin

LCNB large-core needle biopsy

LCO left coronary ostium; low cardiac output

LCOS low cardiac output syndrome

LCP Legg-Calvé-Perthes [syndrome]; long-chain polysaturated [fatty acid]; lymphocyte cytosol polypeptide

LCPD Legg-Calvé-Perthes disease

LCPS Licentiate of the College of Physicians and Surgeons

LCQ Learning Climate Questionnaire

LCR late cutaneous reaction; lifetime clinical record; ligase chain reaction; locus control region; long control region

Lcr low calcium response

LCRB locus control region beta

LCRI limit cycle reciprocal interaction

LCRUS Leigh Clinical Research Unit Study

LCrv retroventral lateral cortex

LCS cerebrospinal fluid [L. *liquor cerebrospinalis*]; laboratory of computer science; laparoscopic coagulating shear; left coronary sinus; Leydig cell stimulation; lichen chronicus simplex; life care service; Life Closure Scale; longest common substring; low constant suction; low continuous suction; lymphocyte culture supernatants

LCSB Liaison Committee for Specialty Boards

LCSC local community service centre

LCSD left cardiac sympathetic denervation

LCSG Lung Cancer Study Group

lcSSc limited cutaneous systemic sclerosis

LCST low critical solution temperature

LCSW licensed clinical social worker

LCT laser dynamic compliance measurement technique; liquid crystal thermography; liver cell tumor; long-chain triglyceride; lymphocytotoxicity; lymphocytotoxin

LCt₅₀ median lethal vapor or aerosol concentration

LCTA lymphocytotoxic antibody

LCU laparoscopic contact ultrasonography; life change unit

LCV Lake Clarendon virus; lecithovitellin; leukocytoclastic vasculitis; lymphocytic choriomeningitis virus

LCWI left cardiac work index

LCX left circumflex [coronary artery]

LCXB left [coronary] circumflex branch

LD label dictionary; labor and delivery; laboratory data; labyrinthine defect; lactate dehydrogenase; Lafora disease; laser Doppler; learning disability; learning disorder; left deltoid; Legionnaires' disease; lethal dose; levodopa. L-dopa; light differentiation; limited disease; linear dichroism; linear discriminate; linguodistal; linkage disequilibrium; lipodystrophy; liver disease; living donor; loading dose; Lombard-Dowell [agar]; longitudinal diameter; low density; low dose; Lyme disease; lymphocyte defined; lymphocyte depletion

L-D Leishman-Donovan [body]

L/D light/darkness ratio

L&D labor and delivery

LD₁ isoenzyme of lactate dehydrogenase found in the heart, erythrocytes, and kidneys

LD₂, LD₃ isoenzymes of lactate dehydrogenase found in the lungs

LD₄ isoenzyme of lactate dehydrogenase found in the liver

LD₅ isoenzyme of lactate dehydrogenase found in the liver and muscles

LD₅₀ median lethal dose

LD₅₀/₃₀ a dose that is lethal for 50% of test subjects within 30 days

LD₁₀₀ lethal dose in all exposed subjects

Ld *Leishmania donovani*

LDA laser Doppler anemometry; Learning Disabilities Association of America; left dorsoanterior; linear discriminant analysis; low density area; low disease activity; lymphocyte-dependent antibody

LDAC low-dose cytosine arabinoside
LDAR latex direct agglutination reaction
LDB lamb dysentery bacillus; Legionnaires' disease bacillus; Location Database
LDC lactose digestion capacity; limited assistance dialysis center; lymphoid dendritic cell; lysine decarboxylase
L-dC L-deoxycytidine
LDCC lectin-dependent cellular cytotoxicity
LDCF lymphocyte-derived chemotactic factor
LDCI low-dose continuous infusion
LDCMC Lady Davis Carmel Medical Center
LdCPV *Lymantria dispar* cypovirus
LDCT late distal cortical tubule
LDD late dedifferentiation; light-dark discrimination; liquefy, digest, and discharge
LDDB London Dysmorphology Database
LDDE low-dose dobutamine echo
LDER lateral view dual-energy radiography
LD-EYA Lombard-Dowell egg yolk agar
LDF laser Doppler flowmetry; laser Doppler flux, laser Doppler fluxometry; limit dilution factor
LDFA linear discrimination functional analysis
LDG lactic dehydrogenase; lingual developmental groove
L-dG L-deoxyguanosine
LDH lactate dehydrogenase; low-dose heparin
LDHA lactic dehydrogenase A
LDHB lactic dehydrogenase B
LDHC lactic dehydrogenase C
LDHSPS Low-Dose Heparin Stroke Prevention Study
LD im lethal intramuscular dose
LD ip lethal intraperitoneal dose
LDL loudness discomfort level; low-density lipoprotein
LDLA low-density lipoprotein apheresis
LDL A low-density lipoprotein receptor class A
LDL B low-density lipoprotein receptor class B
LDL-C, LDL-c low-density lipoprotein−cholesterol complex
LDL/HDL low-density lipoprotein/high-density lipoprotein ratio
LD$_{Lo}$ lowest lethal dose
LDLP low-density lipoprotein
LDLR, LDL-R low-density lipoprotein receptor; Low-Density Lipoprotein Receptor Mutation Database
LDM lactate dehydrogenase, muscle; limited dorsal myeloschisis
LDMF latissimus dorsi myocutaneous flap
LD-NEYA Lombard-Dowell neomycin egg yolk agar
L-DOPA, L-dopa levodopa [levo-3, 4-dihydroxyphenylalanine]
LDP left dorsoposterior; lumbodorsal pain

LDQ Leeds Dyspepsia Questionnaire
LDR labor, delivery, recovery; lifetime data repository; low dose rate
LDRI leukotriene D4 receptor inhibitors
LDRPS labor-delivery-recovery-postpartum suite
LDRS labor-delivery-recovery suite
LDS Licentiate in Dental Surgery; lightweight decontamination system; Lipids in Diabetes Study; locked door seclusion
LDSc Licentiate in Dental Science
LDT left dorsotransverse
LDUB long double upright brace
LDUH low-dose unfractionated heparin
LDV lactate dehydrogenase−elevating virus, lactic dehydrogenase virus; large dense-cored vesicle; laser Doppler velocimetry; lateral distant view; Le Dantec virus; Lordsdale virus
LE lactate extraction; law enforcement; left ear; left eye; leukocyte elastase; leukoerythrogenic; life expectancy; linkage equilibrium; live embryo; Long Evans [rat]; low exposure; lower extremity; lupus erythematosus
LEA lower extremity amputation; lumbar epidural anesthesia
LEB lower extremity bypass
LEADER Lightweight Epidemiological Advanced Detection and Emergency Response System
LEAF layman education and activation system
LEAP Lower Extremity Amputation Prevention [program]
LEAV Leanyer virus
LEBV Lebombo virus
LEC leprosy elimination campaign; leukoencephalitis; long Evans cinnamon [rat]; low energy cardioversion; lower esophageal contractility
LECP low-energy charged particle
LED light-emitting diode; lowest emitting dose; lupus erythematosus disseminatus
LEDC low-energy direct current
LEDV Lednice virus
LEE locus of enterocyte effacement
LEED low-energy electron diffraction
LEEDS low-energy electron diffraction spectroscopy
LEEP left end-expiratory pressure; loop electrosurgical excision procedure
LEER likelihood equivalent error
LEET Low-Energy Endotak Trial
LEF late expression factor; leflunomide; leukokinesis-enhancing factor; lupus erythematosus factor; lymphoid-enhanced binding factor; lymphoid enhancer factor

Leg legal; legislation
LEHPZ lower esophageal high-pressure zone
LEHR lifetime electronic health record
LeIF leukocyte interferon
LEIS low-energy ion scattering
LEL lower explosive limit; lowest effect level
LELC lymphoepithelioma-like carcinoma
LEM lateral eye movement; Leibovitz-Emory medium; leukocyte endogenous mediator; light electron microscope; light emission microscopy; limited esophagomyotomy; low-electrolyte meal
LEMA least error matrix analysis
LEMO lowest empty molecular orbital
LEMS Lambert-Eaton myasthenic syndrome
LEN Level of Expressed Needs [questionnaire]
Lenit lenitive
LENT late effect to normal tissues
LEOPARD lentigines, electrocardiogram abnormalities, ocular hypertelorism, pulmonary stenosis, genital abnormalities, retardation of growth, and deafness [syndrome]
LEP laboratory of enteric pathogens; lethal effective phase; lipoprotein electrophoresis; low egg passage; lower esophageal pressure
Lep leptotene
LEPC local emergency planning committee
L_EPN effective perceived noise level
LEPR leptin receptor
Leq loudness equivalent
LER laparoscopic endoscope-holder robot; lysozomal enzyme release
LERG local electroretinogram
LERS learning from examples based on rough sets
LES Lambert-Eaton syndrome; Lawrence Experimental Station [agar]; Life Experiences Survey; lifestyle evaluation system; local excitatory state; Locke egg serum; low excitatory state; lower esophageal sphincter; lupus erythematosus, systemic
Les lesion
LESD Letterer-Siwe disease
LES-Dx Layered Expression Scanning, Diagnostic
LESP lower esophageal sphincter pressure
LESS lateral electrical spine stimulation
LESSD lupus erythematosus–specific skin disease
LESTR leukocyte-derived seven-transmembrane domain receptor
LET lidocaine, epinephrine, tetracaine [solution]; linear energy transfer; Losartan Effectiveness and Tolerability [study]

LETD lowest effective toxic dose
LETS large external transformation sensitive [protein]; Leiden Thrombophilia Study
LEU leucine; leucovorin; leukocyte equivalent unit
Leu, leu leucine
Leuc leukocyte
Leu-CAM leukocyte cell adhesion molecule
LeuRS leucyl ribonucleic acid synthetase
LEUT leucine transport
LEV levamisole
LEW Lewis [rat]
L/ext lower extremity
LF labile factor; lactoferrin; laryngofissure; Lassa fever; latex fixation; left foot; left forearm; lethal factor; leukotactic factor; ligamentum flavum; limit of flocculation; long frequency; low fat [diet]; low flow; low forceps; low frequency; lymphatic filariasis
L/F Latin female
Lf lactoferrin; limit of flocculation; low frequency
LFA left femoral artery; left frontal craniotomy; left frontoanterior; leukocyte function–associated antigen; leukotactic factor activity; logical framework analysis; low-friction arthroplasty; lymphocyte function–associated antigen
LFAB lipid-associated formation of amphotericin B
LFB luxol fast blue [stain]
LFBMA lattice function biologic movement artifacts
LFC living female child; low fat and cholesterol [diet]
LFD lactose-free diet; large for date [fetus]; late fetal death; lateral facial dysplasia; least fatal dose; local field potential; low-fat diet; low-fiber diet; low forceps delivery
LFE local frequency estimation; low-frequency enhancement
LFER linear free-energy relationship
LFH left femoral hernia
LFHL low-frequency hearing loss
LFL left frontolateral; leukocyte feeder layer; lower flammable limit; lower frequency limit
LFN lactoferrin
LFO low field open
L-[form] a defective bacterial variant that can multiply on hypertonic medium
LFP left frontoposterior
LFPPV low-frequency positive pressure ventilation
LFPS Licentiate of the Faculty of Physicians and Surgeons
LFR lymphoid follicular reticulosis

LFS lateral facet syndrome; latest finishing shift; Li-Fraumeni syndrome; limbic forebrain structure; liver function series

LFSE ligand field-stabilizing energy

LFT latex fixation test; latex flocculation test; left frontotransverse; liver function test; low-frequency tetanus; low-frequency transduction; low-frequency transfer; lung function test

LFU lipid fluidity unit

LFV large field of view; Lassa fever virus; low-frequency ventilation

LFx linear fracture

LG lactoglobulin; lamellar granule; laryngectomy; lateral gastrocnemius; left gluteal; Lennox-Gastaut [syndrome]; leucylglycine; linguogingival; lipoglycopeptide; liver graft; low glucose; lymphatic gland

Lg large; leg

LGA large for gestational age; left gastric artery; low-grade astrocytoma

LGALS lecithin, galactoside-binding, soluble

LGB Landry-Guillain-Barré [syndrome]; lateral geniculate body; lymphoglandular body

LGBS Landry-Guillain-Barré syndrome

LGBT lesbian, gay, bisexual, or transgender

LGBTQIA+ lesbian, gay, bisexual, transgender, queer [or questioning], intersex, asexual, plus everything on gender/sexuality spectrum words cannot yet describe

LGD limb girdle dystrophy; limit grid displacement; low-grade dysplasia

LGE Langat encephalitis

LGF lateral giant fiber

LGH lactogenic hormone

LGI large glucagon immunoreactivity; low gastrointestinal; lower gastrointestinal

LGIB low gastrointestinal bleeding

LGIC ligand-gated ion channel

LGL large granular leukocyte; large granular lymphocyte; Lown-Ganong-Levine [syndrome]

LGL-NK large granular lymphocyte–natural killer

LGM left gluteus medius

3LGM three-level graph-based model

LGMD limb-girdle muscular dystrophy

LGN lateral geniculate nucleus; lateral glomerulonephritis

LGP labioglossopharyngeal

LGS Langer-Giedion syndrome; Lennox-Gastaut syndrome; limb-girdle syndrome

LGSIL low-grade squamous intraepithelial lesions

LGSS low-grade stromal sarcoma

LGT late generalized tuberculosis

LGTI lower genital tract infection

LGTV Langat virus

LGV large granular vesicle; lymphogranuloma venereum

LGVHD lethal graft-versus-host disease

LgX lymphogranulomatosis X

LH late healing; lateral habecular [nucleus]; lateral hypothalamic [syndrome]; lateral hypothalamus; left hand; left heart; left hemisphere; left hyperphoria; liver homogenate; long handled; loop of Henle; lower half; lues hereditaria; lung homogenate; luteinizing hormone; Lyon hypertensive [rat]

L/H lung/heart ratio

LHA lateral hypothalamic area; lay health advisor; left hepatic artery; low height for age

LHB long head of biceps; luteinizing hormone beta chain

LHBV left heart blood volume

LHC Langerhans cell histiocytosis; left heart catheterization; left hypochondrium; light-harvesting complex; Local Health Council

LHCA laparoscopic hepatectomy by curettage and aspiration

LHCGR luteinizing hormone–choriogonadotropin receptor

LHD lateral head displacement [sperm]; left heart disease

LHe liquid helium

LHEG local health care executive group

LHF left heart failure

LHFA lung Hageman factor activator

LHG left hand grip; localized hemolysis in gel

LHI laboratory for health care informatics; lipid hydrocarbon inclusion; local health jurisdiction

LHIPS Local Heparin Infusion Pre-Stenting [trial]

LHIS lipomatous hypertrophy of interatrial septum

LHL left hepatic lobe

LHM lysuride hydrogen maleate

LHMP Life Health Monitoring Program

LHN lateral hypothalamic nucleus

LHNCBC Lister Hill National Center for Biomedical Communication

LHOF laparoscopically harvested omental flap

LHON Leber hereditary optic neuropathy

LHP lifetime health plan

LHPZ low high-pressure zone

LHR leukocyte histamine release; lifetime health record; lymph node homing receptor

L-hr lumen-hour

LHRF luteinizing hormone–releasing factor

LHRH, LH-RH luteinizing hormone—releasing hormone

LHRHR luteinizing hormone—releasing hormone receptor

LHS left-hand side; left heart strain; left heelstrike; library of health sciences; Losartan Hemodynamic Study; Lung Heart Study; lymphatic hematopoietic system

LHT left hypertropia; Lifestyle Heart Trial

LHV left hepatic vein

LI first stage of syphilis; labeling index; lactose intolerance; lacunar infarct; lamellar ichthyosis; Langerhans islet; large intestine; *Leptospira icterohaemorrhagiae*; linguoincisal; link interface; lithogenic index; low impulsiveness

LI, LII, LIII first, second, third stage of syphilis

L&I liver and iron

Li blood group system; labrale inferius; lithium

L-I late inspiratory

LIA Laser Institute of America; left iliac artery; leukemia-associated inhibitory activity; lock-in amplifier; lymphocyte-induced angiogenesis; lysine iron agar

LIAF laser-induced arterial fluorescence; lymphocyte-induced angiogenesis factor

LIAFI late infantile amaurotic familial idiocy

Lib one pound [L. *libra*]

LIBC latent iron-binding capacity

LIC left internal carotid [artery]; left interventricular coronary [artery]; limiting isorrheic concentration; link interface connector; liver iron concentration; local intravascular coagulation

Lic licentiate

LICA left internal carotid artery

LICM left intercostal margin

LicMed Licentiate in Medicine

LICS left intercostal space

LICU laparoscopic intracorporeal ultrasound

LID large intraluminal density; late immunoglobulin deficiency; lymphocytic infiltrative disease

LIF laser-induced fluorescence; left iliac fossa; left index finger; leukemia-inhibiting factor; leukocyte inhibitory factor; leukocytosis-inducing factor; light-induced fluorescence

LIFE lifestyle intervention, food, and exercise program; Losartan Intervention for Endpoint Reduction in Hypertension [trial]; lung imaging fluorescence endoscope

LIFO last in, first out

LIFR leukemia inhibitory factor receptor

LIFT late intervention following thrombolysis; lymphocyte immunofluorescence test

Lig ligament; ligation

LIH left inguinal hernia

LIHA low impulsiveness, high anxiety

LIHFE Living With Heart Failure [questionnaire]

LIHPS local infusion of heparin prior to stenting

LIJ left internal jugular [vein]

LILA low impulsiveness, low anxiety

LILT low-intensity laser therapy

LIM line isolation monitor

Lim limit, limited

LIMA left internal mammary artery

LIME Leeds interactive medical education

LIMIT Laboratory for Integrated Medical Interface Technology; Leicester Intravenous Magnesium Intervention Trial

LIMIT-AMI Double Blind, Placebo-Controlled, Multicenter Angiographic Trial of RhuMAb CD 18 in Acute Myocardial Infarction

LIMITS Liquemin in Myocardial Infarction During Thrombolysis with Saruplase [trial]

LIMM lethal infantile mitochondrial myopathy

LIN linear statistical classifier

lin liniment

LINAC linear accelerator

LINC laboratory instrumentation computer

LINE long interspersed repetitive element

Linim liniment

LIO left inferior oblique

LIP lipase; lipocortin; lithium-induced polydipsia; lower inflection point; lymphoid/lymphocytic interstitial pneumonitis

Lip lipoate

LIPA line probe assay

LIPB lipase B

LIPD lipase D

LIPID Long-Term Intervention with Pravastatin in Ischemic Disease [trial]

LipoMM lipomyelomeningocele

LIPOX lipid oxidation; lipoxygenase

LIPP laser-induced pressure pulse

LIPS Lescol Intervention Prevention Study

LIPV left inferior pulmonary vein; Lipovnik virus

LIQ low inner quadrant

Liq liquid [L. *liquor*]

Liq dr liquid dram

Liq oz liquid ounce

Liq pt liquid pint

Liq qt liquid quart

LIR left iliac region; left inferior rectus

LIRBM liver, iron, red bone marrow

LIS laboratory information system; lateral intercellular space; learning and intelligent system; left intercostal space; library

LISA information service; lissencephaly; lobular in situ; locked-in syndrome; low intermittent suction; low ionic strength

LISA Lescol in Severe Atherosclerosis [trial]; less-invasive surgical approach; Library and Information Science Abstracts

LISF linear least square fit

LISP List Processing Language

LISREL linear structural relations

LISS less invasive stabilization system; low-ionic-strength saline

LISU library and information statistics unit

Li/SVO lithium silver vanadium oxide

LIT Leiden Intervention Trial; leukocyte immunization therapy; liver infusion tryptose; liver-intestinal transplantation; local immune therapy; Lopressor Intervention Trial

LITA left internal thoracic artery; Library and Information Technology Association

LITE low-intensity treadmill exercise

LITT laser-induced interstitial thermotherapy; laser-induced thermal therapy; laser-induced thermography/thermotherapy

LIU liver injury units

LIV left innominate vein; louping ill virus

Liv live, living

LIV-BP leucine, isoleucine, and valine-binding protein

LIVC left inferior vena cava

LIVE Left Ventricular Hypertrophy: Indapamide vs. Enalapril [trial]

LIVEN linear inflammatory verrucous epidermal nevus

LIVH laparoscopic incisional/ventral hernia

LJ Lowenstein-Jensen [medium]

LJAV Landjia virus

LJI List of Journals Indexed [in Index Medicus]

LJM limited joint mobility; Lowenstein-Jensen medium

LJNV Lanjan virus

LJV La Joya virus

LK lamellar keratoplasty; Landry-Kussmaul [syndrome]; left kidney; lichenoid keratosis; lymphokine

Lkc leukocyte

Lkcs leukocytes

LKKS liver, kidneys, spleen

LKM liver-kidney microsomal [antibody]

LKP lamellar keratoplasty

LKS Landau-Kleffner syndrome; liver, kidneys, spleen

LKSB liver, kidney, spleen, bladder

LKV laked kanamycin vancomycin [agar]

LL large lymphocyte; lateral lemniscus; left lateral; left leg; left lower; left lung; lepromatous; lepromatous leprosy; lipoprotein

lipase; loudness level; lower lid; lower limb; lower lip; lower lobe; lumbar length; lymphocytic lymphoma; lymphoid leukemia; lysolecithin

LLA left lung apex; limulus lysate assay; lipid-lowering agent

LLAEP long latency auditory evoked potential

LLam lumbar laminectomy

LLAT left lateral; lysolecithin aminotransferase

L lat left lateral

LLB left lateral border; long leg brace

LLBCD left lower border of cardiac dullness

LLC laparoscopic laser cholecystectomy; Lewis lung carcinoma; link layer controller; liquid-liquid chromatography; long-leg cast; lymphocytic leukemia

LLCC long-leg cylinder cast

LLCD link layer controller detector

LLC-MK1 rhesus monkey kidney cells

LLC-MK2 rhesus monkey kidney cells

LLC-MK3 *Cercopithecus* monkey kidney cells

LLC-RK1 rabbit kidney cells

LLD left lateral decubitus; leg length discrepancy; limb length discrepancy; lipid-lowering drug; long-lasting depolarization; lower limit of detectability

LLE left lower extremity

LLETZ large loop excision of the transformation zone

LLF Laki-Lorand factor; late-life forgetfulness; left lateral femoral; left lateral flexion

LLI leg length inequality; low-level interface

LLL late luminal loss; left lower lid; left liver lobe; left lower leg; left lower lobe

LLLE lower lid, left eye

LLLT low reactive level laser therapy

LLM localized leukocyte mobilization

LLMSE linear least mean square error

LLN lower limit of normal

LLNA local lymph node assay

LLO *Legionella*-like organism; listeriolysin O; lower limb orthosis

LLP late luteal phase; long-lasting potentiation

LLPV left lower pulmonary vein

LLQ left lower quadrant; low-level question

LLR large local reaction; left lateral rectus; left lumbar region; ligation linked reaction; long intergenic region; long latency reflex

LLRE lower lid, right eye

LLS lazy leukocyte syndrome; Level of Living Survey; linear least squares; long leg splint; low-level segmentation

LLSB left lower scapular border; left lower sternal border

LLSF linear least squares fit

LLSV Llano Seco virus

LLT left lateral thigh; lowest level term; low-level light therapy; lysolecithin

LLV lymphatic leukemia virus

LLV-F lymphatic leukemia virus, Friend associated

LLVP left lateral ventricular preexcitation

LLWC long leg walking cast

LLX left lower extremity

LLZ left lower zone

LLZ-TB lower lung zone tuberculosis

LM labiomental; lactic acid mineral [medium]; lactose malabsorption; laminin; laryngeal mask; laryngeal melanosis; laryngeal muscle; lateral malleolus; left main [coronary artery]; left marginal [coronary artery]; left median; legal medicine; lemniscus medialis; leptomeningeal; Levenberg-Marquardt [algorithm]; Licentiate in Medicine; Licentiate in Midwifery; light microscope, light microscopy; light minimum; lincomycin; lingual margin; linguomesial; lipid mobilization; liquid membrane; *Listeria monocytogenes*; living male; localized movement; longitudinal muscle; lower motor [neuron]; lung metastases; lymphatic metastases

L/M Latin male

Lm *Listeria monocytogenes*; lower midline; lumen

L/m liters per minute

LMA laryngeal mask airway; left main [coronary] artery; left mentoanterior; limbic midbrain area; liver cell membrane auto-antibody

LMB Laurence-Moon-Biedl [syndrome]; left main bronchus; leiomyoblastoma; leukomethylene blue

LMBB Laurence-Moon-Bardet-Biedl [syndrome]

LMBS Laurence-Moon-Biedl syndrome

LMC large motile cell; lateral motor column; left main coronary [artery]; left middle cerebral [artery]; living male child; lymphocyte-mediated cytotoxicity; lymphomyeloid complex

LMCA left main coronary artery; left middle cerebral artery

LMCAD left main coronary artery disease

LMCAO left marginal coronary artery occlusion

LMCC Licentiate of the Medical Council of Canada

LMCL left midclavicular line

LMD lipid-moiety modified derivative; local medical doctor; low-molecular-weight dextran; lumbar microdiscotomy

LMDS locally multiply damaged site

LMDX low-molecular-weight dextran

LME left mediolateral episiotomy; leukocyte migration enhancement; longitudinal mixed effects

LMed&Ch Licentiate in Medicine and Surgery

LMF left middle finger; lymphocyte mitogenic factor

Lm/ft² lumens per square foot

LMG lethal midline granuloma; lingual mucosal graft

LMH lipid-mobilizing hormone

Lmh lumen hour

LMHI Liga Medicorum Homeopathica Internationalis

LMI leukocyte migration inhibition

LMIF leukocyte migration inhibition factor

L/min liters per minute

LMK low molecular weight kininogen

LML large and medium lymphocytes; left mediolateral; left middle lobe

LMM *Lactobacillus* maintenance medium; laser microbeam microdissection; lentigo maligna melanoma; light meromyosin

Lm/m² lumens per square meter

LMMG low molecular mass G [protein]

LMMH low molecular mass heparin

LMN lower motor neuron

LMNL lower motor neuron lesion

LMO living modified organism; localized molecular orbital

LMP large multifunctional protease; last menstrual period; latent membrane potential; left mentoposterior; lumbar puncture

LMPS lethal multiple pterygium syndrome

LMR left medial rectus; localized magnetic resonance; longitudinal medical record; lymphocytic meningopolyradiculitis

LMRCP Licentiate in Midwifery of the Royal College of Physicians

LMRP local medical review policy

LMS laboratory information management system; laser marker system; lateral medullary syndrome; least mean square; left main stem [coronary artery]; leiomyosarcoma; Licentiate in Medicine and Surgery

Lms lumen-second

LMS HPF least means square high-pass filter

LMSSA Licentiate in Medicine and Surgery of the Society of Apothecaries

LMT left main trunk; left mentotransverse; leukocyte migration technique; Licensed Massage Therapist

LMV larva migrans visceralis

LMW low molecular weight

Lm/W lumens per watt
LMWD low-molecular-weight dextran
LMWH low-molecular-weight heparin
LMWP low-molecular-weight proteinuria
LMWT low molecular weight
LMZ left midzone
LN labionasal; laminin; Lesch-Nyhan [syndrome]; lipoid nephrosis; Lisch nodule; low necrosis; lung nodule; lupus nephritis; lymph node; Lyon normotensive [rat]
LN₂ liquid nitrogen
L/N letter/numerical [system]
Ln lymph node; natural logarithm
LNAA large neutral amino acid
LNBx lymph node biopsy
LNC Legal Nurse Consultant; lymph node cell
LNCC Legal Nurse Consultant, Certified
lncRNA long non-coding radionuclide angiography
LND lymph node dissection
LNDS lymph node–negative dataset
LNE lymph node enlargement
LNF laparoscopic Nissen fundoplication
Lng-IUD levonorgestrel-releasing intrauterine device
LNG-IUS levonorgestrel-releasing intrauterine system
LNH large number hypothesis
LNKS low natural killer syndrome
LNL lymph node lymphocyte
LNLS linear-nonlinear least squares
LNM lymph node metastasis
LNMC lymph node mononuclear cell
LNMP last normal menstrual period
LNNB Luria-Nebraska Neuropsychological Battery
LNP large neuronal polypeptide
LNPF lymph node permeability factor
LNS lateral nuclear stratum; Lesch-Nyhan syndrome
LNV last normal vertebra
LO lateral oblique; linguo-occlusal; lipooxygenase; lumbar orthosis; lysyl oxidase
5-LO 5-lipooxygenase
LOA leave of absence; Leber optic atrophy; left occipitoanterior
LOAEL lowest observed adverse effect level
LOB loss of balance
LOC laxative of choice; level of consciousness; liquid organic compound; locus of control; loss of consciousness
LOCA low osmolarity contrast agent
Lo cal low calorie
Lo calc low calcium
LOCAT Lopid Coronary Angiography Trial
LOCF last observation carried forward

Lo CHO low carbohydrate
Lo chol low cholesterol
LOCM low molecular contrast medium
LOCS laryngoonychocutaneous syndrome; lens opacities classification system
LOD laparoscopic ovarian drilling; limit of detection; line of duty; log odds ratio
LOF lofexidine
LOFD low-outlet forceps delivery
LOG lipoxygenase
LOG, LoG laplacian of gaussian [imaging]
Log logarithm
LOGI low glycemic index
LOGIC laryngeal and ocular granulations in children of the Indian subcontinent [syndrome]
LOH loop of Henle; loss of heterozygosity
LOHF late-onset hepatic failure
LOI level of incompetence; level of injury; limit of impurities; loss of imprinting
LOIH left oblique inguinal hernia
Lo K low potassium
LOKD late-onset Krabbe disease
LOKV Lokern virus
LOL left occipitolateral
LOM left otitis media; ligament of Marshall; limitation of motion; loss of motion
LOMC laser optical memory card
LOMIR-MCT-IL Lomir [Isradipine] Multicenter Study in Israel
LOMSA left otitis media suppurativa acuta
LOMSC, LOMSCh left otitis media suppurativa chronica
Lo Na low sodium
Long longitudinal
LONIR Laboratory of Neuro-Imaging Resources
LOO leave one out
LOP leave on pass; left occipitoposterior
LOPAIR long path infrared [alarm]
LOPP chlorambucil, vincristine, procarbazine, prednisolone
LOPS length of patient's stay
LOQ limit of quantification; lower outer quadrant
LOR limit of reporting; long open reading frame; lorazepam; loricrin; loss of righting reflex
Lord lordosis, lordotic
LORETA low-resolution brain electromagnetic tomography
LORF long open reading frame
LOS length of stay; Licentiate in Obstetrical Science; lipo-oligosaccharide; low cardiac output syndrome; lower [o]esophageal sphincter
LOS(P) lower [o]esophageal sphincter

LOT lateral olfactory tract; left occipito-transverse; Long-Term Outcome After Thrombolysis [study]; lysis onset time
Lot lotion
LOV large opaque vesicle; loviride
LOWBI low-birth-weight infant
LOX liquid oxygen; lysyl oxidase
LOXL lysyl oxidase−like
LP labile peptide; labile protein; laboratory procedure; lactic peroxidase; lamina propria; laryngopharyngeal; late potential; latency period, latent period; lateralis posterior; lateral plantar; lateral posterior; lateral pylorus; latex particle; *Legionella pneumophila*; leukocyte poor; leukocytic pyrogen; levator palatini; levator palpebrae; lichen planus; ligamentum patellae; light padding; light perception; lingua plicata; linear predictive; linear programming; linguopulpal; lipoprotein; liver plasma; longitudinal propagation; loss of privileges; low potency; low power; low pressure; low protein; lumbar puncture; lumboperitoneal; lung parenchyma; lymphocyte predominant; lymphoid plasma; lymphomatoid papulosis
L/P lactate/pyruvate ratio; liver plasma [concentration]; lymph/plasma ratio
Lp lipoprotein; sound pressure level
L$_p$ path length
LPA latex particle agglutination; left pulmonary artery; lipoprotein A; lysophosphatidic acid
Lp(a) lipoprotein A
LPAI low-pathogenic avian influenza
LPAM L-phenylalanine mustard
LPB, Lp(b) lipoprotein B
LPBP low-profile bioprosthesis
LPC laser photocoagulation; late positive component; leukocyte-poor cell; linear predictive coding; lipocortin; longitudinal primary care [program]; lysophosphatidylcholine
LPCh lateroposterior choroidal
LPCM low-placed conus medullaris
LP/cm line pairs per centimeter
LPCT late proximal cortical tubule
LPD Lovelace Patient Database; low-protein diet; luteal phase defect; lymphoproliferative disease
LPDF lipoprotein-deficient fraction
LPDS lymph node−positive dataset
LPE lipoprotein electrophoresis; liquid phase epitaxy; lysophosphatidylethanolamine
LPF leukocytosis-promoting factor; leukopenia factor; lipopolysaccharide factor; localized plaque formation; low-pass filter; low-power field; lymphocytosis-promoting factor

Lpf low-power field
LPFB left posterior fascicular block
LPFN low-pass filtered noise
LPFS low-pass filtered signal
LPG left paracolic gutter; lipophosphoglycan
LPH lactase-phlorizin hydrolase; left posterior hemiblock; lipotropic pituitary hormone
LPHA local public health agency
LPHAS limb/pelvis hypoplasia/aplasia syndrome
LPHD lymphocyte-predominant Hodgkin disease
LPHL lymphocyte-predominant Hodgkin lymphoma
LPI left posterior-inferior; lysinuric protein intolerance
LPIFB left posteroinferior fascicular block
LPIH left posteroinferior hemiblock
LPK liver pyruvate kinase
LPL left precordial lead; lethal−potentially lethal; lichen planus−like lesion; lipoprotein lipase; local probability of lesion; lymphoplasmacytic lymphoma
LPLA lipoprotein lipase activity
LPM lateral pterygoid muscle; leverage and parallelepiped mechanism; liver plasma membrane
Lpm lines per minute; liters per minute
Lp/mm line pairs per millimeter
LPN Licensed Practical Nurse
LPO lactoperoxidase; left posterior oblique; light perception only; lipid peroxidation
LPOHH large paraesophageal hiatus hernia
LPOp lipid peroxidation potential
LPP large plaque parapsoriasis; lateral pterygoid plate
LPPH late postpartum hemorrhage
LPR lactate-pyruvate ratio; laryngopharyngeal reflux; late-phase reaction
Lpro longitudinal prospective [trial]
LPS lateral premotor system; levator palpebrae superioris; linear profile scan; link power status; lipase; lipopolysaccharide; Lovastatin Pravastatin Study; low pain sensitivity
Lps liters per second
LPSR lipopolysaccharide receptor
LPT Language Proficiency Test; lipotropin
LPTP Laboratory Proficiency Testing Program [AOAC program]
LPV lapine parvovirus; left portal view; left pulmonary veins; lopinavir
LPVP left posterior ventricular preexcitation
LPV/RTV lopinavir/ritonavir
LPW lateral pharyngeal wall
Lpw lumens per watt
LPX, Lp-X lipoprotein-X
LPyV lymphotropic polyomavirus

LQ linear quadratic; longevity quotient; lordosis quotient; lower quadrant

LQS Lexicon Query Service Specifications

LQT long QT [syndrome]

LQTS long QT syndrome

LR labeled release; laboratory references; laboratory report; labor room; lactated Ringer's [solution]; large reticulocyte; latency reaction; latency relaxation; lateral rectus; lateral retinaculum; left hand; left handed; left rotation; level of recommendation; level of risk; light reaction; light reflex; likelihood ratio; limb reduction; limit of reaction; livedo reticularis; local recurrence; logistic regression; low renin; lymphocyte recruitment

L-R left to right

L/R left/right ratio

LR[+] positive likelihood ratio

LR[−] negative likelihood ratio

L&R left and right

Lr lawrencium; limes reacting dose [least amount of toxin that will produce a reaction]

L$_r$ limes reacting dose [least amount of toxin that will produce a reaction]

LRA local relevance aggregation; low right atrium

LRC learning resource center; lipid research clinic; lower rib cage

LRC-CDPT Lipid Research Clinics Coronary Drug Project Trial

LRC-CPPT Lipid Research Clinics Coronary Primary Prevention Trial

LRCMB Laboratory of Retinal Cell and Molecular Biology

LRC-MFS Lipid Research Clinics Mortality Follow-Up Study

LRCP Licentiate of the Royal College of Physicians; low-risk chest pain

LRCS Licentiate of the Royal College of Surgeons

LRCSE Licentiate of the Royal College of Surgeons, Edinburgh

LRD living related donor

LRDT living related donor transplant

LRE lamina rara externa; leukemic reticuloendotheliosis; lymphoreticuloendothelial

LREC language resources and evaluation

LREH low renin essential hypertension

LRES long-range evaluation system

LRes limited resuscitation

Lretro longitudinal retrospective

LRF latex and resorcinol formaldehyde; liver residue factor; luteinizing hormone−releasing factor

LRG leucine-rich glycoprotein

LRH likelihood ratio for heterogeneity; luteinizing hormone−releasing hormone

LRI lamina rara interna; Learning Retinal Implant [system]; lower respiratory illness/ infection; lymphocyte reactivity index

LRL lower rate limit

LRLT living related donor transplantation

LRM left radical mastectomy; logistic regression model

LRMP last regular menstrual period

LRN Laboratory Response Network; lateral reticular nucleus; low-risk neonatal

LROP lower radicular obstetrical paralysis

LRP lichen ruber planus; linear resolution pattern; lipoprotein receptor−related protein; long-range planning

LRPC Long-Range Planning Committee

Lr-PET low-resolution positron emission tomography

LRQ lower right quadrant

LRR labyrinthine righting reflex; leucine-rich repeat; light reflection rheography; local regional recurrence; locoregional recurrence; locoregional relapse; lymph return rate

LRS laboratory results; lactated Ringer solution; lateral recess stenosis; lateral recess syndrome; low rate of stimulation; lumboradicular syndrome

LRSB lower right sternal border

LRSDS long-range standoff-detection system

LRSF lactating rat serum factor; liver-regenerating serum factor

L-Rsh, L-R shunt left-right shunt

LRSS late respiratory systemic syndrome

LRT lateral reticular nucleus; living related transplant; local radiation therapy; long terminal repeat; Lovastatin Restenosis Trial; lower respiratory tract

LRTI lower respiratory tract illness; lower respiratory tract infection

LRV Lato River virus; left renal vein; *Leishmania* RNA virus

LRYGBP laparoscopic Roux-en-Y gastric bypass

LS lateral septum; lateral suspensor; leader sequence; learning system; least; left sacrum; left septum; left side; legally separated; Leigh syndrome; leiomyosarcoma; length of stay; Leriche syndrome; Letterer-Siwe [disease]; Licentiate in Surgery; lichen sclerosis; life sciences; light scanning; light scattering; light sensitive, light sensitivity; light sensor; light sleep; Likert score; liminal sensation; linear scanning; linear scleroderma; lipid synthesis; liver and spleen; long sleep; longitudinal section; longitudinal study; Lowe syndrome; low-sodium [diet]; lower strength; lumbar spine; lumbosacral; lung surfactant; lymphosarcoma

L-S Letterer-Siwe [disease]; lipid-saccharide

L:S lecithin/sphingomyelin ratio

L/S lactase/sucrase ratio; lecithin/sphingomyelin ratio; lipid/saccharide ratio; longitudinal section; lumbosacral

L&S liver and spleen

LSA left sacroanterior; left subclavian artery; leukocyte-specific activity; leukocyte-specific antigen; Licensed Surgical Assistant; lichen sclerosus et atrophicus; lymphosarcoma

LS&A lichen sclerosus et atrophicus

LSAH Longitudinal Study of Astronaut Health

LSANA leukocyte-specific antinuclear antibody

LSA/RCS lymphosarcoma/reticulum cell sarcoma

LSB least significant bit; left sternal border; left scapular border; long spike burst; lower sternal border; lumbar sympathetic block

LSBE low-segment Barrett esophagus

LS-BMD lumbar spine bone mineral density

LSC last sexual contact; late systolic click; least significant change; left side colon cancer; left subclavian; lichen simplex chronicus; liquid scintillation counting; liquid-solid chromatography; locus subcoeruleus

LSc local scleroderma

LScA left scapuloanterior

LSCL lymphosarcoma cell leukemia

LSCM laser scanning confocal microscopy

LScP left scapuloposterior

LSCS lower segment cesarean section

LSCT lung cancer screening test

LSCVP left subclavian central venous pressure

LSD laryngeal sound discrimination; least significant difference; least significant digit; low-sodium diet; lysergic acid diethylamide

LSD-25 lysergic acid diethylamide

LSDIS large-scale distributed information system

LSE least squares error; left sternal edge

LSect longitudinal section

LSEM loaned self-measurement

LSEP left somatosensory evoked potential; lumbosacral somatosensory evoked potential

LSER linear solvation energy relationship

LSF linear spread function; low saturated fat; lymphocyte-stimulating factor

LSFB least squares forward backward

LSG labial salivary gland; losigamone

LSGP leukocyte sialoglycoprotein

LSH laparoscopic supracervical hysterectomy; lutein-stimulating hormone; lymphocyte-stimulating hormone

LSHTM London School of Hygiene and Tropical Medicine

LSI large-scale integration; latent semantic indexing; life satisfaction index; List of Serials Indexed; lumbar spine index

LSIL low-grade squamous intraepithelial lesion

LSK liver, spleen, kidneys

LSKM liver-spleen-kidney megaly

LSL left sacrolateral; left short leg; lymphosarcoma leukemia

LSM laser scanning microscopy; late systolic murmur; least square matching; least square mean; lymphocyte separation medium; lysergic acid morpholide

LSN large-scale networking; left substantia nigra; Licensed School Nurse

LSNWG Large Scale Networking Working Group

LSO lateral superior olive; left salpingo-oophorectomy; left superior oblique; lumbosacral orthosis

LSP left sacroposterior; linguistic string project; liver-specific protein; lymphocyte-specific protein

LSp life span

L-Spar asparaginase (Elspar)

LSP-MLP linguistic string project medical language processor

LSPV left superior pulmonary vein

LSR lanthanide shift reagent; laser skin resurfacing; lecithin/sphingomyelin ratio; left superior rectus; liver/spleen ratio

LSRA low septal right atrium

LSRO Life Sciences Research Office

LSS latest starting shift; Life Span Study; life support station; liver-spleen scan; lumbar spinal stenosis; lumbosacral spine

LSSA lipid-soluble secondary antioxidant

LS-SEDUHS Longitudinal Study on Socio-Economic Differences in Utilization of Health Services

LS-SEHD Longitudinal Study on Socio-Economic Health Differences

LSSP-PCR low-stringency single specific primer polymerase chain reaction

LST lateral spinothalamic tract; lateral spreading tumor; left sacrotransverse; leishmanin skin test; life-sustaining treatment

LSTAT life support for trauma and transport

LSTL laparoscopic tubal ligation

LSU lactose-saccharose-urea [agar]; life support unit

LSV lateral sacral vein; left subclavian vein; lesser saphenous vein; Lone Star virus; longitudinal sound velocity

LSVC left superior vena cava

LSVT large-scale vocabulary test; left saphenous vein thrombophlebitis

LSWA large amplitude slow wave activity

LT heat-labile toxin; laboratory technologist; laboratory technology; laminar tomography; Laplace transform; laryngeal tube; left; left thigh; left thoracic; less than; lethal time; lethal toxin; leukotriene; Levin tube; levothyroxine; light; line termination; liver transplantation; long term; low temperature; lumbar traction; lymphocytic thyroiditis; lymphocytotoxin; lymphotoxin; syphilis [lues] test

L-T3 ʟ-triiodothyronine

L-T4 ʟ-thyroxine

Lt left; light; low tension

LTA leukotriene A; lipoate transacetylase; lipotechoic acid; local tracheal anesthesia; long-term archives; lost-time accident

LTAC long-term acute care

L-TAP Lipid Treatment Assessment Project

LTAS lead tetraacetate Schiff

LTB larparoscopic tubal banding; laryngotracheobronchitis; leukotriene B

LTBI latent tuberculosis infection

LTBMC long-term bone marrow culture

LTC large transformed cell; leukotriene C; lidocaine tissue concentration; long-term care; lysed tumor cell

L1TC level 1 trauma center

LTCF long-term care facility

LTCIC, LTC-IC long-term culture-initiating cell

LTCS low transverse cervical section

LTD Laron-type dwarfism; laterodorsal tegmental [nucleus]; leukotriene D; long-term [cortical] depression; long-term disability

LTE laryngotracheoesophageal; leukotriene E

LT-ECG long-term electrocardiography

LTF lactotransferrin; lateral tegmental field; lipotropic factor; lymphocyte-transforming factor

LTFU lost to follow-up

LTG lamotrigine; long-term goal; low-tension glaucoma

LTH lactogenic hormone; local tumor hyperthermia; low temperature holding; luteotropic hormone

LTI lupus-type inclusion

LTK laser thermokeratoplasty; leukocyte tyrosine kinase

Lt lat left lateral

LTLT low temperature, long time

LTM lean tissue mass; long-term memory

LTMs leukotriene-modifying agents

LTN lateral telangiectatic nevus

LTNP long-term nonprogressor

LTO₂ long-term oxygen therapy

LTOT long-term oxygen therapy

LTP laryngotracheoplasty; lateral thigh perforator; Learning Technologies Project; leukocyte thromboplastin; lipid transfer protein; long-term potentiation; ʟ-tryptophan

LTPA leisure-time physical activity

LTPP lipothiamide pyrophosphate

LTR laryngotracheal reconstruction; location transactivating region; long terminal repeat

LTRA leukotriene receptor antagonist; long-term repopulating ability

LTS laboratory tests; least trimmed squares; long-term survival/survivor

LTST low-temperature stabilization technology

LTT lactose tolerance test; leucine tolerance test; limited treadmill test; lymphocyte transformation test

LTV lung thermal volume

LTW Leydig cell tumor in Wistar rat

LTX liver transplantation

LU left upper; loudness unit; Lupron; lytic unit

L&U lower and upper

Lu lutetium

LUC large unstained cell; luciferase

LUCL lateral ulnar collateral ligament

LUE left upper extremity

LUF lesion underdose factor; luteinized unruptured follicle

LUFS luteinized unruptured follicle syndrome

LUKV Lukuni virus

LUL left upper eyelid; left upper limb; left upper lobe; left upper lung

Lumb lumbar

LUMD lowest usual maintenance dose

LUMO lowest unoccupied molecular orbital

LUMPS liver unit management protocol system

LUNA laparoscopic uterine nerve ablation

LUO left ureteral orifice

LUOQ left upper outer quadrant

LUP left ureteropelvic; low urethral pressure

LUPV left upper pulmonary vein

LUQ left upper quadrant

LURD living unrelated donor

LUS laparoscopic ultrasound; lower uterine segment

LUSB left upper scapular border; left upper sternal border

LUT look-up table

LUTO lower urinary tract obstruction

LUTS lower urinary tract symptoms

LUV large unilamellar vesicle

LUZ left upper zone

LV laryngeal vestibule; latent virus; lateral ventricle; lecithovitellin; left ventricle, left ventricular; Lentivirus, leucovorin; leukemia virus; leukosis virus; live vaccine; live virus;

livedo reticularis; low voltage; low volume; lumbar vertebra; lung volume; lupus vulgaris; lyssavirus

Lv brightness or luminance; leave

LVA left ventricular aneurysm; left vertebral artery

LVAD left ventricular assist device

LV$_{ap}$ apical aspect of left ventricle

L-variant a defective bacterial variant that can multiply on hypertonic medium

LVAS left ventricular assist system

LV$_{bas}$ lateral basilar left ventricle

LVBP left ventricular bypass pump

LVC low-viscosity cement

LVCS low vertical cesarean section

LVD left ventricular dysfunction

LVd latent viroid; left ventricle, distal

LVDD left ventricular diastolic dimension

LVDd left ventricular diastolic dimension; left ventricular dimension in end diastole

LVDI left ventricular dimension

LVDP left ventricular developed pressure; left ventricular diastolic pressure

LVDT linear variable differential transformer

LVDV left ventricular diastolic volume

LVE left ventricular ejection; left ventricular enlargement

LVED left ventricular end diastole

LVEDA left ventricular end-diastolic area

LVEDC left ventricular end-diastolic circumference

LVEDD left ventricular end-diastolic diameter; left ventricular end-diastolic dimension

LVEDI left ventricular end-diastolic volume index

LVEDP left ventricular end-diastolic pressure

LVEDV left ventricular end-diastolic volume

LVEF left ventricular ejection fraction

LVEJT left ventricular ejection time

LVEP left ventricular ejection pressure; left ventricular end-diastolic pressure; low-voltage electric pulse

LVESD left ventricular end-systolic diameter; left ventricular end-systolic dimension

LVESV left ventricular end-systolic volume

LVESVI left ventricular end-systolic volume index

LVET left ventricular ejection time; low-volume eye test

LVETI left ventricular ejection time index

LVF left ventricular failure; left ventricular function; left visual field; low-voltage fast; low-voltage foci

LVFP left ventricular filling pressure

LVFT$_2$ left ventricular slow filling time

LVFW left ventricular free wall

LVG left ventriculogram

LVH large vessel hematocrit; left ventricular hypertrophy

LVI left ventricular insufficiency; left ventricular ischemia; lymphovascular invasion

LVID left ventricular internal dimension

LVIDd left ventricle internal dimension in diastole

LVID$_d$ left ventricle internal dimension in end diastole

LVIDs left ventricle internal dimension in systole

LVID$_s$ left ventricle internal dimension in end systole

LVIV left ventricular inflow volume

LVL large-volume lipoplasty; left vastus lateralis

LVLG left ventrolateral gluteal

LVM left ventricular mass; left ventricular mass index

LVMF left ventricular minute flow

LV$_{mid}$ midanterior left ventricle

LVN Laguerre-Volterra network; lateral ventricular nerve; lateral vestibular nucleus; Licensed Visiting Nurse; Licensed Vocational Nurse

LVO left ventricle outflow

LVOH left ventricle outflow [tract] height

LVOT left ventricular outflow tract

LVOTG left ventricular outflow tract gradient

LVOTO left ventricular outflow tract obstruction

LVOV left ventricular outflow volume

LVP large volume parenteral [infusion]; left ventricular pressure; levator veli palatini; lysine-vasopressin

LVp left ventricle, proximal

LVPFR left ventricular peak filling rate

LVP$_{max}$ maximum left ventricular pressure

LVP$_{min}$ minimum left ventricular pressure

LVPW left ventricular posterior wall

LVQ learning vector quantization

LVR loviride

LVRD left ventricular replacement device

LVRS lung volume reduction surgery

LVS laryngovideostroboscopy; left ventricular strain; live vaccine strain

LVs left ventricular system

LVSEMI left ventricular subendocardial myocardial ischemia

LVSI left ventricular systolic index; lymphovascular space invasion

LVSO left ventricular systolic output

LV-SO left ventricular site of origin

LVSP left ventricular systolic pressure

LVST lateral vestibulospinal tract

LVSV left ventricular stroke volume

LVSW left ventricular stroke work

LVSWI left ventricular stroke work index

LVT left ventricular tension; levetiracetam; lysine vasotonin

LVV left ventricular volume; Le Veen valve; live varicella vaccine; live varicella virus

LVW left ventricular wall; left ventricular work

LVWI left ventricular work index

LVWM left ventricular wall motion

LVWT left ventricular wall thickness

LW lacerating wound; lateral wall; Lee-White [method]

L&W, L/W living and well

Lw lawrencium [obsolete]

LWA low weight for age

LWBS leaving without being seen

LWCT Lee-White clotting time

LWK large white kidney

LWP lateral wall pressure

LWS Lowry-Wood syndrome

LX local irradiation; lower extremity; lymphatic metastases cannot be assessed

Lx larynx; latex; lower extremity; lux

L-XRF L x-ray fluorescence

LXT left exotropia

LY lactoalbumin and yeastolate; lymphocyte

Ly a T-cell antigen used for grouping T lymphocytes into different classes

LyD lysis deficiency

LYDMA lymphocyte-detected membrane antigen

LYES liver yang exuberance syndrome

LYG lymphomatoid granulomatosis

LYM lymph nodes

Lym, lymph lymphocyte, lymphocytic

LyNeF lytic nephritic factor

Lyo lyophilized

LYP lactose, yeast, peptone [agar]; lower yield point

LYS, Lys lysine; lysodren

lys lysine

LySLk lymphoma syndrome leukemia

Lyso-PC lysophosphatidyl phosphatidylcholine

lytes electrolytes

LYZ lysozyme

LZM, Lzm lysozyme

M blood factor in the MNS blood group system; chin [L. *mentum*]; concentration in moles per liter; death [L. *mors*]; dullness [of sound, Lat. *mutitas*]; macerate; macroglobulin; macroscopic magnetization vector; magnetization; magnification; male; malignant; married; masculine; mass; massage; maternal contribution; matrix; mature; maximum; mean; meatus; median; mediator; medical, medicine; medium; mega; megohm; membrane; memory; mental; mesial; metabolite; metanephrine; metastases; meter; methionine; methotrexate; *Micrococcus*; *Microspora*; minim; minute; mitochondria; mitosis; mix, mixed, mixture; mobility; molar [permanent tooth, solution]; molarity; mole; molecular; moment of force; monkey; monocyte; month; morgan; morphine; mother; motile; mouse; mucoid; mucous; multipara; murmur; muscle; muscular response to an electrical stimulation of its motor nerve; *Mycobacterium*; *Mycoplasma*; myeloma or macroglobulinemia [component]; myopia; strength of pole; thousand [L. *mille*]

M- mega- [10^6]

M0 leukemia with large granular blasts and negative myeloperoxidase; no distant tumor metastases; no metastases; no tumor metastases

M1 breast tumor, no distant metastases; distant metastases; distant tumor metastases; leukemia with poorly differentiated myeloblasts; primary motor area

1M, 2M, 3M, 4M, 5M first, second, third, fourth, fifth metatarsal

M₁ mitral component [first heart sound]; mitral first [sound]; myeloblast; slight dullness

M2 breast tumor, distant metastases; leukemia with myeloblasts with differentiation and Auer rods

2-M 2-microglobulin

M₂ dose per square meter of body surface; marked dullness; promyelocyte

M3 leukemia with hypergranular promyelocytes and multiple Auer rods

3-M [syndrome] initials for Miller, McKusick, and Malvaux, who first described the syndrome

M/3 middle third

M₃ absolute dullness; myelocyte at the third stage of maturation

M4 leukemia monoblastic differentiation

M₄ myelocyte at the fourth stage of maturation

M5 monoblastic leukemia

M₅ metamyelocyte

M6 erythroleukemia with dyserythropoiesis and megaloblastosis

M₆ band form in the sixth stage of myelocyte maturation

M7 megakaryoblastic leukemia

M₇ polymorphonuclear neutrophil

M/10 tenth molar solution

M/100 hundredth molar solution

m electron rest mass; electromagnetic moment; magnetic moment; magnetic quantum number; male; mass; median; melting [temperature]; metastable; meter; milli-; minim; minimum; minute; molality; molar [deciduous tooth]; mutated

μ lowercase Greek letter mu; chemical potential; electrophoretic mobility; heavy chain of immunoglobulin M; linear attenuation coefficient; magnetic moment; mean; micro; micrometer; micron; mutation rate; permeability

m⁻¹ per meter

m² square meter

m³ cubic meter

m₈ spin quantum number

MA macrophage aggregate; malignant arrhythmia; management and administration; mandelic acid; Martin-Albright [syndrome]; masseter; Master of Arts; maternal age; matrix; maximum amplitude; mean arterial; mechanical activity; medial amygdaloid; medical assistance; medical audit; medical authorization; mega-ampere; megaloblastic anemia; megestrol acetate; membrane antigen; menstrual age; mental age; mentum anterior; metatarsus adductus; meter-angle; methacrylic acid; microadenoma; microagglutination; microalbuminuria; microaneurysm; microscopic agglutination; Miller-Abbott [tube]; milliampere; mitochondrial antibody; mitogen activation; mitotic apparatus; mixed agglutination; mobile agent; moderately advanced; monoamine; monoarthritis; monoclonal antibody; motor area; movement artifacts; moving average; multiple action; muscle activity; mutagenic activity; myelinated axon; myoclonic absences

MA-104 embryonic rhesus monkey kidney cells

MA-111 embryonic rabbit kidney cells

MA-163 human embryonic thymus cells

MA-184 newborn human foreskin cells

M/A male, altered [animal]; mood and/or affect

Ma mass of atom

mA, ma milliampere; meter-angle

mÅ milliangstrom

ma milliampere

μA microampere

MAA macroaggregated albumin; maleylacetoacetic acid; Medical Assistance for the Aged; melanoma-associated antigen; methacrylic acid; microphthalmia (or anophthalmos) with associated anomalies; moderate aplastic anemia; monoarticular arthritis

MAAB male assigned at birth

MAAC maximum allowable actual charges

MAACL Multiple Affect Adjective Check List

MAAGB Medical Artists Association of Great Britain

MAAP multiple arbitrary amplicon profiling

MAAS Multicenter Anti-Atherosclerosis Study; Multicenter Antiatheroma Study

MAB, MAb, mAB maintained intentional bias; monoclonal antibody

m-AB *m*-aminobenzamide

MABIS Munich and Berlin Infarction Study

MABP mean arterial blood pressure

Mabs, mABs, mAbs monoclonal antibodies

MAC MacConkey [broth]; magnetic authentication code; major ambulatory category; malignancy-associated changes; maximum aerobic capacity; maximum allowable concentration; maximum allowable cost; medical alert center; membrane attack complex; message authentication code; midarm circumference; minimum alveolar concentration; minimum antibiotic concentration; mitral annular calcium; modulator of adenylate cyclase; monitored anesthesia care; multiaccess catheter; *Mycobacterium avium* complex

MACAS Marburg Cardiomyopathy Study

MacCAT-CR MacArthur Competence Assessment Tool for Clinical Research

MACCEs major adverse cardiac and cerebral events

MACDP Metropolitan Atlanta Congenital Defects Program

MACE main adverse coronary event; major adverse cardiac events; major cardiac event; Mayo Asymptomatic Carotid Endarterectomy [trial]

MAC-ei minimum alveolar concentration, endotracheal intubation

MACEmed Middleware Architecture Committee for Education in Medicine

macer maceration

MACH machine activity; Mortality Assessment in Congestive Heart Failure [study]

mAChR muscarinic acetylcholine receptor

MacMV Maclura mosaic virus

MACR mean axillary count rate

mACR muscarinic acetylcholine receptor

MACRA Medicare Access and CHIP Reauthorization Act

macro macrocyte, macrocytic; macroscopic

MACS maximum aortic cusp separation; Multicenter AIDS Cohort Study; myristoylated alanine-rich protein kinase C substrate

MACT maximum achievable control technology

MACTAR McMaster-Toronto arthritis and rheumatism [questionnaire]

MACV Machupo virus

MAD major affective disorder; mandibuloacral dysplasia; master accession database; maximum allowable dose; mean axis direction; median absolute deviation; methylandrostenediol; mind-altering drug; minimum average dose; mitotic arrest defective; mucosal atomization device; multiple autoimmune disorder; myoadenylate deaminase

mAD, MADA muscle adenylate deaminase; myoadenylate deaminase

MADAM Moexipril as Antihypertensive Drug After Menopause [study]

mADAM mouse A disintegrin and A metalloprotease

MadCAM mucosal addressin cell adhesion molecule

MADD Mothers Against Drunk Driving; multiple acyl-CoA dehydrogenase deficiency

MADDS monoacetyldiaminodiphenylsulfone

MADGE microliter array diagonal gel electrophoresis

MADIT Multicenter Automatic Defibrillator Implantation Trial

MADIT/CES Multicenter Automatic Defibrillator Implantation Trial Cost Effectiveness Study

MADPA Medicaid Antidiscriminatory Drug Pricing and Patient Benefit Restoration Act

MADRS Medicare Automated Data Retrieval System; Montgomery-Asberg Depression Rating Scale

MADT morphology alteration and disintegration test

MADU methylaminodeoxyuridine

MADV Madrid virus

MAE mean absolute error; medical air evacuation; medication administration error; 2-methylaminoethanol; moves all extremities; multilingual aphasia examination; myoclonic astatic epilepsy

MAF macrophage activation factor; macrophage agglutinating factor; maximum atrial fragmentation; minimum audible field; minor allele frequency; mouse amniotic fluid

MAFD manic affective disorder

MAFF Ministry of Agriculture, Fisheries and Food

MAFH macroaggregated ferrous hydroxide

MAFI MedicAlert Foundation International

MAG mercaptoacetyltriglycerine; multi-tumor aberrant growth; myelin-associated glyco-protein

Mag magnesium

mAg minor antigen

mag large [L. *magnus*]; magnification

mag cit magnesium citrate

MAGE melanoma antigen

MAGF male accessory gland fluid

MAggF macrophage agglutination factor

MAGIC Magnesium in Cardiac Arrest [trial]; Magnesium in Coronaries [trial]; microprobe analysis generalized intensity correction; mouth (or mucosal) and genital ulceration with inflamed cartilage [syndrome]

MAGICA Magnesium in Cardiac Arrhythmia [trial]

magn large [L. *magnus*]; magnification

MAGP microfibril-associated glycoprotein

MAGPIE Magnesium Sulfate Compared with Placebo in Pre-Eclampsia [study]

MAGUK membrane-associated guanylate kinase

MAGV Maguari virus

MagV mag virus

MAH macronodular adrenal hyperplasia

mAH, mA-h milliampere-hours

MAHA microangiopathic hemolytic anemia

MAHH malignancy-associated humoral hypercalcemia

MAHI, MAHIV medically acquired human immunodeficiency [virus]

MaHR major hematologic response

MAHST Multicenter Austrian Hemodilution Stroke Trial

MaHV Macropodid herpesvirus

MAI Medication Appropriateness Index; microscopic aggregation index; miscarriage after infertility; movement assessment of infants; multilevel assessment instrument; *Mycobacterium avium* infection; *Mycobacterium avium-intracellulare*

MAIDS mouse acquired immunodeficiency syndrome

MAIESTRO The Michael Reese Hospital Institute of Technology Expert System for Stroke

MAIN medication induced, autoimmune, infectious, and neoplastic

MAIPA monoclonal antibody−specific immobilization of platelet antigens

MAIR-IR multiple attenuated internal reflexion infrared [spectroscopy]

MAIS manual axial in-line stabilization; mild androgen insensitivity syndrome

MAJIC Mayo Japan Investigation on Chronic Total Occlusion

MAKA major karyotypic abnormality

MAL malemide; midaxillary line; motor activity log

Mal malate; malfunction; malignancy

mal malaise; male; malposition

Mal-BSA maleated bovine serum albumin

MALD matrix-assisted laser desorption

MALDI matrix-assisted laser desorption/ionization

MALDI-MS matrix-assisted laser desorption/ionization mass spectrometry

MALDI-TOF matrix-assisted laser desorption/ionization time of flight

MALG Minnesota antilymphoblast globulin

MALiMET Master List of Medical Indexing Terms

MALLS multiangle laser light scattering

MALS magnetic alignment and light scattering

MALT male, altered [animal]; mucosa-associated lymphoid tissue; Munich Alcoholism Test

MALTOMA mucosal associated lymphoid tissue lymphoma

MALV Malakal virus

MAM median age at menarche; metabolically active mass; methylazoxymethanol

mam milliampere-minute; myriameter

M+Am compound myopic astigmatism

6-MAM monoacetyl-morphine

MAMA medical application multimedia authoring; monoallelic mutation analysis; monoclonal antimalignin antibody; Mothers Against Misuse and Abuse

MAM Ac methylazoxymethanol acetate

MAMC mean arm muscle circumference

mA-min, ma-min milliampere-minute

Mammo mammogram, mammography

MAN mannose; manual endoscopic instrument

Man mannose

man manipulate

MANA mannosidase alpha

MANB mannosidase beta

ManBP mannan-binding protein

mand mandible, mandibular

MANET mobile ad-hoc network

manifest manifestation

manip manipulation

MANOVA multivariate analysis of variance

MAN-6-P mannose-6-phosphate

MANU manufactured object

MANV Manzanilla virus

MAO Master of the Art of Obstetrics; maximal acid output; monoamine oxidase

MAOA monoamine oxidase A

MAOB monoamine oxidase B

MAOI monoamine oxidase inhibitor

MAP malignant atrophic papulosis; mandibular angle plane; maturation-activated protein; maximal aerobic power; maximum a posteriori; mean airway pressure; mean aortic pressure; mean arterial pressure; Medical Audit Program; megaloblastic anemia of pregnancy; memory algorithm processor; mercapturic acid pathway; methyl acceptor protein; methylacetoxy-progesterone; methylaminopurine; microtubule-associated protein; minimum audible pressure; mitogen-activated protein; modified atmosphere packaging; moment angle plotter; monophasic action potential; motor [nerve] action potential; mouse antibody production; multiphasic algorithmic protocol; multiple antigen peptide; muscle action potential; mussel adhesive protein

MAPA muscle adenosine phosphoric acid

MAPC migrating action potential complex

MAPCA major aortopulmonary collateral artery

MAPE mean absolute percentage error

MAPF microatomized protein food

MAPHY Metoprolol Atherosclerosis Prevention in Hypertension [study]

MAPI microbial alkaline protease inhibitor; Millon Adolescent Personality Inventory

MAPK mitogen-activated protein kinase

MAPK-K mitogen-activated protein kinase kinase

MAPKP mitogen-activated protein kinase phosphatase

MAPP multiple asynchronous parallel processing

MAPPET Management Strategy and Prognosis of Pulmonary Embolism Trial

MAPREC mutant analysis by polymerase chain reaction and restriction enzyme cleavage

MAPS Make a Picture Story [test]; Micro-AIDS Processing System; morphokinetic algorithms to predict success; Multidimensional Affect and Pain Survey; Multivessel Angioplasty Prognosis Study

MAPT microtubule-associated protein tau

MAPV Mapputta virus; mean area—peak value

MAR main admissions room; marasmus; marrow; matrix attachment region; maximal

aggregation ratio; mean atrial rate; medication administration record; microanalysis reagent; minimal angle resolution; mixed antiglobulin reaction; multiple aberration region; multivariate autoregressive [model]

mar margin; marker

MARAV Maraba virus

MARC machine-readable catalog/cataloging; Multicenter Asthma Research Collaboration; multifocal and recurrent choroidopathy

MARCKS myristoylated alanine-rich protein C kinase substrate

MarHV Marmomid herpesvirus

MARIAC Magnetic Resonance Image Analysis Research Centre

MarMV Maracuja virus

MARS magnetic anchor retinal stimulation; medical archival system; Medical Article Record System; methionyl-transfer ribonucleic acid synthetase; Mevinolin Atherosclerosis Regression Study; Missouri Automated Radiology System; mobile autonomous robot software; molecular adsorbent recirculating system; molecular adsorbents system; Monitored Atherosclerosis Regression Study; mouse antirat serum; multivariate adaptive regression spline

MARSA methicillin-aminoglycoside—resistant *Staphylococcus aureus*

MAR/SAR matrix attachment region/scaffold attachment region

MART multiplicative algebraic reconstruction technique

MARV Marburg virus

mar(X) marker X [chromosome]

MAS macrophage activation syndrome; magic angle spinning; Manifest Anxiety Scale; marker-assisted selection; maximum average score; McCune-Albright syndrome; meconium aspiration syndrome; medical administrative services; medical advisory service; medical audit study; meiosis activation sterol; mesoatrial shunt; milk-alkali syndrome; milliampere-second; minor axis shortening; mitral aortic septum; mobile arm support; monoclonal antibodies; Morgagni-Adams-Stokes [syndrome]; motion analysis system; motor assessment scale; multiagent system; multiple access server; myoclonic astatic seizures

mA-s, mas milliampere-second

MASA Medical Association of South Africa; mental retardation, aphasia, shuffling gait, adducted thumbs [syndrome]; mutant allele specific amplification

MASC Multidimensional Anxiety Scale for Children

masc masculine; mass concentration

MASCIS Multicenter Animal Spinal Cord Injury Study

MAS-ECMO meconium aspiration syndrome extracorporeal membrane oxygenation

MASER microwave amplification by stimulated emission of radiation

MASH mobile Army surgical hospital; multiple automated sample harvester

MASK Medical Anatomy Segmentation Kit

masl meters above sea level

MASS Medicine, Angioplasty, or Surgery Study

mass massage

massc mass concentration

MAST Managing Anticoagulation Services Trial; medical antishock trousers; Michigan Alcohol Screening Test; military antishock trousers; motion artifact suppression technique

mast mastectomy; mastoid

MAST-E Multicentre Acute Stroke Trial-Europe

MAST-I Multicenter Acute Stroke Trial-Italy

MASU mobile Army surgical unit

MAT manual arts therapist; Master of Arts in Technology; mean absorption time; medial axis transform; medical assistance team; medical augmentation team; medication-assisted treatment; methionine adenosyltransferase; microagglutination test; minimal access technique; multifocal atrial tachycardia; multiple agent therapy

Mat, mat maternal; mature

MATC maximum allowable toxicant concentration

MATCH Matching Alcoholism Treatment to Client Heterogeneity

MatD maternal disomy

MatDp maternal duplication

MATE Medicine vs. Angiography for Thrombolytic Exclusions [trial]

mat gf maternal grandfather

mat gm maternal grandmother

MATH Modern Approach to Treatment of Hypertension [study]

MATIS Mathematics Tools Integration System

MATSA Marek-associated tumor-specific antigen

MATTIS Multicenter Aspirin and Ticlopidine Trials After Intracoronary Stenting

MATTUS Minimal Access Therapy Training Unit-Scotland

MATV Matucare virus

MAU multiattribute utility

MAUS Mammography Attitudes and Usage Study

MAUT multiattribute utility theory

MAV mechanical auditory ventricle; minimal alveolar ventilation; minimum apparent viscosity; movement arm vector; myeloblastosis-associated virus

MAVD mixed aortic valve disease

MAVERIC Midlands Trial of Empirical Amiodarone vs. Electrophysiological Guided Intervention and Cardioverter Implant in Ventricular Arrhythmias

MAVIS mobile artery and vein imaging system

MAVR mitral and aortic valve replacement

MAX maxadilan

max maxilla, maxillary; maximum

MaxDu maximum duration

MaxEP maximum esophageal pressure

MAYV Mayaro virus

MB Bachelor of Medicine [L. *Medicinae Baccalaureus*]; buccal margin; General Modeling Bayesian Fitting; isoenzyme of creatine kinase containing M and B subunits; mammillary body; Marsh-Bender [factor]; maximum breathing; medulloblastoma; megabyte; mesiobuccal; methyl bromide; methylene blue; microbiologic assay; multibacillary; muscle balance; myocardial band

Mb megabase; megabit; million bases; mouse brain; myoglobin

mb millibar

μ$_B$ Bohr magneton

μb microbar

MBA methylbenzyl alcohol; methyl bovine albumin

MBAC Member of the British Association of Chemists

MBAR myocardial beta adrenergic receptor

mbar millibar

μbar microbar

MBAS methylene blue active substance

MBB modified barbiturate buffer

MBBG metabromobenzylguanidine

MBBS Medicinae Baccalaureus/Bachelor of Surgery

MBC male breast cancer; maximal bladder capacity; maximal breathing capacity; memory B cell; metastatic breast cancer; methyl-1-(butylcarbamoyl)-2-benzimidazole-carbamate; methylthymol blue complex; microcrystalline bovine collagen; minimum bactericidal concentration; moving blood cells

MB-CK creatine kinase isoenzyme containing M and B subunits

MBCL monocytoid B-cell lymphoma

MbCO carbon monoxy myoglobin

MBCR Molecular Biology Computational Resource

MBCS medical billing and coding specialist

MBD Marchiafava-Bignami disease; maximum bactericidal dilution; metabolic bone disease; methylene blue dye; methyl-binding domain; minimal brain damage; minimal brain dysfunction; Morquio-Brailsford disease

MBDG mesiobuccal developmental groove

MBE medium below elbow [cast]

MBEC mouse brain endothelial cell

MBF medullary blood flow; mesenteric blood flow; muscle blood flow; myocardial blood flow

MBFC medial brachial fascial compartment

MBFLB monaural bifrequency loudness balance

MbFV mite-borne filamentous virus

MBG Marburg [disease]; mean blood glucose; morphine-benzedrine group

MBH medial basal hypothalamus

MBH₂ reduced methylene blue

MBHI Millon Behavioral Health Inventory

MBHO managed behavioral health care organization

MBHR mesh-based hernia repair

MBI Maslach Burnout Inventory; maximum blink index

MBK methyl butyl ketone

MBL mannose-binding lectin; Marine Biological Laboratory; menstrual blood loss; minimum bactericidal level

MBLA methylbenzyl linoleic acid; mouse-specific bone-marrow−derived lymphocyte antigen

MbLV mite-borne latent virus

MBM meat and bone meal; mineral basal medium

MBNOA Member of the British Naturopathic and Osteopathic Association

MBO management by objectives; mesiobuccoocclusal

MBO₂ oxymyoglobin

MBOV Mboke virus

MBP major basic protein; maltose-binding protein; management by policy; mannose-binding protein; mean blood pressure; melitensis, bovine, porcine [antigen]; mesiobuccopulpal; myelin basic protein

MBPM modified backward Prony method

MBPS multigated blood pool scanning

Mbps megabits per second; myeloblastic syndrome

MBq megabecquerel

MBR methylene blue, reduced

MBRT methylene blue reduction time

MBS Martin-Bell syndrome; media broadband service; modified barium swallow

MBSA methylated bovine serum albumin

MBSI multichannel blind system identification

MBT maternal blood type; mercaptobenzothiazole; meridian-based therapy; mixed bacterial toxin; myeloblastin

MBTA modeling better treatment advice

MBTH 3-methyl-2-benzothiazoline hydrazone

MBTI Myers-Briggs type indicator

MBVT Munich and Berlin Trial for Sustained Ventricular Tachyarrhythmias

MC mass casualties; mast cell; Master of Surgery [L. *Magister Chirurgiae*]; maximum concentration; Medical Corps; medium chain; medullary cavity; medullary cyst; megacoulomb; melanocortin; melanoma cell; menstrual cycle; Merkel cell; mesiocervical; mesocaval; metacarpal; methyl cellulose; microcephaly; microcholecystectomy; microcirculation; microscopic colitis; midcapillary; mineralocorticoid; mini-catheterization; minimal change; mitomycin C; mitotic cycle; mitral commissurotomy; mixed cellularity; mixed cryoglobulinemia; monkey cell; mononuclear cell; mucous cell; musculocutaneous; myocardial channeling; myocarditis

M/C male, castrated [animal]

M-C mineralocorticoid

M&C morphine and cocaine

Mc megacurie; megacycle

Mₑ mitral closure

mC millicoulomb

mc millicurie

μC microcoulomb; first concept; second concept

μc microcurie

MCA major coronary artery; Maternity Center Association; mean cell area; medical care administration; Medicines Control Agency; methylcholanthrene; microchannel architecture; middle cerebral artery; monoclonal antibody; mucinlike carcinoma-associated antigen; multichannel analyzer; multiple congenital anomaly

MCAB monoclonal antibody

MCAD medium chain acyl-CoA dehydrogenase

MCAF monocyte chemotactic and activating factor

MCA/MR multiple congenital anomaly/mental retardation (intellectual disability) [syndrome]

MCAO middle cerebral artery occlusion

MCAR mixed cell agglutination reaction

MCARE managed care

MCAS middle cerebral artery syndrome

MCAT medical chemical advisory team; medical college admission test; middle cerebral artery thrombosis; Multimedia Cardiac Angiogram Tool; myocardial contrast appearance time

MCAV Macaua virus

MCB master cell bank; membranous cytoplasmic body; monochlorobimane

McB McBurney [point]

mCBF mean cerebral blood flow

MCBIT Munich Coronary Bypass Intervention Trial

MCBM muscle capillary basement membrane

MCBR minimum concentration of bilirubin

MCBS Medicare Current Beneficiary Survey

MCBV minimum conditional bias/variance

MCBW mass casualty biological weapon

MCC mean corpuscular hemoglobin concentration; measles control campaign; medial cell column; Medical Council of Canada; medical information communication control-ler; metacarpal-carpal; metacerebral cell; metastatic cord compression; microcalcification cluster; microcrystalline cellulose; microcrystalline collagen; midstream clean catch; minimum complete-killing concentration; muco-cutaneous candidiasis; mutated in colorectal cancer

MC-C metacarpal-carpal

MCCA mean common carotid artery; Medicare Catastrophic Care Act; Medicare Catastrophic Coverage Act

MCCD minimum cumulative cardiotoxic dose

MCCI medical care component of the consumer price index; medical cost-control initiative

MCCPI medical care component of the consumer price index

MCCU mobile coronary care unit

MCD magnetic circular dichroism; mast cell degranulation; mean cell diameter; mean central dose; mean corpuscular diameter; mean of consecutive differences; Medicaid competition demonstration; medical concepts dictionary; medullary collecting duct; medullary cystic disease; metacarpal cortical density; minimal cerebral dysfunction; minimal change disease; multiple carboxylase deficiency; muscle carnitine deficiency

MCDI Minnesota Child Development Inventory

MCDK multicystic dysplastic kidney

MCDNP medullary cystic disease/nephrolithiasis disease

MCDP mast cell degranulating peptide

MCDU mercaptolactate-cysteine disulfiduria

MCE maximum credible event; medical care evaluation; military clinical engineering; multicystic encephalopathy; multiple cartilaginous exostosis; myocardial contrast echocardiography

MCES medical care evaluation study; multiple cholesterol emboli syndrome

MCF macrophage chemotactic factor; median cleft face; medium corpuscular fragility; method conversion factor; microcomplement fixation; mink cell focus forming; mononuclear cell factor; myocardial contraction force

MCFA medium-chain fatty acid; miniature centrifugal fast analyzer

MCFP mean circulating filling pressure

MCFSR mean circumferential fiber shortening rate

MCG magnetocardiogram; membrane cell graft; membrane coating granule; monoclonal gammopathy

mcg microgram

MCGC metacerebral giant cell

MCGF mast cell growth factor

MCGN mesangiocapillary glomerulonephritis; minimal change glomerulonephritis; mixed cryoglobulinemia with glomerulonephritis

MCGNX mesangiocapillary glomerulonephritis, X-linked

MCH Maternal and Child Health; mean cell hemoglobin; mean corpuscular hemoglobin; medical college hospital; melanin-concentrating hormone; mucous cell hyperplasia; muscle-contraction headache

MCh Master of Surgery [L. *Magister Chirurgiae*]; methacholine

mc-h, mch millicurie-hour

μch microcurie-hour

M-CHAT-R/F Modified Checklist for Autism in Toddlers-Revised, with Follow-up

MCHB Maternal and Child Health Bureau

MCHC maternal/child health care; mean cell hemoglobin concentration; mean corpuscular hemoglobin concentration; mean corpuscular hemoglobin count

MChD Master of Dental Surgery

MCHgb mean corpuscular hemoglobin

MChir Master in Surgery [L. *Magister Chirurgiae*]

MChOrth Master of Orthopaedic Surgery

MChOtol Master of Otology

MCHR Medical Committee for Human Rights

mc-hr millicurie-hour

μC-hr microcurie-hour

MCHS Maternal and Child Health Service

MCI mean cardiac index; methicillin; mild cognitive impairment; molecular connectivity index; mucociliary insufficiency; multiple-casualty incident; muscle contraction interference

MCi megacurie

mCi millicurie

µCi microcurie

MCICU medical coronary intensive care unit

MCID minimum clinically important difference

M-CIDI Munich Composite International Diagnostic Interview

MCi-hr millicurie-hour

µCi-hr microcurie-hour

MCINS minimal change idiopathic nephrotic syndrome

MCK multicystic kidney

MCKD multicystic kidney disease

MCL Macintosh common lisp; mantle cell lymphoma; maximum containment laboratory; maximum contaminant level; medial collateral ligament; midclavicular line; midcostal line; minimal change lesion; mixed culture, leukocyte; modified chest lead; most comfortable loudness; mucocutaneous leishmaniasis; multiple cutaneous leiomyomata; myeloid cell leukemia

MCLC medial collateral ligament complex

MCLNS, MCLS mucocutaneous lymph node syndrome

MClSci Master of Clinical Science

MCM medical core metadata; methylmalonic coenzyme A mutase; minimum capacitation medium; multi-chip module; multicompartmental model

MCMC Markov Chain Monte Carlo [method]

MCMI Millon Clinical Multiaxial Inventory

MCMM Monte Carlo multiple minimum [method]

MCMV murine cytomegalovirus

MCN maternal child nursing; minimal change nephropathy; mixed cell nodular

MCNS minimal change nephrotic syndrome

MCO managed care organization; medical care organization; multichannel option; multicystic ovary

MCommH Master of Community Health

mcoul millicoulomb

µcoul microcoulomb

MCOV Marco virus; modified covariance

MCP major capsid protein; maximum closure pressure; maximum contraction pattern; medical command physician; melanocortin receptor; melphalan, cyclophosphamide, and prednisone; membrane cofactor protein; metacarpophalan-

geal; metoclopramide; mitotic-control protein; monocyte chemotactic protein; Monte Carlo program; mucin clot prevention

MCP-1 monocyte chemotactic protein 1

MCPA Member of the College of Pathologists, Australasia

MCPH metacarpophalangeal

MCPJ metacarpophalangeal joint

MCPP Medical Cannabis Pilot Program; metacarpophalangeal pattern profile; metacarpophalangeal profile

mCPP meta-chlorophenylpiperazine

MCPPP metacarpophalangeal pattern profile plot

MCPS Member of the College of Physicians and Surgeons

Mcps megacycles per second

MCPT Monte Carlo photon transport

MCQ multiple-choice question

MCR massive cortical reorganization; melanocortin receptor; message competition ratio; metabolic clearance rate; myotonia congenita, recessive type

5-MCR 5-methylchrysene

mcr minor breakpoint cluster region

MCRA Member of the College of Radiologists, Australasia

MCRD monolithic controlled release device

MCRE mother-child relationship evaluation

MCRglc cerebral metabolic rate for glucose

MCRI Multifactorial Cardiac Risk Index

mCRPC metastatic castration-resistant prostate cancer

MCS malignant carcinoid syndrome; managed care system; massage of the carotid sinus; mechanical circulatory support; medical computing services; Meharry Cohort Study; mesocaval shunt; method of constant stimuli; methylcholanthrene sarcoma; microculture and sensitivity; middle coronary sinus; Miles-Carpenter syndrome; minimally conscious state; Minnesota Coronary Survey; moisture-control system; multicenter study; multiple chemical sensitivity; multiple cloning site; multiple combined sclerosis; myocardial contraction state

MC & S microscopy, culture, and sensitivity

mc/s megacycles per second

MCSA Moloney cell surface antigen

MCSD minimum clinically significant difference

MCSDS Marlowe-Crowne Social Desirability Scale

MCSDT Minnesota Coronary Survey Dietary Trial

MCSF, (M)-CSF macrophage colony−stimulating factor

MCSP Member of the Chartered Society of Physiotherapists

mCSP, MCSPG melanoma-specific chondroitin sulfate proteoglycan

McSPI Multicenter Study of Perioperative Ischemia

MCSW male commercial sex worker

MCT manual cervical traction; mean cell thickness; mean cell threshold; mean circulation time; mean corpuscular thickness; medial canthal tendon; medium-chain triglyceride; medullary carcinoma of thyroid; medullary collecting tubule; microtoxicity test; microwave coagulation therapy; microwave computed tomography; minimal common tagset; multiple compressed tablet

µCT micro-computed tomography

MCTC metrizamide computed tomography cisternography

MCTD mixed connective tissue disease

MCTF mononuclear cell tissue factor

MC/TF multiple choice/true-false

MCU malaria control unit; maximum care unit; micturating cystourethrography; motor cortex unit; multipoint control unit

MCUG micturating cystogram

MCV Malvaceous chlorosis virus; mean cell volume; mean clinical value; mean contour value; mean corpuscular volume; measles-containing vaccine; median cell volume; meningococcal conjugate vaccine; molluscum contagiosum virus; motor conduction velocity; myelocytomatosis virus

MCV4 tetravalent meningococcal conjugate vaccine

MCx main circumflex [artery]

MCyR major cytogenic response

MD Doctor of Medicine; magnesium deficiency; main duct; maintenance dose; major depression; malate dehydrogenase; malignant disease; malrotation of duodenum; manic depressive; Mantoux diameter; Marek disease; maternal deprivation; maximum dose; mean deviation; Meckel diverticulum; mediastinal disease; medical department; Medical Design [brace]; mediodorsal; medium dosage; mendelian dominant gene; Meniere disease; meningococcal disease; Menkes disease; mental deficiency; mental depression; mesiodistal; methyldifluoroarsine; Miller-Dieker [syndrome]; Minamata disease; minimum dose; mitral disease, mixed diet; moderate disability; molecular diagnostics; molecular dynamics; monocular deprivation; movement disorder; multidrug; multiple deficiency; muscular dystrophy; mutual information; myelodysplasia; myocardial damage; myocardial disease; myotonic dystrophy

Md mendelevium

md median

MDA malondialdehyde; manual dilation of anus; mass drug administration; methylene dianiline; 3,4-methylenedioxyamphetamine; minimal deviation adenocarcinoma; moderate disease activity; monodehydroascorbate; motor discriminative acuity; Müllerian duct anomaly; multivariant discriminant analysis; mutation detection enhancement; right mentoanterior

MDα megadalton

MDAC multiple-dose activated charcoal; multiplying digital-to-analog converter

MDACC M.D. Anderson Cancer Center

MDAD mineral dust airway disease

MDAP Machover Draw-A-Person [test]

MDB medulloblastoma; Mental Deterioration Battery

MDBDF March of Dimes Birth Defect Foundation

MDBK Madin-Darby bovine kidney [cell]

MDC macrophage-derived chemokine; major diagnostic categories; metalloprotease disintegrin cysteine; Metoprolol in Dilated Cardiomyopathy [trial]; minimum detectable concentration; monocyte-depleted mononuclear cell; Multicenter Dilated Cardiomyopathy [trial]

mDC mature dendritic cell

MDCK Madin-Darby canine kidney

MDCR Miller-Dieker [syndrome] chromosome region

MDCT multidetector computed tomography

MDCV Mojui Dos Campos virus

MDD major depressive disorder; mean daily dose; medical data dictionary; medical device directives; minimal detectable dose; monitored drug dictionary

MDDC monocyte-derived dendritic cell

MDDL medical device data language

MDDS Malmö Diet and Disease Study; medical diagnostic decision support

MDE major depressive episode; major duct excision; minimum defibrillation energy; molecular distance edge

MDEBP mean daily erect blood pressure

MDEG mammalian degenerin

MDentSc Master of Dental Science

MDEV medical device

MDF mean dominant frequency; myocardial depressant factor

MDFA multiple developmental field anomalies

MDFC multidirectional flow chamber
MDFD map-dot-fingerprint dystrophy
MDG mean diastolic gradient; methyladenine deoxyribonucleic acid glycosylase
MDGF macrophage-derived growth factor
MDGs Millennium Development Goals
MDH malate dehydrogenase; medullary dorsal horn
MDHR maximum determined heart rate
MDHV Marek disease herpesvirus
MDI manic-depressive illness; metered-dose inhaler; methylene diphenyl diisocyanate; Michelson Doppler imager; multidirectional instability; multiple daily injection; multiple document interface; multiple dosage insulin; Multiscore Depression Inventory
MDIA multidimensional interaction analysis
MDI-A metered-dose inhaler with aerochamber
MDI-DED metered-dose inhaler with delivery-enhancement device
MDIPT Multicenter Diltiazem Postinfarction Trial
MDIS medical diagnostic imaging support; medical diagnostic imaging system
MDIT mean disintegration time
MDK midkine
MDL minimum description length; minimum detection limit
MDLIS molecular diagnostic laboratory information system
MDLS Miller-Dieker lissencephaly syndrome
MDM medical decision making; mid-diastolic murmur; minor determinant mix; monocyte-derived macrophage
MDMA methylenedioxymethamphetamine
MD-MPH Doctor of Medicine−Master of Public Health
MDMU medical devices for military use
mdn median
MDNB mean daily nitrogen balance; metadinitrobenzene
MDNCF monocyte-derived neutrophil chemotactic factor
MDNV Maiden virus
MDO minimum detectable object
MDOPA, mdopa methyldopa
MDOV Monte Dourado virus
MDP manic-depressive psychosis; maximum diastolic potential; maximum digital pulse; methylene diphosphate; microsomal dipeptidase; minimum distending pressure; muramyldipeptide; muscular dystrophy, progressive; right mentoposterior
MDPD maximum daily permissible dose
MD-PhD combined degree in medicine and science

MDPIT Multicenter Diltiazem Postinfarction Trial
MDPK myotonic dystrophy protein kinase
MDQ memory deviation quotient; Menstrual Distress Questionnaire; minimum detectable quantity
MDR median duration of response; medical device regulation; minimum daily requirement; multidrug resistance/resistant
mdr multidrug resistance
MDRD Modification of Diet in Renal Disease [study]
MDRE multidrug-resistant *Enterococcus*
MDREF multidrug-resistant enteric fever
MDRP multidrug resistance protein
MDRS Mattis Dementia Rating Scale
MDRSP multidrug-resistant *Streptococcus pneumoniae*
MDR TB multidrug resistance in tuberculosis
MDR-TB multidrug-resistant tuberculosis
MDRV Mill Door virus
MdRV *Musca domestica* reovirus
MDS Master of Dental Surgery; maternal deprivation syndrome; medical data screening; medical data source; medical data system; medical device system; mesonephric duct system; microdilution system; milk drinker's syndrome; Miller-Dieker syndrome; minimum dataset; monophasic damped sine; Mood Disorders Service; morpheme database; multidimensional scaling; myelodysplastic syndrome; myocardial depressant substance
MDS+ minimum dataset (plus)
MDS/AML myelodysplastic syndrome and acute myeloblastic leukemia
MDSBP mean daily supine blood pressure
MDSC muscle-derived stem cell
MD/SC multidrug/short course
MDS-HC ACP minimum dataset home-care assessment clients protocol
MDSO mentally disturbed sex offender
MDSP multiple diagnostic services program
MDSS medical decision support system
MDT maggot debridement therapy; mast [cell] degeneration test; mean dissolution time; median detection threshold; multidisciplinary team; multidrug therapy; right mentotransverse
MDTP multidisciplinary treatment plan
MDTR mean diameter/thickness ratio
MDUO myocardial disease of unknown origin
MDV Main Drain virus; Marek disease virus; mean dye velocity; mucosal disease virus; multidose vial
MDW monophasic defibrillation waveform
MDX Medical Internet Exchange

MDY month, date, year
Mdyn megadyne
ME macular edema; malic enzyme; manic episode; maximum effort; maximum entropy; median eminence; medical education; medical examiner; meningoencephalitis; menopause educator; mercaptoethanol; metabolic energy; metabolic equivalent; metabolism; metamyelocyte; microembolism; microenvironment; middle ear; mouse embryo; mouse epithelial [cell]; muscle examination; myalgic encephalomyelitis; myoclonic epilepsy; myoelectric; myoepithelial
M/E myeloid/erythroid ratio
M+E, M&E monitoring and evaluation
2-ME 2-mercaptoethanol
Me menton; methyl
μE microelectrode
MEA male-enhanced antigen; Medical Exhibition Association; mercaptoethylamine; monoethanolamine; multi-electrode array; multiple endocrine abnormalities; multiple endocrine adenomatosis
3MeA 3-methyladenine
MEAC Measles Elimination Advisory Committee
mEAD monophasic action potential early afterdepolarization
MEADOW Method Alternative: Distal Occlusion and Wash-out in Saphenous Vein Graft [study]
MEA-I multiple endocrine adenomatosis type I
MEANS modular electrocardiogram analysis system
MEAP multiphasic environmental assessment procedure
meas measurement
MEAV Meaban virus
MEB Medical Evaluation Board; muscle-eye-brain [disease]
MeB methylene blue
ME-BH medial eminence of basal hypothalamus
MEBS muscle-eye-brain syndrome
MeBSA methylated bovine serum albumin
MEC mammary epithelial cell; median effective concentration; middle ear canal; middle ear cell; minimum effective concentration; mobile examination center
mec meconium
MECA methylcholanthrene
MECC mini extracorporeal circulation
MeCCNU methylchloroethylcyclohexylnitrosourea
MECG mixed essential cryoglobulinemia
MECM Midwest Ethics Committee Network

MECP methyl-CpG-binding protein
MECTA mobile electroconvulsive therapy apparatus
MECY methotrexate and cyclophosphamide
MED median erythrocyte diameter; medical; medical electronic desktop; Medical Entities Dictionary; medication, medicine; minimum effective dose; minimum erythema dose; multiple epiphyseal dysplasia
MED$_{50}$ median effective dose for mild cognitive impairment of the exposed population
med medial; median; medication; medicine, medical; medium
MEDAC multiple endocrine deficiency, Addison disease, candidiasis [syndrome]
MEDAL Medical Algorithms [project]
MED-ART Medical Automated Records Technology
MEDAS medical emergency decision-assistance system
MEDCEN medical center
MEDCOM medical command
MEDDAC medical department activity
MedDRA Medical Dictionary for Regulatory Activities
MedDX medical diagnosis
MEDEVAC, Medevac medical evacuation
MEDEX, Medex extension of physician [Fr. *médicin extension*]
MEDIC multiecho data image combination
medic military medical corpsman
Medi-Cal Medicaid in California
MEDICO Medical International Cooperation
MEDICS Medway Integrated Care Support
MED-IDDM multiple epiphyseal dysplasia–insulin dependent diabetes mellitus
MEDIGATE Medical Examination Direct Iconic and Graphic Augmented Test Entry
MEDIHC Military Experience Directed Into Health Careers
MedIndEx medical indexing expert
MEDINFO medical informatics
MEDIPP medical district-initiated planning program
MEDIPRO medical district-initiated peer review organization
MEDIS-DC Medical Information System Development Center
MEDIX medical data interchange
MED-LAN medical center with local area network
MedLAN Medical Local Area Network
MEDLARS Medical Literature Analysis and Retrieval System
MedLEE Medical Language Extraction and Encoding

MedPAC Medicare Payment Advisory Commission

MEDPAR medical provider analysis and review

MEdREP Medical Education Reinforcement and Enrichment Program

MEDRIS Medical Records Interface or Input System

MEDS minimum emergency dataset; Mortality in Emergency Department Sepsis [score]

meds medications

MEDScD Doctor of Medical Science

MEDSTATS Medical Statistics Expert System

Med-surg medicine and surgery

MEdSYNDIKATE Synthesis of Distributed Knowledge Acquired from Medical Text

Med Tech medical technologist, medical technology

MED-TEP Medical Treatment Effectiveness Program

MEE measured energy expenditure; methylethyl ether; middle ear effusion; multilocus enzyme electrophoresis

MEES medical element engineering and simulation

MEF maximal expiratory flow; middle ear fluid; midexpiratory flow; migration enhancement factor; mouse embryo fibroblast

MEF$_{50}$ mean maximal expiratory flow

MEFR maximal expiratory flow rate

MEFV maximal expiratory flow volume

MEG magnetoencephalogram, magnetoencephalography; megakaryocyte; Megestrol; mercaptoethylguanidine; multifocal eosinophilic granuloma

MeG methylguanine

meg megacycle; megakaryocyte; megaloblast

Meg-CSA megakaryocyte colony-stimulating activity

MEGD minimal euthyroid Graves disease

mEGF mouse epidermal growth factor

MEGG mucosal electrogastrogram

MegMV Megakepasma mosaic virus

MEGS Montefiore endovascular graft system

Megs maternally expressed genes

MEGX monoethylglycinexylidide

mEH membrane-bound epoxide hydrolase

MEHP Metoprolol in Elderly Hypertensive Patients [study]

MEI master encounter index; maximally exposed individual; Medicare economic index

MEIA microparticle enzyme immunoassay

MEII minimum essential information infrastructure

MEK methylethylketone

MEL melphalan; metabolic equivalent level; miniature electromechanical latch; mouse erythroleukemia

mel melanoma; melena

MELAS mitochondrial encephalomyopathy, lactic acidosis, and strokelike symptoms [syndrome]

MEL B melarsoprol

MELC murine erythroleukemia cell

mel-CSPG melanoma-specific chondroitin sulfate proteoglycan

MELD model for end-stage liver disease

MELD/PELD Model for End-Stage Liver Disease/Pediatric End-Stage Liver Disease

MELODHY Metoprolol Low Dose in Hypertension [study]

MELV Melao virus

MEM macrophage electrophoretic mobility; malic enzyme, mitochondrial; minimal Eagle medium; minimal essential medium

memb membrane, membranous

MEME Metathesaurus Enhancement and Maintenance Environment

MEmerg Nsg Master in Emergency Nursing

MEM-FBS minimal essential medium with fetal bovine serum

MEMR multiple exostoses-mental retardation [syndrome]

MEMRs middle ear muscle reflexes

MEMS medication event monitoring system; microelectromechanical system

MEN meningitis; multiple endocrine neoplasia

men meningeal; meningitis; meniscus; menstruation

MEND Medical Education for National Defense

MENG magnetoenterography

MEN-I multiple endocrine neoplasia, type I

MENT maximum entropy [algorithm]

ment mental, mentality

MENTOR Medtronic Wiktor Hepamed Stent Trial

MEO malignant external otitis

5-MeODMT 5-methoxy-*N,N*-dimethyl-tryptamine

MeOH methyl alcohol

MEOS microsomal ethanol oxidizing system

MEP maximum expiratory pressure; mean effective pressure; mepiridine; minimum error point; mitochondrial encephalopathy; molecular electrostatic potential; motor end plate; motor evoked potential

mep meperidine

6-MeP 6-mercaptopurine

MEPAS mobility-assist for paralyzed, amputee, and spastic patients

MEPC miniature end plate current

6-MeP-dR 6-mercaptopurine deoxyriboside

M-Epi epicardium and M regions

MEPP miniature end plate potential

MEPS Medical Expenditure Panel Survey

MEPS-IC Medical Expenditure Panel Survey-Insurance Component

mEQ, mEq, meq milliequivalent

mEq/L milliequivalents per liter

MER mean ejection rate; medical emergency room; Merck Index Online; methanol extraction residue; microelectrode recording; murmur/energy ratio

MERB Medical Examination and Review Board

MERC multiple ejaculation, resuspension, and centrifugation

MERCATOR Multicenter European Research Trial With Cilazapril After Angioplasty to Prevent Transluminal Coronary Obstruction and Restenosis

MERFF myoclonus epilepsy with ragged red fibers

MERG macular electroretinogram

MERIT Medical Records, Images, Texts Information Exchange

MERIT-HF Metoprolol Controlled-Release Randomised Intervention Trial in Heart Failure

MERRF myoclonus epilepsy with ragged red fibers [syndrome]

MERRLA myoclonus epilepsy, ragged red fibers, lactic acidosis [syndrome]

MERS Middle East respiratory syndrome; mild encephalitis/encephalopathy with reversible splenial lesion; Multiagency Electronic Regulatory Submission

MERS-CoV Middle East respiratory syndrome coronavirus [emerged in 2012]

MES maintenance electrolyte solution; maximal electroshock; maximal electroshock seizures; microembolic signal; Minitran Efficacy Study; multiple endocrine syndrome; myoelectric signal

Mes mesencephalic, mesencephalon

MESA Marshfield Epidemiologic Study Area; Multi-Ethnic Study of Atherosclerosis; myoepithelial sialadenitis

Mesc mescaline

MESCH Multi-Environment Scheme

MESF molecules of equivalent soluble fluorochrome

MeSH Medical Subject Headings

MESNA [sodium 2-]mercaptoethanesulfonate

MESOR midline estimating statistic of rhythm

MesPGN mesangial proliferative glomerulonephritis

MESS mangled extremity severity score

MEST Medical Equipment Technical Society; mouse ear swelling test

MESV murine embryonic stem cell virus

MET maximal exercise test; metabolic equivalent of the task; metastasis, metastatic; methionine; midexpiratory time; modality examination terminal; multistage exercise test

Met methionine

met metallic; methionine

META medical editors trial accounting; medical editors trial amnesty; Metathesaurus; 3-methacryloyloxyethyl trimellitate anhydride

Meta Metathesaurus

metab metabolic, metabolism

metas metastasis, metastatic

Met-Enk methionine-enkephalin

METEOR managing end-to-end operations

METH methicillin

Meth methedrine

meth methyl

Met-Hb, met-Hb, metHb methemoglobin

MeTHF methyltetrahydrofolic acid

Met-hGH *N*-methionyl recombinant human growth hormone

MetMb metmyoglobin

METR miniature electronic temperature recorder

METS Medical Equipment Technical Society; metabolic equivalents

MetS metabolic syndrome

mets metastases

METT maximum exercise tolerance test

MEU maximum expected utility

MEURI Monitored Emergency Use of Unregistered Interventions [framework]

MEV maximum exercise ventilation; mevalonate; minimal excursionary ventilation; murine erythroblastosis virus

MeV measles virus; megaelectron volts

mev megaelectron volts

MEWD, MEWDS multiple evanescent white dot syndrome

MEXIS Metoprolol and Xamoterol Infarction Study

MF magnetic field; magnification factor; maximal force; mean field; meat free; medium frequency; megafarad; membrane filler; merthiolate formaldehyde; metacarpal fusion; microfibril; microfilament; microflocculation; microscopic factor; mid frequency; midcavity forceps; mitochondrial fragments; mitogenic factor; mitomycin-fluorouracil; mitotic figure; mucosal fluid; multifactorial; multiplication factor; mutation frequency; mycosis fungoides; myelin figure; myelofibrosis; myocardial fibrosis; myofibrillar

M&F male and female; mother and father

M:F, M/F male/female ratio

Mf maxillofrontale

mF millifarad

mf microfarad; microfilaria

µF, µf microfarad

MFA Master of Fine Arts; mean field annealing; metabolic flux analysis; monofluoroacetate; multifocal functional autonomy; multiple factor analysis

MFAQ Multidimensional Functional Assessment Questionnaire

MFAT multifocal atrial tachycardia

MFB medial forebrain bundle; metallic foreign body; multiple feedback

MFC mean fluorescence channel; medical follow-up clinic; minimal fungicidal concentration

MFCM Master, Faculty of Community Medicine

MFCV muscle fiber conduction velocity

MFD mandibulofacial dysostosis; methylphenidate; midforceps delivery; milk-free diet; minimum fatal dose; multiple fractions per day

mfd microfarad

MFG magnetic field gradient; minimumdistance frontal gyrus

MFH malignant fibrous histiocytoma

MFH-B malignant fibrous histiocytoma of bone

MFHom Member of the Faculty of Homeopathy

MFI male factor infertility; malleable facial implant; mean fluorescence intensity; Multidimensional Fatigue Inventory; multi-facility integration

MFID multielectrode flame ionization detector

M-FISH multiplex fluorescence in situ hybridization

MFL myofibril

m flac membrana flaccida

MFLOPS, Mflops megaflops [million floating points per second]

MFM magnetic force microscopy

MFO medium frequency oscillator; mid field open; mixed function oxidase

MFOM Master, Faculty of Occupational Medicine

MFP monofluorophosphate; myofascial pain

M-FPIA monoclonal fluorescence polarization immunoassay

MFPR multifetal pregnancy reduction

MFR mean flow rate; mucus flow rate

MFRPS Manufactured Food Regulatory Program Standards

MFS Marfan syndrome; Medicare fee schedule

MFSS Medical Field Service School

MFST Medical Field Service Technician

MFT multifocal atrial tachycardia; muscle function test

MFTA molecular field topology analysis

MFUN molecular function

MFUS Manitoba Follow-up Study

MFV maximal flow-volume [loop]

MFW multiple fragment wounds

MG maintenance goal; Marcus Gunn [pupil]; margin; mean gradient; medial gastrocnemius; membranous glomerulonephritis; menopausal gonadotropin; mesiogingival; methylglucoside; methylguanidine; monoclonal gammopathy; monoglyceride; mucous granule; muscle group; myasthenia gravis; myoglobin

M3G morphine-3-glucuronide

Mg magnesium

m^{7G} 7-methylguanosine

mg milligram

µg microgram

mγ milligamma

µγ microgamma

MGA 3-methylglutaconicaciduria; Master of General Administration; medical gas analyzer; melengestrol acetate

MgATP magnesium adenosine triphosphate

MGB medial geniculate body; myoglobin

MGBG methylglyoxal bis(guanylhydrazone)

MGC Mammalian Gene Collection; medical genetics center; medical genetics clinic; megacolon; minimal glomerular change

MgC magnocellular neuroendocrine cell

MGCE multifocal giant cell encephalitis

MGCN megalocornea

MGCR meningioma chromosome region

MGCRB Medicare Geographic Classification Review Board

MGD maximal glucose disposal; Microbial Germplasm Database; mixed gonadal dysgenesis; Mouse Genome Database; multiglandular disease

mg/dL milligrams per deciliter

MGDS Member in General Dental Surgery

MGEIR Mouse Gene Expression Information Resource

MGES multiple gated equilibrium scintigraphy
MGF macrophage growth factor; maternal grandfather
MGG May-Grünwald-Giemsa [staining]; molecular and general genetics; mouse gamma-globulin; multinucleated giant cell
MGGH methylglyoxal guanylhydrazone
MGH Massachusetts General Hospital
mgh milligram-hour
MGHL medial glenohumeral ligament
MGI magnetically guided intubation
MGIT mycobacterial growth indicator tube
mg/kg milligrams per kilogram
μg/kg micrograms per kilogram
MGL minor glomerular lesion
Mgl myoglobin
mg/L milligrams per liter
μg/L micrograms per liter
mGluR metabotropic glutamate receptor
MGM maternal grandmother; meningioma
mgm milligram
MGMA Medical Group Management Association
MGMT methylguanine-deoxyribonucleic acid methyltransferase
mgmt management
MGN medial geniculate nucleus; membranous glomerulonephritis
MGP marginal granulocyte pool; marginating granulocyte pool; membranous glomerulonephropathy; mucin glycoprotein
MGPS hereditary [Montreal] giant platelet syndrome
MGR modified gain ratio; multiple gas rebreathing
mgr milligram
MGS metric gravitational system; modified Gram-Schmidt orthogonalization
MGSA malignant growth stimulatory activity
MGT medical guideline technology; multiple glomus tumors
MGUS monoclonal gammopathies of undetermined significance
MGV mean gray value
MGW magnesium sulfate, glycerin, and water
mGy milligray
μGy microgray
MH malignant histiocytosis; malignant hyperpyrexia; malignant hypertension; malignant hyperthermia; mammotropic hormone; mannoheptulose; marital history; medial hypothalamus; medical history; melanophore-stimulating hormone; menstrual history; mental health; mental hygiene; moist heat; monosymptomatic hypochondriasis; murine hepatitis; mutant hybrid; *Mycobacterium haemophilum*; myohyoid

mH millihenry
μH microhenry
MHA major histocompatibility antigen; May-Hegglin anomaly; Mental Health America; Mental Health Association; methemalbumin; microangiopathic hemolytic anemia; microhemagglutination; middle hepatic artery; mixed hemadsorption; Mueller-Hinton agar
MHAM multiple hamartoma
MHAQ Modified Health Assessment Questionnaire
M-HART Montreal Heart Attack Readjustment Trial
MHA-TP microhemagglutination—*Treponema pallidum*
MHAUS Malignant Hyperthermia Association of the United States
MHB maximum hospital benefit; Mueller-Hinton base
MHb methemoglobin; myohemoglobin
MHBSS modified Hank balanced salt solution
MHC major histocompatibility complex; mental health care; mental health center; mental health clinic; myosin heavy chain
MHCS Mental Hygiene Consultation Service
MHCU mental health care unit
MHD maintenance hemodialysis; mean hemolytic dose; mental health department; minimization of hypersurface distance; minimum hemolytic dilution; minimum hemolytic dose
MHDI Minnesota Health Data Institute
MHDP methylene hydroxydiphosphonate
MHDPS Mental Health Demographic Profile System
M-HEART Multi-Hospital Eastern Atlantic Restenosis Trial
MHFT Munich Mild Heart Failure Trial
MHG metropolitan health group
mHg millimeter of mercury
μHg micron of mercury
MHHP Minnesota Heart Health Program
MHHS Minnesota Heart Health Survey
MHI malignant histiocytosis of intestine; Mental Health Index; Mental Health Inventory; minor head injury
MHIQ McMaster health index questionnaire
MHL medial hypothalamic lesion
MHLC Multidimensional Health Locus of Control
MHLS metabolic heat load stimulator
MHN massive hepatic necrosis; mental health nurse; Mohs hardness number; morbus hemolyticus neonatorum

MHO microsomal heme oxygenase

mho reciprocal ohm, siemens unit

MHP 1-mercuri-2-hydroxypropane; hemiplegic migraine; maternal health program; medical center health plan; metropolitan health plan; monosymptomatic hypochondriacal psychosis; multiskilled health practitioner

MHPA mild hyperphenylalaninemia

MHPG 3-methoxy-4-hydroxyphenyl-glycol

MHR major histocompatibility region; malignant hyperthermia resistance; maternal heart rate; maximal heart rate; methemoglobin reductase

MHRA Medicines and Health Care Products Regulatory Agency

MHRI Mental Health Research Institute

MHS major histocompatibility system; malignant hyperthermia in swine; malignant hyperthermia syndrome; malignant hypothermia susceptibility; Milan hypertensive [rat]; Minnesota Heart Survey; modified hybrid sign; multiple health screening; multihospital system

MHSA microaggregated human serum albumin

MHSS Military Health Services System

MHT mixed hemagglutination test

MHTS Multiphasic Health Testing Services

MHV magnetic heart vector; middle hepatic vein; mouse hepatitis virus; murine hepatitis virus

MHW mental health worker

MHx medical history

MHyg Master of Hygiene

MHz megahertz

MI magnetic-guided intubation; maturation index; medical illustrator; medical informatics; medical inspection; melanophore index; membrane integrity; menstruation induction; mental illness; mental institution; mercaptoimidazole; mesioincisal; metabolic index; microinvasion; microsatellite instability; migration index; migration inhibition; mild irritant; minimally invasive; mitotic index; mitral incompetence; mitral insufficiency; mononucleosis infectiosa; morphology index; motility index; mutual information; myocardial infarction; myocardial ischemia; myoinositol

MI, M-I first meiotic metaphase

mi mile

MIA missing in action

MIAMI Metoprolol in Acute Myocardial Infarction [study]

MIAS Mammographic Image Analysis Society

MIAs multiinstitutional arrangements; medically indigent adults

MIB management information base; Medical Impairment Bureau; Medical Information Bureau; minimally invasive biopsy

MIBG, mIBG metaiodobenzylguanidine

MIBI methoxyisobutyl isonitrile

MIBiol Member of the Institute of Biology

MIBK methylisobutyl ketone

MIBT methyl isatin-beta-thiosemicarbazone

MIC maternal and infant care; maximum inhibitory concentration; maximum insufflation capacity; mean inhibitory concentration; medical intensive care; Medical Interfraternity Conference; methyl isocyanate; microinvasive carcinoma; microscopy; minimal inhibitory concentration; minimal isorrheic concentration; minocycline; model immune complex; mononuclear inflammatory cell; morphologic, immunologic, and cytogenic

MICA mean internal carotid artery

MICAB minimally invasive coronary artery bypass surgery

MICABG minimally invasive coronary artery bypass graft

MICAM maturation index for colostrum and mature milk

MICC mitogen-induced cellular cytotoxicity

MICCAI Medical Image Computing and Computer-Assisted Intervention

MICG macromolecular insoluble cold globulin

MICN mobile intensive care nursing

MICOL Multicenter Italian Study of Cholesterol

MICR methacholine inhalation challenge response

MICRA Medical Injury Compensation Reform Act

MICRO Medical Information Collecting Robot

micro microcyte, microcytic; microscopic

microbiol microbiology

microCi microcurie

microg microgram

MICRO-HOPE Microalbuminuria, Cardiovascular and Renal Outcomes—Heart Outcomes Prevention Evaluation

MICS microincision cataract surgery; Myocardial Infarction Cost Study

MICST Ministry of Industry, Commerce, Science, and Technology

MICT mobile intensive care technician

MICU medical intensive care unit; mobile intensive care unit

MICUP management of intensive care unit and patients

MicV micropia virus

MID maximum inhibiting dilution; mesioincisodistal; midinfarct dementia; minimum infective dose; minimum inhibitory dose; minimum irradiation dose; multiinfarct dementia; multiple indicator dilution; multiple ion detection

mid middle

MIDA myocardial ischemia dynamic analysis

MIDAS medical image display and analysis system; Medical Information Data Analysis System; metal ion−dependent adhesion site; microphthalmia, dermal aplasia, sclerocornea [syndrome]; Multicenter Isradipine Diuretic Atherosclerosis Study; Myocardial Infarction Data Acquisition System [study]

MIDCAB minimally invasive direct coronary artery bypass

MIDS Management Information Decision System

midsag midsagittal

MIDSPAN Middle-Aged Span of Life Study

MIDV Middelburg virus

MIE minimally invasive esophagectomy

MIEMIS model for investment and evaluation of medical information system

MIF macrophage migration inhibitory factor; maximum inspiratory flow; maximum inspiratory force; melanocyte[-stimulating hormone] inhibiting factor; merthiolate-iodine-formaldehyde [method]; microimmunofluorescence; midinspiratory flow; midline interhemispheric fusion; migration inhibitory factor; mixed immunofluorescence; müllerian inhibiting factor

MIFC merthiolate-iodine-formaldehyde concentration

MIFR maximal inspiratory flow rate

MIFT microinjection fallopian transfer

MIG measles immune globulin; Medicare Insured Groups; message implementation guideline; Mitochondria Interest Group; monokine induced by interferon gamma

MIg malaria immunoglobulin; measles immunoglobulin; membrane immunoglobulin

mIg membrane-anchored immunoglobulin

mIgM membrane-anchored immunoglobulin M

MIGT multiple inert gas elimination technique

MIH Master of Industrial Health; migraine with interval headache; minimal intermittent heparin [dose]; moderate induced hypothermia

MIHA Maternal and Infant Health Assessment; minor histocompatibility antigen [also spelled MiHA]

MIHR Management of Intellectual Property in Health Research and Development

MII, M-II second meiotic metaphase

MIIO minimally invasive intraoperative osteosynthesis

MIKA minor karyotype abnormalities

MIKE mass-analyzed ion kinetic energy

MIL mean intercept length analysis

MILESTONE Multicenter Iloprost European Study on Endangeitis

MILIS Multicenter Investigation of the Limitations of Infarct Size

MILP mitogen-induced lymphocyte proliferation

MILS medication information leaflet for seniors

MILT medical laboratory technician

MILT-AD medical laboratory technician associate degree

MILT-C medical laboratory technician certificate

MIM Mendelian Inheritance in Man; message information model; Multilateral Initiative in Malaria

MIMC multivane intensity modulation compensator

MIMI minimalist immediate mechanical intervention

MIMIC multivane intensity modulation compensation

MIMOSA medical image management in an open system architecture

MIMR minimal inhibitor mole ratio

MIMS medical information management system; medical inventory management system; Migraine and Myocardial Ischemia Study

MIMyCa maternally inherited disorder with adult-onset myopathy and cardiomyopathy

MIN medial interlaminar nucleus; medical information network; multiple intestinal neoplasia

min mineral; minim; minimal, minimum; minor; minute

μin microinch

MINA monoisonitrosoacetone

MinDu minimum duration

MINIA monkey intranuclear inclusion agent

MINPHIS Made in Nigeria Primary Healthcare and Hospital Information System

MINSAT minimum cost satisfiability

MINT Myocardial Infarction with Novastan and Tissue Plasminogen Activator Study

MINV Minnal virus

MIO metal-induced oxidation; minimum identifiable odor; modular input/output

MiO microorchidism

MION monocrystalline iron oxide

MIOP magnetic iron oxide particle

MIOS Myocardial Infarction Onset Study

MIP macrophage inflammatory protein; major intrinsic protein; maximum inspiratory pressure; maximum-intensity pixel; maximum-intensity projection; mean incubation period; mean intravascular pressure; Medical Informatics Programme; middle interphalangeal; minimal inspiratory pressure; minimally invasive parathyroidectomy; minimally invasive procedure

mIP minimum-intensity projection

Mip macrophage infectivity potentiator, macrophage infectivity promoter

MIPA macrophage inflammatory protein alpha

MIPB macrophage inflammatory protein beta

MIPcor coronary maximum-intensity projection

MIPO minimally invasive plate osteosynthesis

MIPP maximum-intensity pixel projection

MIPPO minimally invasive percutaneous plate osteosynthesis

MIPS Martinsried Institute for Protein Sequences; mean index procedure sum; merit-based incentive pay [system]; millions of instructions per second; Munich Information Center for Protein Sequences; myocardial isotope perfusion scan

MIR main immunogenic region; multiple isomorphous replacement

MIRACL myocardial ischemia reduction with aggressive cholesterol lowering

MIRC microtubuloreticular complex

MIRD medical internal radiation dose

MIRL medical imaging research laboratory; membrane inhibitor of reactive lysis

MIRMO Medical Information Resources Management Office

miRNA micro−ribonucleic acid

MIRON Medical Information Resources on the Net

MIROW Modeling of Immunization Registry Operations Workgroup

MIRP myocardial infarction rehabilitation program

MIRRACLE Myocardial Infarction Risk Recognition and Conversion of Life-Threatening Events into Survival [trial]

MIRS mean index resuscitation sum

MIRSA Multicenter International Randomized Study of Angina Pectoris

MIRU myocardial infarction research unit

MIRU-VNTR mycobacterial interspersed repetitive-unit variable-number tandem repeat

MIRV Mirim virus

MIS management information system; manager of information system; medical information service; medical information system; meiosis-inducing substance; minimally invasive surgery; motor index score; müllerian inhibiting substance

MiSAD Milan Study on Atherosclerosis and Diabetes

MISC multi−interface sensor controlled

MIS-C multisystem inflammatory syndrome in children

misc miscarriage; miscellaneous

MISCHF management to improve survival in congestive heart failure

MISG modified immune serum globulin

MISHAP microcephalus, imperforate anus-syndactyly, hamartoblastoma, abnormal lung lobulation, polydactyly [syndrome]

MISI multiple input−single input

MISJ Medical Instrument Society of Japan

MISNES Multicenter Italian Study on Neonatal Electrocardiography and Sudden Infant Death Syndrome

MISS medical image-sharing system; Medical Interview Satisfaction Scale; minimally invasive spinal surgery; Modified Injury Severity Scale

MIST Management of Influenza in the Southern Hemisphere Trials; Medical Information Service by Telephone; Mibefradil Ischemia Suppression Trial; minimally invasive surgery and intervention technology; Multicenter Israndipine Salt Trial

MISU Maternal Interview of Substance Abuse

MIT magnetic induction tomography; male impotence test; marrow iron turnover; Massachusetts Institute of Technology; mean input time; melodic intonation therapy; metabolism inhibition test; miracidial immobilization test; mitomycin; monoiodotyrosine

mit mitral

MITF microphthalmia-associated transcription factor

MITI Myocardial Infarction Triage and Intervention [Project]

MITIS Modular Integrated Transplant Information System

MITO mitomycin

Mito C mitomycin C

MITRA Maximal Individual Therapy in Acute Myocardial Infarction

MITT minimally invasive thermal therapy; Myers introduction to type

mIU milli−International Unit; one-thousandth of an International Unit

µIU one-millionth of an International Unit

MIVAP minimally invasive video-assisted parathyroidectomy

MIVAT minimally invasive video-assisted thyroidectomy
MIVD mobile interactive videodisk
MIWC mercurial insensitive water channel
mix, mixt mixture
MJ Machado-Joseph [disease]; marijuana; megajoule
mJ, mj millijoule
μ**J** microjoule
MJA mechanical joint apparatus
MJAD Machado-Joseph Azorean disease
MJD Machado-Joseph disease; Mseleni joint disease
MJI moral judgment interview
MJRT maximum junctional recovery time
MJT Mead Johnson tube
MK megakaryocyte; monkey kidney; myokinase
Mk monkey
mkat millikatal
μ**kat** microkatal
mkat/L millikatals per liter
MKB medical knowledge database; megakaryoblast
MKC monkey kidney cell
MKF MEDLINE Knowledge Finder
m-kg meter-kilogram
MKHS Menkes kinky hair syndrome
MkK monkey kidney
MkL megakaryoblastic leukemia
MKMD Molecular Knowledge of Metabolic Diseases
MKP monobasic potassium phosphate
MKS, mks meter-kilogram-second
MKSAP medical knowledge self-assessment program
MKT mean kinetic temperature
MKTC monkey kidney tissue culture
MKV killed measles vaccine
ML Licentiate in Medicine; Licentiate in Midwifery; malignant lymphoma; mandibular line; marked latency; markup language; maximum likelihood; medial lemniscus; median load; mediolateral; mesiolingual; middle lobe; midline; molecular layer; motor latency; mucolipidosis; mucosal leishmaniasis; multiple lentiginosis; muscular layer; myeloid leukemia
M/L monocyte/lymphocyte ratio
M-L Martin-Lewis [medium]
mL millilambert; milliliter
ml milliliter
μ**L** microliter
MLA left mentoanterior; medical laboratory assistant; Medical Library Association; mesiolabial; monocytic leukemia, acute
mLa millilambert

MLAA Medical Library Assistance Act
MLAB Multilingual Aphasia Battery
MLAC minimum local anesthetic concentration
MLAEB midlatency auditory evoked potential
MLAEP midlatency auditory evoked potential
MLaI mesiolabioincisal
MLAP mean left atrial pressure
MLaP mesiolabiopulpal
MLB microlaryngobronchoscopy; monaural loudness balance
MLb macrolymphoblast
MLBP mechanical low back pain
MLBPNN multilayer back propagation neural network
MLBW moderately low birthweight
MLC midline catheter; minimum lethal concentration; mixed leukocyte culture; mixed ligand chelate; mixed lymphocyte concentration; mixed lymphocyte culture; morphine-like compound; multilamellar cytosome; multileaf collimator; myelomonocytic leukemia, chronic; myosin light chain
MLCCHF Multicenter Lisinopril Captopril Congestive Heart Failure [study]
MLCK myosin light chain kinase
MLCN multilocular cystic nephroma
MLCO Member of the London College of Osteopathy
MLCP myosin light-chain phosphatase
MLCQ Modified Learning Climate Questionnaire
MLCT metal-to-ligand charge transfer
MLD manual lymph drainage; masking level difference; mean luminal diameter; median lethal dose; metachromatic leukodystrophy; minimal lesion disease; minimum luminal diameter; minimum lethal dose
MLD$_{50}$ median lethal dose
mL/dL milliliters per deciliter
MLE maximum likelihood estimation; maximum likelihood estimator; midline episiotomy
MLEE multilocus enzyme electrophoresis
MLEI most likely exposed individual
MLEL malignant lymphoepithelial lesion
MLEM, ML-EM maximum likelihood expectation maximization
MLF medial longitudinal fasciculus; morphine-like factor
MLFF multilayer feed forward
MLG mesiolingual groove; mitochondrial lipid glycogen
MLGN minimal lesion glomerulonephritis
ML-H malignant lymphoma, histiocytic

MLI mesiolinguoincisal; mixed lymphocyte interaction

ML I, II, III, IV mucolipidosis I, II, III, IV

MLL mixed lineage leukemia; multi-level logistic

mL/L milliliters per liter

MLLT1 mixed lineage leukemia translocated to 1

MLLT2 mixed lineage leukemia translocated to 2

MLM map of local minima; medical liability monitor; medical logic module

MLN manifest latent nystagmus; membranous lupus nephropathy; mesenteric lymph node; motilin

MLNS minimal lesion nephrotic syndrome; mucocutaneous lymph node syndrome

MLO mediolateral oblique; mesiolinguoocclusal; *Mycoplasma*-like organism

MLP left mentoposterior; match list position; maximum lifespan potential; medical language processing; mesiolinguopulpal; microsomal lipoprotein; midlevel practitioner; multilayer perception; multilocus probe

ML-PDL malignant lymphoma, poorly differentiated lymphocytic

MLR mean length response; middle latency response; mineralocorticoid receptor; mixed lymphocyte reaction; multilinear regression; multivariate linear regression

MLRD microgastria—limb reduction defects [association]

MLS maximum length sequence; maximum likelihood estimator; mean lifespan; median lifespan; median longitudinal section; microphthalmia—linear skin defects [syndrome]; middle lobe syndrome; mouse leukemia virus; multilevel scheme; multiple line scan; myelomonocytic leukemia, subacute

MLS-ART multilevel scheme algebraic reconstruction

MLSB mid—left sternal border; migrating long spike burst

MLSI multiple line scan imaging

MLT left mentotransverse [L. *mento-laeva transversa*]; mean latency time; median lethal time; medical laboratory technician

MLT-AD medical laboratory technician associate degree

MLT(ASCP) Medical Laboratory Technician certified by the American Society of Clinical Pathologists

MLTC mixed leukocyte-trophoblast culture; mixed lymphocyte tumor cell

MLT-C medical laboratory technician certificate

MLTI mixed lymphocyte target interaction

MLU mean length of utterance

MLV Moloney leukemia virus; Mono Lake virus; multilaminar vesicle; murine leukemia virus

MLVAR amphotropic receptor for murine leukemia virus

MLVDP maximum left ventricular developed pressure

mlx millilux

MM macromolecule; Maëlzels metronome; major medical [insurance]; malignant melanoma; manubrium of malleus; Marshall-Marchetti [procedure]; Master of Management; mathematic morphology; medial malleolus; mediastinal mass; medical management; megamitochondria; melanoma metastasis; meningococcal meningitis; menstrually related migraine; metastatic melanoma; methadone maintenance; minimal medium; mismatched; molecular mechanics; morbidity and mortality; mucous membrane; multiple model; multiple myeloma; muscularis mucosae; myeloid metaplasia; myelomeningocele

M&M morbidity and mortality

mM millimolar, millimole; mini-MEDLINE

mm methylmalonyl; millimeter; mucous membrane; muscles

mm² square millimeter

mm³ cubic millimeter

mμ millimicron

μM micromole, micromolar

μm micrometer; micromilli-

μ/μ mass attenuation coefficient

MMA mastitis, metritis, agalactia [syndrome]; maxillomandibular advancement; medical management analysis; medical materials account; methylmalonic acid; methylmethacrylate; middle meningeal artery; minor morphologic aberration; monomethyladenosine; monomethylarsonic acid

MMAA mini microaggregates of albumin

MMAD mass median aerodynamic diameter

MMAP mean maternal arterial blood pressure

MMAS Massachusetts Male Aging Study; modified motor assessment scale

MMATP methadone maintenance and aftercare treatment program

MMC Materials Microcharacterization Collaboratory; mechanical myocardial channeling; migrating myoelectric complex; minimum medullary concentration; mitomycin C; mucosal mast cell

mμc millimicrocurie

μμC micromicrocurie [picocurie]

MMCI Multiskilled Medical Certification Institute

MMCO Medicaid managed care organization

MMD mass median diameter; minimum morbidostatic dose; moyamoya disease; myotonic muscular dystrophy

MMDB Molecular Modeling Database

MMDDI mutual molecular dataset diversity index

MMDTSD multiscale morphologic derivative transform-based singularity detector

MME mini mental examination; M-mode echocardiography; mobile medical equipment; mouse mammary epithelium

MMED Master of Medicine

MMEF maximum midexpiratory flow

MMEFR maximum midexpiratory flow rate

MMEP microcephaly, microphthalmia, electrodactyly, prognathism [syndrome]; multimicroelectrode plate

MMF maxillomandibular fixation; maximum midexpiratory flow; mean maximum flow; Member of the Medical Faculty; mycophenolate mofetil

μμF micromicrofarad [picofarad]

MMFF Merck molecular force field

MMFR maximal midflow rate; maximum mid-expiratory flow rate

MMFV maximum mid-respiratory flow volume

MMG mean maternal glucose

mμg millimicrogram

μmg micromilligram [nanogram]

μμg micromicrogram [picogram]

MMH monomethylhydrazine

mm Hg millimeters of mercury

μm Hg micrometer of mercury

mm H₂O millimeters of water

MMI macrophage migration inhibition; man-machine interface; master member index; maximum medical improvement; methylmercaptoimidazole; mucous membrane irritation

MMIF macrophage migration inhibition factor

MMIH megacystis, microcolon, intestinal hypoperistalsis [syndrome]

MMIHS megacystis, microcolon, intestinal hypoperistalsis syndrome

MMIRG Multicenter Myocardial Ischemia Research Group

MMIS Medicaid management information system

MML medical markup language; Moloney murine leukemia; monomethyllysine; myelomonocytic leukemia

mM/L millimoles per liter

MMLV Moloney murine leukemia virus; Montana myotis leukoencephalitis virus

MMM 3-M syndrome; marginal metallophilic macrophage; microsome-mediated mutagenesis; myelofibrosis with myeloid metaplasia; myelosclerosis with myeloid metaplasia

μmm micromillimeter

μmμ meson

MMMF manmade mineral fibers

MMMM megalocornea, macrocephaly, motor and mental retardation [syndrome]

MMMSE Modified Mini-Mental State Exam

MMMT malignant mixed müllerian tumor

MMN mismatch negativity; morbus maculosus neonatorum; multiple mucosal neuroma

MMNC marrow mononuclear cell

MMNCB multifocal motor neuropathy with conduction block

MMNN multimodular neural network

MMO medical management office; methane monooxygenase

MMOA maxillary mandibular odontectomy alveolectomy

MMOB Molecular Modeling Database

M-mode motion mode

MMoL myelomonoblastic leukemia

mmol millimole

μmol micromole, micromolar

mmol/L millimoles per liter

MMP matrix metalloproteinase; maximum maintained pressure; muscle mechanical power

4-MMPD 4-methoxy-*m*-phenylenediamine

MMPI matrix metalloproteinase inhibitor; Minnesota Multiphasic Personality Inventory

MMPNC Medical Maternal Program for Nuclear Casualties

mmpp millimeters partial pressure

MMPR methylmercaptopurine riboside

MMPS Medicare Mortality Predictor System

MMR major molecular response; mass miniature radiography; masseter muscle rigidity; maternal mortality rate; measles-mumps-rubella [vaccine]; megalocornea−mental retardation [syndrome]; mild mental retardation; mobile mass x-ray; mono-methylrutin; multimodal reasoning; myocardial metabolic rate

MMRB mouth-to-mouth rescue breathing

MMRS Mosoriot Medical Record System

MMRV measles, mumps, rubella, varicella [vaccine]

MMS mass mammographic screening; Master of Medical Science; methyl methane sulfonate; Mini Mental State [Examination]

mμs millimicrosecond

MMSA Master of Midwifery, Society of Apothecaries

MMSc Master of Medical Science

MMSE Mini Mental State Examination

mm/sec millimeters per second

MMSP malignant melanoma of soft parts

mm st muscle strength

MMT alpha-methyl-*m*-tyrosine; manual muscle test; microcephaly, mesobrachydactyly, tracheoesophageal fistula [syndrome]; mitochondrial membrane potential; mouse mammary tumor

MMTA methylmetatyramine

MMTB multimedia textbook

MMTP methadone maintenance treatment program

MMTT Multicenter Myocarditis Treatment Trial

MMTV mouse mammary tumor virus

MMU medical maintenance unit; mercaptomethyl uracil

mmu millimass unit

MMuLV Moloney murine leukemia virus

MMV mandatory minute ventilation; mandatory minute volume; Medicines for Malaria Venture

MMVD mixed mitral valve disease

MMVF man-made vitreous fiber

MMVT monomorphic ventricular tachy-cardia

MMWR Morbidity and Mortality Weekly Report

MMWV modulated Morlet wavelet transform vector sum

MN a blood group in the MNS blood group system; malignant nephrosclerosis; Master of Nursing; maternal newborn; median nerve; meganewton; melena neonatorum; melanocytic nevus; membranous nephropathy; membranous neuropathy; mesenteric node; metanephrine; micronucleated; micronucleus; midnight; mononuclear; motor neuron; mucosal neurolysis; multinodular; myoneural

M&N morning and night

M/N neutered, male [veterinary medicine]

Mn manganese; monocyte

mN millinewton; millinormal

mn modal number

μN nuclear magneton

MNA maximum noise area

MNAP mixed nerve action potential; multi-neuron acquisition processor

MNB mannosidase beta; multinucleated blastomere; murine neuroblastoma

5-MNBA 5-mercapto-2-nitrobenzoic acid

MNBCCS multiple nevoid basal cell carcinoma syndrome

MNC mononuclear cell

MNCD mild neurocognitive disorder

MNCV median nerve conduction velocity; motor nerve conduction velocity

MND minimum necrosing dose; minor neurologic dysfunction; modified neck dissection; motor neuron disease

MNER multichannel neural ensemble recording

mng morning

MNG/CRD/DA multinodular goiter, cystic renal disease, digital anomalies [syndrome]

MNGIE myo-, neuro-, gastrointestinal encephalopathy

MNH maternal and neonatal health

MNJ myoneural junction

MNK Menkes syndrome

MNL marked neutrophilic leukocytosis; maximum number of lamellae; mononuclear leukocyte

MN/m^2 meganewtons per square meter

mN/m millinewton per meter

MNMS myonephropathic metabolic syndrome

MNNG *N*-methyl *N'*-nitro-*N*-nitrosoguanidine

MNP micellar nanoparticle; mononuclear phagocyte

MNPJSS Misener Nurse Practitioner Job Satisfaction Scale

MNPV multiple nucleopolyhedrovirus

MNR marrow neutrophil reserve; multiple nucleoside resistance

MNRH may not require hospitalization

MNS medial nuclear stratum; Melnick-Needles syndrome; Milan normotensive [rat]; moesin

Mn-SOD manganese-superoxide dismutase

MNSs blood group system consisting of groups M, N, and MN

MNTBV Manitoba virus

MNTD maximum nontoxic dose

MNTV Minatitlan virus

MNU *N*-methyl-*N*-nitrosourea

MO macroorchidism; manually operated; Master of Obstetrics; Master of Osteopathy; medical officer; mesio-occlusal; metastases, zero; mineral oil; minute output; modeling object; molecular orbital; monofunctional; monooxygenase; month; morbid obesity

MO$_2$ myocardial oxygen

Mo Moloney [strain]; molybdenum; monoclonal

M$_o$ mitral opening

MΩ megohm

mo mode; month; morgan

mΩ milliohm

μ$_o$ permeability of vacuum

μΩ microhm
MOA monoamine oxidase
MoA mechanism of action
MoAb, moab monoclonal antibody
MOANS Mayo's Older Americans Normative Studies
MOAT multispecific organic anion transporter
MOB mobility [scale]
mob, mobil mobility, mobilization
MOBS Moebius syndrome
MOBV methylhydroxy-benzovesamicol; Mobala virus
MOC maximum oxygen consumption; metronidazole, omeprazole, clarithromycin; multiple ocular coloboma
MOCA Montreal Cognitive Assessment; 4,4′-methylene-bis(2-chloroaniline)
MOCHA Multicenter Oral Carvedilol in Heart Failure Assessment
MOCV *Molluscum contagiosum* virus
MOD magnetic optic disc; maturity-onset diabetes; medical officer of the day; mesio-occlusodistal
mod moderate, moderation; modification
MODE 3-methoxy-*o*-demethyl-encainide
MODED microcephaly-oculo-digito-esophageal—duodenal [syndrome]
modem modulator/demodulator
MOD/F multiple organ dysfunction/failure
MODM maturity-onset diabetes mellitus
MODS medically oriented data system; multiple organ dysfunction syndrome
MODV Modoc virus
MODY maturity-onset diabetes of the young
MOF marine oxidation/fermentation; meta object facility; methotrexate, Oncovin, and fluorouracil; multiple organ failure
MoF moment of force
MOFE multiple organ failure in the elderly
MOFS multiple organ failure syndrome
MOG myelin-oligodendrocyte glycoprotein
MO&G Master of Obstetrics and Gynaecology
MOH Medical Officer of Health; Ministry of Health
MOHSAIC Missouri Health Strategic Architectures and Information Cooperative
MOI master object index; maximum oxygen intake; mechanism of injury; multiplicity of infection
moi multiplicity of infection
MOIVC membranous obstruction of the inferior vena cava
MOJUV Moju virus
MOKV Mokola virus
MOL method of limits; molecular

mol mole; molecular, molecule
molc molar concentration
molfr mole fraction
mol/kg moles per kilogram
mol/L moles per liter
mol/m³ moles per cubic meter
mol/s moles per second
mol wt molecular weight
MOM milk of magnesia; mucoid otitis media
MoM multiples of the median
MOMA 3,4-methylenedioxidemethylamphetamine; methylhydroxymandelic acid
MOMEDA mobile medical data
MOMHR metal-on-metal hip resurfacing
MoMLV, Mo-MLV Moloney murine leukemia virus
MOMO macrosomia, obesity, macrocephaly, ocular abnormalities [syndrome]
MO-MOM mineral oil and milk of magnesia
MOMP major outer membrane protein
MOMS multiple organ malrotation syndrome
Mo-MSV Moloney murine sarcoma virus
MOMX macroorchidism—marker X chromosome [syndrome]
MON monensin; Mongolian [gerbil]
MONET multiwavelength optical network
MONICA monitoring trends and determinants in cardiovascular diseases
mono monocyte; mononucleosis
MONT montelukast
MOOKP modified osteo-odonto-keratoprosthesis
MOOSE meta-analysis of observational studies in epidemiology
MOOW Medical Officer of the Watch
MOP major organ profile; medical outpatient; memory organization packet
8-MOP 8-methoxypsoralen
MOPD microcephalic osteodysplastic primordial dwarfism
MOPEG 3-methoxy-4-hydroxyphenylglycol
MOPFC medial and orbital prefrontal cortex
MOPP mechlorethamine, Oncovin, procarbazine, prednisone; mission-oriented protective posture [clothing]
MOPS 3-morpholino-propanesulfonic acid
MOPV monovalent oral poliovirus vaccine; Mopeia virus
mOPV monovalent oral poliovirus vaccine
mOR matched odds ratio
Mor, mor morphine
MORAC mixed oligonucleotides primed amplification of complementary DNA
MORC Medical Officers Reserve Corps
MORD magnetic optical rotatory dispersion

MORFAN mental retardation, pre- and post-natal overgrowth, remarkable face, acanthosis nigricans [syndrome]

morphol morphology

mort, mortal mortality

MORV Moriche virus

MOS mechanism of stroke deducer; medial orbital sulcus; medical outcomes study; metal oxide sensor; microsomal ethanol-oxidizing system; mitral opening snap; Moloney murine sarcoma; myelofibrosis osteosclerosis

mOs milliosmole

mos mosaic

MOSA Medical Officers of School Association

MOSES Morbidity and Mortality After Stroke–Eprosartan vs. Nitrendipine for Secondary Prevention [study]

MOSF multiple organ system failure

MOSFET metal oxide semiconductor field effect transistor

mOsm, MOsm milliosmole

mOsm/kg milliosmoles per kilogram

MOST Mode Selection Trial; mother of super twins

MOSV Mossuril virus

MOT motile sperm; mouse ovarian tumor

Mot, mot motor

MOTA Manitoba oculo-tricho-anal [syndrome]

MOTNAC Manual of Tumor Nomenclature and Coding

MOTSA multiple overlapping thin slab acquisition

MOTT medical observation type table; mycobacteria other than tuberculosis

MOU memorandum of understanding

MOUS multiple occurrence of unexplained symptoms

MOV metal-oxide varistor; minimal occlusive volume; molluscum-like poxvirus

MoV mottle virus

MOVC membranous obstruction of inferior vena cava

MoVd mottle viroid

MOVIES Monongahela Valley Independent Elders Survey

MOX moxalactam

MP macrophage; maintained protocol; malignant pyoderma; matrix protein; maximum parsimony; mean pressure; mechanical processing; median posterior; Medical Psychologist; megapascal; melphalan and prednisone; melting point; membrane potential; menstrual period; mentum posterior; mercaptopurine; mesenteric panniculitis; mesial pit; mesiopulpal; metacarpophalangeal; metalloproteinase; metal particulate; metaphalangeal; metatarsophalangeal; methylphosphonate; methylprednisolone; Mibelli porokeratosis; middle phalanx; moist pack; moment preserving; monophasic; monophosphate; motion profile; motor potential; mouthpiece; movement protein; mucopolysaccharide; multiparous; multiprogrammable pacemaker; muscle potential; mycoplasmal pneumonia; myocardial perfusion

3-MP 3-mercaptopropionate

M6P mannose-6-phosphate

6-MP 6-mercaptopurine

8-MP 8-methylpsoralen

M&P managerial and professional

mp melting point; millipond

μP microprocessor

MPA main pulmonary artery; Master of Public Administration; mean pulmonary artery; medial preoptic area; Medical Procurement Agency; medroxyprogesterone acetate; mercaptopropionic acid; metaphosphoric acid; methylprednisolone acetate; micropipette aspiration; microscopic polyarteritis; minor physical anomaly; multiple project assurance

MPa megapascal

μPa micropascal

M-PACT Mayo-Physician Alliance for Clinical Trials

MPAP, mPAP mean pulmonary arterial pressure

MPAS mild periodic acid–Schiff

mPa/s millipascal per second

M-PATHY Multicenter Pacing Therapy for Hypertrophic Cardiomyopathy; Multicenter Study of Pacing Therapy for Hypertrophic Cardiomyopathy

MPB male pattern baldness; meprobamate; microdissected paraffin block

MPBA maxillary protractor bow appliance

MPC marine protein concentrate; marker for prostatic cancer; maximum permissible concentration; mean plasma concentration; meperidine, promethazine, and chlorpromazine; metallophthalocyanine; metapyrocatechase; minimum mycoplasmacidal concentration; model predictive control

MPCA microbial pest control agent

MPCh medio-posterior choroidal

MPCO micropolycystic ovary syndrome

MPCP mean pulmonary capillary pressure

MPCUR maximum permissible concentration of unidentified radionucleotides

MPD main pancreatic duct; matched peripheral dose; maximum permissible dose; mean population doubling; membrane potential difference; minimal perceptible difference;

minimal phototoxic dose; multiparametric color composite display; multiple personality disorder; myeloproliferative disease; myofascial pain dysfunction

MPDS mandibular pain dysfunction syndrome; medical priority dispatch service; myofascial pain dysfunction syndrome

MPE malignant proliferation of eosinophils; maximum permissible exposure; maximum possible error; Medicaid program evaluation; most probable event

MPEAK multispeak

MPEC multipolar electrocoagulation

MPED minimum phototoxic erythema dose

MPEH methylphenylethylhydantoin

MPEP Model Performance Evaluation Program

MPF maturation promoting factor; mean power frequency; minimally processed foods; M-phase promoting factor

MPG magnetopneumography; mercaptopropionylglycine; methyl green pyronine; 3-methylpurine deoxyribonucleic acid glycosylase; monthly prescribing guide

MPGM monophosphoglycerate mutase

MPGN membranoproliferative glomerulonephritis

MPGR multiple planar gradient recalled

MPH macroporous hydrogel; male pseudohermaphroditism; Master of Public Health; microtiter plate hybridization; milk protein hydrolysate

MPharm Master of Pharmacy

MPHD multiple pituitary hormone deficiencies

mphot milliphot

MPHR maximum predicted heart rate

MPhysA Member of Physiotherapists Association

MPI mannose phosphate isomerase; master patient index; maximum permitted intake; maximum point of impulse; message-passing interface; multidimensional pain inventory; Multiphasic Personality Inventory; myocardial performance index; myocardial perfusion imaging

MPIGL General Activity Scale of West Haven–Yale Multidimensional Pain Inventory

MPIIF Interference Scale of West Haven–Yale Multidimensional Pain Inventory

MPI-I/O message-passing interface input/output

MPIP Multicenter Postinfarction Program

MPIPS Pain Severity Scale of West Haven–Yale Multidimensional Pain Inventory

MPJ metacarpophalangeal joint

MPKC management problem-knowledge coupler

MPKUCS Maternal Phenylketonuria Collaborative Study

MPKV Maprik virus

MPL maximum permissible level; medical professional liability; melphalan; mesiopulpolingual; myeloproliferative leukemia

MPLa mesiopulpolabial

MPLS multiprotocol label switching

MPLV myeloproliferative leukemia virus

MPM malignant papillary or pleural mesothelioma; medial pterygoid muscle; minor psychiatric morbidity; mortality prediction model; mortality probability model; multiple primary malignancy; multipurpose meal

MPME (5R,8R)-8-(4-p-methoxy-phenyl)-1-piperazynylmethyl-6-methylergolene

MPMP 10[(1-methyl-3-piperidinyl)-methyl]-1OH-phenothiazine

MPMT Murphy punch maneuver test

MPMV, M-PMV Mason-Pfizer monkey virus

MPN most probable number

MPNST malignant peripheral nerve sheath tumor

MPO maximum power output; minimal perceptible odor; myeloperoxidase

MPOA medial preoptic area

MPOD myeloperoxidase deficiency

MPOV M'Poko virus

MPP massive peritoneal proliferation; massively parallel processor; medical personnel pool; mercaptopyrazide pyrimidine; metacarpophalangeal profile; methyl phenylpyridinium; myelin protein, peripheral

MPPCD Multifactorial Primary Prevention of Cardiovascular Diseases

mppcf millions of particles per cubic foot of air

MPPEC mean peak plasma ethanol concentration

MPPG microphotoelectric plethysmography

MPPH p-tolylphenylhydantoin

MPPN malignant persistent positional nystagmus

MPPT methylprednisolone pulse therapy; mucin-producing pancreatic tumor

MPP$_v$ mean portal vein peak velocity

MPQ McGill Pain Questionnaire

MPQ-SF McGill Pain Questionnaire-Short Form

MPR mannose 6-phosphate receptor; marrow production rate; massive preretinal retraction; maximum pulse rate; multiplanar reconstruction; multiplanar reformation; multiplanar reformatting; myeloproliferative reaction; myocardial perfusion reserve

mPR membrane progestin receptor

MP-RAGE magnetization-prepared rapid gradient-echo

MP-RAGE-WE magnetization-prepared rapid gradient-echo water excitation

MPRD cation-dependent mannose 6-phosphate receptor

mPRF medial pontine reticular formation

MPRG Multicenter Postinfarction Research Group

MPRO mental process

MPRV Mapuera virus

MPS hereditary giant platelet syndrome; meconium plug syndrome; medial premotor system; Member of the Pharmaceutical Society; methylprednisolone; microbial profile system; mononuclear phagocyte system; Montreal platelet syndrome; movement-produced stimulus; mucopolysaccharide, mucopolysaccharidosis; multidimensional pain scale; multiphasic screening; mushroom poisoning site; myocardial perfusion scintigraphy; myofascial pain syndrome

mps meters per second

m-PSA mutated prostate-specific antigen

MPS-H/I-S mucopolysaccharidosis, Hurler-Scheie type

MPS I mucopolysaccharidosis I

MPS I-H mucopolysaccharidosis I, Hurler type

MPS II mucopolysaccharidosis II

MPS III mucopolysaccharidosis III

MPS IIIA mucopolysaccharidosis III, type A

MPS IIIB mucopolysaccharidosis III, type B

MPS IIIC mucopolysaccharidosis III, type C

MPS IIID mucopolysaccharidosis III, type D

MPS I-S mucopolysaccharidosis I, Scheie type

MPS IV mucopolysaccharidosis IV

MPS IVA mucopolysaccharidosis IV, type A

MPS IVB mucopolysaccharidosis IV, type B

MPS V mucopolysaccharidosis V

MPS VI mucopolysaccharidosis VI

MPSoSIS mucopolysaccharidosis

MPSS methylprednisolone sodium succinate; Music Performance Stress Survey

MPSV myeloproliferative sarcoma virus; meningococcal polysaccharide vaccine

MPsyMed Master of Psychological Medicine

MPT mean peak torque; Michigan Picture Test; mitochondrial permeability transition; multiple particle tracking

MPTP 1-methyl-4-phenyl-1,2,3,6-tetrahydropyridine; mitochondrial permeability transition pore

MPT-R Michigan Picture Test, Revised

MPU Medical Practitioners Union

MPV main portal vein; mean platelet volume; mitral valve prolapse

MpV *Micromonas pusilla* virus

MPVP mean pulmonary venous pressure

MPXV monkeypox virus

MPZ myelin protein, zero

MQ memory quotient; motor quotient

M-Q move quality

MQC microbiologic quality control

MQFD medical quality function deployment

MQIS Medicare quality indicator system

MQL Medical Query Language

MQNB ^{11}C-labeled methyl quinuclidinyl-benzylate

MQOV Mosqueiro virus

MQSA Mammography Quality Standards Act

MQSM molecular quantum similarity measures

MQSPR model-based quantitative structure-property relationship

MR Maddox rods; magnetic resistance; magnetic resonance; mandibular reflex; mannose resistant; may repeat; measles and rubella; medial raphe; medial rectus [muscle]; medical record; medical release; medium range; megaroentgen; mental retardation; metabolic rate; Metathesaurus relational file; methemoglobin reductase; methyl red; mineralocorticoid receptor; mitral reflux; mitral regurgitation; modulation rate; molar refraction; molecular response; mortality rate; mortality ratio; multicentric reticulohistiocytosis; multiregression; muscarinic receptor; muscle receptor; muscle relaxant; myocardial revascularization

M&R measure and record

M/R measles/rubella [vaccine]

M$_2$R muscarinic cholinergic receptor

MR4 Malaria Research and Reference Reagent Resource Center

Mr relative molar mass

M$_r$ relative molecular mass

mR, mr milliroentgen

m/r mass attenuation coefficient; modified release

μR, μr microroentgen

MRA magnetic resonance angiography; main renal artery; marrow repopulation activity; medical record analysis/analyst; medical records administrator; mesenteric resistance artery; mid right atrium; multivariate regression analysis

MRAB machine-readable archives in biomedicine

MRAC model reference adaptive control

mrad millirad

MRAP alpha-2-macroglobulin receptor−associated protein; maximal resting anal pressure; mean right atrial pressure

MRAS main renal artery stenosis

MRB multiply resistant bacteria

MRBC monkey red blood cell; mouse red blood cell

MRBF mean renal blood flow

MRC magnetic resonance cholangiography; maximum recycling capacity; Medical Registration Council; Medical Research Council; Medical Reserve Corps; methylrosaniline chloride; modular robot control

MRCAS medical robotics and computer-assisted surgery

MRC/BHF Medical Research Council, British Heart Foundation Heart Protection Study

MRC CFAS Medical Research Council Cognitive Function and Ageing Study

MR-CISS magnetic resonance constructive interference in steady state

MRCNS methicillin-resistant coagulase-negative staphylococci

MRCOA Medical Research Council Trial in Older Adults

MRCP magnetic resonance cholangiopancreatography; Member of the Royal College of Physicians; movement-related cortical potential

MRCS Member of the Royal College of Surgeons

MRD magnetic resonance diffusion; maximum rate of depolarization; measles-rinderpest-distemper [virus group]; medical records department; minimal reacting dose; minimal renal disease; minimal residual disease

mrd millirutherford

MRDD mentally retarded (intellectually disabled)/developmentally disabled

MRDI medical records document imaging

MR-DTI magnetic resonance diffusion tensor imaging

MRE magnetic resonance elastography; maximal resistive exercise; maximal respiratory effectiveness; Microbiological Research Establishment

MREC mismatch repair enzyme cleavage

MREI mean rate ejection index

mrem millirem

mrep milliroentgen equivalent physical

MRF Markov random field; medical record file; melanocyte [stimulating hormone] releasing factor; mesencephalic reticular formation; midbrain reticular formation; mitral regurgitant flow; moderate renal failure; monoclonal rheumatoid factor; müllerian regression factor; muscle regulatory factor

mRF monoclonal rheumatoid factor

MRFC mouse rosette-forming cell

MRFIT Multiple Risk Factor Intervention Trial

MRFM magnetic resonance force microscopy

MRFT modified rapid fermentation test

MRH melanocyte-stimulating hormone−releasing hormone; multicentric reticulohistiocytosis

MRHA mannose-resistant hemagglutination

mrhm milliroentgens per hour at one meter

MRI machine-readable identifier; magnetic resonance imaging; magnetic resonance interferometry; medical records information; medical reengineering initiative; Medical Research Institute; moderate renal insufficiency

M-RIA monoclonal radioimmunoassay

MRIF melanocyte [stimulating hormone] release-inhibiting factor

MRIH melanocyte [stimulating hormone] release-inhibiting hormone

MRIPHH Member of the Royal Institute of Public Health and Hygiene

MRISM magnetic resonance imaging simulation

MRK Mayer-Rokitansky-Küster [syndrome]

MR-K mannose-resistant *Klebsiella*-like [hemagglutinin]

MRKH Mayer-Rokitansky-Küster-Hauser [syndrome]

MRL Malaria Reference Laboratory; maximum residue limit; medical records librarian; Medical Research Laboratory

MRM magnetic resonance mammography; modified radical mastectomy

MRMIB Managed Risk Medical Insurance Board

MRMT Minnesota Rate of Manipulation Test

MRN magnetic resonance neurography; malignant renal neoplasm; medical record number; Mind Research Network

mRNA messenger ribonucleic acid

mRNA/R messenger ribonucleic acid receptor

mRNP messenger ribonucleoprotein

MRO master reference oscillator; medical review officer; minimal recognizable odor; muscle receptor organ

MROD Medical Research and Operations Directorate

MRP mean resisting potential; medical reimbursement plan; medical removal protection; multidrug resistance−associated protein; mutual recognition process

MR-PET Magnetic Resonance vs. Positron Emission Tomography [study]

MRR marrow release rate

MRS magnetic resonance spectroscopy; Mania Rating Scale; medical receiving station; medical record summary; Melkersson-Rosenthal syndrome

MRSA methicillin-resistant *Staphylococcus aureus*

MRSB mid−right sternal border

MRSD mental retardation, skeletal dysplasia [syndrome]

MRSE methicillin-resistant *Staphylococcus epidermidis*

MRSH Member of the Royal Society of Health

MRSI magnetic resonance spectroscopy imaging; methicillin-resistant staphylococcal infection

MRSO metathesaurus relational source

MRSX X-linked mental retardation

MRT magnetic resonance tomography; maximum relaxation time; median range score; median reaction time; median recognition threshold; median relapse time; medical radiation technology/technologist; medical records technician; medical response team; methyltryptophan; milk ring test; muscle response test

MRTC myelin-peptide reactive T cell

MRTS message routing and translation system

MRU magnetic recognition unit; mass radiography unit; magnetic resonance urography; meningococcal reference unit; minimal reproductive unit; *Mycobacterium* reference unit

MR/UR Medical Review and Utilization Program

MRV magnetic resonance venography; mammalian orthoreovirus; minute respiratory volume; Mitchell river virus; mixed respiratory vaccine

mRV morphological right ventricle

MRVP mean right ventricular pressure; methyl red, Voges-Proskauer [medium]

MRW multiresolution wavelet

MRWT multiresolution wavelet transform

MRX mental retardation, X-linked

MRXA X-linked mental retardation−aphasia syndrome

MRXS X-linked mental retardation syndrome

MS Maffuci syndrome; magnesium sulfate; maladjustment score; mandibular series; mannose sensitive; Marfan syndrome; margin of safety; Marie-Strümpell [syndrome]; mass spectrometry; Master of Science; Master of Surgery; maternal serum; mean score; mean square; mechanical stimulation; Meckel syndrome; mediastinal shift; medical services; medical staff; medical student; medical supplies; medical survey; melanonychia striata; Menkes syndrome; menopausal syndrome; mental status; metabolic syndrome; microscope slide; *Microsporida*; midseptal; minimal support; mitral sounds; mitral stenosis; mobile surgical; modal sensitivity; moderately susceptible; modified sphygmomanometer; molar solution; molecular substitution; Mongolian spot; morning stiffness; morphine sulfate; morphosyntactic; mosaic virus; motile sperm; mucosubstance; multiple sclerosis; Münchausen syndrome; muscle shortening; muscle strength; musculoskeletal; myelosarcoma; myoclonic seizures

3MS modified mini-mental state examination

Ms murmurs; microsphere

ms millisecond

m/s meters per second

m/s² meters per second squared

μs microsecond

MSA magnetic resonance angiography; major serologic antigen; major soluble antigen; male-specific antigen; mammary serum antigen; mannitol-salt agar; medical savings account; Medical Services Administration; membrane-stabilizing action; membrane-stabilizing activity; metropolitan statistical area; microsomal anti-antibody; mitotic spindle apparatus; molecular shape analysis; morphologic sequential approach; mouse serum albumin; multiple sequence alignment; multiple system atrophy; muscle sympathetic activity; myosis-specific antibody

MSAA multiple sclerosis−associated agent

MSA-C multiple system atrophy with predominant cerebellar ataxia

MSAD multiple scan average dose

MSAEFI Monitoring System for Adverse Events Following Immunisation

MSAFP, MS-AFP maternal serum alpha-fetoprotein

MSAM Master of Science in Administrative Medicine

MSAN medical student's admission note

MSAP mean systemic arterial pressure

MSA-P multiple system atrophy with predominant parkinsonism

MSB Master of Science in Bacteriology; mid small bowel; most significant bit

MSBC maximum specific binding capacity

MSBLA mouse-specific B-lymphocyte antigen

MSC magnitude-squared coherence; major septic complication; marrow stromal cell; Medical Service Corps; Medical Staff Corps;

mesenchymal stem cell; midsystolic click; Multimedia SuperCorridor; multispecialty clinic

MSc Master of Science

MScD Master of Dental Science

MScMed Master of Science in Medicine

MScN Master of Science in Nursing

MSCP mean spherical candle power

MSCRAMM Microbial Surface Components Recognizing Adhesive Matrix Molecules

MSCU medical special care unit

MSD Material Safety Data; mean square deviation; mean square displacement; membrane-spanning domain; midsagittal diameter; mild sickle cell disease; minimal systolic displacement; most significant digit; multiple sulfatase deficiency; musculoskeletal dynamic

MSDC Mass Spectrometry Data Centre

MSDI Martin Suicide Depression Inventory

MSDS material safety data sheet

MSE mean squared error; medical screening examination; medical support equipment; mental status examination; mental status expert; muscle-specific enolase

mse mean square error

MSEA Medical Society Executives Association

msec millisecond

m/sec meters per second

μsec microsecond

MSEL Materials Science and Engineering Laboratory; myasthenic syndrome of Eaton-Lambert

MSEP mean square error of prediction

MSER mean systolic ejection rate

MSES medical school environmental stress

MSF macrophage slowing factor; macrophage spreading factor; malignant senescent forgetfulness−meconium-stained fluid; Médicins sans Frontières [Doctors Without Borders]; Mediterranean spotted fever; melanocyte-stimulating factor; modified sham feeding; multiple sequence format

MSG molecular supergraph; monosodium l-glutamate; motion-sensitizing gradient

MSGQ medical student graduation questionnaire

MSGV mouse salivary gland virus

MSH medical self-help; melanocyte-stimulating hormone; melanophore-stimulating hormone; message header; Multicenter Study of Hydroxyurea

MSHA mannose-sensitive hemagglutination; Mine Safety and Health Administration

MSHIF melanocyte-stimulating hormone−inhibiting factor

MSHR melanocyte-stimulating hormone receptor

MSHRF melanocyte-stimulating hormone−releasing factor

MSHRH melanocyte-stimulating hormone−releasing hormone

M-SHRSP malignant stroke-prone spontaneously hypertensive rat

MSHSC multiple self-healing squamous carcinoma

MSHT Mount Sinai Hypertension Trial

MSHyg Master of Science in Hygiene

MSI magnetic source imaging; medium-scale integration; microsatellite instability

MS I, II, III, IV medical student—first, second, third, and fourth year

MSIC mechanically sensitive ion channels

MSIM medical systems infrastructure modernization

MSIS multistate information system

MSIT Multisource Interference Task

MSJ meatal stapedial joint

MSK medullary sponge kidney; Memorial Sloan-Kettering; mitogen-activated S6 kinase; musculoskeletal

MSKCC Memorial Sloan-Kettering Cancer Center

MSKP Medical Sciences Knowledge Profile

MSL midsternal line; multiple symmetric lipomatosis

MSLA morphosynthetic lexical ambiguity; mouse-specific lymphocyte antigen

MSLIS Master of Science in Library and Information Science

MSLL multifocal signal loss lesion

MSLR mixed skin cell leukocyte reaction

MSLS Marinesco−Sjögren-like syndrome

MSLT Multicenter Selective Lymphadenectomy Trial; multiple sleep latency test

MSM medium-size molecule; men who have sex with men; midsystolic murmur; mineral salts medium

MSMA monosodium methanearsonate

MSMAID machine, suction, monitor, airway equipment, intravenous line, drugs

MSMB microseminoprotein beta

MSMI Multicenter Study of Myocardial Ischemia

MS/MS tandem mass spectrophotometry

MSN main sensory nucleus; Master of Science in Nursing; mildly subnormal; moiesin

MSNet Mass Spectrometry Network

MSO management services organization; medial superior olive; medical staff organization

MSOF multiple systems organ failure

MSOP medical school objectives project

MSOS Medication Safety Officers Society

MSP macrophage stimulating protein; maximum squeeze pressure; median sagittal plane; Medicare secondary payer; methylation-specific polymerase chain reaction; microseminoprotein; Münchausen syndrome by proxy

msp muscle spasm

MSPB microseminoprotein beta

MSPGN mesangial proliferative glomerulonephritis

MSPH Master of Science in Public Health

MSPhar Master of Science in Pharmacy

MSPN medical student's progress note

MSPQ Modified Somatic Perception Questionnaire

MSPS myocardial stress perfusion scintigraphy

MSPT Master of Science in Physical Therapy

MSPV Malpais Spring virus

MSQ mental status questionnaire; mini sleep questionnaire; Minnesota satisfaction questionnaire

MSR macrophage scavenger receptor; magnetically shielded room; Member of the Society of Radiographers; mitro-sterno regurgitation; monosynaptic reflex; muscle stretch reflex

MSRI mixed serotonin reuptake inhibitor

MSRPP Multidimensional Scale for Rating Psychiatric Patients

MSRT Minnesota Spatial Relations Test

MSS Marinesco-Sjögren syndrome; Marshall-Smith syndrome; massage; Medical Superintendents' Society; Medicare Statistical System; mental status schedule; minor surgery suite; motion sickness susceptibility; mucus-stimulating substance; multiple sclerosis susceptibility; muscular subaortic stenosis

mss massage

MSSA methicillin-sensitive *Staphylococcus aureus*

MSSE methicillin-sensitive *Staphylococcus epidermidis*; multiple sclerosis self-efficacy scale; multiple self-healing squamous epithelioma

MSSG multiple sclerosis susceptibility gene

MSSI multislice spectroscopic imaging

MSSMI Multicenter Study of Silent Myocardial Ischemia

MSSVD Medical Society for the Study of Venereal Diseases

MST maximal stimulation test; mean survival time; mean swell time; mercaptopyruvate sulfurtransferase; Montenegro skin test; multiple

subpial transections; muscle-sparing thoracotomy; myeloproliferative syndrome, transient

MSTD mean seminiferous tubule diameter

M-Step maximization step

MSTh mesothorium

MSTI multiple soft tissue injuries

MSTP Medical Scientist Training Program; medical student training program

MSTS Musculoskeletal Tumor Society

MsTT microsphere encapsulated tetanus toxoid

MSU maple sugar/syrup urine; medical studies unit; midstream specimen of urine; midstream urine; monosodium urate; myocardial substrate uptake

MSUD maple syrup urine disease

MSurg Master of Surgery

MSV maximum sustained level of ventilation; mean scale value; mean spatial velocity; Moloney sarcoma virus; monkey sarcoma virus; Muir Springs virus; murine sarcoma virus

mSv millisievert

MSVC maximal sustained ventilatory capacity

MSW male sex worker; Master of Social Welfare; Master of Social Work; medical social worker; multiple stab wounds

MSWT modified shuttle walk test

MSWYE modified sea water yeast extract

MT magnetization transfer; malaria therapy; malignant teratoma; mammary tumor; mammilothalamic tract; manual traction; Martin-Thayer [plate, medium]; mastoid tip; maximal therapy; mechanotransduction; medial thalamus; medial thickness; medical technologist; medical therapy; medical transcriptionist; melatonin; membrana tympani; mesangial thickening; metallothionein; metatarsal; Metathesaurus methoxytryptamine; methyltransferase; methyltyrosine; microtome; microtomography; microtubule; mid trachea; minimal touch; minimum threshold; mitochondrial toxicity; Monroe tidal drainage; more than; motor threshold; movement time; Muir-Torre [syndrome]; multi-input threshold; multiple tics; multitest; mural thrombus/thrombosis; muscles and tendons; muscle test; music therapy; *Mycobacterium tuberculosis*

M-T macroglobulin-trypsin

M&T *Monilia* and *Trichomonas*

Mt megatonne; *Mycobacterium tuberculosis*

mt mitochondrial

3-MT 3-methoxytyramine

MTA malignant teratoma, anaplastic; medical technical assistant; medical technology assessment; medullary type adenocarcinoma;

metatarsus adductus; methadone to abstinence; multithreaded architecture; myoclonic twitch activity

mTA meta-tyramine

MTAC mass transfer area coefficient

MTACR multiple tumor-associated chromosome region

MTAD membrana tympana auris dextrae

MTAL medullary thick ascending limb

MTAP methylthioadenosine phosphorylase

MTAS membrana tympana auris sinistrae

MT(ASCP) Medical Technologist certified by the American Society of Clinical Pathologists

MTase methyltransferase

MTB methylthymol blue; Michelin tire baby [syndrome]; *Mycobacterium tuberculosis*

Mtb *Mycobacterium tuberculosis*

MTBE meningeal tick-borne encephalitis; methyltertiary butyl ether

MTBF mean time between (or before) failures

mTBI mild traumatic brain injury

MTBM mean time between maintenance

MTBN modifiable temporal belief network

MTBV Marituba virus

MTC magnetization transfer contrast; mass transfer coefficient; maximum tolerated concentration; maximum toxic concentration; medical test cabinet; medical training center; medullary thyroid carcinoma; metatarsocuneiform; mitomycin C

mTCR monoclonal T-cell receptor

MTCT mother-to-child transmission

MTD maximum tolerated dose; mean total dose; metastatic trophoblastic disease; Midwife Teacher's Diploma; minimal topological difference; Monroe tidal drainage; multidrug therapy; multiple tic disorder; *Mycobacterium tuberculosis* direct test

MTDDA Minnesota Test for Differential Diagnosis of Aphasia

MT-DN multitest, dermatophytes and *Nocardia* [plate]

mtDNA mitochondrial DNA

MTDT modified tone decay test

MTE main timing event; monophasic truncated exponential

mTERF mitochondrial transcription termination factor

MTET modified treadmill exercise test

MTF maximum terminal flow; medical treatment facility; modular tube feeding; modulation transfer function; Musculoskeletal Transplant Foundation

mTF mitochondrial transcription factor

MTg mouse thyroglobulin

MTGA multiple time graphic analysis

MTGua 7-methyl-6-thioguanine

MTGuo 7-methyl-6-thioguanosine

MTH mithramycin

MTh motor threshold

MTHF, mTHF 5,10-methylene tetrahydrofolate

5-MTHF 5-methyl-tetrahydrofolate

MTHFR 5,10-methylene tetrahydrofolate reductase

MTI malignant teratoma, intermediate; maximum tolerable intensity; minimum time interval; model tag image; molecular topological index; moving target indicator

MTIA Medical Training Institute of America; Medical Transcription Industry Alliance

MTL mantle zone lymphoma; medial temporal lobe

MTLE mesial temporal lobe epilepsy

MTLP metabolic toxemia of late pregnancy

MTM medication therapy management; Thayer-Martin, modified [agar]; myotubular myopathy

MT-M multitest, mycology [plate]

MT-MMP membrane-type metalloproteinase

MTMX myotubular myopathy, X-linked

MTO medical technical officer; medical transport officer

MTOC microtubule organizing center; mitotic organizing center

MTOP Medical Treatment Outcomes Project

mTOR mammalian target of rapamycin

MTOS Major Trauma Outcomes Study

MTP maximum tolerated pressure; medial tibial plateau; median time to progression; metatarsophalangeal; micropayment transfer protocol; microsomal triglyceride transfer protein; microtubule protein

MT1PA metallothionein-1 pseudogene-A

MTPD mean trabecular plate density

MTPJ metatarsophalangeal joint

Mt-PK myotonic protein kinase

MTPS mean trabecular plate separation

MTPT mean trabecular plate thickness

MTQ methaqualone

MTR magnetization transfer ratio; maximum tracking rate; Meinicke turbidity reaction; 5-methylthioribose; methyltetrahydrofolate: L-homocysteine *S*-methyltransferase

MTRV Matruh virus

MTS magnetization transfer contrast; mechanical testing machine; Medicare transaction system; menopausal transition; mesial temporal sclerosis; methotrexate; methylphenidate transdermal system; Mohr-Tranebjaerg syndrome; multicellular tumor spheroid; musculotendinous structure

MTST maximal treadmill stress test

MTT malignant teratoma, trophoblastic; maximal treadmill test; meal tolerance test; mean transit time; methyl-thiazol-diphenyl-tetrazolium; mirror tracing test; mitochondrial tetrazolium salt; mucous transport time; Myocarditis Treatment Trial

mTTI modified tension-time index

MTU malignant teratoma, undifferentiated; medical therapy unit; methylthiouracil

MtuRRF *Mycobacterium tuberculosis* ribosome recycling factor

MTV mammary tumor virus; metatarsus varus; Mibuna temperate virus; mild tigré virus; mouse mammary tumor virus

MTX methotrexate

MT-Y multitest yeast [plate]

MTZ microthermal zone

MU measurement uncertainty; megaunit; mescaline unit; methyluric [acid]; monitor unit [radiotherapy]; Montevideo unit; motion unsharpness; motor unit; mouse unit

Mu Mache unit

mU milliunit

mu mouse unit

μU microunit

MUA manipulation under anesthesia; middle uterine artery; motor unit activity

MUAP motor unit action potential

MUC maximum urinary concentration; mucilage; mucin; mucosal ulcerative colitis

muc mucilage; mucous, mucus

MUCV Mucambo virus

MUD matched unrelated donor; meal-unrelated dyspepsia; minimum urticarial dose

MUDV Mudjinbarry virus

MUE motor unit estimated

MUFA monounsaturated fatty acids

MUG 4-methyl-umbelliferyl-β-d-glucuronide

MUGA multiple gated acquisition

MUGEx multigated blood pool image during exercise

MUGR multigated blood pool image at rest

MuHV Murid herpesvirus

mulibrey muscle-liver-brain-eye [nanism, dwarfism]

MULO multipurpose overboot

mult multiple

Multi-CSF multi-colony-stimulating factor

MultiODA multivariable optimal discriminant analysis

multip multiparous

MULV Muleshoe virus

MuLV, MuLv murine leukemia virus

MUMPS Massachusetts General Hospital Utility Multi-Programming System

MuMTv murine mammary tumor virus

MUNV Munguba virus

MUN(WI) Munich Wistar [rat]

MUO myocardiopathy of unknown origin

MUP major urinary protein; maximal urethral pressure; motor unit potential

mUPD maternal uniparental disomy

MUPIBAC Mupirocin in Prevention of Relapses of Wegener Granulomatosis by Elimination of Nasal Bacterial *Staphylococcus aureus* Carriage

mUPID maternal uniparental isodisomy

MUPIT Martinez Universal Perineal Interstitial Template Mural

MUPS medically unexplained physical symptoms

MURAD Moscow-Ulm Radiation Accident Clinical History Database

MURC measurable undesirable respiratory contaminants

MURCS müllerian duct aplasia, cervico-thoracic somite dysostosis [association]

MurNAc *N*-acetylmuramate

MURP Master of Urban and Regional Planning

MURV Murre virus; Murutucu virus

MUS medically unexplained symptoms; mouse urologic syndrome; muscinol

musc muscle, musculature, muscular

MUSCAT MUSIC Criteria for Stent Implantation Using the Controlled Angioplasty Technology Catheter

MUSE medicated uretheral system for erection

MUSIC Measuring the Usability of Systems in Context; Multicenter Ultrasound During Stent Implantation in Coronary Arteries [study]; Multicenter Ultrasound Stent in Coronary Artery Disease [study]; Multicentre Ultrasound Study in Coronaries; multiple signal classification; musculoskeletal intervention center

MUST medical unit, medication use studies; Medical Unit Self-Contained and Transportable; Multicenter Stent Study; Multicenter Stents Ticlodipine [study]; Multicenter Ultrasound Study with Ticlid; Multicenter Unsustained Tachycardia [trial]

MUST-EECP Multicenter Study of Enhanced External Counterpulsation

MUSTIC multisite stimulation in cardiac insufficiency; multisite stimulation in cardiomyopathy

MUSTPAC medical ultrasound three-dimensional portable with advanced communication

MUSTT Multicentre Unstable Tachycardia Trial; Multicenter Unsustained Tachycardia Trial

MUT mutagen

mut mutation

MUU mouse uterine unit

MuV mumps virus

MUWU mouse uterine weight unit

MUX multiplex

MV maturation value; measles virus; mechanical ventilation; megavolt; methotrexate/vinblastine; microvascular; microvillus; Microvirus, microvirus; minute ventilation; minute virus; minute volume; mitral valve; mixed venous; molar volume; mosaic virus; mottle virus; multivessel; myeloblastosis virus; veterinary physician [L. *Medicus Veterinarius*]

Mv mendelevium

mV, mv millivolt

μV microvolt

MVA mechanical ventricular assistance; mevalonic acid; mitral valve area; modified vaccinia virus Ankara; Modified Virus Ankara; motor vehicle accident

MV·A megavolt-ampere

mV·A millivolt-ampere

MVAD mechanical ventricular assist device

mval millival

MVB manual ventilation bag; microvascular bleeding; multivesicular body

MVC maximum voluntary contraction; minute virus of canines [veterinary medicine]; model view controller; motor vehicle crash; multivane collimator; muscle vasoconstriction; myocardial vascular capacity

MVD Doctor of Veterinary Medicine; microvascular decompression; microvessel density; mitral valve disease; multivessel coronary disease

MVd mosaic viroid

MVE maximum velocity envelope; mitral valve echo; mitral valve excursion; Murray Valley encephalitis

MVEC microvascular endothelial cell

MVEV Murray Valley encephalitis virus

MVF mitral valve flow

MVH massive vitreous hemorrhage

MVI mitral valve insufficiency; multivalvular involvement; multivitamin infusion

MV-HIS multi-vendor hospital information system

MVK mevalonate kinase

MVL mitral valve leaflet

MVLS mandibular vestibulolingual sulcoplasty

MVM microvillose membrane; minute virus of mice

MVMT movement

MVN medial ventromedial nucleus; microvascular network

MVO maximum venous outflow; mitral valve opening or orifice

MVO2, MVO₂ myocardial oxygen consumption

MVOA mitral valve orifice area

mVOC mycological volatile organic compound

MVP microvascular pressure; mitral valve prolapse; Multivitamin and Probucol [trial]

MVPP mustine, vinblastine, procarbazine, prednisone

MVPS Medicare Volume Performance Standards; mitral valve prolapse syndrome

MVP-SC mitral valve prolapse-systolic click [syndrome]

MVPT Motor-Free Visual Perception Test

MVR massive vitreous reaction; microvitreoretinal; minimal vascular resistance; mitral valve replacement

MVRI mixed virus respiratory infection

MVS mitral valve stenosis; multivendor service; multivoxel spectroscopy

mV·s millivolt-second

MVSR Monthly Viral Statistics Report

MVT mesenteric venous thrombosis; multi-attribute value theory

mvt movement

MVTR moisture vapor transmission rate

MVV maximal voluntary ventilation

MW Mallory-Weiss [syndrome]; mean weight; megawatt; microwave; middleware; Minot–von Willebrand [syndrome]; molecular weight; multiple window

mW milliwatt

μW microwatt

MWA moving window averaging

MWAPI M [language] windowing application programmer interface

MWAV Manawa virus

MWB modified whole blood

mWb milliweber

MWCB master working cell bank

MWCO molecular weight cut off

MWD maximum walking distance; microwave diathermy; molecular weight data; molecular weight distribution

MWI modified Williams index

MWL mental workload

m-WMFT modified Wolf motor function test

MWP mean wedge pressure

MWS Marden-Walker syndrome; midwall shortening; Moersch-Woltman syndrome; Muckle-Wells syndrome

MWSP multi wall stereo projection

MWSR multiple window spatial registration

MWT myocardial wall thickness

6-MWT 6-minute walk test

MWTA Medical Waste Tracking Act

MwV Manawatu virus

MX matrix; metastases not assessed; methylxanthine

Mx extension of physician; maxwell; metastases not assessed

MXA morphometric x-ray absorptiometry

MXIP maximum inspiratory pressure

MXV Mexico virus

M$_{xy}$ transverse magnetization

My myopia; myxedema

my mayer

MYBC myosin-binding protein C

MYBH myosin-binding protein H

MYBP myosin-binding protein

MycDB *Mycobacterium* Database

Myco *Mycobacterium*

Mycol mycology, mycologist

MyD myotonic dystrophy

MYEL myelogram

Myel myelocyte

myel myelin, myelinated

MYF myogenic factor

MyG myasthenia gravis

MYH heavy chain myosin

MYHC heavy chain cardiac myosin

MYHCA heavy chain cardiac myosin alpha

MYKV Mykines virus

MYL light chain myosin

MyMD myotonic muscular dystrophy

MYO myoglobin

Myop myopia

mYPAS modified Yale Preoperative Anxiety Score

MYW modified Yule-Walker [technique]

MYX myxoma

MYXV myxoma virus

MZ mantle zone; mezlocillin; monozygotic

M$_z$ longitudinal magnetization

m/z mass/charge ratio

MZA monozygotic twins raised apart

MZM marginal zone macrophage

MZT monozygotic twins raised together

N

N asparagine; Avogadro number; blood factor in the MNS blood group system; loudness; nasal; nasion; nausea; negative; neomycin; neper; nerve; neuraminidase; neurology; neuropathy; neutron number; newton; nicotinamide; nifedipine; nitrogen; nodule; normal; nucleocapsid; nucleoprotein; nucleoside; nucleus; number; number in sample; number of molecules; number of neutrons in an atomic nucleus; population size; radiance; refractive index; signal size; spin density; uppercase Greek letter nu

N0 no breast tumor regional lymph node metastases

0.02N one-fiftieth normal

0.1N one-tenth normal

0.5N one-half normal

N1 breast tumor metastases to ipsilateral axillary lymph nodes; normal subject

N 1 to 12 cranial nerves 1 to 12

2N double normal

N2 breast tumor metastases to ipsilateral axillary lymph nodes attached to each other or to other structures

N/2 one-half normal

N3 breast tumor metastases to ipsilateral internal mammary lymph nodes

N/10 one-tenth normal

N/50 one-fiftieth normal

N95 NIOSH-certified mask that filters at least 95% of airborne particles

n amount of substance expressed in moles; born [L. *natus*]; haploid chromosome number; index of refraction; nerve; neuter; neutron; neutron night; nostril; number; number density; number of density of molecule; principal quantum number; refractive index; rotational frequency; sample size

ν lowercase Greek letter nu; degrees of freedom; frequency; kinematic velocity; neutrino

n- nano- $[10^{-9}]$

2n haploid chromosome; diploid

3n triploid

4n tetraploid

NA Avogadro constant or number; nalidixic acid; Narcotics Anonymous; network administrator; neuraminidase; neurologic age; neutralizing antibody; neutrophil antibody; nicotinic acid; Nomina Anatomica; non-A [hepatitis virus]; nonadherent; noradrenalin; not admitted; not applicable; not available; nuclear antibody; nucleic acid; nucleoside analogue; nucleus ambiguus; numerical aperture; nurse's aide; nursing assistant; nursing auxiliary

N/A not applicable

Na Avogadro number; sodium

nA nanoampere

NAA *N*-acetyl aspartate; naphthaleneacetic acid; neutral amino acid; neutron activation analysis; neutrophil aggregation activity; nicotinic acid amide; no apparent abnormalities

NAACCR North American Association of Central Cancer Registries

NAACLS National Accrediting Agency for Clinical Laboratory Sciences

NAACOG Nurses Association of the American College of Obstetricians and Gynecologists

NAA/Cr *N*-acetyl aspartate/creatine ratio

NA-AAF *N*-acetoxy-*N*-acetylaminofluorene

NAAP *N*-acetyl-4-amino-phenazone

NAAQS national ambient air quality standard

NAASO North American Association for the Study of Obesity

NAAT nucleic acid amplification testing

NAB novarsenobenzene; neutralizing antibody

NABP National Association of Boards of Pharmacy

NABPLEX National Association of Boards of Pharmacy Licensing Examination

NAC *N*-acetylcysteine; National Asthma Center; National Audiovisual Center; neuroimaging analysis center; Noise Advisory Council

NaC sodium channel

NACAA National Association of Clean Air Agencies

NACCHO National Association of County and City Health Officials

NACCT North American Congress of Clinical Toxicology

NaC/DEG sodium channel and degenerin

NACDS North American Clinical Dermatological Society

NACED National Advisory Council on the Employment of the Disabled

nAch nicotinic acetylcholine

NAcHPZ 4-*N*-acetyl hydrazinophthalazin-1-one

nAChR nicotinic acetylcholine receptor

NACHRI National Association of Children's Hospitals and Related Institutions

NACI New Applications for Coronary Interventions; New Approaches to Coronary Interventions

NACI DCA New Approaches to Coronary Interventions Directional Coronary Atherectomy [study]
NaCl sodium chloride
NACNEP National Advisory Council on Nurse Education and Practice
NACNS National Association of Clinical Nurse Specialists
NACOR National Advisory Committee on Radiation
NACOSH National Advisory Committee on Occupational Safety & Health
NACPTAR North American Cerebral Percutaneous Transluminal Angioplasty Registration [study]
Nacq number of acquisitions
NACS neonate adaptive capacity to stimulus
NACSAP National Alliance Concerned with School-Age Parents
NACT National Alliance of Cardiovascular Technologists
NAD neutrophil actin dysfunction; new antigenic determinant; nicotinamide adenine dinucleotide; nicotinic acid dehydrogenase; no abnormal discovery; no active disease; no acute distress; no apparent distress; no appreciable disease; normal axis deviation; not done; nothing abnormal detected
NAD⁺ oxidized nicotinamide adenine dinucleotide
NaD sodium dialysate
NADA National Acupuncture Detoxification Association; New Animal Drug Application
NADABA *N*-adenoxyldiaminobutyric acid
NADAC national drug acquisition cost
NaDC sodium dicarboxylate cotransporter
NADG nicotinamide adenine dinucleotide glycohydrolase
NADH nicotinamide adenine dinucleotide-tetrazolium reductase; reduced nicotinamide adenine dinucleotide
NADL National Association of Dental Laboratories
NADMWP National Association of Disease Management and Wellness Professionals
NADNP National Academy of Dermatology Nurse Practitioners
NaDodSO₄ sodium dodecyl sulfate
NADONA/LTC National Association of Directors of Nursing Administration/Long Term Care
NADP National Association of Dental Plans; nicotinamide adenine dinucleotide phosphate
NADP⁺ oxidized form of nicotinamide adenine dinucleotide phosphate

NADPH reduced nicotinamide adenine dinucleotide phosphate
NADR National AIDS Demonstration Research; noradrenalin
NADS National Alcohol and Other Drugs Survey [Canada]
NADSA National Adult Day Services Association
NAE net acid excretion
NaE, Naₑ exchangeable body sodium
NaE1ATP sodium-enzyme-adenosine triphosphate complex
NAED National Academies of Emergency Dispatch
NAEL no adverse effect level
NAEMD National Academy of Emergency Medical Dispatch
NAEMSP National Association of Emergency Medical Services Physicians
NAEMT National Association of Emergency Medical Technicians
NAEP National Asthma Education Program
NAEPP National Asthma Education and Prevention Program
NaERC sodium efflux rate constant
NAF nafcillin; National Amputation Foundation; National Ataxia Foundation; net acid flux; neural adaptive filter; nipple aspirate fluid
NAFAC National Association for Ambulatory Care
NAFD Nager acrofacial dysostosis
NAFEC National Association of Freestanding Emergency Centers
NAFL nonalcoholic fatty liver
NAFLD nonalcoholic fatty liver disease
NAFTA North American Free Trade Agreement
NAG *N*-acetyl-D-glucosaminidase; narrow-angle glaucoma; nonagglutinable
NAGA *N*-acetyl-alpha-D-galactosaminidase
NAGO neuraminidase and galactose oxidase
NAGS *N*-acetylglutamate synthetase
NAH 2-hydroxy-3-naphthoic acid hydrazide
NAHA National Association of Health Authorities
NAHC National Advisory Heart Council
NAHCS National Association of Health Center Schools
NAHDO National Association of Health Data Organizations
NAHG National Association of Humanistic Gerontology
NAHH National Alliance for Hispanic Health

NAHHH National Association of Hospital Hospitality Houses

NAHI National Athletic Health Institute

NAHMOR National Association of Health Maintenance Organization Regulators

NAHN National Association of Hispanic Nurses

NAHPA National Association of Hospital Purchasing Agents

NAHQ National Association for Healthcare Quality

NAHSA National Association for Hearing and Speech Action

NAHSE National Association of Health Services Executives

NAHTM National Association of Healthcare Transport Management

NAHU National Association of Health Underwriters

NAHUC National Association of Health Unit Coordinators

NAHV non-A hepatitis virus

NAI NASA Astrobiology Institute; net acid input; no accidental injury; no acute inflammation; nonadherence index

NAIC National Association of Insurance Commissioners

NAIP National Association of Inpatient Physicians; neuronal apoptosis inhibitory protein

NAIR nonadrenergic inhibitory response

Na,K-ATPase sodium-potassium adenosine triphosphatase

NAL nonadherent leukocyte; Novell Applications Launcher

NALBOH National Association of Local Boards of Health

NALD neonatal adrenoleukodystrophy

NALT nasal-associated lymphoid tissue

NALTH National Association of Long Term Hospitals

NAM *N*-acetylmuramic acid; natural actomyosin; nucleoside analogue mutation; nucleoside-associated mutation

NAMA National Alliance of Methadone Advocates

naMCI nonamnestic mild cognitive impairment

NAMCIC National Academic Medical Center Information Consortium

NAMCR National Association of Managed Care Regulators

NAMCS National Ambulatory Medical Care Survey

NAME National Association of Medical Examiners; nevi, atrial myxoma, myxoid neurofibroma, ephelides [syndrome]

NAMH National Association for Mental Health

NAMI National Alliance for the Mentally Ill; National Alliance on Mental Illness

NAMIS Nifedipine Angina Myocardial Infarction Study

NAMN nicotinic acid mononucleotide

NAMP National Alliance for Mental Patients

NAMRU Navy Medical Reserve Unit

NAMSS National Association Medical Staff Services

NANA *N*-acetyl neuraminic acid

NANB non-A, non-B [hepatitis]

NANBH non-A, non-B hepatitis

NANBHV non-A, non-B hepatitis virus

NANBNC non-A, non-B, non-C [hepatitis virus]

NANC nonadrenergic noncholinergic

NAND non-Alzheimer neuropsychiatric disease

NANDA North American Nursing Diagnosis Association

NANN National Association of Neonatal Nurses

NANPA North Alabama Nurse Practitioner Association

NAOO National Association of Optometrists and Opticians

NAOP National Alliance for Optional Parenthood

NAP nasion, point A, pogonion [facial profile]; nerve action potential; network access point; neurotoxin-associated protein; neutrophil-activating peptide; neutrophil alkaline phosphatase; nodular adrenocortical pathology; nucleic acid phosphatase; nucleosome assembly protein

NAP-1 *Clostridium difficile* strain; North American pulsed-field gel electrophoresis type 1

NAPA *N*-acetyl-*p*-aminophenol; *N*-acetyl procainamide

NAPCA National Air Pollution Control Administration

NAPCRG North American Primary Care Research Group

NAPDP National Association of Prepaid Dental Plans

NAPE *N*-acyl-phosphatidylethanolamine

NaPG sodium pregnanediol glucuronide

NAPGCM National Association of Professional Geriatric Care Managers

NAPH naphthyl; National Association of Public Hospitals; nicotinamide adenine dinucleotide phosphate

NAPHS National Association of Psychiatric Health Systems

NAPHSIS National Association for Public Health Statistics and Information Systems

NAPHT National Association of Patients on Hemodialysis and Transplantation

NAPL nucleosome assembly protein—like

NAPM National Association of Pharmaceutical Manufacturers

NAPN National Association of Physicians' Nurses

NAPNAP National Association of Pediatric Nurse Associates and Practitioners

NAPNES National Association for Practical Nursing Education and Services

NAPP nerve agent pyridostigmine pretreatment

NAPPH National Association of Private Psychiatric Hospitals

NAPPS nerve agent pyridostigmine pretreatment set

NAPQI N-acetyl-p-benzoquinone imine

NAPS12 NLRP12-associated periodic syndrome

NAPT National Association for the Prevention of Tuberculosis

NAQAP National Association of Quality Assurance Professionals

NAR nasal airway resistance; no action required; nutrient adequacy ratio

NARA Narcotics Addict Rehabilitation Act; National Association of Recovered Alcoholics

NARAL National Abortion Rights Action League

NARC narcotic; nucleus arcuatus

NARCF National Association of Residential Care Facilities

narco narcotic, narcotic addict; drug enforcement agent

NARD National Association of Retail Druggists

NARES nonallergic rhinitis-eosinophilia syndrome

NARF National Association of Rehabilitation Facilities

NARHC National Association of Rural Health Clinics

NARIC National Rehabilitation Information Center

NARL no adverse response level

NARMA nonlinear autoregressive moving average

NARMAX nonlinear autoregressive moving average with exogenous [input]

NARMH National Association for Rural Mental Health

NARP neuropathy, ataxia, retinitis pigmentosa [syndrome]

NARS National Acupuncture Research Society

NARSAD National Alliance for Research on Schizophrenia and Depression

NARSD National Alliance for Research on Schizophrenia and Depression

NARX nonlinear autoregressive model with exogenous input

NAS Narcotics Assistance Section; nasal; National Academy of Sciences; National Association of Sanitarians; neonatal abstinence syndrome; neonatal airleak syndrome; network-attached storage; neuroallergic syndrome; neurobehavioral assessment scale [sedation scoring]; no abnormality seen; no added salt; non-*albicans* species; normalized alignment score; Normative Aging Study

NASBA nucleic acid sequence—based amplification

NASCET North American Symptomatic Carotid Endarterectomy Trial

NASCIS National Acute Spinal Cord Injury Study

NASE National Association for the Study of Epilepsy

NASEAN National Association for State Enrolled Assistant Nurses

NASH N-acryloxysuccinimide; nonalcoholic steatohepatitis

NASHS National Adolescent Student Health Survey

NaSIMM National Study of Internal Medicine Manpower

NASM Naval Aviation School of Medicine

NASMD National Association of State Medicaid Directors

NASMHPD National Association of State Mental Health Program Directors

NASN National Association of School Nurses

NAS-NRC National Academy of Science-National Research Council

NASPE North American Society for Pacing and Electrophysiology

NASPE/BPEG North American Society of Pacing and Electrophysiology—British Pacing and Electrophysiology Group

NASPHV National Association of State Public Health Veterinarians

NASS National Accident Sampling System; North American Spine Society

NASTI nonacute soft tissue injury

NASV Nasoule virus

NASW National Association of Social Workers

NAT *N*-acetyltransferase; natal; nateglinide; neonatal alloimmune thrombocytopenia; network address translation; no action taken; nonaccidental trauma; nucleic acid testing

NaT sodium tartrate

Nat native; natural

NATCO North American Transplant Coordinator Organization

Natr sodium [L. *natrium*]

NATSAL National Survey of Sexual Attitudes and Lifestyles

NAVAPAM National Association of Veterans Affairs Physician Ambulatory Care Managers

NAVEL naloxone, atropine, Valium, epinephrine, lidocaine

NAVL nerve, artery, vein, lymphatic

NAZC neutrophil azurocidin

NB nail bed; naïve Baues [algorithm]; needle biopsy; neuro-Behçet [syndrome]; neuroblastoma; neurometric battery; new Ballard [score]; newborn; nitrous oxide–barbiturate; normoblast; note well [L. *nota bene*]; nutrient broth

nb newborn; note well [L. *nota bene*]

NBA neuron-binding activity

NBAC National Bioethics Advisory Committee

NBAT neutral and basic amino acid transporter

NBC network-based computing; non-battle casualty; nuclear, biologic, chemical

NBCC National Board for Certified Counselors; nevoid basal cell carcinoma

NBCCS nevoid basal cell carcinoma syndrome

NBCIE nonbullous congenital ichthyosiform erythroderma

NBCOT National Board for Certification in Occupational Therapy

NBC-PC nuclear, biologic, chemical protective cover

NBCRS nuclear, biologic, chemical reconnaissance system

NBD neurogenic bladder dysfunction; no brain damage; nucleotide-binding domain

NBF no breastfeeding; nucleotide-binding fold

NBI neutrophil bactericidal index; no bone injury; non-battle injury

NBIC neonatal bedside interface controller

NBICU newborn intensive care unit

NBL neuroblastoma

NBM no bowel movement; normal bone marrow; normal bowel movement; nothing by mouth

nBM nucleus basalis of Meynert

nbM newborn mouse

nbMb newborn mouse brain

NBME National Board of Medical Examiners; normal bone marrow extract

NBMPR nitrobenzylmercaptopurine riboside

NBMPR-P nitrobenzylmercaptopurine riboside phosphate

NBN newborn nursery

NBNA National Black Nurses Association

NBO non-bed occupancy

NBOME National Board of Osteopathic Medical Examiners

NBP needle biopsy of prostate; neoplastic brachial plexopathy; no bone pathology; nonbacterial prostatitis; nucleic acid binding protein

NBPME National Board of Podiatric Medical Examiners

NBRC National Board for Respiratory Care

NBRS Neurobiologic Risk Scale

NBRT National Board for Respiratory Therapy

NBS *N*-bromosuccinimide; National Bureau of Standards; neuroblastoma suppressor; nevoid basal cell carcinoma syndrome; newborn bovine serum; Nijmegen breakage syndrome; no bacteria seen; normal blood serum; normal bowel sounds; normal brain stem; nystagmus blockage syndrome

NBSS National Breast Screening Study

NBT Nature-Based Therapy; nitroblue tetrazolium; non–tumor bearing; normal breast tissue

NBTE nonbacterial thrombotic endocarditis

NBTNF newborn, term, normal, female

NBTNM newborn, term, normal, male

NBT PABA *N*-benzoyl-L-tyrosyl paraaminobenzoic acid

NBTS National Blood Transfusion Service

n-Bu n-butyl

NBV Nelson Bay orthoreovirus

NBW normal birth weight

NC continuous nebulization; nasal cannula; nasal clearance; natural cytotoxicity; near card; neck complaint; neonatal cholestasis; nephrocalcinosis; nerve conduction; neural crest; neurocysticercosis; neurologic check; nevus comedonicus; night call; nitrocellulose; no casualty; no change; no charge; no complaints; noise criterion; noncardiac; noncirrhotic; noncontributory; normal cell; normal control [group]; normocephalic; normocytoplasmic; nose clamp; nose cone; not calculated; not completed; not cultured; nucleocapsid; nucleocytoplasmic; nurse counselor; nursing coordinator

N:C, N/C nuclear/cytoplasmic ratio
nC nanocoulomb
nc nanocurie; not counted
NCA National Certification Agency; National Credentialing Agency [for Laboratory Personnel]; neurocirculatory asthenia; neutrophil chemotactic activity; nodulocystic acne; noncompartmental analysis; noncontractile area; nonspecific cross-reacting antigen; nuclear cerebral angiogram
NCa normal calcium
n-CAD negative coronoradiographic documentation
NCADD National Council on Alcoholism and Drug Dependence
NCADI National Clearinghouse for Alcohol and Drug Information
NCAE National Council for Alcohol Education
NC-AFM non−contact mode atomic force microscopy
NCAH National Commission on Allied Health
NCAI National Coalition for Adult Immunization
NCAL National Center for Assisted Living
NCAM neural cell adhesion molecule
NCAMI National Committee Against Mental Illness
NCAMLP National Certification Agency for Medical Laboratory Personnel
NcAMP nephrogenous cyclic adenosine monophosphate
N-CAP Nifedipine Gastrointestinal Therapeutic System Circadian Anti-Ischemic Program
NC/AT normal cephalic atraumatic
NCATS National Center for Advancing Translational Sciences; Nursing Child Assessment Teaching Scale
NCAUR National Center for Agricultural Utilization Research
NCBA National Caucus and Center on Black Aging
NCBF noncovalent bond finder
NCBI National Center for Biotechnology Information
NCBTMB National Certification Board for Therapeutic Massage & Bodywork
NCC National Certification Corporation; neural crest cells; New Computational Challenges Program; noncoronary cusp; nursing care continuity
ncc noncoronary cusp
NCCAM National Center for Complementary and Alternative Medicine
NCCAOM National Certification Commission for Acupuncture and Oriental Medicine

NCCBH National Council for Community Behavioral Healthcare
NCCDC National Center for Chronic Disease Control
NCCDPHP National Center for Chronic Disease Prevention and Health Promotion
NCCEA Neurosensory Center Comprehensive Examination for Aphasia
NCCH National Council of Community Hospitals
NCCHC National Commission on Correctional Health Care
NCCIP National Center for Clinical Infant Program
NCCL noncarious cervical lesions
NCCLS National Committee for Clinical Laboratory Standards
NCCLVP National Coordinating Committee on Large-Volume Parenterals
NCCMERP National Coordinating Council for Medication Error Reporting and Prevention
NCCMHC National Council for Community Mental Health Centers
NCCMP noncompaction cardiomyopathy
NCCN National Comprehensive Cancer Network
NCCP noncardiac chest pain
NCCPA National Commission on Certification of Physician Assistants
NCCPC-R Noncommunicating Children's Pain Checklist-Revised
NCCRA National Colorectal Cancer Research Alliance
NCCS National Coalition for Cancer Survivorship
NCCT National Center for Competency Testing; noncontrast computed tomography
NCCTG North Central Cancer Treatment Group
NCCU newborn convalescent care unit
NCD National Commission on Diabetes; neurocirculatory dystonia; neurocognitive disorder; nitrogen clearance delay; noncommunicable disease; normal childhood disorder; not considered disabling
NCDA National Council on Drug Abuse
ncDCIS noncomedo-type ductal carcinoma in situ
NCDS National Child Development Study
NCDV Nebraska calf diarrhea virus
NCE Na^+/Ca^{2+} exchange; negative contrast echocardiography; new chemical entity; nonconvulsive epilepsy; normochromatic erythrocyte
NCEH National Center for Environmental Health

NCEP National Center for Environmental Protection; National Cholesterol Education Program

NCEPOD National Confidential Enquiry into Peri-Operative Deaths [study]

NCES National Childhood Encephalopathy Study; Netherlands Cost-Effectiveness Study

NCF neutrophil chemotactic factor; Nurses Christian Fellowship

NCFA Narcolepsy and Catalepsy Foundation of America

NCF(C) neutrophil chemotactic factor (complement)

NCG nanochannel glass

NCH National Claims History; nursing care hours

NCHA National Community Hearing Association

NCHC National Coalition on Health Care; National Council of Health Centers

NCHCA National Commission for Health Certifying Agencies

NCHCT National Center for Health Care Technology; noncontrast helical computed tomography

NCHD National Claims History Database

NCHECR National Centre in HIV Epidemiology and Clinical Research

NCHGR National Center for Human Genome Research [now National Human Genome Research Institute]

NCHLS National Council of Health Laboratory Services

NCHPD National Council on Health Planning and Development

NCHS National Center for Health Statistics

NCHSR National Center for Health Services Research

NCHSTE National Consortium on Health Science and Technology Education

NCI National Cancer Institute; noncriterion ischemic [animal]; nuclear contour index; nursing care integration

nCi nanocurie

NCIB National Collection of Industrial Bacteria

NCIC National Cancer Institute of Canada

NCIC CTG National Cancer Institute of Canada Clinical Trial Group

NCID National Center for Infectious Diseases

NCI DIS 2D National Cancer Institute Drug Information System for Two-Dimensional Substructure Searching

NCIH National Council for International Health

NCIHC National Council on Interpreting in Health Care

NCIMB National Collection of Industrial and Marine Bacteria

NCIPC National Center for Injury Prevention and Control

NCIRS National Cancer Incidence Reporting System; National Centre for Immunisation Research and Surveillance

NC-IUB Nomenclature Committee of the International Union of Biochemistry

NC-IUBMB Nomenclature Committee of the International Union of Biochemistry and Molecular Biology

NCJ needle catheter jejunostomy

NCKHEkg note chemistry and hematology, laboratory values, and electrocardiographic findings

NCL neuronal ceroid-lipofuscinosis; noncoronary leaflet; nucleolin

NCLEX-RN National Council Licensure Examination for Registered Nurses

NCM nailfold capillary microscopy; nurse case manager

N/cm^2 newtons per square centimeter

NCMC natural cell-mediated cytotoxicity

NCMH National Committee for Mental Health

NCMHI National Clearinghouse for Mental Health Information

NCMI National Committee Against Mental Illness

NCN National Cardiovascular Network; National Council of Nurses

NCNPC Northern Colorado Nurse Practitioner Coalition

NCNR National Center for Nursing Research

NCOA National Council on Aging

NCO/CIC National Coordinating Office for Computing, Information, and Communication

NCoR, N-CoR nuclear receptor compressor

NCoV novel coronavirus

2019-nCoV 2019 novel coronavirus [initial name for SARS-CoV-2]

NCP neurocybernetic prosthesis; Nijmegen Classification of Pain; noncollagen protein

NCPA National Community Pharmacists Association

N-CPAP, n-CPAP nasal continuous positive airway pressure

NCPDP National Council for Prescription Drug Programs

NCPE noncardiac pulmonary edema

NCPF National Collection of Pathogenic Fungi; noncirrhotic portal fibrosis

NCPH noncirrhotic portal hypertension

NCPI National Clearinghouse for Primary Care Information

NCPIE National Council on Patient Information and Education

NCPIM National Commission to Prevent Infant Mortality

NCPP National Collaborative Perinatal Project

NCPPB National Collection of Plant Pathogenic Bacteria

NCQA National Committee for Quality Assurance

NCR National Research Council; neutrophil chemotactic response; no carbon required; noncoding region; normotensive control rat; nuclear/cytoplasmic ratio

NCRND National Committee for Research in Neurological Diseases

NCRP National Council on Radiation Protection and Measurements

NCRR National Center for Research Resources

NCRSP National Congenital Rubella Surveillance Programme

NCRV National Committee for Radiation Victims

NCS National Collaborative Study; neocarcinostatin; nerve conduction study; neurocutaneous syndrome; newborn calf serum; no concentrated sweets; noncircumferential stenosis; noncoronary sinus; nystagmus compensation syndrome

NCSA National Center for Supercomputing Applications; National Computational Science Alliance

NCSBN National Council of State Boards of Nursing

NCSE nonconvulsive status epilepticus

NCSI number of combined spherical irradiation

NCSN National Certified School Nurse; National Council for School Nurses

NCT neural crest tumor

NCTC National Cancer Tissue Culture; National Collection of Type Cultures

NCTR National Center for Toxicological Research

NCV nerve conduction velocity; noncholera vibrio

NCVHS National Committee on Vital and Health Statistics

NCVIA National Childhood Vaccine Injury Act

NCVS nerve conduction velocity study

NCX sodium-calcium exchanger

NCYC National Collection of Yeast Cultures

ND Doctor of Naturopathy; nasal deformity; natural death; Naval Dispensary; neonatal death; neoplastic disease; neurologic deficit; neuropsychologic deficit; neurotic depression; neutral density; new drug; Newcastle disease; newly dead; nocturnal dip; no data; no disease; nondetectable; nondiabetic; nondiagnostic; nondisabling; normal delivery; normal development; Norrie disease; nose drops; not detected, not determined; not diagnosed; not done; nurse's diagnosis; nutritionally deprived

N/D no defects; not done

N&D nodular and diffuse

N$_D$, n$_D$ refractive index

Nd neodymium

n$_D$ refractive index

NDA National Dental Association; New Drug Application; no data available; no detectable activity; no detectable antibody

NDAC no data accepted

NDATUS National Drug and Alcoholism Treatment Unit Survey

NDBA N-nitrosodibutylamine

NDC National Data Communications; national drug classification; National Drug Code; National Drug Council; Naval Dental Clinic; nicotine dependence center; nondifferentiated cell

NDCD National Drug Code Directory

NDCG Nursing Development Conference Group

NDD no dialysis days

NDDIC National Digestive Diseases Information Clearinghouse

NDDG National Diabetes Data Group

NDE near-death experience; nondestructive evaluation; nondiabetic extremity

NDEC nursing diagnosis extension and classification

NDEKF node-decoupled extended Kalman filtering

NDEV Ndelle virus

NDF neutrophil diffraction factor; new dosage form; no diagnostic findings; no disease found

NDFDA nonadecafluoro-n-decanoic acid

NDGA nordihydroguaiaretic acid

NDHPCCB nondihydropyridine calcium channel blocker

NDHS National Diet-Heart Study

NDI nephrogenic diabetes insipidus

NDIC National Diabetes Information Clearinghouse

NDIR nondispersive infrared analyzer

NDL nipple ductal lavage

NDM naturalistic decision making

NDMA nitrosodimethylamine

NDMR nondepolarizing muscle relaxant

nDNA nuclear deoxyribonucleic acid

NDNQI National Database of Nursing Quality Indicators

NDP net dietary protein; nucleoside diphosphate

NDPK nucleoside diphosphate kinase

NDPKA nucleoside diphosphate kinase A

NDPKB nucleoside diphosphate kinase B

NDR neonatal death rate; normal detrusor reflex

NDRC National Defense Research Committee

NDRF NeuroD-related factor; neutrophil-derived relaxing factor

NDRI National Disease Research Interchange

NDS Naval Dental School; neurologic deficit score; new drug submission; normal dog serum; Novell Directory Services

NDSB Narcotic Drugs Supervisory Board

NDSSC National Dietary Survey of School Children

NDST *N*-deacetylase *N*-sulfotransferase

NDT neurodevelopmental treatment; noise detection threshold; nondestructive test, nondestructive testing

NDTI National Disease and Therapeutic Index

NDTM National Database of Telemedicine

NDUV Ndumu virus

NDV Newcastle disease virus; Nyando virus

NDVI normalized difference vegetation index

Nd/YAG, Nd-YAG neodymium-yttrium-aluminum garnet

NE national emergency; nausea and emesis; necrotic enteritis; necrotizing enterocolitis; neonatal encephalopathy; nephropathia epidemica; nerve ending; nerve excitation; neuroendocrine; neuroendocrinology; neuroepithelium; neurologic examination; neutropenic enterocolitis; neutrophil elastase; niacin equivalent; no effect; no excision; no excitation; no exposure; nocturnal exacerbation; nonelastic; nonendogenous; noninvasive evaluation; norepinephrine; not elevated; not enlarged; not equal; not evaluated; not examined; not exposed; nuclear extract; nurse executive; nutcracker esophagus

Ne neon

NEA neoplasm embryonic antigen; no evidence of abnormality

NEA-BC Nurse Executive Advanced-Board Certified

NEAR National Emergency Airway Registry

NEAS nonerythroid alpha spectrin

NEAT Neurohumoral Effects in Acute Myocardial Infarction of Trandolapril [study]; nonexercise activity thermogenesis

NEB nebulin; neuroendocrine body; neuroepithelial body

NE-BC Nurse Executive−Board Certified

NEC National Electrical Code; necrotizing enterocolitis; neuroendocrine cell; neuroendocrine convertase; no essential changes; non-effect concentration; nonesterified cholesterol; not elsewhere classified or classifiable; nursing ethics committee

NECHI Northeastern Consortium for Health Information

NECR noise-effective count rate

NECT nonenhanced computed tomography

NED no-effect dose; no evidence of disease; no expiration date; normal equivalent deviation

NEDEL no epidemiologically detectable exposure level

NEDSS National Electronic Disease Surveillance System

NEDV North End virus

NEE needle electrode examination

NEEE Near East equine encephalomyelitis

NEEM negative effect erasing method

NEEP negative end-expiratory pressure

NEET Nordic Enalapril Exercise Trial

NEF, NeF nephritic factor

NEFA nonesterified fatty acid

NEFH heavy polypeptide of neurofilament protein

NEFL light polypeptide of neurofilament protein

NEFM medium polypeptide of neurofilament protein

neg negative

NEGF neurite growth-promoting factor

NEHA National Environmental Health Association

NEHE Nurses for Environmental Health Education

NEHEP National Eye Health Education Program

NEI National Eye Institute

NEISS National Electronic Injury Surveillance System

NEISS-AIP National Electronic Injury Surveillance System-All Injury Program

NEJ neuroeffector junction

NEJM *New England Journal of Medicine*

NEL non-effect level; no evidence of leukemia

NeLH National Electronic Library for Health

NEM nemaline; *N*-ethylmaleimide; no evidence of malignancy

nem nutritional milk unit [Ger. *Nahrungs Einheit Milch*]

NEMA National Eclectic Medical Association

nema nematode

NEMAS Nursing Education Modular Authoring System

NEMC-PCR New England Medical Center Posterior Circulation Registry

NEMD nonspecific esophageal motor dysfunction

NEMS nine equivalents of nursing manpower use score

Neo neomycin; neoplasm or neoplastic

neo neoarsphenamine

NEP needle exchange program; negative expiratory pressure; nephrology; neutral endopeptidase; no evidence of pathology

nep nephrectomy

NEPA National Environmental Policy Act

Neph nephron; nephritis; nephrosis

NEPHGE nonequilibrated pH gradient electrophoresis

NEPV Nepuyo virus

NEQ noise equivalent quantum

NEQAS National External Quality Assessment Scheme

NERHL Northeastern Radiological Health Laboratory

NER no evidence of recurrence; nucleotide excision repair

ner nervous

NERD no evidence of recurrent disease; nonerosive reflux disease

NERO noninvasive evaluation of radiation output

NERSC National Energy Research Scientific Computing Center

NES night eating syndrome; not elsewhere specified

NESH Network for Ecosystem Sustainability and Health

NESO Northeastern Society of Orthodontists

NESP novel erythrocyte stimulating protein; Nurse Education Support Program

NEST nonsurgical embryonic selective thinning; Nuclear Emergency Search Team

NET nasoendotracheal tube; nerve excitability test; neuroectodermal tumor; neuroemotional technique; neuroendocrine tumor; norepinephrine transporter

NETI nasotracheal endotracheal intubation

NETRHA North-East Thames Regional Health Authority [study]

NETS National Eye Trauma System; Network for Employers for Traffic Safety

NETT National Emphysema Treatment Trial

NETV Netivot virus

NEU, Neu neuraminidase

neu neurilemma

NeuN neuronal nucleus

neur, neuro, neurol neurology, neurologic, neurologist

neuropath neuropathology

neut neuter, neutral; neutrophil

NEVADA Numerical Evaluation of Variance and Dependence Simulation

NEWDILTIL New Diltiazem vs. Tildiem [study]

NEX number of excitations

NEXT New European XT Stent Registry

NEXUS National Emergency X-Radiography Utilization Study

NEY neomycin egg yolk [agar]

NEYA neomycin egg yolk agar

NF nafcillin; National Formulary; nephritic factor; neurofibromatosis; neurofilament; neutral fraction; neutrophilic factor; noise factor; normal flow; not filtered; not found; nuclear factor; nucleolar frequency [number of nucleoli per 100 nuclei]

nF nanofarad

NF1 neurofibromatosis type I; neurofibromin gene; nuclear factor 1

NF2 neurofibromatosis type II

NFA National Fire Academy; near-fatal asthma; nuclear factor A

NFAIS National Federation of Advanced Information Services

NFAR no further action required

N-FAS neurogenic fetal akinesia sequence

NFAT, NF-AT nuclear factor of activated T [cells]

NFATp preexisting subunit of nuclear factor of activated T [cells]

NFB National Federation of the Blind; National Foundation for the Blind; nonfermenting bacteria

NFBM normalized fractional brownian motion

NFC National Fertility Center

NFCE near-fatal choking episode

NFCS Nationwide Food Consumption Survey

NFD neurofibrillary degeneration

NFDR neuro-facio-digito-renal [syndrome]

NFE nonferrous extract

NFG normal fasting glucose

NFH heavy polypeptide of neurofilament protein; nonfamilial hematuria

NFHD no fetal heart disease

NFI near field imaging

NFIC National Foundation for Ileitis and Colitis

NFID National Foundation for Infectious Diseases

NFIRS National Fire Incident Reporting System

NFJ Naegeli-Franceschetti-Jadassohn [syndrome]

NFK nuclear factor kappa

NFKB, NF-kB, NF-κB nuclear factor kappa B [of pre−B cell]

NFL nerve fiber layer; neurofilament protein, light polypeptide

NFLD nerve fiber layer defect

NFLPN National Federation of Licensed Practical Nurses

NFM neurofilament protein, medium polypeptide

NFMA nonfunctioning pituitary macroadenoma

NFMD National Foundation for Muscular Dystrophy

NFNA National Flight Nurses Association

NFND National Foundation for Neuromuscular Diseases

NFNID National Foundation for Non-Invasive Diagnostics

NFNS, NF-NS neurofibromatosis-Noonan syndrome

NFP natural family planning; no family physician; not for profit; nurse-family partnership

NFRCD Newfoundland rod-cone dystrophy

NFS National Fertility Study; network file system; neural foraminal stenosis; no fracture seen

NFT neurofibrillary tangle; no further treatment

NFTD normal full-term delivery

NFTT neurogenic failure to thrive

NFV nelfinavir

NFW nursed fairly well

NFX nuclear factor X

NG nasogastric; *Neisseria gonorrhoeae*; neoplastic growth; new growth; nitroglycerin; nodose ganglion; no growth; not given

N/G nasogastric

Ng *Neisseria gonorrhoeae*

ng nanogram

NGA nutrient gelatin agar

NGAL neutrophil gelatinase-associated lipocalin

NGAST Nimodipine German-Austrian Stroke Trial

NGAV Ngaingan virus

NGBE neuraminidase/beta-galactosidase expression

NGC National Guidelines Clearinghouse; nerve guidance conduit; nucleus reticularis gigantocellularis

NgCAM neuron glial cell adhesion molecule

NGF nerve growth factor

NGFA nerve growth factor alpha

NGFB nerve growth factor beta

NGFG nerve growth factor gamma

NGFIA nerve growth factor−induced clone A

NGFIC nerve growth factor−induced clone C

NGFR nerve growth factor receptor

NGGR nonglucogenic/glucogenic ratio

NGI nuclear globulin inclusion

NGL neutral glycolipid

ng/mL nanograms per milliliter

NGNA National Gerontological Nursing Association

NGO nongovernmental organization

NGOV Ngoupe virus

NGPA nursing grade point average

NGR narrow gauze roll; nasogastric replacement

NGS next-generation software; normal goat serum

NGSA nerve growth−stimulating activity

NGSF nongenital skin fibroblast

NGT nasogastric tube; nominal group technique; normal glucose tolerance

NGU nongonococcal urethritis

NGVL National Gene Vector Laboratories

NH natriuretic hormone; Naval Hospital; neonatal hemochromatosis; neonatal hepatitis; neurologically handicapped; nocturnal hypoventilation; node of His; nonhuman; nursing home

N(H) proton density

NHA National Health Association; National Healthcareer Association; nonspecific hepatocellular abnormality; nursing home administrator

NHAAP National Heart Attack Alert Program

NHAMCS National Hospital Ambulatory Medical Care Survey

NHANES National Health and Nutrition Examination Survey

NHB National Health Board

NHBCD non−heart-beating cadaver donor

NHBE normal human bronchial epithelial [cell]

NHBPCC National High Blood Pressure Coordinating Committee

NHBPEP National High Blood Pressure Education Program

NHC National Health Council; neighborhood health center; neonatal hypocalcemia; nonhistone chromosomal [protein]; nursing home care

NHCMQ multistate nursing home case mix and quality

NHCP nonhistone chromosomal protein

NHCS National Health Care Survey

NHD non-Hodgkin disease; normal hair distribution
NHDC National Hansen's Disease Center
NHDF neonatal human dermal fibroblast; normal human diploid fibroblast
NHDL non−high-density lipoprotein
NHDS National Health Data System; National Hospital Discharge Survey
NHE National Health Expenditure; nonhemolytic enterotoxin; sodium-hydrogen exchanger
NHE 1 to 6 sodium-hydrogen exchangers, isoforms 1 to 6
NHEFS National Epidemiologic Follow-up Study
NHES National Health Examination Survey
NHF National Health Federation; National Heart Foundation; National Hemophilia Foundation; nonimmune hydrops fetalis; normal human fibroblast
NHG normal human globulin
NHGB net hepatic glucose balance
NHGJ normal human gastric juice
NHGRI National Human Genome Research Institute
NHH neurohypophyseal hormone
NHHCS National Home and Hospice Care Survey
NHI National Heart Institute; nuclear hepatobiliary imaging
NHIC National Health Information Council [Canada]
NHIF National Head Injury Foundation
NHIS National Health Interview Survey
NHIS-YRB National Health Interview Survey−Your Risk Behavior
NHK normal human kidney
NHL nodular histiocytic lymphoma; non-Hodgkin lymphoma
NHLA National Health Lawyers Association
NHLBI National Heart, Lung, and Blood Institute
NHLBI-ICD National Heart, Lung and Blood Institute Implantable Cardioverter Defibrillator [trial]
NHLBI II National Heart, Lung and Blood Institute Type II [study]
NHLBI-PTCA National Heart, Lung, and Blood Institute Percutaneous Transluminal Coronary Angioplasty [registry]
NHLBITS National Heart, Lung, and Blood Institute Twin Study
NHLI National Heart and Lung Institute
NHML non-Hodgkin malignant lymphoma
NHMRC National Health and Medical Research Council
NHP National Hypertension Project; nonhemoglobin protein; nonhistone protein;

normal human pooled plasma; Nottingham Health Profile; nursing home placement
NHPC National Health Planning Council
NHPCO National Hospice and Palliative Care Organization
NHPF National Health Policy Forum
NHPIC National Health Planning Information Center
NHPP nonhomogeneous poison processes
NHPPD nursing hours per patient-day
NHPPN National Health Professions Placement Network
NHQRA Nursing Home Quality Reform Act
NHR net histocompatibility ratio
NHRA Nursing Home Reform Act
NHRC National Health Research Center
NHS Nance-Horan syndrome; Nasu-Hakola syndrome; National Health Service; National Hospice Study; natural history; normal horse serum; normal human serum; Nurses' Health Study
NHS-1 First Natural History Study
NHS-2 Second Natural History Study
NHSAS National Health Service Audit Staff
NHSC National Health Service Corps
NHS CCC National Health Service Centre for Coding and Classification
NHSIA National Health Service Information Authority
NHSR National Hospital Service Reserve
NHSTD National Health Service Training Division
NHT nonpenetrating head trauma; Nurses for a Healthier Tomorrow
NHTSA National Highway Traffic Safety Administration
NHVR normalized hepatic vascular resistance
NI neuraminidase inhibition; neurologic improvement; neutralization index; no information; noise index; noninducible; not identified; not isolated; nucleus intercalatus; nursing informatics
NIA National Institute on Aging; nephelometric inhibition assay; neuroleptic-induced akathisia; niacin; no information available; Nutritional Institute of America
nia niacin
NIAAA National Institute on Alcohol Abuse and Alcoholism
NIADDK National Institute of Arthritis, Diabetes, Digestive, and Kidney Diseases
NIAID National Institute of Allergy and Infectious Diseases
NIAMDD National Institute of Arthritis, Metabolism, and Digestive Diseases

NIAMS National Institute of Arthritis and Musculoskeletal and Skin Diseases

NIAP National Information Assurance Partnership

NIB National Institute for the Blind

NIBIB National Institute of Biomedical Imaging and Bioengineering

NIBP noninvasive blood pressure

NIBSC National Institute for Biological Standards and Control

NIC National Influenza Center; National Informatics Centre; neonatal intensive care; network interface card; neurogenic intermittent claudication; neurointensive care; newborn intensive care; nursing interim care; nursing interventions classification

NICD National Information Center on Deafness

NICE National Institute for Health and Clinical Excellence

NICHCY National Dissemination Center for Children with Disabilities; National Information Center for Children and Youth with Disabilities

NIC-HFH Nephrology Information Center at Henry Ford Hospital

NICHHD National Institute of Child Health and Human Development

NICHSR National Center on Health Services Research; National Information Center on Health Services Research and Health Care Technology

NICOLE Nisoldipine in Coronary Artery Disease in Leuven

NICS nebulized inhaled corticosteroid

NICT new information and communication technology

NICU neonatal intensive care unit; neurointensive care unit; neurologic intensive care unit; neurosurgical intensive care unit; nonimmunologic contact urticaria

NID national immunization day; nidogen; no identifiable disease; nonimmunologic disease; not in distress; number of intervals to fulfill detection

NIDA National Institute on Drug Abuse

NIDCD National Institute on Deafness and Other Communication Disorders

NIDCR National Institute of Dental and Craniofacial Research

NIDD non–insulin-dependent diabetes

NIDDK National Institute of Diabetes and Digestive and Kidney Diseases

NIDDM non–insulin-dependent diabetes mellitus

NIDDY non–insulin-dependent diabetes in the young

NIDM National Institute for Disaster Mobilization

NIDR National Institute of Dental Research

NIDRR National Institute on Disability and Rehabilitation Research

NIDS nonionic detergent soluble

NIDSEC Nursing Information and Data Set Evaluation Center

NIEHS National Institutes of Environmental Health Sciences

NIEPS noninvasive electrophysiological study

NIF negative inspiratory force; neutrophil immobilizing factor; nonintestinal fibroblast

Nig non-immunoglobulin

nig black [L. *niger*]

NIGMS National Institute of General Medical Sciences

NIH National Institutes of Health; neointimal hyperplasia

NIHAS Northern Ireland Health and Activity Survey

NIHL noise-induced hearing loss

Ni-Hon-San Nipponese in Honolulu and San Francisco [dataset]

NIHR National Institute for Health Research

NIHS National Institute of Hypertension Studies

NIH-SS National Institutes of Health Stroke Scale

NII National Information Infrastructure; National Insurance Institute

NIIC National Injury Information Clearinghouse

NII-HIN National Information Infrastructure-Health Information Network

NIIS National Institute of Infant Services

NIL noise interference level

NILT Nursing Intervention Lexicon and Taxonomy

NIMBY not in my backyard

N-IMF nipple–inframammary fold distance

NIMH National Institute of Mental Health

NIMP National Intern Matching Program

NIMR National Institute for Medical Research

NIMS National Infant Mortality Surveillance

NINCDS National Institute of Neurological and Communicative Disorders and Stroke

NINCDS/ADRDA National Institute of Neurological and Communicative Diseases and Stroke/Alzheimer's Disease and Related Disorders Association

NINDB National Institute of Neurological Diseases and Blindness

NINDS National Institute of Neurological Disorders and Stroke

NINDS-TPAST National Institute of Neurological Disorders and Stroke-Tissue Plasminogen Activator Stroke Trial

NIOSH National Institute for Occupational Safety and Health

NIOSHTIC National Institute for Occupational Safety and Health Technical Information Center

NIP National Immunization Program; negative inspiratory pressure; nipple; no infection present; no inflammation present; nonimmigrant patient

NIP AAm *N*-isopropylacrylamide

NIPALS nonlinear iterative partial least square

NIPH National Institute of Public Health

NIPPV noninvasive positive pressure ventilation

NIPS neuroleptic-induced Parkinson syndrome; noninvasive programmed stimulation

NIPTS noise-induced permanent threshold shift

NIR near infrared; New Intravascular Rigid Stent Trial

nIR non−insulin resistance

NIRA nitrite reductase; Nursing Incentives Reimbursement Award

NIRB non-institutional review board

NIRCA nonisotopic ribonuclease cleavage assay

NIRD nonimmune renal disease

NIRF near-infrared fluorescent

NIRMP National Intern and Resident Matching Program

NIRNS National Institute for Research in Nuclear Science

NIRS near-infrared spectroscopy; normal inactivated rabbit serum

NIRVANA NIR Primo Stent Vascular Advanced North America [trial]

NIS National Immunization Survey; nationwide inpatient sample; near-infrared intracranial spectroscopy; network information system; *N*-iodosuccinimide; no inflammatory signs; nursing information system

NI-SIG nursing informatics special interest group

NISO National Information Standards Organization

NISSO Netherlands Institute for Social Sexological Research

NIST National Institute of Standards and Technology

NIT National Intelligence Test; Nutrition Intervention Trial

nit nitrous

NITA National Telecommunications and Information Administration

NITD non−insulin-treated disease

nitro nitroglycerin

NIV nodule-inducing virus; noninvasive ventilation

NIW nursing intensity weights

NIWG Nursing Informatics Workshop Group

NJ nasojejunal; neighbor joining

nJ nanojoule

NFJS Naegeli-Franceschetti-Jadassohn syndrome

NJLV Naranjal virus

NJPC National Joint Practice Commission

NK Commission on Anatomical Nomenclature [Ger. *Nomenklatur Kommission*]; natural killer [cell]; neurokinin; not known

n/k not known

NK2 neurokinin 2

NKA neurokinin A; no known allergies

nkat nanokatal

NKB neurokinin B

NKC nonketotic coma; Northwest Kidney Centers

NKCA natural killer cell activity

NKCF natural killer cytotoxic factor

NKDA no known disabilities; no known drug allergies; nonketotic diabetic acidosis

NKE sodium $[Na^+]$/potassium $[K^+]$ exchange

NKF National Kidney Foundation

NKFA no known food allergies

NKF-KDOQ National Kidney Foundation Kidney Disease Outcomes Quality Initiative

NKH nonketogenic hyperglycemia; nonketotic hyperosmotic

NKHA nonketotic hyperosmolar acidosis

NKHS nonketotic hyperosmolar syndrome; normal Krebs-Henseleit solution

NKMA no known medication allergies

NKN neurokinin

NKNA neurokinin A

NKNAR neurokinin A receptor

NKNB neurokinin B

NKOV Nkolbisson virus

NKP North Karelia Project

NKSF natural killer cell stimulatory factor

NKTR natural killer−triggering receptor

NL natural language; neural lobe; neutral lipid; no direct link; nodular lymphoma; normal; normal libido; normal limits

nL nanoliter

nl normal

NLA National Leukemia Association; neuroleptoanesthesia; normal lactase activity

nLAG nuclear localized β-galactosidase

NLANR National Laboratory for Applied Network Research

NLB needle liver biopsy

NLD nasolacrimal duct; necrobiosis lipoidica diabeticorum

NLDL normal low-density lipoprotein

NLDO nasolacrimal duct obstruction

NLE neonatal lupus erythematosus

Nle norleucine

NLEA Nutrition Labeling and Education Act

NLF nasolabial fold; neonatal lung fibroblast; nonlactose fermentation

NLG natural language generation

NLH National Library for Health; nodular lymphoid hyperplasia

NLK neuroleukin

NLL nonlymphoblastic leukemia

NLLS nonlinear least squares

NLM National Library of Medicine; noise level monitor

NLMC nocturnal leg muscle cramp

NLMS National Longitudinal Mortality Study

nLMS normalized least mean square

NLN National League for Nursing; no longer needed

NLNE National League for Nursing Education

NLP natural language processing; neurolinguistic programming; no light perception; nodular liquefying panniculitis; normal light perception; normal luteal phase

NLR nucleotide oligomerization domain (NOD)-like receptor

NLRA National Leukemia Research Association

NLS Names Learning Test; National Longitudinal Surveys; neonatal lupus syndrome; Neu-Laxova syndrome; nonlinear least squares; normal lymphocyte supernatant; nuclear localization signal

NLSC National Longitudinal Survey of Children

NLSCY National Longitudinal Survey of Children and Youth

NLSQ nonlinear least square

NLT normal lymphocyte transfer; not later than; not less than; novel liver-specific transporter protein; nucleus lateralis tuberis

nlt not later than; not less than

NLTCS National Long-Term Care Survey

NL2SOL nonlinear least square algorithm

NLUS natural language understanding system

NLX naloxone; nephrolithiasis, X-linked

NM near miss; neomycin; neuromedical; neuromedin; neuromuscular; neuronal microdysgenesis; neuronal mode; neutrophil migration; nictitating membrane; nitrogen mustard; nocturnal myoclonus; nodular melanoma; nodules with microcalcifications; nonmotile; normetanephrine; not malignant; not measurable, not measured; not mentioned; not motile; nuclear medicine; nurse manager; nurse/midwife

N-m newton-meter

N&M nerves and muscles; night and morning

N/m newtons per meter

N × m newton meters

N/m² newtons per square meter

nM nanomolar

nm nanometer; night and morning [L. *nocte et mane*]

NMA National Malaria Association; National Medical Association; neurogenic muscular atrophy; *N*-nitroso-*N*-methylalanine

nMA nondominant motor area

NMAC National Medical Audiovisual Center

NM(ASCP) Technologist in Nuclear Medicine certified by the American Society of Clinical Pathologists

NMB neuromedin B; neuromuscular blockade; neuromuscular blocking; neuromuscular blocker/blocking

NMBA neuromuscular blocking agent

NMBR neuromedin B receptor

NMC National Medical Care; Naval Medical Center; neuromuscular control; nonmotor condition; nucleus reticularis magnocellularis

NMCC nasal mucociliary clearance

NMCES National Medical Care Expenditure Survey

NMCUES National Medical Care Utilization and Expenditure Survey

NMD neuromyodysplasia; neuronal migration disorder; nitroglycerin-mediated dilation

NMDA *N*-methyl-D-aspartate

NMDAR *N*-methyl-D-aspartate receptor

NmDG *N*-methyl-D-glutamine

NMDS Nursing Minimum Data Set

NMDSN Nursing Minimum Data Set for the Netherlands

NME National Medical Enterprises; neuromyeloencephalopathy; new molecular entity

NMEP neurogenic motor evoked potential

NMES National Medical Expenditure Survey; neuromuscular electrical stimulation

NMF *N*-methylformamide; National Medical Fellowships; National Migraine Foundation; nonmigrating fraction

NMFF Northwestern Medical Faculty Foundation

NMFI National Master Facility Inventory

NMHCA National Mental Health Consumers Association

NMI no mental illness; normal male infant

NMIBC non–muscle invasive bladder cancer

NMIHS National Maternal and Infant Health Survey

NMIN New Mexico Institute of Neuroimaging

NMIS nursing management information system

NMJ neuromuscular junction

NML nodular mixed lymphoma

NMM nodular malignant melanoma

NMMDS nursing management minimum dataset

NMN nicotinamide mononucleotide; normetanephrine

NMNRU National Medical Neuropsychiatric Research Unit

nmol nanomole

nmol/L nanomoles per liter

NMOR nemadione oxidoreductase; *N*-nitrosomorpholine

NMOS N-type metal oxide semiconductor

NMOSD neuromyelitis optica spectrum disorder

NMP normal menstrual period; nuclear matrix protein; nucleoside monophosphate

NMPC nonlinear model predictive control

NMPCA nonmetric principal component analysis

NMPTP *N*-methyl-4-phenyl-1,2,3,6-tetrahydropyridine

NMR national medical resources; neonatal mortality rate; nictitating membrane response; nuclear magnetic resonance

NMRC NeuroMuscular Research Center

NMRD nuclear magnetic relaxation dispersion

NMRDC Naval Medical Research and Development Command

NMRI Naval Medical Research Institute; nuclear magnetic resonance imaging

NMRL Naval Medical Research Laboratory

NMRS nuclear magnetic resonance spectroscopy

NMRU Naval Medical Research Unit

NMS Naval Medical School; neuroleptic malignant syndrome; neuromuscular spindle; *N*-methylscopolamine; normal mouse serum; Norwegian Multicenter Study

N·m/s newton meters per second

NMSC nonmelanoma skin cancer

NMSE normalized mean square error

NMSIDS near-miss sudden infant death syndrome

NMSS National Multiple Sclerosis Society; National Mycobacterial Surveillance System

NMT neuromuscular tension; neuromuscular transmission; *N*-methyltransferase; *N*-myristoyltransferase; no more than; nuclear medicine technology or technologist

NMTCB Nuclear Medicine Technology Certification Board

NMTD nonmetastatic trophoblastic disease

NMTS neuromuscular tension state; nuclear matrix-targeting signal

NMU neuromuscular unit; nitrosomethy-lurea

NMV New Minto virus

NN nearest neighbor; neonatal; neural network or net; neural network; neuronavigation; nevocellular nevus; normal nutrition; normally not notifiable; nourished; nuclear/nuclear [ratio]; nurse's notes

N/N normocytic/normochromic [anemia]

nN nanonewton

nn nerves; new name

NN-A nearest neighbor algorithm

NNAS neonatal narcotic abstinence syndrome

NNBA National Nurses in Business Association

NNC National Nutrition Consortium

NNCA Navy Nurse Corps Association

NND neonatal death; New and Nonofficial Drugs; nonspecific nonerosive duodenitis

NNDC National Naval Dental Center

NNDSS National Notifiable Diseases Surveillance Scheme; National Notifiable Diseases Surveillance System

NNE neonatal necrotizing enterocolitis; nonneuronal enolase; normalized noise energy

NNEB National Nursery Examination Board

NNG nonspecific nonerosive gastritis

NNH number needed to harm

NNHS National Nursing Home Survey

NNI noise and number index

NN-IMF internipple–inframammary fold distance

NNIS National Nosocomial Infection Surveillance

NNIWG National Nursing Informatics Work Group

NNJ neonatal jaundice

NNK neural network Kubicek [equation]

NNLIT North Norwegian Lidocaine Intervention Trial

NN/LM National Network of Libraries of Medicine

NNM neonatal mortality

NNMC National Naval Medical Center

NNMT nicotinamide *N*-methyltransferase; Norwegian Nifedipine Multicenter Trial

NNN Novy-MacNeal-Nicolle [medium]

NNNMU *N*-nitroso-*N*-methylurethane

NNO no new orders

nNOS neuronal nitric oxide synthase

n nov new name [L. *nomen novum*]

NNP neonatal nurse practitioner; nerve net pulse

nnp nearest neighbor pair

NNQ number needed to quit

NNR new and nonofficial remedies

NNRTI nonnucleoside reverse transcriptase inhibitor

NNS neural network Sramek [equation]; nicotine nasal spray; nonneoplastic syndrome

NNSA National Nurses Society on Addiction

NNS III Third Nationwide Nutritional Survey

NNT nuclei nervi trigemini; number needed to treat

NNU neonatal unit

NNVAWI Nursing Network on Violence Against Women International

NNWI Neonatal Narcotic Withdrawal Index

NO narcotics officer; nitric oxide; nitrous oxide; none obtained; nonobese; nurse's office

No nobelium

No, no number

NOA National Optometric Association; nitro-L-arginine; nonobstructive azoospermia; Nursing Organization Alliance

NOABX no antibiotics

NOAEL no observed adverse effect level

NOAH New York Online Access to Health

NOAPP National Organization of Adolescent Pregnancy and Parenting

N$_{obs}$ number of observations

NOBT nonoperative biopsy technique

NOC *N*-nitroso compound; not otherwise classified; nursing outcomes classification

NOCDQ nursing organizational climate description questionnaire

Noct. at night [L. *nocte*]

NOD Naito-Oyanagi disease; National Organization on Disability; nodular melanoma; nonobese diabetic [mouse]; notify of death; nucleotide oligomerization domain

NOE naso-orbital ethmoid [fracture]; nuclear Overhauser effect

NOEC no observed effect concentration

NOEL no observed effect level

NOES National Occupational Exposure Survey

NOESY nuclear Overhauser effect spectroscopy

NOF National Osteopathic Foundation; National Osteoporosis Foundation

NOFT nonorganic failure to thrive

NOHS National Occupational Hazards Survey

NOII nonocclusive intestinal ischemia

NOK next of kin

NOL nitric oxide level

NOLAV Nola virus

NOM nonoperative management

nom dub a doubtful name [L. *nomen dubium*]

NOMI nonocclusive mesenteric infarction

NOMID neonatal-onset multisystem inflammatory disease

NONMEM nonlinear mixed effects model

NONPF National Organization of Nurse Practitioner Faculties

non-REM non−rapid eye movement

non repetat do not repeat [L. *non repetat*]

NOP not otherwise provided for

NOPHN National Organization for Public Health Nursing

NOR Neurologic Outcome Research; noradrenaline; normal; nortriptyline; nucleolar organizer region

NORA Nordic Research on Aging

NORASEPT North American Sepsis Trial

NORC National Opinion Research Center

NORD National Organization for Rare Disorders

NORDIL Nordic Diltiazem [study]

NORDUnet Nordic Countries Network

NOR-EPI norepinephrine

NORIF nonstimulated oocyte retrieval in (office) fertilization

norleu norleucine

NORM naturally occurring radioactive material

norm normal

NORML National Organization for the Reform of Marijuana Laws

NORMS National Occupational Respiratory Mortality System

NOR-P1 NOR-P1 carcinoma masses

NORV Northway virus

NOS network operating system; Newcastle-Ottawa scale; nitric oxide synthetase; non−organ specific; not on staff; not otherwise specified

NOs nitric oxide synthetase

NOSAC nonsteroidal antiinflammatory compound

NOSE nanomechanical olfactory sensor

NOSER Newton's one-step error reconstructor

NOSIC Neurologic Outcome Scale for Infants and Children

NOSIE Nurses' Observation Scale for Inpatient Evaluation

NOSTA Naval Ophthalmic Support and Training Activity

NOT neuro-organizational testing; nocturnal oxygen therapy

NOTB National Ophthalmic Treatment Board

NOTES natural orifice transluminal endoscopic surgery

NOTT Nocturnal Oxygen Therapy Trial

NOV Nodamura virus; Novantrone

NoV norovirus

NOVA Nurses Organization of Veterans Affairs

nov n new name [L. *novum nomen*]

NOVS National Office of Vital Statistics

nov sp new species [L. *novum species*]

NOW network of workstations

NOWIS North Wurttemberg Infarction Study

NOWS neonatal opioid withdrawal syndrome

NO$_x$ nitrogen oxide

NP 4-hydroxy-3-nitrophenylacetyl; nasopharyngeal, nasopharynx; natriuretic peptide; near point; necrotizing pancreatitis; neonatal perinatal; nerve palsy; neuritic plague; neuropathic pain; neuropathology; neuropeptide; neurophysin; neuropsychiatry; new patient; newly presented; Niemann-Pick [disease]; nitrogen-phosphorus; nitrophenol; nitroprusside; no pain; no pressure; nonpalpable; nonparalytic; nonpathogenic; nonphagocytic; nonpracticing; no progress or progression; normal plasma; normal pressure; nosocomial pneumonia; not palpable; not perceptible; not performed; not pregnant; not present; not protected; nucleoplasmic; nucleoprotein; nucleoside phosphorylase; nurse practitioner; nursed poorly; nursing procedure; proper name [L. *nomen proprium*]

N-P need persistence

Np neper; neptunium; neurophysin

np nucleotide pair

NPA nasopharyngeal airway; nasopharyngeal aspirate; National Pharmaceutical Association; National Pituitary Agency; near point accommodation; negative predictive accuracy; Nurse Practice Act

NPα nail-patella [syndrome]

nPA lanoteplase

NPACI National Partnership for Advanced Computational Infrastructure

NPA-NIHHDP National Pituitary Agency—National Institutes of Health Hormone Distribution Program

N$_{par}$ number of parameters

NPAT nonparoxysmal atrial tachycardia

NPB nodal premature beat; nonprotein bound; nucleolus precursor bodies

NPBF nonplacental blood flow

NPBV negative pressure body ventilator

NPC nasopharyngeal carcinoma; National Pharmaceutical Council; near point of convergence; neuroparacoccidioidomycosis; nodal premature contractions; nonparenchymal [liver] cell; nonphysician clinician; nonproductive cough; nuclear pore complex; nucleus of posterior commissure; Nurse Practitioner, Certified; nursing protocol consultant

NPCα nasopharyngeal carcinoma

NPCE National Phlebotomy Certification Examination

NPCP National Prostatic Cancer Project; non—*Pneumocystis carinii* pneumonia

NPCRDC National Primary Care Research and Development Centre

NP-CRN nonpolypoid colorectal neoplasia

NP cult nasopharyngeal culture

NPD narcissistic personality disorder; natriuretic plasma dialysate; negative pressure device; Niemann-Pick disease; nightly peritoneal dialysis; nitrogen-phosphorus detector; nonpathologic diagnosis; normal protein diet

NPDB National Practitioner Data Bank

NPDC neurofibromatosis, pheochromocytoma, duodenal carcinoid [syndrome]

NPDL nodular poorly differentiated lymphocytic

NPDR nonproliferative diabetic retinopathy

NPDS National Poison Data System

NPE neurogenic pulmonary edema; neuropsychologic examination; no palpable enlargement; normal pelvic examination

NPF nasopharyngeal fiberscope; National Parkinson Foundation; National Pharmaceutical Foundation; National Provider File; National Psoriasis Foundation; neuronal population function; no predisposing factor

NPFT Neurotic Personality Factor Test

NPGA niched Pareto algorithm

NPH nephrophthisis; neutral protamine Hagedorn (insulin) [obsolete]; normal pressure hydrocephalus; nucleus pulposus herniation

NPhA National Pharmaceutical Association

NPHCE national personal health care expenditures

NPHDO Nadroparin Posthospital Discharge in Orthopedics [study]

NPHE natural phenomenon

NPHF Nurse Practitioner Healthcare Foundation

NP HRF nasal pool histamine-releasing factor

NPHS National Population Health Survey; Northwick Park Heart Study

NPhx nasopharynx

NPI Narcissistic Personality Inventory; National Provider Identifier; neuropsychiatric institution; neuropsychiatric inventory; no present illness; nuclear polymorphism index; nucleoplasmic index

NPIC neurogenic peripheral intermittent claudication

NPII Neonatal Pulmonary Insufficiency Index

NPI-NH Neuropsychiatric Inventory–Nursing Home

NPIP *N*-nitrosopiperidine

NPI-Q Neuropsychiatric Inventory Questionnaire

NPJT nonparoxysmal atrioventricular junctional tachycardia

NPK neuropeptide K

nPKC novel protein kinase C

NPL National Physics Laboratory; neoproteolipid

NPM nonpacemaker [cells]; nothing per mouth

NPN neural Petri net; nonprotein nitrogen

NPO nothing by mouth [L. *nil per os*]; nucleus preopticus

NPO/HS nothing by mouth at bedtime [L. *nil per os hora somni*]

NPOS nurses professional orientation scale

NPP nitrophenylphosphate; normal pool plasma; nucleus tegmenti pedunculopontinus; Nurse Practitioner, Psychiatric

NPPase nucleotide pyrophosphatase

NPPC Nursing Professional Practice Council

NPPE negative pressure pulmonary edema

NPPH nucleotide pyrophosphohydrolase

NPPNG nonpenicillinase-producing *Neisseria gonorrhoeae*

NP polio nonparalytic poliomyelitis

NPPV noninvasive positive-pressure ventilation

NPR net protein ratio; normal pulse rate; nucleoside phosphoribosyl

nPR nuclear progestin receptor

NPRI nicardipine prolonged-release implant

NPRL Navy Prosthetics Research Laboratory

NPS nail-patella syndrome; nasopharyngeal secretion; National Pharmaceutical Services;

National Pharmaceutical Stockpile; neonatal progeroid syndrome; Neuropathic Pain Scale; noise power spectrum

NPSA normal pilosebaceous apparatus

NPSH nonprotein sulhydryl [group]

NPT nasal provocation test; neoprecipitin test; nocturnal penile tumescence; normal pressure and temperature; sodium phosphate transport

NPTR National Pediatric Trauma Registry

NPU net protein utilization

NPUAP National Pressure Ulcer Advisory Panel classification

NPUI nursing process utilization inventory

NPV negative predictive value; negative pressure value; negative pressure ventilation; net present value; nuclear polyhidrosis virus; nucleus paraventricularis

NPWH Nurse Practitioners in Women's Health

NPWT negative pressure wound therapy

NPY neuropeptide Y

NPYR neuropeptide Y receptor; nitrosopyrrolidine

N pyr nitrosopyrrolidine

NQA nursing quality assurance

NQF National Quality Forum

NQMI non–Q-wave myocardial infarction

NQO NAD(P)H:quinone oxidoreductase

4NQO 4-nitroquinoline 1-oxide

NQR nuclear quadruple resonance; reduced nicotinamide adenine dinucleotide quinine reductase

NR do not repeat [L. *non repetatur*]; nerve root; neural retina; neutral red; noise reduction; no radiation; no reaction; no recurrence; no refill; no report; no respiration; no response; no result; nonmatch response; nonreactive; nonrebreathing; nonresponder; nonretarded; normal range; normal reaction; normotensive rat; not readable; not recorded; not reported; not resolved; nurse; nursing [service]; nutrition ratio; Reynold's number

N/R not remarkable

N$_R$ Reynold's number

NR50 neutral red 50%

nr near

NRA nitrate reductase; nucleus retroambigualis

NRAEMT Nationally Registered Advanced Emergency Medical Technician

NRASMC neonatal rat aortic smooth muscle cell

NRB nonrejoining break; nursing reference base

NRBC National Rare Blood Club; normal red blood cell; nucleated red blood cell

NRbc nucleated red blood cell

NRC National Red Cross; National Research Council; National Response Center; normal retinal correspondence; not routine care; Nuclear Regulatory Commission

NRCAM National Resource for Cell Analysis and Modeling

NrCAM neuron glial cell–related cell adhesion molecule

NRCC National Registry in Clinical Chemistry; National Research Council of Canada

NRCL nonrenal clearance

NRDC Natural Resources Defense Council

NRDL Naval Radiological Defense Laboratory

NREE nonresting energy expenditure

NREH normal renin essential hypertension

NREM non–rapid eye movement

NREMT National Registry of Emergency Medical Technicians

NREMT-P nationally registered emergency medical technician-paramedic

NREN National Aeronautics and Space Administration Research and Engineering Network

NRF Neurosciences Research Foundation; normal renal function

NRFC nonrosette-forming cell

NRFD not ready for data

NRG nursing resources grouping

NRGC nucleus reticularis gigantocellularis

NRH nodular regenerative hyperplasia

NRHA National Rural Health Association

NRHS National Runners' Health Study

NRI nerve root involvement; nerve root irritation; nonrespiratory infection

NRICR National Registry of Inhospital Cardiopulmonary Resuscitation

NRIV Ngari virus

NRK normal rat kidney

NRL national reference laboratory; nucleus reticularis lateralis

NRM National Registry of Microbiologists; no regular medications; normal range of motion; nucleus reticularis magnocellularis

NRMI National Registry of Myocardial Infarction

NRMP National Resident Matching Program

NRMSE normalized root mean square error

nRNA nuclear ribonucleic acid

nRNP nuclear ribonucleoprotein

NROM normal range of motion

NRP nucleus reticularis parvocellularis

NRPB National Radiological Protection Board

NRPC nucleus reticularis pontis caudalis

NRPG nucleus reticularis paragigantocellularis

NRR net reproduction rate

NRRC National Rotavirus Reference Centre

NRRL Northern Regional Research Laboratory

NRS Neurobehavioral Rating Scale; normal rabbit serum; normal reference serum; Norman-Roberts syndrome; numerical rating scale

NRSA National Research Service Award

NRSCC National Reference System in Clinical Chemistry

NRSCL National Reference System for the Clinical Laboratory

NRSFPS National Reporting System for Family Planning Services

NRT near real time; networking research team; nicotine replacement therapy; nucleus reticularis thalami

NRTI nucleoside reverse transcriptase inhibitor

NRU neutral red uptake; nursing research unit

NRV nucleus reticularis ventralis

NRVR normalized renal vascular resistance

NS natural science; necrotizing sialometaplasia; Neosporin; nephrosclerosis; nephrotic syndrome; nervous system; Netherton syndrome; neurologic surgery, neurosecretion; neurosecretory; neurosurgery; neurosyphilis; neurotic score; nodular sclerosis; noise/signal [ratio]; nonsmoker; nonspecific; nonstimulation; nonstructural; nonsymptomatic; Noonan syndrome; normal saline; normal serum; normal sodium; Norwegian scabies; no sample; no sequelae; no shear; nosocomial sinusitis; no specimen; not seen; not significant; not specified; not sufficient; not symptomatic; nuclear sclerosis; nursing services; Nursing Sister

N/S noise/signal ratio; normal saline

Ns nasospinale; nerves

ns nanosecond; nonspecific; no sequelae; no specimen; not significant; nylon suture

NSA National Stroke Association; Neurological Society of America; Neurosurgical Society of America; Niger seed agar [medium]; nonsurgical sperm aspiration; normal serum albumin; no salt added; no significant abnormality; no significant anomaly; number of signals averaged

nsa no salt added

NSABP National Surgical Adjuvant Breast and Bowel Project

NSAD no signs of acute disease

NSAE non-serious adverse event; non-supported arm exercise

NSAI nonsteroidal antiinflammatory

NSAIA nonsteroidal antiinflammatory agent

NSAID nonsteroidal antiinflammatory drug

NSAM Naval School of Aviation Medicine

NSAS National Survey of Ambulatory Surgery

NSC neurosecretory cell; no significant change; nonservice connected; non−small cell; nonspecific suppressor cell; normal child with short stature

nsc nonservice connected; no significant change

NSCC National Society for Crippled Children

NSCD non−service connected disability

NSCLC non−small cell lung cancer

NSCS night shift call system

NSCT National Society of Cardiovascular Technologists

NSD *N*-acetylneuraminic acid storage disease; Nairobi sheep disease; neonatal staphylococcal disease; neurosecretory dysfunction; night sleep deprivation; nominal single dose; nominal standard dose; normal standard dose; no significant defect; no significant deficiency; no significant deviation; no significant difference; no significant disease; normal spontaneous delivery

NSDUH National Survey on Drug Use and Health

NSDV Nairobi sheep disease virus

NSE neuron-specific enolase; nonspecific esterase; normal saline enema

nsec nanosecond

NSEP needle and syringe exchange program; nuclease-sensitive element protein

NSERC Natural Sciences and Engineering Research Council

NSF National Science Foundation; National Service Framework; nephrogenic systemic fibrosis; nodular subepidermal fibrosis

NSFNET National Science Foundation Network

NSFTD normal spontaneous full-term delivery

NSG neurosecretory granule

nsg nursing

NSGA nondominated sorting genetic algorithm

NSGC National Society of Genetic Counselors

NSGCT nonseminomatous germ cell tumor

NSGCTT nonseminomatous germ cell tumor of the testis

NSG Hx nursing history

NSGI nonspecific genital infection

NSH National Society for Histotechnology

NSHD nodular sclerosing Hodgkin disease

NSHG National Study of Health and Growth

NSHL nonsyndromic hearing loss

NSHPT neonatal severe hyperparathyroidism

NSI negative self-image; neurosensory impairment; no signs of infection/inflammation; non−syncytium inducing

NSIAD nephrogenic syndrome of inappropriate antidiuresis

NSICU neurosurgical intensive care unit

NSIDS near sudden infant death syndrome

NSILA nonsuppressible insulin-like activity

NSILP nonsuppressible insulin-like protein

NSIVCD nonspecific intraventricular conduction delay

NSJ nevus sebaceus of Jadassohn

NSK nonsquamous keratin

NSM neurosecretory material; neurosecretory motor neuron; nonantigenic specific mediator; nutrient sporulation medium

N·s/m² newton-seconds per square meter

NSMR National Society for Medical Research

NSN nephrotoxic serum nephritis; nicotine-stimulated neurophysin; non−special needs

NSNA National Student Nurses' Association

NSND nonsymptomatic and nondisabling

NSO Neosporin ointment; nucleus supraopticus; Nursing Standard Online

NSP neuron-specific protein; neurotoxic shellfish poisoning; nonstructural protein; nuclear shuttle protein; nurse scheduling problem

NSPB National Society for the Prevention of Blindness

NSPECT normal single photon emission computed tomography

NSPH neonatal severe hyperparathyroidism

NSPN neurosurgery progress note

NSPORT nurse-sensitive patient outcome research team

NSQ Neuroticism Scale Questionnaire; not sufficient quantity

NSR nasal septal reconstruction; nonspecific reaction; normal sinus rhythm; no sign of recurrence; not seen regularly

NSR/M no sign of recurrence or metastases

NSS Nordic Sleep Survey; normal saline solution; normal size and shape; not statistically significant; nutrition support services

NSSQ Norbeck social support questionnaire

NSSTT nonspecific ST and T [wave]

NST neospinothalamic; nonshivering thermogenesis; nonstress test; nutritional support team

NSTACS non–ST-segment elevation acute coronary syndromes
NSTC National Science and Technology Council
NSTEMI non–ST-segment elevation myocardial infarction
NSTI necrotizing soft tissue infection
NST-ICF nonstationary ionic channel current fluctuations
NSTT nonseminomatous testicular tumor
NSU neurosurgical unit; nonspecific urethritis
NSurg neurosurgery, neurosurgeon
NSV nonspecific vaginitis/vaginosis
NSVD normal spontaneous vaginal delivery
NSVR normalized systemic vascular resistance
NSVT nonsustained ventricular tachycardia
NSX neurosurgical examination
nsy nursery
NT nasotracheal; neotetrazolium; neurotensin; neurotoxin; neurotrophic; neutralization test; nicotine tartrate; nontender; nontumoral; normal temperature; normal tissue; normotensive; nortriptyline; not tested; N-terminal [fragment]; nourishment taken; nuchal translucency; nuclear transfer; nucleation time; nucleotidase; nucleotide; numbness and tingling
N&T nose and throat
NT-3 neurotrophin 3
5′NT 5′-nucleotidase
Nt amino terminal
nt nucleotide
NTA natural thymocytotoxic autoantibody; nitrilotriacetic acid; Nurse Training Act
NTAB nephrotoxic antibody
NTAV Ntaya virus
NTBI non–transferrin bound iron
NTBR not to be resuscitated
NTC neotetrazolium chloride
NTCC National Type Culture Collection
NTCP noninvasive transcutaneous cardiac pacing; normal tissue complication probability
NTCT negative temperature coefficient thermistor
NTD 5′-nucleotidase; neural tube defect; nitroblue tetrazolium dye; noise tone difference
NTDB National Trauma Data Bank
NTDDS nerve-targeting drug-delivery system
NTE neuropathy target esterase; neurotoxic esterase; no toxic effect level; not to exceed
NTF neurotrophic factor; normal throat flora
NTFOM normal tissue complication-based figure of merit
NTG nitroglycerin; nitrosoguanidine; nontoxic goiter; normal triglyceridemia

NTGO nitroglycerin ointment
NTGS National Tuberculosis Genotyping Service
Nth normothermia
NTHH nontumorous, hypergastrinemic hyperchlorhydria
NTHi nontypable *Haemophilus influenzae*
NTI nonthyroid illness
NTIA National Telecommunications and Information Administration
NTIG nontreated immunoglobulin
NTIRE non-thermal irreversible electroporation
NTIS National Technical Information Service
NTKR neurotrophic tyrosine kinase receptor
NTL near-total laryngectomy; nonthoracotomy lead; nortriptyline; no time limit
NTLI neurotensin-like immunoreactivity
NTM nontuberculous mycobacteria
NTMI nontransmural myocardial infarction
NTN nephrotoxic nephritis
NTNH nontoxic, nonhemagglutinating
NTO nontarget organism
NTON National Transparent Optical Network
NTOS neurogenic thoracic outlet syndrome
NTP narcotic treatment program; National Toxicology Program; nitroprusside; nonthrombopenic purpura; normal temperature and pressure; 5′-nucleotidase; sodium nitroprusside
NT&P normal temperature and pressure
NTPPH nucleoside-triphosphate pyrophosphohydrolase
NTR negative therapeutic reaction; nitroreductase; nontranslated region; normotensive rat; nutrition
ntr nutrition
NTRC National Toxins Research Center
NTS nasotracheal suction; nephrotoxic serum; neurotensin; nicotine transdermal system; nontropical sprue; nucleus tractus solitarius
NTSS National Tuberculosis Surveillance System
NTT near-total thyroidectomy
NTU Navy Toxicology Unit
N-TUL internal tumescent ultrasound liposculpture
NTV nerve tissue vaccine
NTVR normal transvalvular regurgitation
nt wt net weight
NTX naltrexone
NTZ normal transformation zone
NU name unknown
nU nanounit
nu nude [mouse]
NUAPS National Unstable Angina Pectoris Study
NUBS nonuniform rational B-spline

NUC nonspecific ulcerative colitis; sodium urate crystal
Nuc nucleoside
nuc nucleated
NUCARE nursing care research
nucl nucleus
NUD nonulcer dyspepsia; nursing utilization database
NUG necrotizing ulcerative gingivitis
NUGV Nugget virus
NUI number user identification
NUIS non-urgent information system
nullip nulliparous
vm nanometers
NUMA nonuniform memory access; nuclear mitotic apparatus
numc number concentration
NUPV nucleopolyhedrovirus
NURB Neville upper reservoir buffer
Nut nutrition
NUTRIC nutrition risk in the critically ill
NUV near ultraviolet
NV nausea and vomiting; necrosis virus; negative variation; neovascularization; next visit; nonveteran; normal value; Norwalk virus; not vaccinated; not venereal; not verified; not volatile
N&V nausea and vomiting
Nv naked vision
nv new variant
NVA near visual acuity
NVB neurovascular bundle
NVCA National Venereology Council of Australia
nvCJD new variant Creutzfeldt-Jakob disease
NVD nausea, vomiting, and diarrhea; neck vein distention; neovascularization of the disk; neurovesicle dysfunction; nonvalvular disease; normal vaginal delivery; no venereal disease; Newcastle virus disease; number of vessels diseased
N/V/D nausea, vomiting, diarrhea
NVDRS National Violent Death Reporting System
NVE native valve endocarditis
NVG neovascular glaucoma; night vision goggles; nonventilated group
NVIm *N*-vinyl imidazole

NVL no visible lesion
NVM neovascular membrane; nonvolatile matter
NVP nevirapine; *N*-vinyl pyrrolidone
NVPO National Vaccine Program Office
NVS neurologic vital signs; nutritionally variant streptococci
NVSN New Vaccine Surveillance Network
NVSS National Vital Statistics System; normal variant short stature
NVTS normal volunteer telephone screening
NW naked weight; nasal wash
nW nanowatt
NWB nonweightbearing
NWCL New World cutaneous leishmaniasis
NWDA National Wholesale Druggists Association
NWM nucleotide weight matrix
NWR normotensive Wistar rat
NWTS National Wilms Tumor Study
NWTSG National Wilms Tumor Study Group
NX naloxane; no evidence of lymph node metastases; no evidence of breast tumor lymph node metastases
Nx no evidence of lymph node metastases; no evidence of breast tumor lymph node metastases
NXG necrobiotic xanthogranuloma
ny nystagmus
NYAV Nyabira virus
NYC New York City [medium]
NYD not yet diagnosed; not yet discovered
NYHA New York Heart Association
NYHAFC New York Heart Association Functional Class
NYMV Nyamanini virus
NYQAS New York Quality Assurance System
nyst nystagmus
NYV New York virus
NZ neutral zone; normal zone
NZB New Zealand black [mouse]
NZC New Zealand chocolate [mouse]
NZO New Zealand obese [mouse]
NZR New Zealand red [rabbit]
NZV New Zealand virus
NZW New Zealand white [mouse]

O

O blood type in the ABO blood group; eye [L. *oculus*]; nonmotile strain of microorganisms [Ger. *ohne Hauch*]; no response [pacemaker]; objective findings; observed frequency in a contingency table; obstetrics; obvious; occipital electrode placement; occiput; occlusal; office; often; ohm; old; opening; operator; operon; opium; oral, orally; orange; orderly respirations; ortho-; orthopedics; osteocyte; other; output; ovine [veterinary medicine]; owner [veterinary medicine]; oxygen; pint [L. *octarius*]; uppercase Greek letter omicron; zero

Ω uppercase Greek letter omega; ohm

ω lowercase Greek letter omega; angular velocity

O₂ both eyes; diatomic oxygen; molecular oxygen

O₃ ozone

O125 nonmucinous ovarian tumor antigen

o eye [L. *oculus*]; opening; ovary transplant; pint [L. *octarius*]

ο lowercase Greek letter omicron

ō negative; without

OA [o]esophageal atresia; obstructive apnea; occipital artery; occipito-anterior; occiput anterior; occupational asthma; octanoic acid; ocular albinism; old age; okadaic acid; oleic acid; on admission/arrival; open access; open appendectomy; opiate analgesia; ophthalmic artery; opsonic activity; optic atrophy; oral airway; oral alimentation; organic anion; orotic acid; osteoarthritis; osteoarthrosis; ovalbumin; ovarian antibody; overall assessment; Overeaters Anonymous; oxalic acid

O&A observation and assessment

OA1 ocular albinism type 1

O₂a oxygen availability

OAA Old Age Assistance; Older Americans Act; Opticians Association of America; oxaloacetic acid

OAAD ovarian ascorbic acid depletion

OAAS observer's assessment alertness/sedation scale

OAAV ovine adeno-associated virus

OAdV ovine adenovirus

OAdV-A, B, C ovine adenoviruses A, B, C

OAB old-age benefits; overactive bladder

OABP organic anion binding protein

OA/BVM oral airway/bag-valve-mask

OAC omeprazole, amoxicillin, clarithromycin

OACT occupational activity

OAD obstructive airway disease; organic anionic dye

OADC oleate-albumin-dextrose-catalase

OAE otoacoustic emission

OAF off-axis factor; off-axis ratio; open-air factor; osteoclast activating factor

OAFNS oculo-auriculofrontonasal syndrome

OAG open-angle glaucoma

OAH ovarian androgenic hyperfunction

OAIS Outcomes and Information Set

OAISO overaction of the ipsilateral superior oblique

OAK Kjer optic atrophy

OALF organic acid labile fluid

OALL ossification of anterior longitudinal ligament

OAM Office of Alternative Medicine; outer acrosomal membrane

OAP Office of Adolescent Pregnancy; old-age pension/pensioner; ophthalmic artery pressure; osteoarthropathy; oxygen at atmospheric pressure; precocious osteoarthrosis

OAPP Office of Adolescent Pregnancy Programs

OAR organ at risk; Ottawa ankle rule

OARS Older Americans Research and Service; older Americans resources and services; Optimal Atherectomy Restenosis Study

OAS old-age security; ongoing abuse screening; oral allergy syndrome; osmotically active substance

OASD ocular albinism, sensorineural deafness [syndrome]

OASDHI Old Age, Survivors, Disability and Health Insurance

OASDI Old Age Survivors and Disability Insurance

OASI Old Age and Survivors Insurance

OASIS Older Adults Service and Information System; Organization to Assess Strategies for Ischemic Syndromes; Outcome and Assessment Information Set; Overweight and Seeking Infertility Support

OASP organic acid soluble phosphorus

OAstV ovine astrovirus

OAT *O*-acetyltransferase; Ochanomizu Aspirin Trial; oligoasthenoteratozoospermia; Open Artery Trial; organic anion transporter; ornithine aminotransferase

OATL ornithine aminotransferase-like

OATP1B1 organic anion-transporting polypeptide 1B1

OATR organism attribute

OAV oculoauriculovertebral

OAVS oculoauriculovertebral syndrome

OAVD oculoauriculovertebral dysplasia

OAW oral airways

OB obese [mouse]; obese, obesity; objective benefit; obliterative bronchiolitis; obstetrics, obstetrician; occult bacteremia; occult bleeding; olfactory bulb; oligoclonal band

O&B opium and belladonna

ob obese [mouse]

OBA office-based anesthesia; Office of Biotechnology Activities

OBAD optimal biologically active dose

OBB oriented bounding boxes; own bed bath

OBD organic brain disease

OBCAM opioid-binding cell adhesion molecule

OBE Office of Biological Education

OBET odor-baited entry trap

OBF organ blood flow

OBG, ObG obstetrics and gynecology, obstetrician-gynecologist

OBGS obstetric and gynecologic surgery

OB-GYN, ob-gyn obstetrics and gynecology, obstetrician-gynecologist

obj objective

obl oblique

OBMT omeprazole, bismuth, metronidazole, tetracycline

OBOV Obodhiang virus

OBP odorant-binding protein; ova, blood, parasites

OBR obesity gene receptor

OBRA Omnibus Reconciliation Act

OBS obesity; obstetric service; office-based surgery; organic brain syndrome

Obs observation, observed; obstetrics, obstetrician

obs obsolete

Obst obstetrics, obstetrician

obst, obstr obstruction, obstructed

OBT optimized background therapy

OB-US obstetric ultrasound

OC obstetric conjugate; occlusocervical; [o]esophageal candidiasis; office call; on call; only child; optical colonoscopy; optic chiasma; oral contraceptive; orbicularis oculi; order communication; organ culture; organochlorine; original claim; orofacial cleft; outer canthal [distance]; ovarian cancer; oxygen consumed

O&C onset and course

O/C ornithine/citrulline ratio

OCA obeticholic acid; octylcyanoacrylate; oculocutaneous albinism; olivopontocerebellar atrophy; optical clearing agent; oral contraceptive agent

OCα ovarian carcinoma

OCA1A oculocutaneous albinism type 1a

OCA1B oculocutaneous albinism type 1b

OCA2 oculocutaneous albinism type 2

OCA3 oculocutaneous albinism type 3

OCA4 oculocutaneous albinism type 4

OCAD occlusive carotid artery disease

O₂cap oxygen capacity

OCB obsessive-compulsive behavior

OCBAS Optimal Coronary Balloon Angioplasty vs. Stent [trial]; Optimal Coronary Balloon Angioplasty with Provisional Stenting vs. Primary Stent [trial]

OCBF outer cortical blood flow

OCC object-centered coordinate; oculocerebrocutaneous; oocyte-cumulus complexes; operable case-based reasoning−oriented case; optimal care committee; oral cholecystography; original component complexes

occ occasional; occiput, occipital; occlusion, occlusive; occupation; occurrence

occas occasional

OCCI oblique clear corneal incision

occip occiput, occipital

occl occlusion, occlusive

OCCPR open-chest cardiopulmonary resuscitation

OccTh occupational therapist/therapy

occ ther occupational therapist/therapy

occup occupation, occupational

occup Rx occupational therapy

OCCV object-centered coordinate values

OCD obsessive-compulsive disorder; Office of Child Development; Office of Civil Defense; osteochondritis dissecans; ovarian cholesterol depletion; oxygen cost diagram

OCDD octachlorodibenzo-*p*-dioxin

OCF occipito-frontal

OCG omnicardiogram; oral cholecystogram

OCH oral contraceptive hormone

OCHA Office for the Coordination of Humanitarian Affairs

OCHAMPUS Office of Civilian Health and Medical Programs of the Uniformed Services

OCHS Office of Cooperative Health Statistics

OCIS Oncology Clinical Information System

OCL osteochondrosis latens

OCLC Ohio Computer Library Center; online computer library center

OCM oral contraceptive medication

OCN oculomotor nucleus; oncology certified nurse; osteocalcin

OCOA Online Cytogenetics of Animals

OCP octacalcium phosphate; ocular cicatricial pemphigoid; Onchocerciasis Control Programme; oral case presentation; oral contraceptive pill

OC&P ova, cysts, and parasites

OCPD obsessive-compulsive personality disorder

OCPE office of clinical practice evaluation

OCR oculocardiac reflex; oculocerebrorenal [syndrome]; optical character reader; optical character recognition

oCRF ovine corticotropin-releasing factor

OCRG oxycardiorespirography

oCRH ovine corticotropin-releasing hormone

OCRL oculocerebrorenal [syndrome] of Lowe

OCRS oculocerebrorenal syndrome

OCS occipital condyle syndrome; Ondine's curse syndrome; open canalicular system; oral contraceptive steroid; order communication system; outpatient clinic substation; Oxford Cholesterol Study

OCSD oculocraniosomatic disease

OCSI orthostatic change in shock index

OCSP Oxfordshire Community Stroke Project

OCT object classification test; ocular coherence tomography; optical coherence tomography; optimal cutting temperature; oral cavity tumor; oral contraceptive therapy; organic cation transporter; ornithine carbamoyltransferase; orthotopic cardiac transplantation; outer canthal distance; oxytocin challenge test

O-CT ortho-computed tomography

OCTD overlap connective tissue disease

OCTM open-cavity tympanomastoidectomy

OCU observation care unit

OCV ordinary conversational voice

OD Doctor of Optometry; object dictionary; obtained absorbance; occipital dysplasia; occupational dermatitis; occupational disease; oculodynamic; Ollier disease; on duty; once a day; open drop; optical density; optimal dose; originally derived; out-of-date; outside diameter; overdosage, overdose; right eye [L. *oculus dexter*]

O-D obstacle dominance

OD-1 Organ Disease 1 [study]

OD-2 Organ Disease 2 [study]

O₂D oxygen delivery

ODA office document architecture; open document architecture; overall disease assessment; right occipitoanterior [L. *occipito-dextra anterior*]

ODAC Oncologic Drugs Advisory Committee

ODB opiate-directed behavior

ODBC open database connectivity

ODC oritidine decarboxylase; ornithine decarboxylase; oxygen dissociation curve

Odc ornithine decarboxylase

ODCP ornithine decarboxylase pseudogene

ODD oculodentodigital; oppositional defiant disorder; osteodental dysplasia

OD'd overdosed

ODE Office of Device Evaluation; ordinary differential equation; orphan drug exclusivity

ODED oculo-digito-esophago-duodenal [syndrome]

ODES Oslo Diet and Exercise Study

ODFR oxygen-derived free radical

ODI oxygen desaturation index

ODIF office document interchange format

ODISY Online Deaconess Information System

ODM ophthalmodynamometer, ophthalmodynamometry

ODN oligodeoxyribonucleotide

ODOD oculo-dento-osseous dysplasia

Odont odontogenic

ODP offspring of diabetic parents; open distributed processing; right occipitoposterior [L. *occipito-dextra posterior*]

ODPHP Office of Disease Prevention and Health Promotion

ODQ on direct questioning

ODRV Odrenisrou virus

ODS organized delivery system; original dataset; osmotic demyelination syndrome

ODSG ophthalmic Doppler sonogram

ODT oculodynamic tract; right occipitotransverse [L. *occipito-dextra transversa*]

ODTS organic dust toxic syndrome

ODU optical density unit

ODV optimal diagnostic value

OE on examination; organization engine; orthopedic examination; otitis externa; out-stationed enrollment

O/E observed/expected ratio

O&E observation and examination

Oe oersted

OEE osmotic erythrocyte enrichment; outer enamel epithelium

OEF oil immersion field; oxygen extraction fraction

O₂EI oxygen extraction index

OEIS omphalocele, exstrophy, imperforate anus, spinal defects

OEL occupational exposure limit

OELM optimal external laryngeal manipulation

OEM object exchange model; opposite ear masked; original electronic manufacturer

OEP operational effectiveness program

OEPA Onchocerciasis Elimination Program for the Americas

OER osmotic erythrocyte; oxygen enhancement ratio

O₂ER oxygen extraction ratio

OERP Office of Education and Regional Programming

OERR, OE/RR order entry and results reporting

OES optical emission spectroscopy; oral esophageal stethoscope

oesoph [o]esophagus

OET oral endotracheal tube; oral esophageal tube

O₂Ext oxygen extraction

OF occipitofrontal; opacity factor; open field; optical fundus; orbital fracture; orbitofrontal; osmotic fragility; osteitis fibrosa; output factor; oxidation-fermentation

O/F oxidation-fermentation

OFA oncofetal antigen

OFAGE orthogonal field alternation gel electrophoresis

OFAS Office of Food Additive Safety

OFBM oxidation-fermentation basal medium

OFC occipitofrontal circumference; optical flow constraint; orbitofacial cleft; orbitofrontal cortex; osteitis fibrosa cystica

OFCTAD occipito-facio-cervico-thoraco-abdomino-digital dysplasia

OFD object-film distance; occipital frontal diameter; oro-facial-digital [syndrome]

ofd object-film distance

Off official

OFHA occipitofrontal headache

OFI open and flexible learning

OFM orofacial malformation

OFNE oxygenated fluorocarbon emulsion

OFS optical file system; oscillating field stimulator

OFTT organic failure to thrive

OFUN organism function

OG n-octyl-β-D-glucoside; obstetrics and gynecology; occlusogingival; oligodendrocyte; optic ganglion; orange green; orogastric; overgarment

O&G obstetrics and gynecology

OGC oculogyric crisis

OGD [o]esophago-gastro-duodenoscopy

OGDH oxoglutarate dehydrogenase

OGF ovarian growth factor; oxygen gain factor

OGH ovine growth hormone

OGI oxygen-glucose index

OGIB obscure gastrointestinal bleeding

OGJ [o]esophagogastric junction

OGLA oral glucose-lowering agents

OGNP Obstetrics and Gynecology Nurse Practitioner

OGS oxygenic steroid

OGTT oral glucose tolerance test

OGZN organization

OH hydroxycorticosteroid; obstructive hypopnea; occipital horn; occupational health; occupational history; oligomer hybridization; open heart; orthostatic hypotension; osteopathic hospital; out of hospital; outpatient hospital

17-OH 17-hydroxycorticosteroid

OHA oral hypoglycemic agents

OHAHA ophthalmoplegia, hypotonia, ataxia, hypacusis, athetosis [syndrome]

OHB₁₂ hydroxycobalamin

O₂Hb oxyhemoglobin

OHC occupational health center; outer hair cell; Oxford Haemophilia Centre

5-OHC 5-hydroxycysteine

OHCA out-of-hospital cardiac arrest

OH-Cbl hydroxycobalamin

OHCC hydroxycalciferol; out-of-home child care

OHCOB hydroxycobalamin

OHCS hydroxycorticosteroid

OHD hydroxylase deficiency; hydroxyvitamin D; Office of Human Development; Ondine-Hirschsprung disease; organic heart disease

1,25(OH)₂D₃ 1,25-dihydroxyvitamin D_3

25-OH-D 25-hydroxyvitamin D

OHDA hydroxydopamine

8-OH-dG 8-hydroxy-2'-deoxyguanosine

16-OH-DHAS 16-alpha-hydroxydehydroepiandrosterone sulfate

8-OH-DPAT 8-hydroxy-2-(di-n-propylamino) tetralin

OHDS Office of Human Development Services

OHE optimized zona-free hamster egg-sperm penetration assay; other hospital employee

OHF Omsk hemorrhagic fever

OHFA hydroxy fatty acid

OHFT overhead frame trapeze

OHFV Omsk hemorrhagic fever virus

OHI Occupational Health Institute; operative hypertension indicator; oral hygiene index; Oral Hygiene Instruction

OHIAA hydroxyindoleacetic acid

OHIPD Office of Health Information Programs Development

OHI-S Oral Hygiene Instruction-Simplified

OHL oral hairy leukoplakia

OHMO Office of Health Maintenance Organizations

OHN occupational health nurse; optical nerve head

OHP hydroxyprogesterone; hydroxyproline; occupational health plan; Oregon Health Plan; oxygen under high pressure

17-OHP 17-hydroxyprogesterone

OHPCC Office of High-Performance Computing and Communications

OHR occupational health research; Office of Health Research

OHRP Office for Human Research Protections

OHS obesity hypoventilation syndrome; occipital horn syndrome; occupational health and safety; occupational health service; ocular histoplasmosis syndrome; open heart surgery; Oslo Hypertension Study; ovarian hyperstimulation syndrome

OHSD hydroxysteroid dehydrogenase

OHSR Office of Human Subjects Research

OHSS ovarian hyperstimulation syndrome

OHT ocular hypertension; orthotopic heart transplantation; Oslo Heart Trial

OHTA Office of Health Technology Assessment

5-OHU 5-hydroxyuracil

OI obturator internus; occasional insomnia; opportunistic infection; opsonic index; orgasmic impairment; orientation inventory; orthoiodohippurate; osteogenesis imperfecta; ouabain insensitivity; oxygen intake

O-I outer and inner

OIC opioid-induced constipation; organized indigenous caregiving

OID object identifier; optimal immunomodulating dose; Organism Identification Number; oxygen insufflation device

OIF observed intrinsic frequency; oil immersion field; open internal fixation; Osteogenesis Imperfecta Foundation

OIG Office of the Inspector General

OIH Office of International Health; orthoiodohippurate; ovulation-inducing hormone

OILD occupational immunologic lung disease

oint ointment

OIP organizing interstitial pneumonia

OIR Office of Information Resources; Office of International Research; ongoing implantation rate

OIS object information system; organ injury scale; Oslo Ischemia Study; outpatient information system

OIT organic integrity test

OITAV Oita virus

OJ orange juice

OKC odontogenic keratocyst

OKHV Okhotskiy virus

OKN optokinetic nystagmus

OKOV Okola virus

OKR optokinetic response; Ottawa knee rules

OKS optokinetic stimulus

OKT ornithine ketoacid aminotransferase

OL open label(ed)

ol left eye [L. *oculus laevus*]

OLA left occipitoanterior [L. *occipito-laeva anterior*]; oligonucleotide ligation assay

OLAP online analytical processing

OLAS oligoisoadenylate synthetase

OLB olfactory bulb; open liver biopsy; open lung biopsy

OLBx open lung biopsy

OLC ouabain-like compound

OLD obstructive lung disease; orthochromatic leukodystrophy

OLDMEDLINE Old MEDLARS Online

OLE object linking and embedding

olf olfactory

OLFR olfactory receptor

OLGIH obscure lower gastrointestinal hemorrhage

OLH ovine lactogenic hormone

oLH ovine luteinizing hormone

OLI octree level index

OLIDS open-loop insulin delivery system

OLIV Olifantsvlei virus

OLMC online medical control

OLP left occipitoposterior [L. *occipito-laeva posterior*]

OLR otology, laryngology, and rhinology

ol res oleoresin

OLRx orthotopic liver transplantation

OLS ordinary least square; oubain-like substance

OLT left occipitotransverse; orthotopic liver transplantation

OLVV Oliveros virus

OM obtuse marginal [artery]; obtuse mental; occipitomental; occupational medicine; ocular movement; oculomotor; operations manager; Osborne Mendel [rat]; osteomalacia; osteomyelitis; osteopathic manipulation; otitis media; outer membrane; ovulation method

OMA object management architecture; Official Methods of Analysis [AOAC international program]; omapatrilat

OMAC otitis media, acute catarrhal

OMAS occupational maladjustment syndrome

OMB obtuse marginal branch; Office of Management and Budget

OMC office of managed care; orientation-memory-concentration [test]

OMCH Office of Maternal and Child Health

OMCT Orientation-Memory-Concentration Test

OMD ocular muscle dystrophy; oculomandibulodyscephaly; orbital maxillary disjunction; organic mental disorder; oromandibular dystonia

OMDB object microdatabase

OME office of medical examiner; otitis media with effusions

OMED World Organisation for Digestive Endoscopy [Fr. *Organisation Mondiale d'Endoscopie Digestive*]

OMEGA Ottawa-Madison electron gamma algorithm

OMERACT Outcome Measures in Rheumatoid Arthritis Clinical Trial

OMFAQ Older Americans Resources and Services (OARS) Multidimensional Functional Assessment Questionnaire

OMG object management group; oligodendrocyte-myelin glycoprotein; osteopathic medical school graduate

OMGE World Organization for Gastroenterology [Fr. *Organisation Mondiale de Gastro-Enterologie*]

OMGP oligodendrocyte-myelin glycoprotein

OMH Office of Mental Health

OMI office of medical investigator; old myocardial infarction

OMIA Online Mendelian Inheritance in Animals

OMIM Online Mendelian Inheritance in Man

OML orbitomental line

OMN oculomotor nerve

OMNI Organizing Medical Networked Information

OMOV Omo virus

OMP olfactory marker protein; oligonucleoside methylphosphonate; ornithine monophosphate; orotidine-5′-monophosphatase; outer membrane protein

OMPA octamethyl pyrophosphoramide; otitis media, purulent, acute

OmpA, ompA outer membrane protein A

OMPC, OMPCh otitis media, purulent, chronic

OmpF, ompF outer membrane protein F

OMR oligomycin-resistant; online medical record

OMRT Ontario Association of Medical Radiation Technologists

OMS occupational medical services; organic mental syndrome; otomandibular syndrome

OM&S osteopathic medicine and surgery

OMSA otitis media, suppurative, acute

OMSC otitis media secretory/suppurative chronic

OMT object modeling technique; ocular microtremor; *O*-methyltransferase; ophthalmic medical technician/technologist; osteopathic manipulative therapy

OMV outer membrane vesicle

OMVC open mitral valve commissurotomy

ON occipitonuchal; office nurse; olfactory nucleus; onlay; optic nerve; orthopedic nurse; osteonecrosis; osteonectin; overnight

ONAC Office of Noise Abatement and Control

ONC oncogene; oncology; open network communication; Orthopedic Nurse, Certified; over-the-needle catheter

OND Ophthalmic Nursing Diploma; orbitonasal dislocation; other neurologic disorders

ONE otoneurologic expert system

ONG optic nerve glioma; Orthodontic National Group [UK]

ONMRS onychotrichodysplasia, neutropenia, mental retardation (intellectual disability) syndrome

ONNV o'nyong-nyong virus

ONP operating nursing procedure; orthonitrophenyl

ONPG *o*-nitrophenyl-beta-D-galactopyranoside

ONS Office for National Statistics; Oncology Nursing Society; oral nutritional supplementation

ONSA Organization for Nucleotide Sequencing and Analysis

ONTG oral nitroglycerin

ONTR orders not to resuscitate

OO object oriented; oophorectomy; orbicularis oculi

O&O on and off

OOA object-oriented analysis; outer optic anlage

OOB out of bed

OODB object-oriented database

OODBMS object-oriented database management system

OOG optic oculography

OOH out of hospital

OOH/CA out-of-hospital cardiac arrest

OOHP out-of-hospital program

OOHRT object-oriented health care terminology respository

OOLR ophthalmology, otology, laryngology, and rhinology

OOM, oom oogonial metaphase

OOMM object-oriented matrix model

OON out of network

OOP object-oriented programming

OOR out of room

OORR orbicularis oculi reflex response
OOSE object-oriented software engineering
OOSS Outpatient Ophthalmic Surgery Society
OOW out of wedlock
OOWS objective opiate withdrawal scale
OP occipitoparietal; occipitoposterior; occiput posterior; octapeptide; olfactory peduncle; opening pressure; operation, operative; operative procedure; ophthalmology; opponens pollicis; optic neuritis; organophosphate; oropharynx; orthostatic proteinuria; osmotic pressure; osteoporosis; outpatient; ovine prolactin
O&P ova and parasites
O/P outpatient
Op ophthalmology; opisthocranion
op operation; operator
OPA oligonucleoside phosphoramidate; open procurement agency; *o*-phthaladehyde; optic atrophy; organ procurement agency; oropharyngeal airway; outcome and process assessment; ovine pulmonary adenocarcinoma
OPALS Ontario Prehospital Advanced Life Support [study]
op-amp operational amplifier
OPB osteoporosis-preventing behaviors; outpatient basis
OPC oculopalatocerebral [syndrome]; oligonucleotide purification cartridge; outpatient clinic; overall performance category
OPCA olivopontocerebellar atrophy
OPCAB off-pump coronary artery bypass
OPCD olivopontocerebellar degeneration
OPCOS oligomenorrheic polycystic ovary syndrome
OPCRIT operational criteria
OPCS Office of Population Censuses and Surveys
OPD obstetric prediabetic; once per day; *o*-phenylenediamine; optical path difference; otopalatodigital [syndrome]; outpatient department; outpatient dispensary
o-PDA *o*-phenylenediamine
O'p-DDD mitotane
OpDent operative dentistry
OPDG ocular plethysmodynamography
OPDM oculopharyngodistal myopathy
OPDP Office of Prescription Drug Promotion
OPDS otopalatodigital syndrome
OPF oligo[poly(ethylene glycol) fumarate]
OPG ocular pneumoplethysmography; orthopantomogram; osteoprotegerin; oxypolygelatin
opg opening
OPH obliterative pulmonary hypertension; ophthalmia; organic phosphate

OPH, Oph ophthalmology; ophthalmoscope, ophthalmoscopy
Oph A ophthalmic artery
OPHC Office of Prepaid Health Care
OphD Doctor of Ophthalmology
OPHS Office of Public Health and Science
Ophth ophthalmology
OPI oculoparalytic illusion; Omnibus Personality Inventory
OPIDN organophosphate-induced delayed neuropathy
OPIDP organophosphate-induced delayed polyneuropathy
OPIM other potentially infectious material
OPK object-processing kernel; optokinetic; ovulation predictor kit
OPL other party liability; outer plexiform layer; ovine placental lactogen
OPLINK Ohio Public Library Information Network
OPLL ossification of posterior longitudinal ligament
OPM occult primary malignancy; Office of Personnel Management; ophthalmoplegic migraine
OPMD oculopharyngeal muscular dystrophy
OPMSS Olestra Postmarketing Surveillance Study
OPN ophthalmic nurse; osteopontin
OPO organ procurement organization
OPP osmotic pressure of plasma; oxygen partial pressure
opp opposite
OPPA vincristine, procarbazine, prednisone, Adriamycin
OPPG oculopneumoplethysmography
OPPS outpatient prospective payment system
OPR ongoing pregnancy rate
OPRD opiate receptor delta
OPRK opiate receptor kappa
OPRR Office for Protection from Research Risks
OPRT orotate phosphoribosyltransferase
OPRTase orotate phosphoribosyltransferase
OPS operations; optical position sensor; optimal parameter search; osteoporosis-pseudolipoma syndrome; outpatient service; outpatient surgery
OPSA ovarian papillary serous adenocarcinoma
OpScan optical scanning
OPSEC operations security
OPSI overwhelming postsplenectomy infection

OPSR Office of Professional Standards Review

OPT oligonucleoside phosphorothioate; *o*-phthaldialdehyde; optimal pharmacologic therapy; optimization; outpatient; outpatient treatment; ovulation predictor test

opt best [L. *optimus*]; optician, optics

OPTHD optimal hemodialysis

OPTICUS Optimization with Intracoronary Ultrasound to Reduce Stent Restenosis [trial]

OPTIMAAL Optimal Trial in Myocardial Infarction with Angiotensin II Antagonist Losartan

OPTIME Outcomes of a Prospective Trial of Intravenous Milrinone for Exacerbations

OPTIME CHF Outcomes of a Prospective Trial of Intravenous Milrinone for Exacerbations of Chronic Heart Failure

OPTN organ procurement and transplant network

OPU oocyte pick-up

OPUS Orbofiban in Patients with Unstable Coronary Syndromes [study]

OPV oral polio vaccine; ovine papillomavirus

OPV 1, 2 ovine papillomaviruses 1, 2

OPWL opiate withdrawal

OQAQ Overview Quality Assessment Questionnaire

OR a logical binary relation that is true if any argument is true and false otherwise; odds ratio; [o]estrogen receptor; oil retention; oligomer of resveratrol; open reduction; open repair; operating room; optic radiation; oral rehydration; orbicularis oris; orosomucoid; orthopedic; orthopedic research; ouabain resistant; outwardly rectifying; oxidized radical

O-R oxidation-reduction

O$_R$ rate of outflow

Or orbitale

ORA opiate receptor agonist

ORACLE Overview of the Role of Antibiotics in Curtailing Labor and Early Delivery [trial]

ORALABX oral antibiotics

ORANS Oak Ridge Analytical System

ORB object request broker

ORBC ox red blood cell

ORBIT Oral Glycoprotein IIb/IIIa Receptor Blockade to Inhibit Thrombosis [trial]

ORC oculo-reno-cerebellar [syndrome]; origin recognition complex

ORCA open record for care

orch orchitis

ORCHIDS Office Records Charts Information Data System

OR$_{Cl}$ outwardly rectifying chloride current

ORD optical rotatory dispersion; oral radiation death

ORDS Office of Research, Demonstration, and Statistics

ORE oil retention enema

OREF Orthopedic Research and Education Foundation

ORESTES open reading expressed sequence tags

ORF, orf open reading frame

OR&F open reduction and fixation

ORFV orf virus

Org, org organic

ORGM organism

ORH order header

ORI Office of Research Integrity

ORIA Office of Radiation and Indoor Air

ORIF open reduction with internal fixation

ORIS ophthalmic retrobulbar injection simulator

oriT origin of transfer

ORIV Oriboca virus

OrJ orange juice

ORL otorhinolaryngology

ORLS Oxford Record Linkage Study

ORM object relational mapping; Office of Research and Methodology; orosomucoid; other regulated material; oxygen ratio monitor

ORMC oxygen ratio monitor controller

ORN olfactory receptor neuron; operating room nurse; orthopedic nurse

Orn ornithine

ORNL Oak Ridge National Laboratory

ORO oil red O

OR$_O$ observed odds ratio

OROS oral osmotic; osmotic controlled-release technology

OROV Oropouche virus

ORP operating room personnel; oxidation-reduction potential

ORPM orthorhythmic pacemaker

ORR objective response rate; Office of Refugee Resettlement [DHHS]; overall response rate

ORS olfactory reference syndrome; oral rehydration solution; oral surgery, oral surgeon; Orthopaedic Research Society; orthopedic surgeon, orthopedic surgery; oxygen radical scavengers

ORSA osteoclast resorption stimulating activity; oxacillin-resistant *Staphylococcus aureus*

ORT object relations technique; operating room technician; oral rehydration therapy

OR$_T$ true odds ratio

orth, ortho orthopedic, orthopedics

ORUV 1, 2, 3, 4 Orungo viruses 1, 2, 3, 4
ORW Osler-Rendu-Weber [syndrome]
ORXV Oriximina virus
ORYX outcome research yields excellence
OS left eye [L. *oculus sinister*]; object oriented; occipitosacral; occupational safety; office surgery; oligosaccharide; Omenn syndrome; opening snap; open source; open splenectomy; operating system; Opitz syndrome; oral surgery; ordinal scale; organ-specific; orthognathic surgery; orthopedic surgeon, orthopedic surgery; Osgood-Schlatter [disease]; osteogenic sarcoma; osteosarcoma; osteosclerosis; ouabain sensitivity; overall survival; oxygen saturation
Os osmium
OSA obstructive sleep apnea; Office of Services to the Aging; Optical Society of America; ovarian sectional area
OSACA Osaka Follow-up Study for Ultrasonographic Assessment of Carotid Atherosclerosis
OSAHS obstructive sleep apnea—hypopnea syndrome
OSAI organism-specific antibody index
OSAS obstructive sleep apnea syndrome
OSBP oxysterol binding protein
OSC on-scene coordinator
osc oscillation
OSCAR Olive Oil, Safflower Oil, Canola Oil and Rapeseed Oil [study]; online survey, certification, and reporting system
OSCC oral squamous cell carcinoma
OSCE objective structured clinical examination
OS-CS osteopathia striata—cranial sclerosis [syndrome]
OSDAT Oslo Study Diet and Antismoking Trial
OSE ovarian surface epithelium
OS-EM ordered-subsequent expectation maximization
OSF open software foundation; organ system failure; osteoclast-stimulating factor; outer spiral fiber; overgrowth stimulating factor
OSF/DCE open software foundation/distributed computing environment
OSG Office of the Surgeon General
OSGi open services gateway initiative
OSHA Occupational Safety and Health Administration
OSH Act Occupational Safety and Health Act of 1970
OsHV ostreid herpesvirus
OSI open systems interconnection; owner stopped in [veterinary medicine]

OSIRIS Open Study of Infants at High Risk or with Respiratory Insufficiency: the Role of Surfactants; Optimization Study of Infarct Reperfusion Investigated by ST-Monitoring
OSLER objectively structured long examination record; Offspring of Systemic Lupus Erythematosus Mothers Registry
OSM ovine submaxillary mucin; oxygen saturation meter
Osm osmolarity, osmosis
osm osmole; osmosis, osmotic
OSMED otospondylometaphyseal dysplasia
Osm/kg osmoles per kilogram
Osm/L osmoles per liter
osmol osmole
OSMT Ontario Society of Medical Technologists
O-SP O-specific polysaccharide
OspA outer surface protein A
OSQL object structure query language
OSRC osteosarcoma
OSRD Office of Scientific Research and Development
OSS osseous; over-the-shoulder strap
oss osseous
OSSAV Ossa virus
OST object sorting test; Office of Science and Technology; opioid substitution therapy; osteosarcoma takase cells; Ottawa Stroke Trial
osteo osteoarthritis; osteomyelitis; osteopathy
OSTI Optimal Stent Implantation [trial]
OSTP Office of Science and Technology Policy
OSUK Ophthalmological Society of the United Kingdom
OSV observable state variable
OT objective test; oblique talus; occlusion time; occupational therapist, occupational therapy; ocular tension; office therapy; old term [anatomy]; old tuberculin; olfactory threshold; on treatment; optic tract; orientation test; original tuberculin; ornithine transcarbamylase; orotracheal; orthopedic treatment; otolaryngology; otology; oxytocin; oxytryptamine
Ot otolaryngology
OTA occupational therapy assistant; ochratoxin A; Office of Technology Assessment; ornithine transaminase; Orthodontic Technicians Association [UK]; orthotoluidine arsenite
OTBA open tranaxillary breast augmentation
OTC ornithine transcarbamylase; oval target cell; ovarian tissue culture; over-the-counter; oxytetracycline

OTCD ornithine carbamoyltransferase deficiency

OTD oculotrichodysplasia; oral temperature device; organ tolerance dose

OTE optically transparent electrode

OTF octamer-binding transcription factor; optical transfer function; oral transfer factor; outpatient treatment file

OTFC oral transmucosal fentanyl citrate

OTI ovomucoid trypsin inhibitor

OTIS Organization of Teratology Information Specialists

OTM orthotoluidine manganese sulfate

OTO otology; otorhinolaryngology

OTOF orthogonal time-of-flight

Otol otology, otologist

OTPS other than personal services

OTR Occupational Therapist, Registered; Ovarian Tumor Registry

OTReg Occupational Therapist, Registered

OTRs organ transplant recipients

OTS n-octadecyltrichlorosilane; occipital temporal sulcus; optical tracking system; orotracheal suction

OTSG Office of the Surgeon General

OTSMD Ornithine Transcarbamoylase Structure and Mutation Database

OTT orotracheal tube

OTU olfactory tubercle; operational taxonomic unit

OTW over the wire

OTZ oxathiozolidine

OU observation unit; Oppenheimer-Urbach [syndrome]

ou both eyes together [L. *oculi unitas*]

OUAV Ouango virus

OUB ouabain

OUBIV Oubi virus

OUBR ouabain resistance

OULQ outer upper left quadrant

OUME operative unit of medical herpetology

OUR oxygen uptake rate

OURQ outer upper right quadrant

OURS Oxford University Research Study; oxygen utilization rate study

OURV Ourem virus

OUS overuse syndrome

OUTCLAS Outpatient Coronary Low-Profile Angioplasty Study

OUTI other urinary tract infections

OV oculovestibular; office visit; oncovirus; osteoid volume; outflow volume; ovalbumin; ovary; overventilation; ovulation

Ov ovary

ov ovum

OVA ovalbumin

ova ovariectomy

OVAT Ongoing Violence Assessment Tool

OVC ovarian cancer

OVD occlusal vertical dimension; ophthalmic viscosurgical device

OvDF ovarian dysfunction

OvHV ovine herpesvirus

OVLT organum vasculosum of the lamina terminalis

OVRV Oak-Vale virus

OVSMC ovine vascular smooth muscle cell

OVX ovariectomized

OW once weekly; open wedge; outcome washing; outer wall; oval window; overweight

O/W, o/w oil in water

OWCL Old World cutaneous leishmaniasis

OWI Office of Worksite Initiatives

OW/O overweight and obesity

o/w/o oil in water/oil

OWR Osler-Weber-Rendu [syndrome]; ovarian wedge resection

OWS outerwear syndrome

OX optic chiasma; orthopedic examination; oxacillin; oxalate; oxide; oxytocin

Ox oxygen

ox oxidized

OXA oxaprotiline

OXCHECK Oxford and Collaborators Health Check [trial]

OXIPHOS oxidative phosphorylation

OxLDL, Ox-LDL oxidized low-density lipoprotein

OXMIS Oxford Myocardial Infarction Incidence Study

Oxo oxanosine

8oxoA 8-oxoadenine

8oxoG 8-oxoguanine

OXP oxypressin

OXPHOS oxidative phosphorylation

OXT oxytocin

OXTR oxytocin receptor

OXY oxytocin

OXY, oxy oxygen

OYE old yellow enzyme

OYS Oslo Youth study

oz ounce

oz ap, oz apoth apothecary ounce

OZD optic zone diameter

oz t, oz tr troy ounce

P

P an electrocardiographic wave corresponding to a wave of depolarization crossing the atria; by weight [L. *pondere*]; father [L. *pater*]; near [L. *proximum*]; near point [L. *punctum proximum*]; pain; parietal electrode placement [EEG]; parity; part; partial pressure; *Pasteurella*; paternal; patient; penicillin; penta- [10^{15}]; percent; percussion; perforation; permeability; peta-; pharmacopeia; phenophthalein; phenylalanine; phosphate group; phosphorus; physiology; pig; pint; placebo; plan; plasma; *Plasmodium*; *Pneumocystis*; point; poise; poison, poisoning; polarity; polarization; pole; polymyxin; pons; population; porcelain; porcine; porphyrin; position; positive; posterior; postpartum; power; precipitin; precursor; prednisone; premolar; presbyopia; pressure; primary; primipara; probability; product; progesterone; prolactin; proline; promoter; properdin; propionate; protein; *Proteus*; proximal; *Pseudomonas*; psychiatry; pulmonary; pulse; pupil; radiant power; significance probability; simple programmable [pacemaker]; sound power; weight [L. *pondus*]

φ uppercase Greek letter phi; magnetic flux; osmotic coefficient

Π uppercase Greek letter pi

π lowercase Greek letter pi; the ratio of circumference to diameter

ψ Greek letter psi; wave function

P₁ first parental generation; pulmonic first sound

P.1 gamma variant of SARS-CoV-2 [also called Brazil variant]

P.2 zeta variant of SARS-CoV-2

P₂ pulmonic second sound

P₃ proximal third

P³ primary prevention project

P-50 oxygen half-saturation pressure

P₉₀ 90th percentile

p atomic orbital with angular momentum quantum number 1; freeze preservation; frequency of the more common allele of a pair; momentum; papilla; pathologic; phosphate; pico-; pint; pond; pressure; probability; proton; pulse; pupil; short arm of chromosome; sound pressure

p- para

p̄ after [L. *post*]

p24 HIV antigen

p120 phosphoprotein 120 (kDa)

PA panic attack; pantothenic acid; paralysis agitans; paranoia; parathion; passive aggressive; pathology; patient's advocate; peak amplitude; performance assessment; periarteritis; peridural artery; periodic acid; periodontal abscess; pernicious anemia; perpetual asymmetry; phakic-aphakic; phenylalanine; phenylalkylamine; phosphatidic acid; phosphoarginine; photoallergy; phthalic anhydride; physical abuse; physical activity; physician advisor; physician assistant; pituitary-adrenal; plasma adsorption; plasma aldosterone; plasminogen activator; platelet adhesiveness; platelet aggregation; platelet associated; plicatic acid; polyamine; polyarteritis; polyarthritis; post-aural; posteroanterior; preadipocyte; prealbumin; preamplifier; predictive accuracy; pregnancy associated; presents again; pressure augmentation [respiration]; primary aldosteronism; primary amenorrhea; primary anemia; prior to admission; proactivator; proanthocyanidin; procainamide; professional association; prolonged action; propionic acid; prostate antigen; protective antigen; proteolytic action; prothrombin activity; protrusio acetabuli; pseudoaneurysm; *Pseudomonas aeruginosa*; psychoanalysis; psychogenic aspermia; pulmonary arterial [pressure]; pulmonary artery; pulmonary atresia; pulpoaxial; puromycin aminonucleoside; pyrrolizidine alkaloid; pyruvic acid; yearly [L. *per annum*]

P-A posteroanterior

P(A) probability of event A

P&A percussion and auscultation

Pₐ alveolar pressure; atrial pressure; paternal allele; partial pressure of arterial fluid

PA3 Atrial Pacing Peri-Ablation for Paroxysmal Atrial Fibrillation [trial]

Pa acellular pertussis [vaccine]; atrial pressure; pascal; pathologist, pathology; prealbumin; protactinium; *Pseudomonas aeruginosa*; pulmonary arterial [pressure]

pA picoampere

pa through the anus [L. *per anum*]; yearly [L. *per annum*]

PAA partial agonist activity; phenylacetic acid; phosphonoacetic acid; physical abilities analysis; plasma angiotensinase activity; polyacrylamide; polyacrylic acid; polyamino acid; popliteal artery aneurysm; pyridine acetic acid

PAAI personal access and alert interface

pAAM polyacrylamide

P(A − a)O₂ alveolar-arterial oxygen pressure difference

PAAS panic and anticipatory anxiety scale

PAB para-aminobenzoate; passenger air bags; performance assessment battery; pharmacologic autonomic block; poly(A) binding [protein]; premature atrial beat; purple agar base

Pab abdominal pressure

pAb polyclonal antibody

PABA, pABA para-aminobenzoic acid

PABD predeposit autologous blood donation

PABN polyadenylate-binding protein, nuclear

PABP poly-A binding protein; pulmonary artery balloon pump

PABV percutaneous aortic balloon valvuloplasty

PAC P1 artificial chromosome; paclitaxel; papular acrodermatitis of childhood; parent-adult-child; pericarditis, arthropathy, camptodactyly [syndrome]; phenacetin, aspirin, and caffeine; physical activity [scale]; plasma aldosterone concentration; platelet-associated complement; Policy Advisory Committee; preadmission certification; predictive acquisition cost; premature atrial contraction; product of ambulatory care; pulmonary arterial capacitance; pulmonary artery catheter, pulmonary artery catheterization

pac pachytene

PACAP pituitary adenylate cyclase activating polypeptide

PAC-A-TACH Pacemaker Atrial Tachycardia [trial]

PACC primary ambulatory care center; promoting aphasics' communicative competence

PACCO Pulmonary Artery Catheterization and Clinical Outcomes [study]

PACCS Prospective Army Coronary Calcium Study

PACE Pacing and Clinical Electrophysiology; paired basic amino acid cleaving enzyme; Partnership in Active Continuous Education; Patient Care Expert; People with Arthritis Can Exercise [program]; personalized aerobics for cardiovascular enhancement; population-adjusted clinical epidemiology; Prevention with Low-Dose Aspirin of Cardiovascular Diseases in the Elderly [study]; primary ambulatory care and education; Program of All-inclusive Care for the Elderly; pulmonary angiotensin I converting enzyme

PACI Partnership for Advanced Computational Infrastructure

PACIFIC potential angina class improvement from intramyocardial channels

PACK Prevention of Atherosclerotic Complications with Ketanserin [study]

PACNS primary angiitis of the central nervous system

PA$_{CO}$ mean alveolar gas volume

Pa$_{CO_2}$ partial pressure of carbon dioxide in arterial blood

PACP pulmonary alveolar-capillary permeability; pulmonary artery counterpulsation

PACS picture archiving and communication system; postoperative atrial fibrillation in cardiac surgery

PACS DB picture archiving and communication system database

PACST Putney Auditory Comprehension Screening Test

PACT papillary carcinoma of thyroid; Philadelphia Association of Clinical Trialists; Plasminogen Activator Angioplasty Compatibility Trial; Plasminogen Activator Coronary Angioplasty Trial; precordial acceleration tracing; Prehospital Application of Coronary Thrombolysis [study]; prepaid accountable care term; prescription analyses and cost; Prospective Acute Coronary Syndrome Trial; Pro-urokinase in Acute Coronary Thrombosis [study]

PACU postanesthesia care unit

PACV Pacui virus

PACWP pulmonary arterial capillary wedge pressure

PAD pain and distress; patient surface axis depth; percutaneous abscess drainage; percutaneous automated discectomy; peripheral artery disease; phenacetin, aspirin, and desoxyephedrine; photon absorption densitometry; practitioners accessing data; primary affective disorder; psychoaffective disorder; public access to defibrillation; pulmonary artery diastolic; pulsatile assist device; Pulse Arrhythmia Detection; pulsed amperometric detection

PADI peptidylarginine deiminase

PAD-I Public Access Defibrillation I [trial]

PADL personal activities of daily living

PADP pulmonary artery diastolic pressure

PADPRP, pADPRP polyadenosine diphosphate−ribose polymerase

PADS patient archiving and documentation system

PADSS Postanesthesia Discharge Scoring System

PADUA progressive augmentation by dilating the urethra anterior

PAdV 1 to 5 porcine adenoviruses 1 to 5

PAdV-A, -B, -C porcine adenoviruses A, B, C

PADyC passive arm with dynamic constraints

PAE paradoxic air embolism; parsimony analysis of endemicity; postanoxic encephalopathy; postantibiotic effect; progressive assistive exercise

PAEC porcine aortic endothelial cell

PAED pediatric anesthesia emergence delirium

paed pediatrics

PAEDP pulmonary artery end-diastolic pressure

PAEP progestagen-associated endometrial protein

PAES popliteal artery entrapment syndrome

PAF paroxysmal atrial fibrillation; peroxisomal assembly factor; phosphodiesterase-activating factor; plain abdominal film; platelet-activating factor; platelet-aggregating factor; pollen adherence factor; population-attributable fractions; premenstrual assessment form; progressive autonomic failure; pulmonary arteriovenous fistula; pure autonomic failure

PA&F percussion, auscultation, and fremitus

PAFA priority-based assessment of foot additives

PAF-A platelet-activating factor of anaphylaxis

PAFAC Prevention of Atrial Fibrillation After Cardioversion [study]

PAFAH platelet-activating factor acetylhydrolase

PAFAMS Pan-American Federation of Associations of Medical Schools

PAFD percutaneous abscess and fluid drainage; pulmonary artery filling defect

PAFI platelet-aggregation factor inhibitor

PAFIB paroxysmal atrial fibrillation

PAFIT Paroxysmal Atrial Fibrillation Italian Trial

PAFP pre-Achilles fat pad

PAFra platelet-activating factor receptor antagonist

PAFT Propafenone Atrial Fibrillation Trial

PAG periaqueductal gray [matter]; polyacrylamide gel; pregnancy-associated globulin; proliferation-associated gene; proximal anastomosis graft; pulmonary arteriography

pAg protein A—gold [technique]

PAGA proliferation-associated gene A

PAGE perfluorocarbon-associated gas exchange; polyacrylamide gel electrophoresis

PAGE-IEF polyacrylamine gel electrophoresis isoelectric focusing

PAGIF polyacrylamide gel isoelectric focusing

PAGMK primary African green monkey kidney

PAGOD pulmonary hypoplasia, hypoplasia of pulmonary artery, agonadism, omphalocele/diaphragmatic defect, dextrocardia [syndrome]

PAH para-aminohippurate; phenylalanine hydroxylase; polycyclic aromatic hydrocarbon; predicted adult height; pulmonary alveolar hypoventilation; pulmonary artery hypertension; pulmonary artery hypotension

PAHA para-aminohippuric acid; procainamide-hydroxylamine

PAHCOM Professional Association of Health Care Office Management

PAHO Pan-American Health Organization

PAHP *p*-aminoheptanoylphenone

PAHV Pahayokee virus

PAHVC pulmonary alveolar hypoxic vasoconstrictor

PAI pain assessment inventory; partial androgen insensitivity; pathogenicity island; patient assessment instrument; perforating arterial infarction; plasminogen activator inhibitor; platelet accumulation index; pregnancy after infertility

PAI-1 plasminogen activator inhibitor 1

PAI-2 plasminogen activator inhibitor 2

PAIC procedures, alternatives, indications, and complications

PAICS phosphoribosylaminoimidazole carboxylase

PAID problem areas in diabetes

PAIDS paralyzed academic investigator's disease syndrome; pediatric acquired immunodeficiency syndrome

PAIg platelet-associated immunoglobulin

PAIgG platelet-associated immunoglobulin G

PAIMS Plasminogen Activator Italian Multicenter Study

PAIN pyoderma gangrenosum, aphthous stomatitis, inflammatory eye disease, erythema nodosum

PAIRS Pain and Impairment Relationship Scale

P_airway airway pressure

PAIS partial androgen insensitivity syndrome; phosphoribosylaminoimidazole synthetase; Pravastatin in Acute Ischemic Syndromes [study]; psychosocial adjustment to illness scale

PAIS-SR psychosocial adjustment to illness scale, self-reported

PAIVS Pulmonary Atresia with Intact Ventricular Septum [study]

PAJ paralysis agitans juvenilis

PAK p21-activated kinase; pancreas after kidney [transplantation]

PAKY percutaneous access to kidney

PAKY-RCM percutaneous access to kidney—remote center of motion

PAL pathology laboratory; peptidyl-alpha-hydroxyglycine alpha-amidating lysine phase alteration plane; physical activity level; pointer to text application language; posterior assisted levitation; posterior axillary line; power-assisted lipoplasty; product of activated lymphocytes; pyogenic abscess of the liver

pal palate

PALA *N*-(phosphonacetyl)-L-aspartate

PALF pediatric acute liver failure

PALP placental alkaline phosphatase

palp palpable; palpate, palpation

palpi palpitation

PALS parietolateral lymphocyte sheath; Patient Advocacy and Liaison Service; pediatric advanced life support; prison-acquired lymphoproliferative syndrome

PALV Palyam virus

PAM pancreatic acinar mass; penicillin aluminum monostearate; peptidylglycine alpha-amidating monooxygenase; phenylalaline mustard; physical agent modality; *p*-methoxyamphetamine; postauricular myogenic; potassium-aggravated myotonia; pralidoxime; prearrest morbidity; pregnancy-associated alpha-macroglobulin; primary amebic meningoencephalitis; principles of ambulatory medicine; professions allied to medicine; pulmonary alveolar macrophage; pulmonary alveolar microlithiasis; pulse amplitude modulation; pyridine aldoxime methiodide

PAMC pterygoarthromyodysplasia congenita

2-PAM Cl 2-pralidoxime chloride

PAMD primary adrenocortical micronodular dysplasia

PAME preanesthesia medical examination; primary amebic meningoencephalitis

PAMED Pennsylvania Medical Society

PAMI Primary Angioplasty in Myocardial Infarction [trial]

PAMIE physical and mental impairment of function evaluation

PAMI-No SOS Primary Angioplasty in Myocardial Infarction with No Surgery on Site

PAMP pathogen-associated molecular pattern; pulmonary artery mean pressure

PAMR progressively automated medical record

PAMV Pampa virus

PAN periarteritis nodosa; periodic alternating nystagmus; peroxyacylnitrate; personal area network; polyacrylonitril; polyarteritis nodosa; positional alcohol nystagmus; puromycin aminonucleoside

pan pancreas, pancreatic, pancreatectomy

PanIN pancreatic intraepithelial neoplasia

Panc pancreas or pancreatic

pANCA perinuclear antineutrophil antibodies

P-ANCA perinuclear antineutrophilic cytoplasmic antibody

PAND primary adrenocortical nodular dysplasia

PANDA Paediatric Asthma Education of a New Multidose Dry Powder Inhaler [study]

PANDAS pediatric autoimmune neuropsychiatric disorders associated with streptococcal infection

PANE pediatric ambulance needs evaluation

PANI polyanilide

PANS puromycin aminonucleoside

PANSS Positive and Negative Syndrome Scale

PANSS-EC Positive and Negative Symptom Scale–Excitement Component

PAO peak acid output; periacetabular osteotomy; peripheral airway obstruction; plasma amine oxidase; polyamine oxidase; pulmonary artery occlusion; pustulotic arthroosteitis

PAO₂ alveolar oxygen partial pressure

PAo airway opening pressure; ascending aortic pressure; pulmonary artery occlusion pressure

PaO₂ partial arterial oxygen tension

PAO₂/FIO₂, PaO₂/FiO₂ ratio of alveolar partial pressure of oxygen to fraction of inspired air

PAOD peripheral arterial occlusive disease; peripheral arteriosclerotic occlusive disease

Pao max peak airway pressure

PAOP *p*-aminooctanoylphenone; pulmonary artery occlusion pressure

PaOP pulmonary artery occlusion pressure

PAP pancreatitis-associated protein; Papanicolaou [test]; papaverine; passive-aggressive personality; password authentication protocol; patient assessment program; peak airway pressure; peroxidase antibody to peroxidase; peroxidase-antiperoxidase [method]; phosphoadenosine phosphate; placental acid/alkaline phosphatase; poly-A polymerase; positive airway pressure; primary atypical pneumonia; prostatic acid phosphatase; pulmonary alveolar proteinosis; pulmonary artery pressure; purified alternate pathway

Pap Papanicolaou [test]

pap papilla

PAPC paraxial protocadherin

PAPF platelet adhesiveness plasma factor

papova papilloma polyoma vacuolating agent [virus]

PAPP para-aminopropiophenone; pregnancy-associated plasma protein

PAPPA pregnancy-associated plasma protein A

PAPPC pregnancy-associated plasma protein C

PAPR powered air-purifying respirator

PAPS 3′-phosphoadenosine-5′-phosphosulfate; primary antiphospholipid antibody syndrome

Paps papillomas

Pap sm Papanicolaou smear

PAPUFA physiologically active polyunsaturated fatty acid

pa-pv pulmonary arterial pressure−pulmonary venous pressure

PAPVC partial anomalous pulmonary venous connection

PAPVD partial anomalous pulmonary venous drainage

PAPVR partial anomalous pulmonary venous return

PAQ patient asked questions; Personal Attitudes Questionnaire

PAQLQ Pediatric Asthma Quality-of-Life Questionnaire

PAR parent in semantic hierarchy; participating provider; passive avoidance reaction; percentage abnormal results; perennial allergic rhinitis; photosynthetically active radiation; Physical Activity Recall [questionnaire]; physiologic aging rate; plain abdominal radiograph; platelet aggregation receptor; platelet/aggregate ratio; Policy, Action, and Rational Drug Use; population-attributable risk; population-attribute risk [calculation]; postanesthesia recovery; postanesthesia room; posterior wall or aortic root; primary angioplasty research; Program for Alcohol Recovery; proximal alveolar region; pseudoautosomal region; pulmonary arteriolar resistance

PAR% population-attributable risk percent

par paraffin; paralysis

PAR-2 proteinase-activated receptor inhibitor 2

PARA, Para, para number of pregnancies producing viable offspring

para paraplegic; parathyroid; parathyroidectomy

para 0 nullipara

para 1, para I primipara

para 2, para II secundipara

para 3, para III tripara

para 4, para IV quadripara

PARADIGM Platelet Aggregation Receptor Antagonist Dose Investigation for Perfusion Gain in Myocardial Infarction [study]

PARADISE Platelet IIb/IIIa Antagonism for the Reduction of Acute Coronary Events

Dose Investigation and Safety Evaluation [study]

PARAGON Platelet IIb/IIIa Antagonist for the Reduction of Acute Coronary Syndrome Events in a Global Organization Network [study]

parasit parasitology; parasite, parasitic

parasym parasympathetic

PARAT Prevention of Arterial Restenosis Angiographic Trial

PARC Palo Alto Research Center; Pan-African Rinderpest Campaign

PARCO parallel computing

parent parenteral

pArg poly-L-arginine

PARIS Peripheral Artery Radiation Investigational Study; Persantine Aspirin Reinfarction Study

PARK Postangioplasty Restenosis Ketanserin [study]; Prevention of Angioplasty Reocclusion with Ketanserin

parox paroxysm, paroxysmal

PARP poly(adenosine diphosphate ribose) polymerase

PARR plasma aldosterone/renin activity ratio; postanesthesia recovery room

PARS Personal Adjustment and Role Skills Scale

PART Prevention of Atherosclerosis with Ramipril Therapy [trial]; Probucol Angioplasty Restenosis Trial

PART-1 Predictors of Atherosclerosis Risk and Thrombosis [trial]

PART-2 Predictors of Atherosclerosis Risk and Thrombosis [trial]

PARTNER Peripheral Arterial Disease Response to Taprostene with New Established Response Criteria [trial]

PARTNERS Primary Care Access to Resources, Training, Networks, Education, and Research Services

PARTY prevent alcohol and risk-related trauma in youth

PARU postanesthesia recovery unit

PARV Parana virus

ParVox Parallel Volume Rendering System for Scientific Visualization [trial]

PAS para-aminosalicylate; Paragon Elective or Acute Stent [trial]; Parent Attitude Scale; patient administration system; patient appointments and scheduling; periodic acid−Schiff; peripheral anterior synechia; persistent atrial standstill; Personality Assessment Scale; photoacoustic spectroscopy; phosphatase acid serum; physician-assisted suicide; Polish Amiodarone Study; posterior airway space; preadmission screening; predictive accuracy on survival; pregnancy advisory service; premature atrial stimulus; professional activity study; progressive accumulated stress; pulmonary arterial stenosis; pulmonary artery systolic

Pas, Pa·s, Pa × s pascal-second

PASA para-aminosalicylic acid; polymerase chain reaction amplification of specific alleles; primary acquired sideroblastic anemia; proximal articular set angle

PASAR programmable automatic scanning arrhythmia reversion [algorithm]

PASAR-O orthorhythmic programmable automatic scanning arrhythmia reversion [algorithm]

PASARR preadmission screening and resident review

PASAT Paced Auditory Serial Addition Task

PASB protein-associated strand breaks

PAS-C para-aminosalicylic acid crystallized with ascorbic acid

PASD after diastase digestion

PASE Pacemaker Selection in the Elderly [trial]; physical activity scale for the elderly [evaluation]

PASG pneumatic antishock garment

PASH periodic acid−Schiff hematoxylin; pseudoangiomatous stromal hyperplasia

PASI psoriasis area severity index

PASM periodic acid−silver methenamine

PASP pancreas-specific protein; polymer-assisted solution phase; pulmonary artery systolic pressure

PASS personal alerting safety system; Piracetam in Acute Stroke Study; Postarthroplasty Screening Study [for deep venous thrombosis]; Practical Applicability of Saruplase Study; Prehospital Applicability of Saruplase Study

pass passive

PASSOR Physiatric Association of Spine, Sports, and Occupational Rehabilitation

pass ROM passive range of motion

PAST periodic acid−Schiff technique

Past *Pasteurella*

PASTA partial articular supraspinatus tendon avulsion [lesion]; Percutaneous Ambulatory Stent Trial; polarity-altered spectral-selective acquisition; Primary Angioplasty vs Stent Implantation in Acute Myocardial Infarction [trial]

PAstV porcine astrovirus

PASVR pulmonary anomalous superior venous return

PASW personal assistance service worker

PAT Pain Apperception Test; paroxysmal atrial tachycardia; patient; patient domain; penetrating abdominal trauma; peripheral

arterial tonometry; phenylaminotetrazole; physical abilities test; picric acid turbidity; platelet aggregation test; Polish Amiodarone Trial; polyamine acetyltransferase; postoperative atrial tachycardia; preadmission assessment team; preadmission assessment test; preadmission testing; predictive ability test; pregnancy at term; psychoacoustic test

pat patella; patent; paternal origin; patient

PATAF Prevention of Arterial Thromboembolism in Nonvalvular Atrial Fibrillation [study]; Primary Prevention of Arterial Thromboembolic Processes in Atrial Fibrillation [trial]

PATAV Pata virus

PATCH planned approach to community health

Pat-CIS patient clinical information system

PatDp paternal duplication

PATE Pravastatin Anti-Atherosclerosis Trial in the Elderly; psychodynamic and therapeutic education; pulmonary artery thromboembolism

PATENT Pro-Urokinase and Tissue Plasminogen Activator Enhancement of Thrombolysis [trial]

PATG patient group

PATH pathologic function; pathologic, pathology; pituitary adrenotropic hormone; physicians at teaching hospitals

path pathogenesis, pathogenic; pathologic, pathology

PATHS Prevention and Treatment of Hypertension Study

Patm atmospheric pressure

PATMAN Patient Workflow Management [system]

PAtr pulmonary atresia

PATRIC position and time−resolved ion counting

PATS Poststroke Antihypertensive Treatment Study; Prehospital Administration of Tissue Plasminogen Activator Study; Protection Assessment Test System

PAT-SED pseudoachondroplastic dysplasia

PA-T-SP periodic acid−thiocarbo-hydrazide−silver proteinate

PATV Patois virus

PAU penetrating aortic ulcer; phenol−acetic acid−urea

PAUP phylogenic analysis using parsimony

PAUSE Popliteal Artery Ultrasound Examination [study]

PAV percutaneous aortic valvuloplasty; poikiloderma atrophicans vasculare; posterior arch vein; proportional assist ventilation

PaV Pariacoto virus

Pav airway pressure
P_{ave} mean average pressure during inspiration
PAVEC porcine aortic valve endothelial cell
pavex passive vascular exercise
PAVF pulmonary arteriovenous fistula
PAVM pulmonary arteriovenous malformation
PAVNRT paroxysmal atrioventricular nodal reciprocal tachycardia
pAVP plasma arginine vasopressin
PA-VSD pulmonary atresia with ventricular septal defect
PAW peripheral airways; pulmonary artery wedge
P_{AW}, Paw airway pressure
PAWP pulmonary arterial wedge pressure
PAWS primary withdrawal syndrome
PAX paired box homeotic [family]
PAZ prednisone/azathioprine
PB British Pharmacopeia [*Pharmacopoeia Britannica*]; paraffin bath; paraffin block; paucibacillary; Paul-Bunnell [antibody]; periodic breathing; peripheral blood; peroneus brevis; phenobarbital; phenoxybenzamine; phonetically balanced; pinealoblastoma; Polybrene; polymyxin B; premature beat; pressure breathing; protein binding; punch biopsy; pyridostigmine bromide
P_B barometric pressure
P&B pain and burning; phenobarbital and belladonna
Pb body [surface] pressure; lead [L. *plumbum*]; phenobarbital; presbyopia
PBA polyclonal B-cell activity; pressure breathing assist; prolactin-binding assay; prune belly anomaly; pulpobuccoaxial
PBAC Pharmaceutical Benefits Advisory Committee
PBAL protected bronchoalveolar lavage
PBB polybrominated biphenyl
Pb-B lead in blood
PBC perfusion balloon catheter; peripheral blood cell; phosphocreatine; point of basal convergence; prebed care; primary biliary cirrhosis; progestin-binding complement
PBCC point biserial correlation coefficient
PBCH polymorphic B-cell hyperplasia
PBCL polymorphic B-cell lymphoma
PBCRA progressive bifocal chorioretinal atrophy
PBCV *Paramecium bursaria* chlorella virus
PBD postburn day
PBDE polybrominated diphenyl ether
PBE tuberculin from *Mycobacterium tuberculosis bovis* [Ger. *Perlsucht Bacillen-emulsion*]
PBF pencil beam function [radiotherapy]; peripheral blood flow; placental blood flow;

predominant breast feeding; pulmonary blood flow
PBFE peroxisomal bifunctional enzyme
PBFe protein-bound iron
PBG porphobilinogen
PBGD porphobilinogen deaminase
PBGS, PBG-S porphobilinogen synthase
PBH profiling by hybridization; pulling-boat hands; pyrenabutyric acid hydrazide
PBHB poly-beta-hydroxybutyrate
PBI parental bonding instrument; penile pressure/brachial pressure index; protein-bound iodine
PbI lead intoxication
PBIgG platelet surface-bound immunoglobulin G
PBK phosphorylase B kinase
PBL peripheral blood leukocyte; peripheral blood lymphocyte; problem-based learning
PBLC peripheral blood lymphocyte count; premature birth living child; problem-based learning curriculum
PBLM problem-based learning module
PBLT peripheral blood lymphocyte transformation
PBM pancreatobiliary maljunction; peak bone mass; peripheral basement membrane; peripheral blood mononuclear [cell]; pharmacy benefit manager; placental basement membrane; prescription benefit manager
PBMA poly n-butyl methacrylate
PBMC percutaneous balloon mitral commissurotomy; peripheral blood mononuclear cell; pharmaceutical benefit management company
PBMNC peripheral blood mononuclear cell
PBMV percutaneous balloon mitral valvuloplasty; pulmonary blood mixing volume
PBN α-phenyl-*n-tert*-butylnitrone; paralytic brachial neuritis; peripheral benign neoplasm; polymyxin B sulfate, bacitracin, and neomycin
PBNA partial body neutron activation
PBO penicillin in beeswax and oil; placebo
PBP penicillin-binding protein; platelet basic protein; porphyrin biosynthesis pathway; prostate-binding protein; pseudobulbar palsy; pulsatile bypass pump
PBPC peripheral blood progenitor cell; progressive bulbar palsy of childhood
PBPI penile-brachial pulse index
PBPK physiologically based pharmacokinetic [model]
PBPND progressive bulbar palsy with neural deafness
PBPV percutaneous balloon pulmonary valvuloplasty

PBRN practice-based research network

PBS perfusion-pressure breakthrough syndrome; phenobarbital sodium; phosphate-buffered saline; planar bone scan; primer binding site; protected brush specimen; prune belly syndrome; pulmonary branch stenosis

PBSA phosphate buffered saline [solution]

PBSC peripheral blood stem cell

PBSCT peripheral blood stem cell transplantation

PBSP prognostically bad signs during pregnancy

PBT Paul-Bunnell test; persistent, bioaccumulative, and toxic; phenacetin breath test; piebald trait; profile-based therapy; pulmonary barotrauma

PBT₄ protein-bound thyroxine

PBV predicted blood volume; pulmonary blood volume

PBW posterior bite wing; present breast width

PBX private branch exchange

PBZ personal breathing zone; phenylbutazone; phenoxybenzamine; pyribenzamine

PC avoirdupois weight [L. *pondus civile*]; pacinian corpuscle; packed cells; paper chromatography; paracortex; paramyotonia congenita; parent cell; particulate component; partition coefficient; patch clamp; penicillin; penile carcinoma; pentose cycle; peritoneal cell; personal care; personal computer; pharmacology; phase contrast; pheochromocytoma; phosphate cycle; phosphatidylcholine; phosphorylcholine; photoconduction; physicians' corporation; pill counter; piriform cortex; placebo controlled; plasma concentration; plasma cortisol; plasmacytoma; plasmin complex; plastocyanin; platelet concentrate; platelet count; pneumotaxic center; polycarbonate; polycentric; polyposis coli; poor condition; poor coordination; portacaval; portal cirrhosis; postcoital; posterior cervical; posterior chamber; posterior commissure; posterior cortex; potential complications; preconditioned, preconditioning; precordial; prenatal care; present complaint; primary closure; principal component; printed circuit; procollagen; productive cough; professional corporation; prohormone convertase; prophlogistic corticoid; prostacyclin; prostatic carcinoma; protective cover; protein C; protein convertase; proximal colon; pseudocyst; pubococcygeus; pulmonary capillary; pulmonary circulation; pulmonary compliance; pulmonic closure; Purkinje cell; pyloric canal; pyruvate carboxylase

PC1 first principal component

P꜀ critical pressure

pc parsec; percent; picocurie

p.c. after meals [L. *post cibum*]

p/c presenting complaint

PCA pancreatic carcinoma; para-chloramphetamine; parietal cell antibody; passive cutaneous anaphylaxis; patient care aide; patient care assistant; patient care audit; patient-controlled analgesia; penicillamine; perchloric acid; percutaneous carotid angiography; percutaneous coronary angioplasty; personal care assistant; personal computer advisory; phenylcarboxylic acid; Physicians Corporation of America; plasma catecholamine; plate count agar; polyclonal antibody; porcine coronary artery; porous coated anatomic [prosthesis]; portacaval anastomosis; postconceptional age; postcoronary arrest; posterior cerebral artery; posterior communicating aneurysm; posterior communicating artery; posterior cricoarytenoid; precoronary care area; prehospital cardiac arrest; President's Council on Aging; principal components analysis; procainamide; procoagulant activity; program component area; prostatic carcinoma; protected catheter aspirate; protective concentration level; pyrrolidine carboxylic acid

PcA prostatic adenocarcinoma

PCAD Patent Citation Analysis Database; progression of coronary artery disease

pCAF phasic carotid activation function

PCAPS Primary Care Act Pilot Sites

PCASSO Patient-Centered Access to Secure System Online

PCAST President's Committee of Advisors on Science and Technology; President's Council of Advisors on Science and Technology

PCASYS pattern-level classification automation system

PCAT phosphatidylcholine-cholesterol acyltransferase; primary care assessment tool

PCAV Pacora virus

PCB paracervical block; polychlorinated biphenyl; portacaval bypass; postcoital bleeding; printed circuit board; procarbazine

PcB near point of convergence to the intercentral base line [L. *punctum convergens basalis*]

PC-BMP phosphorylcholine-binding myeloma protein

PCC Pasteur Culture Collection; patient-centered care; percutaneous cecostomy; peripheral cholangiocarcinoma; pheochromocytoma; phosphate carrier compound; plasma catecholamine concentration; platinumcontaining compound; pneumatosis cystoides coli; Poison Control Center; precoronary care; premature chromosome condensation; primary care center/clinic; primary care continuum; primary care curriculum; prospective case control; protein C cofactor

PCc periscopic concave

pcc premature chromosome condensation

PCCA polychlorocycloalkane

PCCC pediatric critical care center

PCCF protein C cofactor

PC CLIN-SIM personal computer clinical simulation

PCCM pediatric critical care medicine; primary care case management; primary care case manager

PCCN Progressive Care Certified Nurse

PCCTEA patient-controlled continuous thoracic epidural analgesia

PCCU post-coronary care unit

PCD pacer-cardioverter-defibrillator; papillary collecting duct; paraneoplastic cerebellar degeneration; paroxysmal cerebral dysrhythmia; percutaneous catheter drainage; pervasive developmental disorder; phosphate-citrate-dextrose; plasma cell dyscrasia; polycystic disease; posterior corneal deposits; postmortem cesarean delivery; premature centromere division; primary ciliary dyskinesia; programmable cardioverter-defibrillator; programmed cell death; prolonged contractile duration; pterin-4a-carbinolamine dehydratase; pulmonary clearance delay

PCDC plasma clot diffusion chamber

PCDD Patient Clinical Data Directory; polychlorinated dibenzodioxin

PCDF polychorinated dibenzofuran

PCDS Patient Care Data Set

PCE patient care encounter; perchloroethylene; physical capacity evaluation; polychromatic erythrocyte; pseudocholinesterase

PCEA patient-controlled epidural anesthesia

pCEA polyclonal carcinoembryonic antigen

PCES patient care evaluation study

PCF peripheral circulatory failure; pharyngoconjunctival fever; platelet complement fixation; posterior cranial fossa; potential coding fragment

pcf pounds per cubic feet

PCFIA particle concentration of fluorescence immunoassay

PCFT platelet complement fixation test

PCG pancreato-cholangiography; paracervical ganglion; phonocardiogram, phonocardiography; pneumocardiogram; postcentral gyrus; preconditioned conjugate gradient; preventive

care group; primate chorionic gonadotropin; pubococcygeus

PCH paroxysmal cold hemoglobinuria; patient care hours; polycyclic hydrocarbon

PCHE pseudocholinesterase

PCHI Partners Community Health Care Incorporated

P²C² HIV Pediatric Pulmonary and Cardiovascular Complications of Human Immunodeficiency Virus Infection [study]; Pediatric Pulmonary and Cardiac Complications of Vertically Transmitted HIV Infection [study]

PCI patient classification index; percutaneous coronary intervention; pneumatosis cystoides intestinales; prophylactic cranial irradiation; protein C inhibitor; prothrombin consumption index

P/CI physical and chemical indicators

pCi picocurie

PCIC Poison Control Information Center

pCi/L picocuries per liter

PC-IRV pressure-controlled inverted ratio ventilation

PCIS Patient-Care Information System; point-of-care information system; postcardiac injury syndrome

PCK phosphoenolpyruvate carboxykinase; polycystic kidney

PCKD polycystic kidney disease

PCL pacing cycle length; packaging cell line; persistent corpus luteum; plasma cell leukemia; posterior chamber lens; posterior cruciate ligament; primary care loan; proximal collateral ligament; pubococcygeal line

PCLI plasma cell labeling index

PCM palliative care management; paracoccidioidomycosis; patient care management; patient care manager; phase contrast microscopy; primary cutaneous melanoma; process control monitor; protein-calorie malnutrition; protein carboxymethylase

PCMB parachloromercuribenzoate

PCMC protein-coated microcrystal

PCMO Principal Clinical Medical Officer

PCMR Pediatric Cardiomyopathy Registry

PC-MRA phase-contrast magnetic resonance angiography

PCMS patient care management system

PCMs patient care management categories

PCMT pacemaker circus movement tachycardia; protein carboxyl-methyltransferase

PCMX parachlorometoxylenol

PCN parent-child nursing; penicillin; pregnenolone-16α-carbonitrile; primary care network; primary care nursing

PCNA proliferating cell nuclear antigen

PCNB pentachloronitrobenzene
PCNL percutaneous nephrostolithotomy
PCNS Pediatric Clinical Nurse Specialist
PCNV postchemotherapy nausea and vomiting; Provisional Committee on Nomenclature of Viruses
PCO parametric clinical observation; patient complains of; polycystic ovary; posterior capsular opacification; predicted cardiac output
P$_{CO}$ partial pressure of carbon monoxide
P$_{CO2}$, pCO$_2$ partial pressure of carbon dioxide
PCOC Primary Care Organization Consortium
PCOD polycystic ovarian disease
PCOM phase-contrast optical method; posterior communicating [artery]
PCON Primary Care Organization Network
PCOS polycystic ovary syndrome
PCOV porcine type C oncovirus
PCP parachlorophenate; patient care plan; pentachlorophenol; 1-(1-phenylcyclohexyl) piperidine; peripheral coronary pressure; persistent cough and phlegm; phencyclidine palmitate; *Pneumocystis carinii* pneumonia; postoperative constrictive pericarditis; primary care physician; primary care provider; prochlorperazine; procollagen peptide; prolylcarboxypeptidase; pulmonary capillary pressure; pulse cytophotometry
PCPA para-chlorophenylalanine; Pest Control Practices Act
PCPB procarboxypeptide B
PCPL pulmonary capillary protein leakage
pcpn precipitation
PCPP poly[di(carboxylatophenoxy)phosphazene]
PC-PTSD Primary Care Posttraumatic Stress Disorder [screening tool]
PCPV pseudocowpox virus
PCQ polychloroquaterphenyl
PCR patient contact record; perinatal clinical record; phosphocreatinine; photoconvulsive response; plasma clearance rate; polymerase chain reaction [test]; postcompression remodeling; prehospital care report; principal component regression; protein catabolism rate
PCr phosphocreatine
P$_{Cr}$ plasma creatinine
pcr protein catabolic rate
PCRA percutaneous coronary rotational atherectomy
PCR-DS polymerase chain reaction–direct sequencing
PCR-ELISA polymerase chain reaction enzyme-linked immunosorbent assay
PCR-ISH polymerase chain reaction in situ hybridization
PCR-MASA polymerase chain reaction mutant allele–specific amplification
PCR-RFLP polymerase chain reaction restriction fragment-length polymorphism
PCR-RH polymerase chain reaction reverse hybridization
PCRS partner counseling and referral service
PCR/SSCP polymerase chain reaction single-stranded conformation polymorphism
PCRV Parry Creek virus; polycythemia rubra vera
PCS palliative care service; patient care system; patient classification system; patient-controlled sedation; patterns of care study; peak change in signal; pelvic congestion syndrome; pharmacogenic confusional syndrome; portacaval shunt; post cardiac surgery; postcardiotomy syndrome; postcholecystectomy syndrome; postconcussion syndrome; postnatal corticosteroids; premature centromere separation; Prevention of Coronary Atherosclerosis Study; primary cancer site; prolonged crush syndrome; proportional counter spectrometry; proximal coronary sinus; pseudotumor cerebri syndrome
pcs preconscious
PCS/ADS patient care system/application development system
PCSM percutaneous stone manipulation
PCSS Perth Community Stroke Study
PCSW personal care service worker
PCT peripheral carcinoid tumor; phase-contrast tomography; plasma clotting time; plasmacrit test; plasmacytoma; polychlorinated triphenyl; porphyria cutanea tarda; portacaval transposition; positron computed tomography; postcoital test; primary care team; procalcitonin; progesterone challenge test; prothrombin consumption time; proximal convoluted tubule
pCT porcine calcitonin
pct percent
PCTI penetrating cardiac trauma index
PCU pain control unit; palliative care unit; patient care unit; primary care unit; progressive care unit; pulmonary care unit
PCV packed cell volume; pneumococcal conjugate vaccine; polycythemia vera; porcine circovirus; postcapillary venule; pressure-control ventilation
PCV7 7-valent pneumococcal conjugate vaccine; heptavalent pneumococcal vaccine
PCV13 13-valent pneumococcal conjugate vaccine

PCVC percutaneous central venous catheter

PCV-M polycythemia vera with myeloid metaplasia

PCW pericanalicular web; personal care worker; primary capillary wedge; pulmonary capillary wedge; purified cell walls

PCWP pulmonary capillary wedge pressure

PCx patient's cardex; periscopic convex

PCZ procarbazine; prochlorperazine

PD Doctor of Pharmacy; Dublin Pharmacopoeia; interpupillary distance; Paget disease; pancreas divisum; pancreatic duct; panic disorder; papilla diameter; paralyzing dose; Parkinson disease; parkinsonian dementia; paroxysmal discharge; pars distalis; patent ductus; patient-day; pediatric, pediatrics; percentage difference; percutaneous discectomy; percutaneous drain; peritoneal dialysis; personal database; personality disorder; pharmacodynamics; phenyldichloroarsine; phosphate dehydrogenase; phosphate dextrose; photodiode; photosensitivity dermatitis; Pick disease; plasma defect; pneumatic dilation; polymeric diet; poorly differentiated; postdischarge; posterior descending; posterior division; postnasal drainage; postural drainage; potential difference; pregnanediol; present disease; pressor dose; prism diopter; problem drinker; program director; progression of disease; progressive disease; proliferative disease; protein degradation; protein diet; proton density; psychotic depression; pulmonary disease; pulpodistal; pulse duplicator; pulse duration; pulsed diastolic; pulsed Doppler; pupil diameter; pupillary distance; pyloric dilator; pyrimidine dimer

P/D proximal to distal

2-PD two-point discrimination

Pd palladium; pediatrics

P_d diastolic pressure

PDA patent ductus arteriosus; patient distress alarm; poorly differentiated adenocarcinoma; portable decontamination apparatus; posterior descending artery; pulmonary disease anemia

PdA pediatric allergy

PDAB para-dimethylaminobenzaldehyde

PD-AB-SAAP pulsed diastolic autologous blood selective aortic arch perfusion

PDAP Palmer drug abuse program

PD/AR photosensitivity dermatitis and actinic reticuloid syndrome

PDAY pathologic determinants of atherosclerosis in youth

PDAY/RFEHA Pathobiological Determinants of Atherosclerosis in Youth/Risk Factors in Early Human Atherogenesis [study]

PDB Paget disease of bone; paradichlorobenzene; patient's database; phosphorus-dissolving bacteria; preventive dental behavior; Protein Data Bank

PDBu phorbol 12,13-dibutyrate

PDC parkinsonism-dementia complex; patient data card; pediatric cardiology; pentadecylcatechol; phosducin; physical dependence capacity; plasma dioxin concentration; preliminary diagnostic clinic; private diagnostic clinic

PdC pediatric cardiology

PDCA plan, do, check, act

PDCD primary degenerative cerebral disease

PD-CSE pulsed Doppler cross-sectional echocardiography

PDD percentage depth dose; pervasive developmental disorder; platinum diamminedichloride [cisplatin]; primary degenerative dementia; primary degenerative disorder; pyridoxine-deficient diet

PDDA poly(dimethyldiallylammonium chloride); power-driven decontamination apparatus

PDDD primary degenerative/deformative disorder

PD DNA pyrimidine dimer deoxyribonucleic acid

PDD-NOS pervasive developmental disorder not otherwise specified

PDDP Poincaré dispersed dot plots

PDDR pseudovitamin D−dependent rickets

PDE paroxysmal dyspnea on exertion; partial differential equation; peritoneal dialysis effluent; phosphodiesterase; physician data entry; progressive dialysis encephalopathy; pulsed Doppler echocardiography

PdE pediatric endocrinology

PDEA phosphodiesterase

PDEAEM poly(diethylaminoethyl methacrylate)

PDEB phosphodiesterase beta

PDEC pancreatic ductal epithelial cell

PD-ECGF platelet-derived endothelial cell growth factor

PDEG phosphodiesterase gamma

PDF parameterized diastolic filling; Parkinson's Disease Foundation; peritoneal dialysis fluid; Portable Document Format; probability density function; pyruvate dehydrogenase

pdf probability density function

PDG parkinsonism-dementia complex of Guam; Pharmacopoeial Discussion Group; phosphogluconate dehydrogenase

PDGA pteroyldiglutamic acid

PDGF platelet-derived growth factor

PDGF-A platelet-derived growth factor A

PDGF-B platelet-derived growth factor B

PDGFR platelet-derived growth factor receptor

PDGFRB platelet-derived growth factor receptor beta

PDGS partial form of DiGeorge syndrome

PD-GXT postdischarge graded exercise test

PDH past dental history; phosphate dehydrogenase; position of the dynamometer handle [test]; progressive disseminated histoplasmosis; pyruvate dehydrogenase

PDHA pyruvate dehydrogenase alpha

PDHa pyruvate dehydrogenase in active form

PDHB pyruvate dehydrogenase beta

PDHC pyruvate dehydrogenase complex

PdHO pediatric hematology-oncology

PdHV perdicid herpesvirus

PDI pain disability index; periodontal disease index; plan-do integration; portal dose image; psychomotor development index

Pdi, P$_{di}$ transdiaphragmatic pressure

PDIE phosphodiesterase

Pdi$_{max}$ maximum transdiaphragmatic pressure

P-diol pregnanediol

PDIS participatory design of information system

PDK primary duck kidney

PDL pancreatic duct ligation; periodontal ligament; poorly differentiated lymphocyte; population doubling level; progressive diffuse leukoencephalopathy

pdl poundal; pudendal

PDLC poorly differentiated lung cancer

PDLD poorly differentiated lymphocytic [lymphoma], diffuse

PDLL poorly differentiated lymphocytic lymphoma

PDLN poorly differentiated lymphocytic [lymphoma], nodular

PDM point distribution model

PDMS pain data management system; patient data management system; pharmacokinetic drug monitoring service; polydimethylsiloxane

PDN prednisone; private duty nurse

pDNA plasmid deoxyribonucleic acid

PdNEO pediatric neonatology

PdNEP pediatric nephrology

PDP pancreatic duct pressure; papular dermatitis of pregnancy; parallel distributed processing; pattern disruption point; peak diastolic pressure; piperidinopyrimidine; plasma display; platelet-derived plasma; postural drainage and chest percussion; primer-dependent deoxynucleic acid polymerase; Product Development Protocol; programmed data processor; proprioceptive dynamic posture (training); Protein Domain Parser

PD&P postural drainage and percussion

PDPD prolonged-dwell peritoneal dialysis

PDPDM protein-deficient pancreatic diabetes mellitus

PDPH postdural puncture headache

PDPI primer-dependent deoxynucleic acid polymerase index

PDQ Personality Diagnostic Questionnaire; physician's data query; Premenstrual Distress Questionnaire; prescreening developmental questionnaire; protocol data query

PDR pediatric radiology; peripheral diabetic retinopathy; physical device representation; *Physicians' Desk Reference*; postdelivery room; primary drug resistance; proliferative diabetic retinopathy

PdR pediatric radiology

pdr powder

PDRB Permanent Disability Rating Board

PDRT Portland Digit Recognition Test

PDS pain-dysfunction syndrome; Paris dosimetry system; paroxysmal depolarizing shift; patient data system; Patient-Doctor Society; pediatric surgery; penile Doppler study; perfusion defect size; peritoneal dialysis system; personnel decontamination station; phobic disorder screen; plasma-derived serum; polydioxanone sutures; postdetermination software; predialyzed serum; progressive deterioration scale; proteodermatan sulfate

PdS pediatric surgery

PDSCs placental-derived stem cells

PDSG pigment dispersion syndrome glaucoma

PDSIP Physician-Delivered Smoking Intervention Project

PDSRS Panic Disorder Self-Rating Scale

PDT percutaneous dilational tracheostomy; photodynamic therapy; population doubling time

PDTC pyrrolidine dithiocarbamate

PDUF pulsed Doppler ultrasonic flowmeter

PDUFA Prescription Drug User Fee Act

PDUR Predischarge Utilization Review

PDUS pulsed Doppler ultrasound

PDV peak diastolic velocity; phocine distemper virus; plasma-derived vaccine

PDVT proximal deep vein thrombosis

PDW platelet distribution width

PDWA proliferative disease without atypia

PDWHF platelet-derived wound-healing factor

PDYN prodynorphin

PE *Edinburgh Pharmacopoeia*; pancreatic extract; paper electrophoresis; partial epilepsy; peak ejection; peak error; pediatric exclusivity; pelvic examination; penile erection; pericardial effusion; peritoneal exudate; pharyngoesophageal; phase-encoded; phenylephrine; phenylethylamine; phenytoin equivalent; phosphatidyl ethanolamine; photographic effect; photosensitive epilepsy; phycoerythrin; physical education; physical engineering; physical examination; physical exercise; physician extender; physiologic ecology; pigmented epithelium; pilocarpine-epinephrine; placental extract; plant engineering; plasma exchange; platinum etoposide; pleural effusion; point of entry; polyethylene; potential energy; powdered extract; preeclampsia; preexcitation; prescription error; present evaluation; pressure equalization; presumptive eligibility; prior to exposure; probable error; processing element; professional engineer; program evaluation; pseudoexfoliation; pulmonary edema; pulmonary embolism; pulmonary embolus; pyrogenic exotoxin

Pe pressure on expiration

PEA patient-controlled epidural anesthesia; pelvic examination under anesthesia; phenylethyl alcohol; phenylethylamine; polysaccharide egg antigen; pulseless electrical activity

PEAAc poly(ethylacrylic acid)

PEACH Physiologic Evaluation After Coronary Hyperemia [trial]

PEAP positive end-airway pressure

PEAR phase-encoded artifact reduction

PEARLA pupils equal and react to light and accommodation

PEAS patient education and activation system; possible estuary-associated syndrome

PEAV Peaton virus

PEBD partial external biliary diversion

PEBG phenethylbiguanide

PEBP patient escorted by police

PEC patient evaluation center; pelvic cramps; peritoneal exudate cell; perivascular epithelioid cell; probability of error in classification; pulmonary ejection click; pyrogenic exotoxin C

PECAM platelet endothelial cell adhesion molecule

PECG pseudo-electrocardiogram

PECHO prostatic echogram

PEComa perivascular epithelioid cell tumor

PECS patient evaluation and conference system; pediatrics evaluation in community setting

PECT positron emission computed tomography

PECTE Pulmonary Embolism Colfarit Trial in the Elderly

PECV porcine enteric calicivirus

PECVD plasma-enhanced chemical vapor deposition

PED palmoplantar ectodermal dysplasia; patient examined by doctor; pediatric emergency department; pink-eyed dilution

PED, ped pediatrics

PEDF pigment epithelium-derived factor

PEDIG Pediatric Eye Disease Investigator Group

PeDS Pediatric Drug Surveillance

PedsQL pediatric quality of life

PEDV porcine epidemic diarrhea virus

PEE phosphate-eliminating enzyme

PEEC pathogen-elicited epithelial chemoattractant

PEEK polyetheretherketone

PEEP positive end-expiratory pressure

PEEP/CPAP positive end-expiratory pressure/continuous positive airway pressure

PEEPrs resistive positive end-respiratory pressure

PEER peer review effectiveness evaluation research

PEF peak expiratory flow; pharyngoepiglottic fold; potential energy function; prediction error filter; Psychiatric Evaluation Form; pulmonary edema fluid

PEFR peak expiratory flow rate

PEFV partial expiratory flow volume

PEG Patient Evaluation Grid; percutaneous endoscopic gastrostomy; pneumoencephalogram, pneumoencephalography; polyethylene glycol

PEG-ADA polyethylene glycol—modified adenine deaminase

PEGASUS Percutaneous Endarterectomy, the Goal of Atherectomy Successfully Guided by Ultrasound [trial]

PEGDA, PEG-DA polyethylene glycol diacrylate

PEGDMA polyethylene glycol dimethacrylate

PEGME polyethylene glycol methyl ether

Pegs paternally expressed genes

PEG-SOD polyethylene glycol superoxide dismutase

PEG-SPA polyethylene glycol succinyl propionate

PEHO progressive encephalopathy, edema-hypsarrhythmia, optic atrophy [syndrome]

PEHPC periodic examination and health-promotion center

PeHV percid herpesvirus

PEI Patient Exit Interview; percutaneous ethanol injection; phosphate excretion index; physical efficiency index; polyethyleneimine
PeIN penile intraepithelial neoplasia
PEIRS pathology expert interpretative reporting system
PEJ percutaneous endoscopic jejunostomy
PEK punctate epithelial kerotopathy
PEL peritoneal exudate lymphocyte; permissible exposure limit
PELA peripheral excimer laser angioplasty
PELCA percutaneous excimer laser coronary angioplasty
PELD pediatric end-stage liver disease
PELF pulse extremely low frequency
PEM pediatric emergency medicine; peritoneal exudate macrophage; polymorphic epithelial mucin; positron emission mammography; precordial electrocardiographic monitoring; prescription event monitoring; primary enrichment medium; probable error of measurement; protein energy malnutrition; pulmonary endothelial membrane
PEMA phenylethylmalonamide
PE_max maximum expiratory pressure
PEMD primary esophageal motility disorder
PEMF pulsed electromagnetic field
PEN pharmacy equivalent name; practitioners entering notes
Pen penicillin
PENK proenkephalin
PEN&PAD practitioners entering notes and practitioners accessing data [system]
PENT phenylethanolamine *N*-methyltransferase
Pent pentothal
PEO polyethylene oxide; progressive external ophthalmoplegia
PEO-PBD polyethylene oxide−polybutadiene
PEO-PLA polyethylene dioxide−polylactic acid
PEP patient education program; Pediatric Education for Paramedics; peptidase; peer evaluation program; phosphoenolpyruvate; pigmentation, edema, and plasma cell dyscrasia [syndrome]; polyestradiol phosphate; pore-forming protein; positive expiratory pressure; postencephalitic parkinsonism; post−endoscopic retrograde cholangiopancreatography [ERCP] pancreatitis; postexposure prophylaxis; preejection period; protein electrophoresis; Psychiatric Evaluation Profile; pudendal evoked potential
Pep peptidase
PEPA peptidase A; prospective evaluation of prognosis in angina
PEPB peptidase B

PEPC peptidase C
PEPc corrected pre-ejection period
PEPCK phosphoenolpyruvate carboxykinase
PEPD peptidase D
PEPE peptidase E
PEPFAR President's Emergency Plan for AIDS Relief
PEPI pre-ejection period index; Postmenopausal Estrogen-Progestin Intervention [trial]
PEPLine Postexposure Prophylaxis Hotline
PEPP Payment Error Prevention Program; positive expiratory pressure plateau; Pregnancy Exposures and Pre-eclampsia Prevention [project]
PEPS peptidase S
PEPT peptide transporter
PEPV penguinpox virus
PER peak ejection rate; periodogram; peritoneum; protein efficiency ratio
per perineal; periodicity, periodic
perc percutaneous
perCP peridinin chlorophyll protein
percus percussion
Perf perfusion or perfusionist
perf perforation
PERFEXT Perfusion, Performance, Exercise Trial
PERG pattern electroretinogram
PERI Psychiatric Epidemiology Research Interview
periap periapical
Perio periodontics
Peritf peritoneal fluid
PERK prospective evaluation of radial keratotomy [protocol]
p-ERK dual phosphorylated extracellular signal−regulated kinase
PERL pupils equal, reactive to light
PERLA pupils equal, reactive to light and accommodation
PERM Prospective Evaluation of Perfusion Markers [study]
PerNET peripheral neuroectodermal tumor
PERP positive end-respiratory pressure
perp perpendicular
PERRLA pupils equal, round, and reactive to light and accommodation
PERS Patient Evaluation Rating Scale; pediatric emergency rating scale
PERT phenol-enhanced reassociation technique; program evaluation review technique
PERV Perinet virus; porcine endogenous retrovirus
PES patient escort service; pharyngoesophageal segment; photoelectron spectroscopy; physical examination syndrome; physicians'

equity services; polyethylene sulfonate; post-extrasystolic; preepiglottic space; preexcitation syndrome; primary empty sella [syndrome]; programmed electrical stimulation; pseudoepileptic seizures; pseudoexfoliation/pseudoexfoliative syndrome; psychiatric emergency services

Pes esophageal pressure

PESDA perfluorocarbon-exposed sonicated dextrose albumin

PESP postextrasystolic potentiation

P$_{es}$/P$_l$max mean esophageal pressure/maximum inspiratory pressure ratio

PESS problem, etiology, signs, and symptoms

Pess pessary

PET paraffin-embedded tissue; peak ejection time; peritoneal equilibrium test; polyethylene terephthalate; polyethylene tube; poor exercise tolerance; positron emission tomography; preeclamptic toxemia; [antimicrobial] preservative effectiveness test [called also AET, APE]; pressure equalization tube; privacy-enhancing technique; progressive exercise test; psychiatric emergency team

PET$_{CO_2}$, P$_{ET}$CO$_2$ end-tidal pressure of carbon dioxide

PETH pink-eyed, tan-hooded [rat]

PET-MRI positron emission tomography magnetic resonance imaging

PETN pentaerythritol tetranitrate

PETQI patient education total quality improvement

petr petroleum

PETRA parameter estimation for the treatment of reactivity application

PETS percutaneous epiphysiodesis using transphyseal screws

PETSc portable extensible toolkit for scientific computation

PETT pendular eye-tracking test; positron emission transverse tomography

PETV Petevo virus

PEU plasma equivalent unit

PEUU polyurethane-urea

PEV peak expiratory velocity; positive effect variegation; pseudoenteritis virus

pev peak electron volts

PEV 2 to 13 porcine enteroviruses 2 to 13

PEV A, B porcine enteroviruses A and B

PEW pulmonary extravascular water

PEWV pulmonary extravascular water volume

PEX presence of exfoliation syndrome

PEx physical examination

Pex peak exercise

PEXG primary exfoliative glaucoma

P$_{ext}$ pressure across external breathing apparatus

PF pair feeding; peak flow; peak frequency; pemphigus foliaceus; perfusion fluid; pericardial fluid; periosteal fibroblast; peritoneal fluid; permeability factor; personality factor; picture frustration [study]; plantar flexion; plasma factor; plasmapheresis; platelet factor; pleural fluid; power factor; primary fibrinolysin; prostatic fluid; protection factor; pterygoid fossa; pulmonary factor; pulmonary function; Purkinje fiber; purpura fulminans; push fluids; pyrozafurin

P-F picture frustration [test]

PF$_{1-4}$ platelet factors 1 to 4

P$_f$ final pressure

Pf *Plasmodium falciparum*

pF picofarad

PFA *p*-fluorophenylalanine; phosphonoformate; probability of false alarm; profunda femoris artery; pulverized fluid ash

PFAS perception of functional ability scale; performic acid−Schiff

PFB perflubron; proportion of fed bugs

PFC pair-fed control [mice]; pancreatic fluid collection; patient-focused care; pelvic flexion contracture; perfluorocarbon; perfluorochemical; pericardial fluid culture; persistent fetal circulation; plaque-forming cell

pFc noncovalently bonded dimer of the C-terminal immunoglobulin of the Fc fragment

PFD pelvic floor disorder; perfluorodecalin; polyostotic fibrous dysplasia; pseudoinflammatory fundus disease

PFDA perfluoro-decanoic acid

PfDNV *Periplanata fuliginosa* densovirus

PFE pelvic floor exercise

PFFD proximal focal femoral deficiency

PFG peak flow gauge; pulsed-field gel electrophoresis

PFGE pulsed-field gel electrophoresis

PFGS phosphoribosyl formylglycinamide synthetase

PFIB perfluoroisobutylene

PFIC progressive familial intrahepatic cholestasis

PFJ patellofemoral joint

PFK phosphofructokinase; 6-phosphofructo-2-kinase

PFKF 6-phosphofructo-2-kinase, fibroblast type

PFKL phosphofructokinase, liver type; 6-phosphofructo-2-kinase, liver type

PFKM phosphofructokinase, muscle type
PFKP phosphofructokinase, platelet type; 6-phosphofructo-2-kinase, platelet type
PFKX 6-phosphofructo-2-kinase X
PFL profibrinolysin
pflops pentaflops [floating points per second]
PFM peak flow meter
PFMT pelvic floor muscle training
PFN partially functional neutrophil; profilin; proximal femoral nail
PFO patent foramen ovale; perfringolysin O; plantar fasciitis orthosis
PFOB perfluorocytylbromide
PFOR pyruvate:ferredoxin oxidoreductase
PFP pentafluorophenol; peripheral facial paralysis; plain film pelvis [x-ray]; platelet-free plasma; pulmonary fibroproliferation
PFPA postfundoplication pseudoachalasia
P-FPIA polyclonal fluorescence polarization immunoassay
PFPS patellofemoral pain syndrome
PFQ personality factor questionnaire
PFR parotid flow rate; particulate filter respirator; peak flow rate; proximal femoral replacement
PFRC predicted functional residual capacity
PFS patellofemoral syndrome; primary fibromyalgia syndrome; progression-free survival; protein-free supernatant; pulmonary function score; pulsatile flow system
PFSH past, family and social history
PFT pancreatic function test; parafascicular thalamotomy; posterior fossa tumor; prednisone, fluorouracil, and tamoxifen; pulmonary function test
PFTBE progressive form of tick-borne encephalitis
PFTL pulmonary function test laboratory
PFU plaque-forming unit; pock-forming unit
pfu plaque-forming unit
PFUI pelvic fracture urethral injury
PFUO prolonged fever of unknown origin
PFV physiologic full value
PFWD pain-free walking distance
PG parallel group; parapsoriasis guttata; paregoric; parotid gland; partial gastrectomy; pentagastrin; pepsinogen; peptidoglycan; percutaneous gastrostomy; Pharmacopoeia Germanica; phase gradient; phosphate glutamate; phosphatidylglycerol; phosphogluconate; pigment granule; pituitary gonadotropin; plasma glucose; plasma triglyceride; polygalacturonate; post graft; postgraduate; postprandial glucose; practice guideline; pregnanediol glucuronide; pregnant; progesterone; prolyl hydrolase; propyl gallate; propylene glycol; Prospect Hill [virus];

prostaglandin; proteoglycan; pulse generator; pyoderma gangrenosum
2PG 2-phosphoglycerate
3PG 3-phosphoglycerate
P$_G$ plasma glucose
Pg gastric pressure; nasopharyngeal electrode placement [EEG]; plakoglobin; plasminogen; pogonion; pregnancy, pregnant; pregnenolone
pg parthenogenic; picogram; pregnant
PGA pancreatogastrostomy; pepsinogen A; phosphoglyceric acid; polyglandular autoimmune [syndrome]; polyglycolic acid; programmable-gain amplifier; prostaglandin A; pteroylglutamic acid
PGA$_{1-3}$ prostaglandins A$_1$ to A$_3$
PGAM monophosphoglycerate mutase
PGAP pilot geriatric arthritis program
PGAS persisting galactorrhea-amenorrhea syndrome; polyglandular autoimmune syndrome
PGAV Pongola virus
PGB progabide; prostaglandin B
PGC primordial germ cell; progastricin
PGCL paragigantocellularis lateralis
PGD phosphogluconate dehydrogenase; phosphoglyceraldehyde dehydrogenase
PGD$_2$ prostaglandin D$_2$
6-PGD 6-phosphogluconate dehydrogenase
PGDH phosphogluconate dehydrogenase
PGDR plasma glucose disappearance rate
PGE platelet granule exract; posterior gastroenterostomy
PGE$_1$ prostaglandin E$_1$
PGE$_2$ prostaglandin E$_2$
PGF phylogenetic footprint
PGF$_{2\alpha}$ prostaglandin F$_{2\alpha}$
PGFT phosphoribosylglycinamide formyltransferase
PGG polyclonal gamma globulin
PGG$_2$ prostaglandin G$_2$
PGH pituitary growth hormone; porcine growth hormone
PGH$_2$ prostaglandin H$_2$
PGHS prostaglandin G/H synthase
PGI phosphoglucose isomerase; potassium, glucose, and insulin
PGI$_2$ prostacyclin [prostaglandin I$_2$]
PGK phosphoglycerate kinase
PGL paraganglioma [syndrome]; persistent generalized lymphadenopathy; phosphoglycolipid; 6-phosphogluconolactonase
PGLN periglandular lymph node
PGlyM phosphoglyceromutase
PGM phosphoglucomutase; phosphoglycerate mutase
PGMA phosphoglycerate mutase A

PGMB phosphoglycerate mutase B
PGMDE postgraduate and continuing medical and dental education
pg/mL picograms per milliliter
PGN proliferative glomerulonephritis
PGNA prompt gamma neutron activation
PGO ponto-geniculo-occipital
PGP phosphoglycerol phosphatase; postgamma proteinuria; prepaid group practice; progressive general paralysis
PGPV pigeonpox virus
PGR progesterone receptor; psychogalvanic response
PgR progesterone receptor
PGS peristent gross splenomegaly; Pettigrew syndrome; plant growth substance; polar grid system; postsurgical gastroparesis syndrome; primary generalized seizures; prostaglandin synthetase
PGSI prostaglandin synthetase inhibitor
PGSR phosphogalvanic skin response
PGT preimplantation genetic testing
PGTC primary generalized tonic-clonic seizures
PGTR plasma glucose tolerance rate
PGTT prednisolone glucose tolerance test
PGU peripheral glucose uptake; postgonococcal urethritis
PGUT phosphogalactose uridyl transferase
PGV proximal gastric vagotomy
PGVS postganglionic vagal stimulation
PGWB Psychological General Well-Being [Index]
PGX prostacyclin
PGY postgraduate year
PGYE peptone, glucose yeast extract
PH Pallister-Hall [syndrome]; papillary hyperplasia; parathyroid hormone; partial hepatectomy; partial hysterectomy; passive hemagglutination; past history; patient history; persistent hepatitis; personal history; pharmaceutical, pharmacist; pharmacopeia; pharmacy; physical history; porphyria hepatica; posterior heel; posterior hypothalamus; prehospital; previous history; primary hyperoxaluria; primary hyperparathyroidism; prostatic hypertrophy; pseudohermaphroditism; public health; pulmonary hypertension; pulmonary hypoplasia
PH1 primary hyperoxaluria type 1
Ph phantom; pharmacopeia; phenyl; Philadelphia [chromosome]; phosphate
Ph^1 Philadelphia chromosome
pH hydrogen ion concentration
pH$_1$ isoelectric point
ph phot

PHA passive hemagglutination assay; peripheral hyperalimentation; phenylalanine; Physician Hospitals of America; phytohemagglutinin; phytohemagglutinin antigen; pseudohypoaldosteronism; public health agency; Public Health Association; pulseheight analyzer
PHA1 pseudohypoaldosteronism type 1
PHA2 pseudohypoaldosteronism type 2
pH$_A$ arterial blood hydrogen tension
pH$_a$ arterial hydrogen ion concentration
PHAC phaclofen
PhAdV pheasant adenovirus
PHAF peripheral hyperalimentation formula
PHAH polyhalogenated aromatic hydrocarbon
PHAL phytohemagglutinin-stimulated lymphocyte
phal phalangeal
PHA-LCM phytohemagglutinin-stimulated leukocyte conditioned medium
Ph+ALL Philadelphia chromosome−positive acute lymphoblastic leukemia
PHA-NSP passive hemagglutination to nonstructural protein
PHAP phytohemagglutinin protein
PHAR pharmacologic substance
phar pharmaceutical; pharmacy; pharynx
Phar C pharmaceutical chemist
PHARM Pharmacist in Heart Failure: Assessment, Recommendation and Monitoring [study]
Pharm pharmacy
pharm pharmacist; pharmacology; pharmacopeia; pharmacy
Pharm B Bachelor of Pharmacy
Pharm D Doctor of Pharmacy
Pharm M Master of Pharmacy
PHASE prehospital arrest survival evaluation
PHAVER pterygia, heart defects, autosomal recessive inheritance, vertebral defects, ear anomalies, radial defects [syndrome]
PHB polyhydroxybutyrate; preventive health behavior; prohibitin
PhB, Phb Pharmacopoeia Britannica
PHBB propylhydroxybenzyl benzimidazole
PHBQ Physicians' Humanistic Behaviors Questionnaire; Post-Hospitalization Behavior Questionnaire
PHC personal health costs; posthospital care; premolar hypodontia, hyperhidrosis, [premature] canities syndrome; primary health care; Primary Healthcare Center; primary hepatic carcinoma; proliferative helper cell; public health center

PHCA profound hypothermic circulatory arrest
PhC pharmaceutical chemist
Ph¹ᶜ Philadelphia chromosome
PHCC primary hepatocellular carcinoma
PHCDM public health computational data model
PHCP prehospital care provider
PHD pathological habit disorder; personal health data; post-heparin plasma diamine oxidase; potentially harmful drug
PhD Doctor of Pharmacy; Doctor of Philosophy
PHE periodic health examination; phenylephrine
Phe phenylalanine
PhEEM photoemission electron microscopy
PHEI prevention and health evaluation informatics
pHEMA polyhydroxyethyl methacrylate
PHEN phenomenon or process
Phen phentermine
Pheo pheochromocytoma; pheophytin
PhEur *Pharmacopeia Europaea*
Ph. Eur. U. European Pharmacopoeia unit
PHEX phosphate-regulating gene with homologies to endopeptidase on X chromosome
PHF paired helical filament; personal hygiene facility
PHFB psyllium husk fiber bar
PHFG primary human fetal glia
PhG Graduate in Pharmacy; *Pharmacopoeia Germanica*
phgly phenylglycine
PHHI persistent hyperinsulinemic hypoglycemia of infancy
PHHP Pawtucket Heart Health Program
PhHV phalacrocoracid herpesvirus
PHI Paraprofessional Healthcare Institute; passive hemagglutination inhibition; past history of illness; personalized health information; phosphine; phosphohexose isomerase; physiologic hyaluronidase inhibitor; prehospital index; protected health information
PhI *Pharmacopoeia Internationalis*
Phi Partnership in Health Information
pHi intracellular hydrogen ion concentration; intramucosal hydrogen ion concentration
PHICOG Philadelphia Cooperative Group
PHIDIAS Laser Photopolymerisation Models Based on Medical Imaging, a Development Improving the Accuracy of Surgery
PHIDS personalized healthcare information delivery system

PHIHM prehospital invasive hemodynamic monitoring
PHIM posthypoxic intention myoclonus
PHIS personal health information seeking
PhIS pharmacy information system
PHK phosphohexokinase; phosphorylase kinase; postmortem human kidney
PHKA phosphorylase kinase alpha
PHKB phosphorylase kinase beta
PHKD phosphorylase kinase delta
PHKG phosphorylase kinase gamma
PHL public health laboratory
PHLA postheparin lipolytic activity
PHLOP polymerase halt—mediated linkage of primers
PHLS Public Health Laboratory Service
PHM peptide histidine methionine; peptidylglycine alpha-hydroxylating mono-oxygenase; posterior hyaloid membrane; public health measures; pulmonary hyaline membrane
PhM Master of Pharmacy; pharyngeal muscle
PhmG Graduate in Pharmacy
PHN paroxysmal noctural hemoglobinuria; passive Heymann nephritis; postherpetic neuralgia; primary health care nurse; proximal humeral nail; public health nurse/nursing
PHO physician-hospital organization
PH₂O partial pressure of water vapor
PHOCUS Primary Health-Oriented Computer Users' System
PhoHV phocid herpesvirus
phos phosphate
PHOX paired mesoderm homeobox [gene]
PHP panhypopituitarism; partial hospitalization program; postheparin phospholipase; prehospital program; prepaid health plan; primary hyperparathyroidism; pseudohypoparathyroidism; psychological health profile
PHPA passive hemolytic plaque assay; *p*-hydroxyphenylacetate
PHPLA *p*-hydroxyphenyllactic acid
pHPPA *p*-hydrophenylpyruvic acid
p-HPPO *p*-hydroxyphenyl pyruvate oxidase
PHPT primary hyperparathyroidism; pseudohypoparathyroidism
pHPT primary hyperparathyroidism
PHPV persistent hyperplastic primary vitreous
PHR parent-held record; peak heart rate; photoreactivity
PHRN Prehospital Registered Nurse
PHS partial hospitalization system; Personal Handphone System; phenylalanine hydrolase stimulator system; Physicians' Health Study;

pooled human serum; posthypnotic suggestion; pseudoprogeria-Hallermann-Streiff [syndrome]; Public Health Service

PHSC pluripotent hematoopoietic stem cell; powdered human stratum corneum

PHS-LAN Personal Handphone System—Local Area Network

PHSM public health and social measures

PHS-PC Personal Handphone System—Personal Computer

pH-stat apparatus for maintaining the pH of a solution

PHT peak height of tension; phenytoin; portal hypertension; pressure half-time; primary hyperthyroidism; pulmonary hypertension

PhTD Doctor of Physical Therapy

PHTLS prehospital trauma life support

PHTN portal hypertension; pulmonary hypertension

PHU population health unit

PHV peak height velocity; perch hyperplasia virus; Prospect Hill virus

PhVWP Pharmacovigilance Working Party

PHX pulmonary histiocytosis X

Phx past history; pharynx

PHY pharyngitis; physical; physiology

PHYLLIS Plaque Hypertension Lipid-Lowering Italian Study

PHYS physiologic function; physiology

PhyS physiologic saline [solution]

phys physical; physician

Phys Ed physical education

physio physiology; physiotherapy

Phys Med physical medicine

PhysPRC Physician Payment Review Commission

PHYS-SPEC physician's specialty

Phys Ther physical therapist/therapy

PHZ phenylhydrazine

PI class I protein; first meiotic prophase; isoelectric point; pacing impulse; package insert; pain intensity; pancreatic insufficiency; parainfluenza; pars intermedia; patient interest; performance indicator; performance index; performance intensity; perinatal injury; periodontal index; permeability index; personal injury; personality inventory; phagocytic index; *Pharmacopoeia Internationalis*; phosphatidylinositol; physically impaired; physiologic index; pineal body; plaque index; plasmin inhibitor; pneumatosis intestinalis; poison ivy; ponderal index; postictal immobility; postinfection; postinfluenza; postinjury; postinoculation; preinduction; premature infant; prematurity

index; preparatory interval; prescribing information; present illness; primary infarction; primary infection; principal investigator; processor interface; product information; proinsulin; prolactin inhibitor; propidium iodide; proportional plus integral; protamine insulin; protease inhibitor; proximal intestine; pulmonary incompetence; pulmonary index; pulmonary infarction; pulmonic insufficiency; pulsatility index

P₁ inspiratory pressure

P&I pneumonia and influenza

Pi inorganic phosphate; parental generation; pressure in inspiration; protease inhibitor

Pᵢ inorganic phosphate

pI isoelectric point

p-I post inspiratory

pi post injection

PIA photoelectric intravenous angiography; plasma insulin activity; preinfarction angina; Psychiatric Institute of America; *R*-phenylisopropyladenosine

PIAA Physician Insurers Association of America

PiAdV pigeon adenovirus

PIAF pharmacologic intervention in atrial fibrillation; prognosis in atrial fibrillation

PIAT Peabody Individual Achievement Test

PIAV Picola virus

PIAVA polydactyly, imperforate anus, vertebral anomalies [syndrome]

PIB periinfarction block

PIBC percutaneous intraaortic balloon counterpulsation

PIBIDS, PIBI(D)S photosensitivity, ichthyosis, brittle hair, impaired intelligence, (possibly decreased fertility), short stature syndrome

PIC pacing in cardiomyopathy; peripherally inserted indwelling central catheter; Personality Inventory for Children; polymorphism information content; preinitiation complex; preinjury condition; prior informed consent

PICA Porch Index of Communicative Abilities; posterior inferior cerebellar artery; posterior inferior communicating artery

PICC percutaneous indwelling central venous catheter; peripherally inserted central catheter

PICD primary irritant contact dermatitis

PICFS postinfective chronic fatigue syndrome

PICNIC Pediatric Investigators Collaborative Network on Infections in Canada

PICO Pimobendan in Congestive Heart Failure [study]; population, intervention, comparison, and outcome

PiCO₂ partial pressure of carbon dioxide in air

PICS Pacing in Cardiomyopathy Study

PICSO pressure-controlled intermittent coronary sinus occlusion

PICSS Patent Foramen Ovale in Cryptogenic Stroke Study

PICTURE Post-intracoronary Treatment Ultrasound Results Evaluation [study]

PICU patient interface control unit; pediatric intensive care unit; pulmonary intensive care unit

PICV Pichinde virus

PiCV pigeon circovirus

PID pain intensity difference; patient identification; patient identity; pelvic inflammatory disease; photoionization detector; picture image directory; plasma iron disappearance; postinertia dyskinesia; preimplantation diagnosis; prolapsed/protruded intervertebral disk; proportional integral derivative; proportional integral-differential control

PIDRA portable insulin dosage-regulating apparatus

PIDS patient identification service; primary immunodeficiency syndrome

PIDT plasma iron disappearance time

PIE postinfectious encephalomyelitis; preimplantation embryo; prosthetic infectious endocarditis; pulmonary infiltration with eosinophilia; pulmonary interstitial emphysema

PIF parotid isoelectric focusing variant; peak inspiratory flow; photoinhibition factor; proinsulin free; prolactin-inhibiting factor; prolactin release-inhibiting factor; proliferation-inhibiting factor; prostatic interstitial fluid

PIFG poor intrauterine fetal growth

PIFR peak inspiratory flow rate

PIFT platelet immunofluorescence test

PIG Polaris Investigator Group; polymeric immunoglobulin

PIGA phosphatidylinositol glycan A

pIgA polymeric immunoglobulin A

PIGF phosphatidylinositol-glycan biosynthesis class F protein

pIgM polymeric immunoglobulin M

pigm pigment, pigmented

PIGO phosphatidylinositol glycan anchor biosynthesis class O

PIGR, PigR polymeric immunoglobulin receptor

PIH periventricular-intraventricular hemorrhage; pheniprazine; phenyl isopropylhydrazine; pregnancy-induced hypertension; prolactin-inhibiting hormone; pseudointimal hyperplasia

PII plasma inorganic iodine; primary irritation index

PI-IBS postinfectious irritable bowel syndrome

PIIgG surface immunoglobulin G

PIIP portable insulin infusion pump

PIIS posterior inferior iliac spine

P$_{ij}$ propagation delay

PI3K, PI-3K phosphatidylinositol-3′-kinase

PIKQ Prolapse and Incontinence Knowledge Questionnaire

PIL patient information leaflet

Pil. pill

PILBD paucity of interlobular bile ducts

PILL Pennebaker Inventory of Limbic Languidness

PILOT Polish Intramural Low Molecular Weight Heparin Outpatient Stent Trial; Preliminary Investigation of Local Therapy

PILP postinfarction late potential

PILS Pilsen Longitudinal Study

PIM penicillamine-induced myasthenia

PI$_{max}$ maximum inspiratory pressure at residual volume

P$_i$max maximum inspiratory pressure

PIMI predictive index for myocardial infarction; psychophysiologic interventions in myocardial ischemia

PIMS patient information management system

PIN patient information network; personal identification number; product identification number; prostatic intraepithelial neoplasia

Pin inflow pressure; initial pressure

PINN proposed international nonproprietary name

PINV postimperative negative variation

PIo₂ partial pressure of inspired oxygen

PION posterior ischemic optic neuropathy

PIOPED Prospective Investigation of Pulmonary Embolism Diagnosis

PIP paralytic infantile paralysis; peak inflation pressure, peak inspiratory pressure; periodic interim payment; piperacillin; Poly Implant Prostheses; posterior interphalangeal; postinfusion phlebitis; pressure inversion point; primary injury prevention; probable intrauterine pregnancy; prolactin-inducible protein; proximal interphalangeal; psychosis, intermittent hyponatremia, polydipsia [syndrome]; Psychotic Inpatient Profile

PI-P phosphatidylinositol-4-phosphate

PIP₂ phosphatidylinositol 4,5-bisphosphate

Pi/PCr inorganic phosphate/creatine phosphate ratio

PIPE persistent interstitial pulmonary emphysema

PIPER Patient Information Projects Register

PIPIDA *p*-isopropylacetanilidoimidodiacetic acid

PIPJ proximal interphalangeal joint

PI-PP phosphatidylinositol-4,5-biphosphate

PIPS patient information protocol system

PIQ Performance Intelligence Quotient

PIR participant inquiry research; post-inhibition rebound; postisometric relaxation; protein identification/information resource

PIRI plasma immunoreactive insulin

PIR-NREF Protein Information or Identification Resource Nonredundant Reference

PIRS plasma immunoreactive secretion; postinfarction risk stratification

PIRTS patient identification for rotational therapy system

PIRV Pirital virus

PIRYV Piry virus

PIS pharmacy information system; preinfarction syndrome; primary immunodeficiency syndrome; Primary Index Score; Provisional International Standard

pIs isoelectric point

PISA proximal isovelocity surface area

PISA-PED Prospective Investigative Study of Acute Pulmonary Embolism Diagnosis

PISCES percutaneously inserted spinal cord electrical stimulation

PISH polymerase chain reaction in situ hybridization

PISI pediatric illness severity index

PISK pressure-induced intralamellar stromal keratitis

PIT pacing-induced tachycardia; patella inhibition test; pericranial injection therapy; picture identification test; pitocin; pitressin; plasma iron turnover

pit pituitary

PITA powered intracapsular tonsillectomy and adenoidectomy

PITAC President's Information Technology Advisory Committee

PITC phenylisothiocyanate

PITR plasma iron turnover rate

PIU polymerase-inducing unit; programmed instruction unit

PIV parainfluenza virus; particle image velocity; polydactyly, imperforate anus, vertebral anomalies [syndrome]; projective image visualization; Puffin Island virus

PIVD protruded intervertebral disk

PIVH peripheral intravenous hyperalimentation; periventricular-intraventricular hemorrhage

PIVKA protein induced by vitamin K absence or antagonism

P/I/X patients, indicators, external bodies

PIXE particle-induced x-ray emission; proton-induced x-ray emission

Pixel picture element

PIXI paternally imprinted X inactivation

PIXV Pixuna virus

PJ pancreatic juice; Peutz-Jeghers [syndrome]

PJB premature junctional beat

PJC premature junctional contractions

pJC Jamestown Canyon virus plasmid

PJIA polyarticular juvenile idiopathic arthritis

PJM positive joint mobilization

PJP pancreatic juice protein

PJRT permanent junctional reciprocating tachycardia

PJS peritoneojugular shunt; Peutz-Jeghers syndrome

PJT paroxysmal junctional tachycardia

PK penetrating keratoplasty; pericardial knock; pharmacokinetics; pig kidney; Prausnitz-Küstner [reaction]; protein kinase; psychokinesis; pyruvate kinase

Pk peak

pK negative logarithm of the dissociation constant; plasma potassium

pK' apparent value of a pK; negative logarithm of the dissociation constant of an acid

pk peck

PKA protein kinase A

PkA prekallikrein activator

pK$_a$ negative logarithm of the acid ionization constant

PKAN pantothenate kinase—associated neurodegeneration [Hallervorden-Spatz disease]

PKAR protein kinase activation ratio

PKase protein kinase

PKB protein kinase B

PKC Permanente Knowledge Connection; problem-knowledge coupler; protein kinase C

PKCA protein kinase C alpha

PKCB protein kinase C beta

PKCE protein kinase C epsilon

PKCG protein kinase C gamma

PKCSH protein kinase C heavy chain

PKCSL protein kinase C light chain

PKCZ protein kinase C zeta

PKD polycystic kidney disease; proliferative kidney disease

PKD-1 polycystic kidney disease gene 1

PKD-2 polycystic kidney disease gene 2

PKDL post—kala-azar dermal leishmaniasis

PKF phagocytosis and killing function

PKG protein kinase G

PKI potato kallikrein inhibitor; protein kinase inhibitor; public key infrastructure

PKK plasma prekallikrein

PKL pyruvate kinase, liver type

PKM protein kinase M; pyruvate kinase, muscle

PKMB pseudoepitheliomatous, keratotic, and micaceous balanitis

PKN parkinsonism

pkn pseudo-knot

PKP penetrating keratoplasty; plakophilin

PK/PD pharmacokinetic/pharmacodynamic

PKPV peacockpox virus

PKR phased knee rehabilitation; Prausnitz-Küstner reaction

Pk/Rr peak respiratory rate

PKS protein kinase sequence

PKT pancreas-kidney transplantation; Prausnitz-Küstner test

PKU phenylketonuria

PKV killed poliomyelitis vaccine

pkV peak kilovoltage

PL *Paenibacillus larvae*; palmaris longus; pancreatic lipase; perception of light; peroneus longus; phospholipase; phospholipid; photoluminescence; placebo; placental lactogen; plantar; plasmalemma; plastic surgery; platelet lactogen; polarized light; posterolateral; preleukemia; programming language; prolactin; prolymphocytic leukemia; pulpolingual; Purkinje layer

3PL 3-point line

Pl poiseuille

P$_L$ transpulmonary pressure

pL picoliter

pl picoliter; placenta; plasma; platelet

PLA peripheral laser angioplasty; phenyl lactate; phospholipase A; phospholipid antibody; placebo therapy; plasminogen activator; platelet antigen; polylactic acid; potentially lethal arrhythmia; procaine/lactic acid; processed lipoaspirate cells; Product License Application; pulp linguoaxial

PLA2 phospholipase A2

PLa pulpolabial

Pla, PLa left atrial pressure

PLAC Pravastatin Limitation in Atherosclerosis in the Coronary Arteries [study]

PLAC-2 Pravastatin, Lipids and Atherosclerosis in the Carotid Arteries [study]

PLAID PLCG2-associated antibody deficiency and immune dysregulation

PLAP placental alkaline phosphatase

PLAT plasminogen activator, tissue type

Plat platelet

PLAU plasminogen activator, urinary

PLAUR plasminogen activator receptor, urokinase type

PLAV Playas virus

PLB parietal lobe battery; phospholamban; phospholipase B; planar lipid bilayer; porous layer bead; posterolateral bundle; pursed-lip breathing

PLC phospholipase C; pityriasis lichenoides chronica; primary liver cancer; primed lymphocyte culture; programmable logic controller; proinsulin-like component; protein-lipid complex; pseudolymphocytic choriomeningitis

PLCC primary liver cell cancer

PLCO postoperative low cardiac output

PLCx posterolateral circumflex branch [of coronary artery]

PLD peripheral light detection; phospholipase D; platelet defect; polycystic liver disease; posterior latissimus dorsi; potentially lethal damage

PLDH plasma lactic dehydrogenase

pLDH parasite-specific lactate dehydrogenase

PLDR potentially lethal damage repair

PLE paraneoplastic limbic encephalopathy; pleura; protein-losing enteropathy; pseudo-lupus erythematosus

PLED periodic lateral epileptiform discharge

PLES parallel-line equal space

PLET polymyxin, lysosome, EDTA, thallous acetate

PLEVA pityriasis lichenoides et varioliformis acuta

PLEXES Pacing Lead Explant with Excimer Sheath [study]

PLF perilymphatic fistula; posterior lung fiber

Plf pleural fluid

PLFD perilunate fracture dislocation

3PLFLS three-point line fixed least squares

PLFS perilymphatic fistula syndrome

PLG plasminogen; polylactic-co-glycolic acid; poly-DL-lactide/glycolide; L-propyl-L-leucyl-glucinamide

PLGA polylactic-glycolic acid

PlGF placental growth factor

PLGL plasminogen-like

P-LGV psittacosis lymphogranuloma venereum

PLH placental lactogenic hormone

PLHP personalized lifetime health plan

PlHV pleuronectid herpesvirus

PLI pancreatic lymphocytic infiltration; paternal leukocyte immunization; professional liability insurance

PL/I programming language I

PLIF posterior lumbar interbody fusion

PLISSIT permission to be sexual, limited information, specific suggestions, intensive therapy

PLL peripheral light loss; phase-locked loop; poly-L-lysine; posterior longitudinal ligament; potential loss of life; pressure length loop; prolymphocytic leukemia

PLLA poly-L-lactic acid

PLM percent labeled mitoses; periodic leg movement; plasma level monitoring; polarized light microscopy

PLMS periodic limb movements during sleep

PLMV posterior leaf mitral valve

PLN peripheral lymph node; phospholamban

PLNA percutaneous lung needle aspiration

PLND pelvic lymph node dissection

PLNT plant

PLO polycystic lipomembranous osteodysplasia

PLOD procollagen-lysine 2-oxoglutarate 5-dioxygenase

PLOF prior level of function

PLOS postoperative length of stay

PLOSA Physiologic Low-Stress Angioplasty [trial]

PLP *Paenibacillus larvae* subsp. *pulvifaciens*; phospholipid; plasma leukapheresis; polypeptide; polystyrene latex particles; posterior lobe of pituitary; proteolipid protein; pyridoxal phosphate

PLPH post—lumbar puncture headache

PLR pupillary light reflex

PLS Papillon-Lefèvre syndrome; partial least square; polydactyly-luxation syndrome; Postsurgery Logiparin Study; preleukemic syndrome; primary lateral sclerosis; prostaglandin-like substance; pulmonary leukostasis syndrome

PLSA posterolateral segment [coronary] artery

PLSD protected least significant difference

PLSR partial least-square regression

PLST progressively lowered stress threshold

Pl Surg plastic surgeon/surgery

PLSV Palestina virus

PLT platelet; primary lymphoma of the thyroid; primed lymphocyte test; primed lymphocyte typing; psittacosis lympho-granuloma venereum trachoma [group]

PLTC Partnership for Long Term Care

PLTP phospholipid transfer protein

plumb lead [L. *plumbum*]

PLUT Plutchnik [scale]

PLV panleukemia virus; panleukopenia virus; partial liquid ventilation; phenylalanine, lysine, and vasopressin; poliomyelitis live vaccine; posterior left ventricle; puma lentivirus

P_LV left ventricular pressure

PLVP peak left ventricular pressure

PLW Prader-Labhart-Willi [syndrome]

PLWA, PLW As person living with acquired immune deficiency syndrome

PLWHA people living with HIV/AIDS

PLWS Prader-Labhart-Willi syndrome

plx plexus

PLZ phenelzine

PLZF promyelocytic leukemia zinc finger

PM after death [L. *post mortem*]; after noon [L. *post meridiem*]; mean pressure; pacemaker; pantomography; papilla mammae; papillary muscle; papular mucinosis; partial meniscectomy; particle mass; particulate matter; patient management; pectinate muscle; pectoralis major [muscle]; perinatal mortality; periodontal membrane; peritoneal macrophage; petit mal epilepsy; photomultiplier; physical medicine; plasma membrane; platelet membrane; platelet microsome; pneumomediastinum; poliomyelitis; polymorph [polymorphonuclear leukocyte]; polymorphic; polymyositis; poor metabolizer; porokeratosis of Mibelli; posterior mitral; postmenstrual; postmortem; power management; premarketing; premenstrual; premolar; premotor; presents mainly; presystolic murmur; pretibial myxedema; preventive maintenance; preventive medicine; primary motivation; process manager; Prony method; prophylactic mastectomy; prostatic massage; protein methylesterase; protocol management; psammomatous meningioma; pterygoid muscle; pterygomaxillary; pubertal macromastia; pulmonary macrophage; pulpomesial; purple membrane

PM_10 particulate matter <10 microns

Pm promethium

pM picomolar

pm picometer

πm pi meson

PMA index of prevalence and severity of gingivitis [P = papillary gingiva, M = marginal gingiva, A = attached gingiva]; papillary, marginal, attached [gingiva]; paramethoxyamphetamine; Pharmaceutical Manufacturers Association; phenylmercuric acetate; phorbol myristate acetate; phosphomolybdic acid; polymethacrylic acid; premarket approval; primary mental abilities; professional medical association; progressive muscular atrophy; pyridylmercuric acetate

PMAA polymethacrylic acid

P(MAA-g-EG) poly[methacrylic acid-grafted poly(ethylene glycol)]

PMAC Pharmaceutical Manufacturers Association of Canada; phenylmercuric acetate; programmable multiaxis controller

PMAS phenylmercuric acetate

P+$_{max}$ peak positive pressure

PMB papillomacular bundle; para-hydroxymercuribenzoate; polychrome methylene blue; polymorphonuclear basophil; polymyxin B; postmenopausal bleeding

PMC paramyotonia congenita; patient management category; percutaneous myocardial channeling; peritoneal mesothelial cell; phenylmercuric chloride; physical medicine clinic; pleural mesothelial click; premature mitral closure; probability of misclassification; pseudomembranous colitis

Pmc mean circulatory pressure

PMCC product-moment correlation coefficient

PMCH pro−melanin-concentrating hormone

PMCHL pro−melanin-concentrating hormone−like

PMC-RIS patient management category relative intensity score

PMCS patient management computer simulation

PMD Pelizaeus-Merzbacher disease; posterior mandibular depth; primary myocardial disease; primary physician; private medicine doctor; programmed multiple development; progressive muscular dystrophy

PMDD premenstrual dysphoric disorder

PMDF proportion of maternal deaths among women of reproductive age

pMDI pressurized metered-dose inhaler

PM/DM polymyositis/dermatomyositis

PMDS peristent müllerian duct syndrome; primary myelodysplastic syndrome

PME pelvic muscle exercise; periodic monitoring examination; phosphomonoester; polymorphonuclear eosinophil; progressive multifocal encephalopathy; progressive myoclonus epilepsy

PMEA 9-(2-phosphomethoxyethyl) adenine

PMEL Pacific Marine Environmental Laboratory

PMF platelet membrane fluidity; progressive massive fibrosis; protein modified fast; proton motive force; pterygomaxillary fossa

pmf proton motive force

PMFC posterior medial frontal cortex

PMG primary medical group

PMGCT primary mediastinal germ cell tumor

PMH past medical history; posteromedial hypothalamus

PMHAB Provincial Mental Health Advisory Board

PMHCNS Psychiatric and Mental Health Clinical Nurse Specialist

PMHNP Psychiatric and Mental Health Nurse Practitioner

PMHR predicted maximum heart rate

PMHx past medical history

PMI pain management inventory; past medical illness; patient master index; patient medication instruction; perioperative myocardial infarction; photon migration imaging; point of maximal impulse; point of maximal intensity; posterior myocardial infarction; postmyocardial infarction; present medical illness; previous medical illness

PMIA *N*-(1-pyrenamethyl)-iodoacetamide

P−$_{min}$ peak negative pressure

PMIS postmyocardial infarction syndrome; PSRO Management Information System

PMK pacemaker

PML peripheral motor latency; polymorphonuclear leukocyte; posterior mitral leaflet; progressive multifocal leukodystrophy; progressive multifocal leukoencephalopathy; prolapsing mitral leaflet; promyelocytic leukemia; pulmonary microlithiasis

PMLD Pelizaeus-Merzbacher−like disease

PMLE polymorphous light eruption

PMM pentamethylmelamine; protoplast maintenance medium

PMMA polymethylmethacrylate

PMMIS Program Management and Medical Information System

PMN polymorphonuclear; polymorphonuclear neutrophil; premanufacture notification

PMNC percentage of multinucleated cells; peripheral blood mononuclear cell

PMNG polymorphonuclear granulocyte

PMNL peripheral blood monocytes and polymorphonuclear leukocytes; polymorphonuclear leukocyte

PMNN polymorphonuclear neutrophil

PMNR periadenitis mucosa necrotica recurrens

PMNSG Pravastatin Multinational Study Group

PMO postmenopausal osteoporosis; principal medical officer

pmol picomole

pmol/L picomoles per liter

PMP pain management program; paramagnetic particle; patient management problems; patient management program; patient medication profile; peripheral myelin protein; peroxisomal membrane protein;

persistent mentoposterior; previous menstrual period

PMPM, pmpm per member per month

PMPS postmastectomy pain syndrome

PMPY per member per year

PMQ phytylmenaquinone

PMR paper medical record; patient meta-record; percutaneous myocardial revascularization; perinatal mortality rate; periodic medical review; physical medicine and rehabilitation; polymyalgia rheumatica; primidone; prior medical record; progressive muscular relaxation; proportionate morbidity/mortality ratio; proton magnetic resonance

PM&R physical medicine and rehabilitation

PMRA Pest Management Regulatory Agency

PMRG Pimobendan Multicenter Research Group; Postmastectomy Rehabilitation Group

PMRS physical medicine and rehabilitation service

31P-MRS, ³¹P-MRS magnetic resonance spectroscopy with phosphorus 31

PMS patient management system; perimenstrual syndrome; periodic movements during sleep; phenazine methosulfate; polydactyly-myopia syndrome; postmarketing surveillance; postmenstrual stress; postmenstrual syndrome; postmeiotic segregation; postmitochondrial supernatant; Pravastatin Multinational Study; pregnant mare serum; premenstrual stress; premenstrual symptoms; premenstrual syndrome; progressive multiple sclerosis; psychotic motor syndrome

PMSC pediatric medical special care; pluripotent myeloid stem cell

PMSF phenylmethylsulfonyl fluoride

PMSG pregnant mare serum gonadotropin

PMSR peptide methionine sulfoxide reductase

PMT pacemaker-modulated tachycardia; parent management training; phenol *O*-methyltransferase; photomultiplier tube; Porteus maze test; premenstrual tension; pyridoxyl-methyl-tryptophan

PMTCT prevention of mother-to-child transmission

PMTDI provisional maximum tolerable daily intake

PMTS premenstrual tension syndrome

PMTT pulmonary mean transit time

PMV paramyxovirus; percutaneous mitral balloon valvotomy; prolapse of mitral valve

pMV prolapse of mitral valve

PMVI peak myocardial video intensity

PMVL polymorphic ventricular tachycardia; posterior mitral valve leaflet

pMVL posterior mitral valve leaflet

PMW pacemaker wires; patient management workstation

PMX paired mesoderm homeobox [gene]

PN papillary necrosis; parenteral nutrition; patient note; penicillin; perceived noise; percussion note; periarteritis nodosa; perinatal; peripheral nerve; peripheral neuropathy; Petri net; phrenic nerve; plaque neutralization; pneumonia; polyarteritis nodosa; polyneuritis; polyneuropathy; polynuclear; positional nystagmus; posterior nares; postnatal; practical nurse; predicted normal; primary nurse; progress note; protease nexin; psychiatry and neurology; psychoneurotic; pyelonephritis; pyridine nucleotide

P&N psychiatry and neurology

P/N positive/negative

P$_{N_2}$ partial pressure of nitrogen

P-5′-N pyridine-5′-nucleosidase

Pn pneumatic; pneumonia

pN positive regional lymph node

pN0 no regional lymph node metastases

pN1 poorly differentiated myeloblasts

pN1a tumor micrometastases [none larger than 0.2 cm]

pN1b tumor metastases to lymph nodes [larger than 0.2 cm]

pN1bi tumor metastases to one to three lymph nodes [from 0.2 to 2.0 cm]

pN1bii tumor metastases to four or more lymph nodes [0.2 to 2.0 cm]

pN1biii tumor metastases beyond lymph node capsule [none larger than 2.0 cm]

pN1biv tumor metastases to lymph nodes [larger than 2.0 cm]

pN2 tumor metastases to ipsilateral axillary lymph nodes

pN3 tumor metastases to ipsilateral mammary lymph nodes

pn pain

PNA Paris Nomina Anatomica; peanut agglutinin; pentose nucleic acid; *p*-nitroaniline

P$_{Na}$ plasma sodium

pNA *p*-nitroaniline

pNa plasma sodium

PNAC parenteral nutrition−associated cholestasis

PNALD parenteral nutrition−associated liver disease

PNAvQ positive-negative ambivalent quotient

PNB perineal needle biopsy; peripheral nerve block; *p*-nitrobiphenyl; premature nodal beat

PNBA *p*-nitrobenzoic acid

PNBT *p*-nitroblue tetrazolium

PNC Pakistan Nursing Council; penicillin; peripheral nucleated cell; pneumotaxic center; premature nodal contracture; primitive neuroendothelial cell

Pnc pneumococcus

PNCA proliferating nuclear cell antigen

PNCB Pediatric Nursing Certification Board

PNCG preconditioned nonlinear conjugate gradient

PND paroxysmal nocturnal dyspnea; partial neck dissection; postnasal drainage; postnasal drip; postnatal death; prenatal diagnosis; principal neutralizing determinant; purulent nasal drainage

PNdb perceived noise decibel

PNDM permanent neonatal diabetes mellitus

PNDS postnasal drip syndrome

PNE peripheral neuroepithelioma; plasma norepinephrine; pneumoencephalography; pseudomembranous necrotizing enterocolitis

PNEM paraneoplastic encephalomyelitis

PNET peripheral neuroepithelioma; primitive neuroectodermal tumor

PNEU, pneu, pneum pneumonia

PneumoADIP Pneumococcal Vaccines Accelerated Development and Introduction Plan

PNF proprioceptive neuromuscular facilitation

PNG penicillin G

PNH paroxysmal nocturnal hemoglobinuria; polynuclear hydrocarbon

PNHA Physicians National Housestaff Association

PNI peripheral nerve injury; postnatal infection; prognostic nutritional index

PNID Peer Nomination Inventory for Depression

PNK polynucleotide kinase; pyridoxine kinase

PNK(H) pyridoxine kinase, high

PNK(L) pyridoxine kinase, low

PNL peripheral nerve lesion; polymorphonuclear neutrophilic leukocyte

PNLA percutaneous needle lung aspiration

PNM perinatal mortality; peripheral dysostosis, nasal hypoplasia, and mental retardation (intellectual disability) [syndrome]; peripheral nerve myelin

PNMK pyridine nucleoside monophosphate kinase

PNMR postnatal mortality risk

PNMT phenyl-ethanolamine-*N*-methyltransferase

PNN polynomial neural network; probabilistic neural network

PNO principal nursing officer

p-NO₂ *p*-nitrosochloramphenicol

PNP pancreatic polypeptide; paraneoplastic pemphigus; para-nitrophenol; peak negative pressure; pediatric nurse practitioner; peripheral neuropathy; pneumoperitoneum; polyneuropathy; predictive value of negative results; psychogenic nocturnal polydipsia; purine nucleoside phosphorylase

P-NP para-nitrophenol

PNPase polynucleotide phosphorylase

PNPB positive−negative pressure breathing

PNPG alpha-*p*-nitrophenylglycerol

PNPP para-nitrophenylphosphate

PNPR positive−negative pressure respiration

PNS paranasal sinuses; paraneoplastic syndrome; parasympathetic nervous system; partial nonprogressive stroke; perinephric stranding; peripheral nerve stimulation; peripheral nervous system; posterior nasal spine; practical nursing student

PNSA partial negative surface area

PNT partial nodular transformation; patient; picture naming task

Pnt patient

Pnthx pneumothorax

PNU protein nitrogen unit

PNUT portable nursing unit terminal

PNVIm poly-*N*-vinyl imidazole

PNVX pneumococcal vaccine

Pnx pneumothorax

pNX regional lymph node tumor metastases cannot be assessed

PNZ posterior necrotic zone

PO by mouth, orally [L. *per os*]; parietal operculum; parietooccipital; period of onset; perioperative; posterior; postoperative; power output; predominant organism; pulse oximetry

PO₂, P$_{O_2}$, pO2 partial pressure of oxygen

Po porion

P$_o$ airway occlusion pressure; open probability; opening pressure

p.o. by mouth, orally [L. *per os*]

p/o postoperative

POA pancreatic oncofetal antigen; phalangeal osteoarthritis; preoptic area; primary optic atrophy

POADS postaxial acrofacial dysostosis syndrome

POAG primary open-angle glaucoma

POA-HA preoptic anterior hypothalamic area

POB penicillin, oil, beeswax; phenoxybenzamine; place of birth

POBA plain-old balloon angioplasty

POBJ physical object

POC particulate organic carbon; persistent organohalogen compound; point of care; polyolefin copolymer; postoperative care; probability of chance; product of conception; proof of concept; pro-opiomelanocortin

POCD postoperative cognitive dysfunction

POCS prescription order communication system; projection onto convex sets

POCT point-of-care testing

POD peroxidase; place of death; podiatry; polycystic ovary disease; pool of doctors; postoperative day; pouch of Douglas; promyelocytic leukemia oncogenic domain

POD1 first postoperative day

POD2 second postoperative day

PODx preoperative diagnosis

POE pediatric orthopedic examination; physician order entry; point of entry; polyoxyethylene; postoperative endophthalmitis; proof of eligibility

POEA polyoxyethylene amine

POEMS Patient-Oriented Evidence that Matters; polyneuropathy, organomegaly, endocrinopathy/edema, monoclonal-protein or monoclonal gammopathy, skin changes or abnormalities [syndrome]

POET physician order entry term

POF pattern of failure; position of function; premature ovarian failure; primary ovarian failure; pyruvate oxidation factor

PofE portal of entry

POFX X-linked premature ovarian failure

POG Pediatric Oncology Group; polymyositis ossificans generalisata

Pog pogonion

POGO percentage of glottic opening

pOH hydroxide ion concentration in a solution

POHI physically or otherwise health impaired

POHS presumed ocular histoplasmosis syndrome

PoHV pongine herpesvirus

PoHV 1, 2, 3 pongine herpesviruses 1, 2, 3

POI Personal Orientation Inventory; piece of information

PoI Pourcelot Index

poik poikilocyte, poikilocytosis

POIS Parkland On-Line Information Systems

pois poison, poisoned, poisoning

POL physician's office laboratory; physicians' online; Pollution Abstracts; polymerase

Pol polymerase

pol polish, polishing

POLA polymerase alpha

pol-GIK Polish Glucose-Insulin-Kalium [study]

polio poliomyelitis

POLIP polyneuropathy, ophthalmoplegiam leukoencephalopathy, intestinal pseudoobstruction [syndrome]

Pol-MONICA Polish Monitoring Trends and Determinants in Cardiovascular Diseases [study]

POLONIA Polish-American Local Lovenox NIR Stent Assessment [study]

Poly polymorphonuclear

poly-A, poly(A) polyadenylic acid

poly-C, poly(C) polycytidylic acid

poly(CPH) poly[1,6-bis(-carboxyphenoxy) hexane]

poly-dA, poly(dA) polydeoxyadenylic acid

poly-G, poly(G) polyguanylic acid

poly-I, poly(I) polyinosinic acid

poly-IC, poly-I:C copolymer of polyinosinic and polycytidylic acids

polys polymorphonuclear leukocytes

poly(SA) poly(sebacic anhydride)

poly-T, poly(T) polythymidylic acid

poly-U, poly(U) polyuridylic acid

POM pain on motion; prescription-only medicine; purulent otitis media

POMC pro-opiomelanocortin

POMONA pregnancy and postpartum, osteoporosis, mastectomy rehabilitation, osteoarthritis, nerve pain, athletic injuries

POMP phase-offset multiplanar; principal outer material protein

POMR problem-oriented medical record

POMS problem-oriented medical synopsis; Profile of Mood States

POMT phenol *O*-methyltransferase

PON paraoxonase; particulate organic nitrogen; Pollution and Toxicology Database

pond by weight [L. *pondere*]; heavy [L. *ponderosus*]

P-one first parental generation

PONV postoperative nausea and vomiting

POOV Poovoot virus

POP diphosphate group; pain on palpation; paroxypropione; pelvic organ prolapse; persistent occipitoposterior; pituitary opioid peptide; plasma osmotic pressure; plaster of Paris; point of presence; polymyositis ossificans progressiva; post office protocol

Pop popliteal; population

POPG population group

POPLA presurgical orthopedics, gingivoperiosteoplasty, and lip adhesion

POPLINE Population Information Online

poplit popliteal

POPNO pain of predominantly neuropathic origin

POPOP 1,4-bis-(5-phenoxazol-2-yl) benzene

POPQ, POP-Q pelvic organ prolapse quantification [system]
POPR preoperative patient representation
POPS patient outcome plans; postoperative pacing study; pulmonary overpressurization syndrome
pops points of presence
POQ Patient Barriers Questionnaire
POR patient-oriented research; physician of record; postocclusive oscillatory response; prevalence odds ratio; problem-oriented record
PORC porphyria, Chester type
PORH postoperative reactive hyperemia
PORP partial ossicular replacement prosthesis
PORT Patient Outcomes Research Teams [study]; Pneumonia Outcomes Research Team; postoperative radiation therapy; postoperative respiratory therapy
PORV Porton virus
PoRV porcine rubulavirus
PoRV-C porcine rotavirus Cowden
PoRV-E/DC9 porcine rotavirus DC-9
POS periosteal osteosarcoma; physician order set; point of service; polycystic ovary syndrome; provider of services; psychoorganic syndrome
pos position; positive
POSC problem-oriented system of charting
POSCH Program on Surgical Control of Hyperlipidemia
POSM patient-operated selector mechanism
pOsm plasma osmolality
POSS persistent object storage system; proximal over-shoulder strap
POSSUM Pictures of Standard Syndromes and Undiagnosed Malformations; Physiological and Operative Severity Score for the Enumeration of Morbidity and Mortality [study]
POST posterior; Predictors and Outcomes of Stent Thrombosis [study]
Post, post posterior
POST-CARG post—coronary artery bypass graft
postgangl postganglionic
POST LAT posterolateral
postop, post-op postoperative
Post Pit posterior pituitary [gland]
postSA postoperative spherical aberration
POT periostitis ossificans toxica; postoperative treatment; precursor onset time
pot potassium; potential
potass potassium
POTS plain-old telephone service; postural orthostatic tachycardia syndrome
POTV Potosi virus; Potiskum virus

PoTV porcine torovirus
POU placenta, ovary, and uterus
Pout outflow pressure
POV physician order verification
PoV portal vein
PO$_2$v venous oxygen pressure
POW Powassan [encephalitis]
powd powder
POWER Patients Online for Wellness, Education and Research
POWV Powassan virus
POX point of exit
PP diphosphate group; pink puffers [emphysema]; near point of accommodation [L. *punctum proximum*]; pacesetter potential; palmoplantar; pancreatic polypeptide; paradoxic pulse; paraplatin; parietal pericardium; parietal pulse; partial pressure; perfusion pressure; peritoneal pseudomyxoma; persisting proteinuria; Peyer patches; photoplethysmography; pinprick; placental protein; placenta previa; planned parenthood; plaque psoriasis; plasma pepsinogen; plasmapheresis; plasma protein; plaster of Paris; polypropylene; polystyrene agglutination plate; population planning; posterior papillary; posterior pituitary; postpartum; postprandial; precocious puberty; preferred provider; primary provider; primer protein; primipara; private practice; proactivator plasminogen; protein phosphatase; protoporphyria; protoporphyrin; proximal phalanx; prudent practices; pseudomyxoma peritonei; pterygoid process; pulmonary pressure; pulse pressure; pulsus paradoxus; purulent pericarditis; pyrophosphatase; pyrophosphate
P-P prothrombin proconvertin
PP1 protein phosphatase type 1
P-5′-P pyridoxal-5′-phosphate
PP$_1$ free pyrophosphate
Pp plateau pressure
pp near point of accommodation [L. *punctum proximum*]; postpartum; postprandial
p-p peak to peak
PPA palpation, percussion, auscultation; pepsin A; phenylpropanolamine; phenylpyruvic acid; Pittsburgh pneumonia agent; plasmid profile analysis; polyphosphoric acid; positive predictive accuracy; posterior margin of pulmonary artery; posterior pulmonary artery; postpartum amenorrhea; postpill amenorrhea; preferred provider arrangement; prescription-pricing authority; primary progressive aphasia; propanolamine; pure pulmonary atresia
PP&A palpation, percussion, and auscultation

PP2A protein phosphatase type 2A

Ppa pulmonary artery pressure

PP2Ac catalytic subunit of protein phosphatase type 2A

PPACK L-propyl-*p*-phenylalanyl-chloromethylketone

PP2A_D dimeric protein phosphatase type 2A

PPAF progressive perivenular alcoholic fibrosis

PPAR peroxisome proliferator activated receptor

PPAS peripheral pulmonary artery stenosis

PPase protein phosphatase

Ppaw pulmonary artery wedge pressure

PPB parts per billion; plasmatic protein binding; platelet-poor blood; pneumococcal pneumonia and bacteremia; positive pressure breathing

PPb postparotid basic protein

ppb parts per billion

PPBP pro-platelet basic protein

PPBS postprandial blood sugar

PPBV Phnom Penh bat virus

PPC patient-physician communication; pentose phosphate cycle; peripheral posterior curve; plasma protein concentration; plasma prothrombin conversion; pneumopericardium; pocket personal computer; posterior parietal cortex; progressive patient care; proximal palmar crease

PP1c protein phosphatase type 1, catalytic subunit

PP2C protein phosphatase type 2C

PPCA plasma prothrombin conversion accelerator; proserum prothrombin conversion accelerator

PPCD polymorphous posterior corneal dystropy

PPCE postproline cleaving enzyme

PPCF peripartum cardiac failure; plasma prothrombin conversion factor

PPCM postpartum cardiomyopathy

PPCRA pigmented paravenous chorioretinal atrophy

PPD packs per day; paraphenylenediamine; percussion and postural drainage; permanent partial disability; phenyldiphenyloxadiazole; pigmented purpuric dermatoses; postpartum day; primary physical dependence; progressive perceptive deafness; purified protein derivative

PPDS phonologic programming deficit syndrome

PPD-S purified protein derivative-standard

PPD-T purified protein derivative stabilized with Tween

PPE palmoplantar erythrodysesthesia; personal protective equipment; polyphosphoric

ester; porcine pancreatic elastase; probabilistic population estimation; pulmonary permeability edema

P_peak peak cycling respiratory pressure

PPES palmar-plantar erythrodysesthesia syndrome

PPET patient-physician encounter table

PPF pellagra preventive factor; phagocytosis promoting factor; phosphonoformate; plasma protein fraction

PPFA Planned Parenthood Federation of America

PPG peristomal pyoderma gangrenosum; phonopneumography; photoelectric plethysmography; photoplethysmography; platelet proteoglycan; portal pressure gradient

ppg picopicogram

PPGA postpill galactorrhea-amenorrhea

PPGB protective protein of beta-galactosidase

PPGF polypeptide growth factor

PPGP prepaid group practice

ppGpp 3′-pyrophosphoryl-guanosine-5′-diphosphate

PPGSS papular-purpuric gloves-and-socks syndrome

PPH past pertinent history; persistent pulmonary hypertension; phosphopyruvate hydratase; postpartum hemorrhage; primary prevention of hypertension; primary pulmonary hypertension; protocollagen proline hydroxylase

pph parts per hundred

pphm parts per hundred million

PPHN persistent pulmonary hypertension of the newborn

PPHP pseudopseudohypoparathyroidism

ppht parts per hundred thousand

PPI partial permanent impairment; patient package insert; patient physiologic image; perceived penile inadequacy; permanent pacemaker insertion; post pacing interval; present pain intensity; proton pump inhibitor; purified porcine insulin

PPi, PP_i inorganic pyrophosphate

PPIA parental presence during induction of anesthesia; Physicians Professional Indemnity Association

PPIase peptidyl-prolyl isomerase

PPID peak pain intensity difference

PPIE prolonged postictal encephalopathy

PPK palmoplantar keratosis; prekallikrein

PPL penicilloyl polylysine; posterior pulmonary leaflet

Ppl intrapleural pressure; pleural pressure

Pplat plateau pressure

PPLO pleuropneumonia-like organism

PPM parts per million; permanent pacemaker; phosphopentomutase; physician practice management; pigmented pupillary membrane; posterior papillary muscle; pulse position modulated

ppm parts per million; pulses per minute

PPMA progressive postmyelitis muscular atrophy

PPMD Provincial Performance Management Database

PPMS Performax's Personal Matrix System; primary progressive multiple sclerosis

PPN partial parenteral nutrition; parameterized Petri net; pedunculopontine nucleus

PPNA peak phrenic nerve activity

PPNAD primary pigmented nodular adrenocortical disease

PPNG penicillinase-producing *Neisseria gonorrhoeae*

PPNTI perioperative peripheral nerve traction injury

PPO platelet peroxidase; preferred provider option; preferred provider organization; protoporphyrin oxidase

P&PO principles and practice of oncology

PPOCD postpartum obsessive-compulsive disorder

PPP pain perception profile; palatopharyngoplasty; palmoplantar pustulosis; pearly penile papules; pentose phosphate pathway; peripheral pulse present; photostimulable phosphor plate; Pickford projective pictures; platelet-poor plasma; pluripotent progenitor; point-to-point protocol; polyphoretic phosphate; porcine pancreatic polypeptide; portal perfusion pressure; Prospective Pravastatin Pooling [project]; protein phosphatase; purified placental protein

PPPA protein phosphatase alpha

PPPBL peripheral pulses palpable both legs

PPPD pylorus-preserving pancreatoduodenectomy

PPPI primary private practice insurance

PPPMA progressive postpolio muscle atrophy

PPPP porokeratosis punctata palmaris et plantaris

PPR patient-provider relationship; pentatricopeptide repeat; percentage of predicted recovery; photoparoxysmal response; physician-patient relationship; physician payment reform; posterior primary ramus; Price precipitation reaction

PPr paraprosthetic

PPRC Physician Payment Review Commission

PPRF paramedian pontine reticular formation; pontine perireticular formation; postpartum renal failure

PP1$_{RG}$ protein phosphatase type 1, regulatory subunit

PPRM Portable Patient Record Model

PPROM preterm premature rupture of fetal membranes

PPRV peste des petits ruminants (ovine rinderpest) virus

PPRWP poor precordial R-wave progression

PPS Paris Prospective Study; pentosan polysulfate sodium; Personal Preference Scale; physician, patient and society; polyvalent pneumococcal polysaccharide; popliteal pterygium syndrome; postpartum sterilization; postperfusion syndrome; postpericardiotomy syndrome; postpolio syndrome; postpump syndrome; prescription preparation system; primary acquired preleukemic syndrome; prospective payment system; prospective pricing system; protein plasma substitute; pulse per second

PPSC Play Performance Scale for Children

PPSH pseudovaginal perineoscrotal hypospadias

PP1$_{SR}$ protein phosphatase type 1, sarcoplasmic reticulum

PPSTH population poststimulus time histogram

PPSV pneumococcal polysaccharide vaccine; pneumococcal vaccine polyvalent

PPSV23 23-valent pneumococcal polysaccharide vaccine

PPT parietal pleural tissue; partial prothrombin time; parts per thousand; parts per trillion; peak-to-peak threshold; pedunculopontine tegmental; Pfeiffer-Palm-Teller [syndrome]; physical performance test; plant protease test; Polyp Prevention Trial; polypurine tract; postpartum thyroiditis; posterior pelvic tilt; preprotachykinin; pressure pain threshold; pulmonary physical therapy; pulmonary platelet trapping

ppt parts per thousand; parts per trillion; precipitate, precipitation; prepared

pptd precipitated

PPTL postpartum tubal ligation

PPTS pyridinium *p*-toluenesulfonate

PPV Parapoxvirus, parapoxvirus; pneumococcal polysaccharide vaccine; porcine parvovirus; positive predictive value; positive pressure ventilation; Precarious Point virus; progressive pneumonia virus; pulmonary plasma volume

PPVr regional pulmonary plasma volume

PPVT Peabody Picture Vocabulary Test

PPVT-R Peabody Picture Vocabulary Test, Revised

PPW patient protective wrap
Ppw pulmonary wedge pressure
PPX protein phosphatase X
PPX1 protein phosphatase X type 1
PPX2 protein phosphatase X type 2
PPY pancreatic polypeptide
PPYLL potentially productive years of life lost
PPyV baboon polyomavirus 2
PQ paraquat; parent questionnaire; permeability quotient; physician's questionnaire; plastoquinone; pronator quadratus; pyrimethamine-quinine
pQCT peripheral quantitative computed tomography
PQI process quality improvement
PQOL Perceived Quality of Life
PQQ pyrroloquinoline quinone
P-QRS QRS P potential
PQRST Probucol Quantitative Regression Swedish Trial; provocative and palliative factors, quality of pain, radiation of pain, severity of pain, timing of pain
PR by rectum [L. *per rectum*]; far point of accommodation [L. *punctum remotum*]; palindromic rheumatism; parallax and refraction; partial reinforcement; partial remission; partial response; particulate respirator; peer review; perfusion rate; peripheral resistance; per rectum; phenol red; photoreaction; photoresist; physical rehabilitation; pityriasis rosea; police report; posterior root; postmyalgia rheumatica; postural reflex; potency ratio; preference record; pregnancy; pregnancy rate; preretinal; pressoreceptor; pressure; prevention; Preyer reflex; proctology; production rate; profile; progesterone receptor; progressive relaxation; progressive resistance; progress report; prolactin; prolonged remission; propranolol; prosthion; protease; protective ratio; protein; public relations; pulmonary regurgitation; pulmonary rehabilitation; pulse rate; pulse repetition; pyramidal response
P-R interval between P wave and beginning of the QRS complex [ECG]
P&R pelvic and rectal; pulse and respiration
Pr praseodymium; prednisolone; presbyopia; primary; prism; production, production rate; productivity; prolactin; prone positioning; propyl
pr far point of accommodation [L. *punctum remotum*]; pair; per rectum; prism
PRA panel-reactive antibody; patient record architecture; percent reactive antibody; phosphoribosylamine; physician recognition award; plasma renin activity; progesterone receptor assay; proximal reference axis

prac, pract practice, practitioner
PRACTICAL Placebo-Controlled Randomized ACE Inhibition Comparative Trial in Cardiac Infarction and Left Ventricular Function
PRAGMATIC pregnancy, rheumatoid arthritis, acromegaly, glucose metabolism disorders, mechanical injury, amyloid, thyroid disease, infectious disease, crystals in gout or pseudogout [mnemonic]
PRAGUE Primary Angioplasty After Transfer of Patients from General Community Hospitals to Catheterization Units with or Without Emergency Thrombolytic Infusion [study]
PrA-HPA protein A hemolytic plaque assay
PRAI pattern recognition and artificial intelligence
PRAISE Prospective Randomized Amlodipine Survival Evaluation
PRAM pressure-recording analytic method
PRAMS Pregnancy Risk Assessment Monitoring System
PRANN prediction recurrent artificial neural network
PRAS pre-reduced anaerobically sterilized; pseudo–renal artery syndrome
PRB basic proline-rich protein; Prosthetics Research Board
pRB, pRb retinoblastoma protein
PRBC packed red blood cells; placental residual blood volume
pRB-P phosphorylated form of retinoblastoma protein
PRBS pseudorandom binary sequence
PRBV placental residual blood volume
PRC packed red cells; peer review committee; phase response curve; plasma renin concentration; professional review committee; proximal row carpectomy
PRCA pure red cell aplasia
pRCA posterior right coronary artery
PRCCT prospective randomized controlled clinical trial
PRCF peak response coarse frequency
PRCG Polak-Ribiere conjugate gradient
PRCoV, PRCV porcine respiratory coronavirus
PRD partial reaction of degeneration; patient reference dossier; physician relations department; Pitt-Rogers-Danks [syndrome]; postradiation dysplasia
PRDBPC prospective randomized double blind placebo controlled
PRDP Provincial Resource Directory Project
PRDS Pitt-Rogers-Danks syndrome
PRE photoreacting enzyme; physician report of examination; pigmented retinal epithelium;

preliminary evaluation; preplacement examination; progressive resistive exercise; prospective randomized evaluation; proton relaxation enhancement

pre preliminary; preparation, prepare; pretreatment

PREA Pediatric Research Equity Act

pre-AIDS pre—acquired immune deficiency syndrome

pre-amp preliminary amplifier

PRECEDE predisposing, reinforcing, and enabling causes in educational diagnosis and evaluation

precip precipitate, precipitated, precipitation

PRECISE Prospective Randomized Evaluation of Carvedilol in Symptoms and Exercise [trial]

pre-CRT Hb prechemoradiotherapy hemoglobin

PRED prednisone

PREDICT Prospective Randomized Evaluation of Diltiazem CD Trial

PREFACE Pravastatin-Related Effects Following Angioplasty on Coronary Endothelium [study]

prefd preferred

PREFER Patient Randomization to Either Femoral or Radial Catheterization [trial]

preg, pregn pregnancy, pregnant

prelim preliminary

prem premature, prematurity

PreMACE prednisone, methotrexate, Adriamycin, cyclophosphamide, etoposide

PREMIS Prehospital Myocardial Infarction Study

pre-mRNA precursor messenger ribonucleic acid

preop, pre-op preoperative

PREP pattern reversal electrical potential; Physician Review and Enhancement Program

PrEP pre-exposure prophylaxis [with Truvada use]

prep, prepd prepare, prepared

pRER peak respiratory exchange ratio

Pres resistive pressure

PRESEP Pediatric Rural Emergency System and Education Project

preserv preservation, preserve, preserved

PRESERVE Prospective Randomized Enalapril Study Evaluating Regression of Ventricular Enlargement

PRESS Percutaneous Retroperitoneal Splenorenal Shunt [study]; point-resolved spectroscopy

press pressure

PREV Pretoria virus

prev prevention, preventive; previous

PREVENT Program in Ex Vivo Vein Graft Engineering via Transfection; Proliferation Reduction Using Vascular Energy Trial; Prospective Randomized Evaluation of the Vascular Effects of Norvasc Trial

PREVMEDU preventive medicine unit

PREZ posterior root entry zone

PRISMA preferred reporting items for systematic reviews and meta-analyses

PRF partial reinforcement; patient report form; peak repetition frequency; perforin; plasma recognition factor; pontine reticular formation; postrepetition frequency; progressive renal failure; prolactin releasing factor; pulse repetition frequency

pRF polyclonal rheumatoid factor

PRFF peak response, fine frequency

PRFLE Prospective Randomized Flosequinan Longevity Evaluation

PRFM platelet-rich fibrin matrix; premature rupture of fetal membranes

PRG phleborheography; purge

PRGS phosphoribosylglycineamide synthetase

PRH past relevant history; postrepetition frequency [Doppler]; prolactin-releasing hormone

PrH propositus hypoglossi

PRHCIT Project for Rural Health Communication and Information Technologies

PRHHP Puerto Rico Heart Health Program

PRHO Pre-registration house officer [UK]

PRI Pain Rating Index; patient review instrument; phosphate reabsorption index; phosphoribose isomerase; placental ribonuclease inhibitor

P-RIA polyclonal radioimmunoassay

PRIAS Packard radioimmunoassay system

PRICE protection, relative rest, ice, compression, elevation

PRICEMM protection, relative rest, ice, compression, elevation, modalities, medication

PRICES physician modalities, rehabilitation, injections, cross-training, evaluation, salicylates; protection, rest, ice, compression, elevation, support

PRIDE Parents Resource Institute for Drug Education; Platelet Aggregation and Receptor Occupancy with Integrilin-A Dynamic Evaluation [study]; Primary Implantable Defibrillator [study]

PRIH prolactin release—inhibiting hormone

PRIM primase

PRIMA Primary Care Information Across Anglia

PRIME preinversion multiecho; Prematriculation Program in Medical Education; Promotion of Reperfusion by Inhibition of Thrombin During Myocardial Infarction Evaluation [study]; Promotion of Reperfusion in Myocardial Infarction Evolution [study]; Prospective Randomized Ibopamine Mortality Evaluation [study]; Prospective Randomized Study of Ibopamine on Mortality and Efficacy in Heart Failure

PRIME-MD Primary Care Evaluation of Mental Disorders

PRIMEROSE probabilistic rule based on rough sets

PRIMEX primary care extender

PRIMI Prourokinase in Myocardial Infarction [trial]

primip primipara

PRINCE prevention of radiocontrast-induced nephropathy evaluation

PRIND prolonged reversible ischemic neurologic deficit

PRINS primed in situ

PRI(S) pain rating intensity score

PRISAM Primary Stenting for Acute Myocardial Infarction [trial]

PRISE Primary Care Sharing the Evidence

PRISM pediatric risk of mortality; Platelet Receptor Inhibition in Ischemic Syndrome Management [study]

PRISM-PLUS Platelet Receptor Inhibition in Ischemic Syndrome Management in Patients Limited by Unstable Signs and Symptoms [study]

PRISMS Prevention of Relapses and Disability by Interferon Beta-1a Subcutaneously in Multiple Sclerosis [study]

PRIST paper radioimmunosorbent test

PRISTINE Praxilene in Stroke Treatment in Northern Europe [study]

PRK photorefractive keratectomy; primary rabbit kidney

PRKAR protein kinase, cyclic adenosine monophosphate dependent, regulatory

PRKAR1A protein kinase, cyclic adenosine monophosphate dependent, regulatory, type 1 alpha

PRKC protein kinase C

PRKCA protein kinase C alpha

PRL, Prl prolactin

PRLR prolactin receptor

PRM phosphoribomutase; photoreceptor membrane; premature rupture of membranes; primary reference material; primidone; protamine

PrM preventive medicine

PRMS percent root mean square

PRMSE percent root mean square error

PRMST progressive resistance muscle strength training

PRN as needed [L. *pro re nata*]; pertactin; Physicians Research Network; polyradiculoneuropathy; prion; protectin

p.r.n. as needed [L. *pro re nata*]

PRNP prion protein

PRNT plaque reduction neutralization test

PRO patient-reported outcomes; peer review organization; physician review organization; professional review organization; pronation; protease; protein

Pro proline; prophylactic; prothrombin

pro protein

PROACT Prolyse in Acute Cerebral Thrombolysis Trial; Prourokinase in Acute Cerebral Thromboembolism [trial]; Prourokinase in Acute Thromboembolic Stroke [trial]

ProACT professionally advanced care team

prob probable

PROBE Prospective, Randomized, Open Blinded Endpoint Trial; Prospective, Randomized, Open Trial with Blinded Endpoint Evaluation

PROC protein C

proc procedure; proceedings; process

PROCAM Prospective Cardiovascular Münster Study

PROC GLM general linear model procedure

proct, procto proctologist, proctology; proctoscopy

prod production, product

PROFET Prevention of Falls in the Elderly Trial

prog progress, progressive

progn prognosis

PROGRESS Perindopril Protection Against Recurrent Stroke Study

proGRP pro-gastrin-releasing peptide

PROH propyl-4-hydrolase

PROHB propyl-4-hydrolase beta

PROLOG Precursor to EPILOG [study]; programming in logic

prolong prolongation, prolonged

PROM passive range of motion; premature rupture of fetal membranes; programmable read-only memory; prolonged rupture of fetal membranes; prosthetic range of motion

PROMIS Patient-Reported Outcomes Measurement Information System; Problem-Oriented Medical Information System

PROMISE Prospective Randomized Milrinone Survival Evaluation [study]

PROMM proximal myotonic myopathy

PROMPTOR-FM probabilistic method of prompting for test ordering in family medicine

pron pronation, pronator
PROP propranolol
ProPAC Prospective Payment Assessment Commission
PRO-PBP pro-platelet basic protein
PROPC professional point of care
proph prophylactic, prophylaxis
proPO prophenoloxidase
ProRS propyl transfer ribonucleic acid synthase
PROS Pediatric Research in Office Settings; protein S
pros prostate, prostatic
PROSIT proteinuria screening and intervention
PROSP protein S pseudogene
PROSPECT Proscar Safety Plus Efficacy Canadian Two-Year Study
PROSPER Prospective Study of Pravastatin in the Elderly at Risk
PROST pronuclear stage transfer
PROSTATE Physicians for Rational Ordering and Screening Tests and Therapeutic Effectiveness
prosth prosthesis, prosthetic
PROTECT Perindopril Regression of Vascular Thickening European Community Trial; Prospective Reinfarction in the Thrombolytic Era: Cardizem-CD Trial
PROTO protoporphyrin; protoporphyrinogen
pro-u-PA proenzyme urokinase plasminogen activator
prov provisional
PROVED Prospective Randomized Study of Ventricular Failure and the Efficacy of Digoxin
PROW Protein Review on the Web
prox proximal
PRP photolyase regulatory protein; physiologic rest position; pityriasis rubra pilaris; platelet-rich plasma; polyribosyl ribitol phosphate; postural rest position; pressure rate product; primary Raynaud phenomenon; progressive rubella panencephalitis; proliferative retinopathy photocoagulation; proline-rich protein; Psychotic Reaction Profile; pulse repetition period
PrP, Prp prion protein
PRPG platelet-rich plasma gel
PRPH peripherin
PRPLND primary retroperitoneal lymph node dissection
PRPP phosphoribosylpyrophosphate
PRPS prostatic secretory protein
PRP peak response phase
PRQ personal resources questionnaire
PRR pattern recognition receptor; proton relaxation rate; pulse repetition rate

PrR progesterone receptor
PRRB Provider Reimbursement Review Board
PRRE pupils round, regular, and equal
PR-RSV Prague Rous sarcoma virus
PRRT peptide receptor radionuclide therapy
PRS Personality Rating Scale; Pierre Robin syndrome; plasma renin substrate; Prieto syndrome; proctorectosigmoidoscopy
PRSIS Prospective Rate Setting Information System
PRT patient record tree; *Penicillium roqueforti* toxin; pharmaceutical research and testing; phosphoribosyl transferase; pivot repeatability test; positional release technique; postoperative respiratory therapy; prospective randomized trial
PrT protein truncation
PRTD proximal renal tubular dysfunction
PRTH pituitary resistance to thyroid hormone
PRTH-C prothrombin time control
PRTN proteinase
PRTS Partington syndrome
PRU peripheral resistance unit
PRUJ proximal radioulnar joint
PRV Paroo River virus; planning organ at risk volume; polycythemia rubra vera; posterior right ventricle; pseudorabies virus; python orthoreovirus
PRVC pressure-regulated volume control
PRVEP pattern reversal visual evoked potential
PRW polymerized ragweed
PRX pseudoexfoliation
Prx prognosis
prx proximal
PRZF pyrazofurin
PS pacemaker syndrome; pain stimulation; paired stimulation; pancreozymin secretin; paradoxic sleep; paralaryngeal space; paranoid schizophrenia; paraspinal; parasympathetic; Parkinson syndrome; parotid sialography; partial saturation; partial seizure; pathologic stage; patient serum; pediatric site [database, Italy]; pediatric surgery; performance status; performing scale; periodic syndrome; phosphate saline; phosphatidyl serine; photosensitivity, photosensitization; photosynthesis; phrenic stimulation; physical status; physiologic saline; phytosterol; pixel size; plastic surgery; polysaccharide; polystyrene; population sample; population spike; Porter-Silber [chromogen]; postcardiotomy shock; posterior synechiae; posterior synechiotomy; posteroseptal; postmaturity syndrome; precursor state; prescription;

presenilin; presenting symptom; pressure sore; pressure support; prestimulus; procedural sedation; programmed symbol; prostatic secretion; protamine sulfate; proteasome; protein S; protein synthesis; Proteus syndrome; P selectin; psychiatric; pulmonary sequestration; pulmonary stenosis; pulse sequence; pyloric stenosis

P&S paracentesis and suction

P/S polisher-stimulator; polyunsaturated/saturated

Ps prescription; *Pseudomonas*; psoriasis

Ps systolic pressure

ps per second; picosecond

pS2 trefoil factor 1

PSA pacemaker system analysis; parasternal short axis; physical sexual abuse; pleomorphic salivary gland adenoma; polar surface area; polyethylene sulfonic acid; polysaccharide adhesin; polysialic acid; posterior spinal artery; power spectrum analysis; primary sampling unit; professional services agreement; progressive spinal ataxia; prolonged sleep apnea; prostate-specific antigen; protein S alpha; pseudoaneurysm; psoriatic arthritis

PS/A polysaccharide adhesin

PsA psoriatic arthritis

Psa systemic blood pressure

PSAAMI Primary Stenting vs. Angioplasty in Acute Myocardial Infarction [trial]

PSAC President's Science Advisory Committee

PSACH pseudoachondrodysplasia

PSAD prostate-specific antigen density; psychoactive substance abuse and dependence

PSAG pelvic sonoangiography

PSAGN poststreptococcal acute glomerulonephritis

PSAn psychoanalysis

PSA-NCAM polysialic acid neuronal cell adhesion molecule

PSAP peak systolic aortic pressure; personal sound amplification product; primary public safety answering point; prosaposin; pulmonary surfactant apoprotein

P/SAT pediatric severity assessment

PSB protected specimen brush; protein S beta

PSbetaG, PSBG pregnancy-specific beta-1-glycoprotein

PSC patient services coordination; peripheral stem cell; Plasma Single Nucleotide Polymorphism Consortium; pluripotential stem cell; Porter-Silber chromogen; posterior subcapsular cataract; primary sclerosing

cholangitis; professional service corporation; prospective studies collaboration; proteasome component; pulse synchronized contractions

PS-CF pancreatic-sufficient cystic fibrosis

PsChE pseudocholinesterase

PSCI Primary Self Concept Inventory

Psci pressure at slow component intercept

PSCM problem space computational model

PSCT peripheral stem cell transplantation

PSD particle size distribution; peptone, starch, and dextrose; percutaneous stricture dilatation; periodic synchronous discharge; phase-sensitive detector; pilonidal sinus disease; poststenosis dilation; pituitary stalk distortion; posterior sagittal diameter; poststroke depression; postsynaptic density; power spectral density; prevention of significant deterioration; Protein Sequence Database; psychological symptoms of dementia; psychosomatic disease

PSDA Patient Self-Determination Act; psychoactive substance abuse and dependence

PSDES primary symptomatic diffuse esophageal spasm

PSE Pain Self-Efficacy [scale]; paradoxic systolic expansion; penicillin-sensitive enzyme; portal systemic encephalopathy; Present State Examination; purified spleen extract

psec picosecond

PSEK progressive symmetric erythrokeratoderma

PSEN1 presenilin 1 gene

PSEN2 presenilin 2 gene

PSEP post−sexual exposure prophylaxis

pseudo-BTX pseudobatrachotoxin

PSF peak scatter factor; peptide supply factor; point spread function; posterior spinal fusion; prostacyclin stabilizing factor; pseudosarcomatous fasciitis

PSG peak systolic gradient; phosphate, saline, and glucose; polysomnogram; pregnancy-specific glycoprotein; presystolic gallop; programmable sound generator

PSGL P selectin glycoprotein ligand

PSGN poststreptococcal glomerulonephritis

PSH past surgical history; postspinal headache

PsHD pseudo−heart disease

PSHV pulmonary syndrome hantavirus

PsHV psittacid herpesvirus

PSI parenting stress inventory; pneumonia severity index; pollutant standard index; posterior sagittal index; problem-solving information; prostaglandin synthetic inhibitor; Psychiatric Society for Informatics; psychological services index; psychosomatic inventory; purified photosystem I

psi pounds per square inch

psia pounds per square inch absolute

PSI-BLAST position-specific iterated basic local alignment search tool

PSICU pediatric surgical intensive care unit

pSIDS partially unexplained sudden infant death syndrome

PSIFT platelet suspension immunofluorescence test

PSIL percentage signal intensity loss; preferred frequency speech interference level

PSIS posterior sacroiliac spine

PSK protein serine kinase

PSL parasternal line; photostimulable luminescence; potassium, sodium chloride, and sodium lactate; prednisolone

PSM patient self-management; patient-specific mortality; personal status monitor; polymerase chain reaction [PCR]-mediated site-directed mutagenesis; presystolic murmur; problem-solving method

psm patient-specific mortality

PSMA prostate-specific membrane antigen; proximal spinal muscular atrophy

PSMed psychosomatic medicine

PSMF protein-sparing modified fast

PSMS Physical Self-Maintenance Scale

PSMT psychiatric services management team

PSN provider service network

PSNR peak signal/noise ratio

PSO pediatric subtraction osteotomy; proximal subungual onychomycosis

PSOs provider-sponsored organizations

PSOM probabilistic self-organizing map

PSP pancreatic spasmolytic peptide; paralytic shellfish poisoning; parathyroid secretory protein; peak systolic pressure; periodic short pulse; Personal and Social Performance; phenolsulfonphthalein; phosphoserine phosphatase; photostimulable phosphor plate; positive spike pattern; posterior spinal process; postsynaptic potential; prednisone sodium phosphate; primary spontaneous pneumothorax; progressive supranuclear palsy; prostatic secretory protein; pseudopregnancy; pulmonary surfactant apoprotein

PspA pneumococcal surface protein A

PSPR particle surface plasmon resonance

PSPS secretory pancreatic stone protein

PSPV psittacinepox virus

PSQ Parent Symptom Questionnaire; Patient Satisfaction Questionnaire

PSQI Pittsburgh sleep quality index

PsqO$_2$ subcutaneous tissue oximetry

PSR pain sensitivity range; perspective surface rendering; portal systemic resistance; posteroseptal right atrium; poststreptococcal reactive arthritis; pressure sore risk assessment; proliferative sickle retinopathy; pulmonary stretch receptor

PSRC Plastic Surgery Research Council

PSRO Professional Standards Review Organization

PSS painful shoulder syndrome; pain sensation score; patient scheduling system; patient stimulation stack; perceived stress scale; performance support system; phenotypic susceptibility score; physiologic saline solution; polystyrene sulfonate; porcine stress syndrome; primary Sjögren syndrome; progressive systemic scleroderma; progressive systemic sclerosis; psoriasis severity scale; Psychiatric Status Schedule; pure sensory stroke

pSS primary Sjögren syndrome

PSSE partial saturation spin echo

PSSS perceived stress support scale

PST pancreatic suppression test; paralytic shellfish toxin; paroxysmal supraventricular tachycardia; patient-specific therapy; penicillin, streptomycin, and tetracycline; penoscrotal transposition; peristimulus time; phenolsulfotransferase; platelet survival time; posterior sinus tympani; poststenotic; poststimulus time; prefrontal sonic treatment; problem-solving therapy; protein-sparing therapy; proximal straight tubule

PSTAF Pilsicainide Suppression Trial of Atrial Fibrillation

PSTE phase space time evolution

PSTF Pedigree Standardization Task Force [former name for Pedigree Standardization Work Group]

PSTH poststimulus time histogram

PSTI pancreatic secretory trypsin inhibitor

PSTN public switched telephone network

PSTV potato spindle tuber virus

PSU patient service unit; photosynthetic unit; primary sampling unit

PSurg plastic surgery

PSV papular stomatitis virus; peak systolic velocity; pressure-support ventilation; Punta Salinas virus

pSV simian vacuolating virus plasmid

PSV23 23-valent pneumococcal polysaccharide vaccine

PSVER pattern shift visual evoked response

PSVT paroxysmal supraventricular tachycardia

PSW positive sharp wave; primary surgical ward; psychiatric social worker

PSWG Pedigree Standardization Work Group

PSWT psychiatric social work training

PSX pseudoexfoliation
Psy psychiatry; psychology
psych psychological, psychology
PSYCHE Psychiatry Educator
psychiat psychiatric, psychiatry
psychoan psychoanalysis, psychoanalytical
psychol psychologic, psychology
psychopath psychopathologic, psychopathology
psychosom psychosomatic
psychother psychotherapy
psy-path psychopathic
Ps-ZES pseudo−Zollinger-Ellison syndrome
PT pain thermometer; pain threshold; pancreatic transplantation; parathormone; parathyroid; paroxysmal tachycardia; part time; patient; pericardial tamponade; permanent and total; phage type; pharmacy and therapeutics; phenytoin; phosphorothioate; photophobia; phototoxicity; physical therapist; physical therapy; physical training; physiotherapy; pine tar; plasma thromboplastin; pluridirectional tomography; pneumothorax; polynomial transform; polyvalent tolerance; position tracking; posterior tibial; posttetanic; posttransfusion; posttransplantation; posttraumatic; preferred term; premature termination; preoperative therapy; preterm; preventive therapy; previously treated; primary tumor; propylthiouracil; protamine; prothrombin time; pseudotumor; psychometric test; psychotherapy; pulmonary thrombosis; pulmonary tuberculosis; pyramidal tract
P&T permanent and total; pharmacy and therapeutics
Pt patient; platinum
pT pertussis toxin; postoperative tumor size
pT0 no evidence of primary tumor
pT1 no visible tumor tissue
pT2 less than 1.5 cm tumor remains
pT3 1.5 to 5.0 cm tumor remains
pT4 more than 5.0 cm tumor remains
pt part; patient; pint; point
PTA pancreatic transplantation alone; parallel tubular arrays; parathyroid adenoma; peak twitch amplitude; percutaneous transluminal angioplasty; peroxidase-labeled antibody; persistent truncus arteriosus; phosphotungstic acid; physical therapy assistant; plasma thromboplastin antecedent; posttraumatic amnesia; pretreatment anxiety; primitive trigeminal artery; prior to admission; prior to arrival; prothrombin activity

PTAB pterygoalar bar
PTAF platelet activating factor
PTAFR platelet activating factor receptor
PTAH phosphotungstic acid hematoxylin
PTAP purified diphtheria toxoid precipitated by aluminum phosphate
PTAT pure tone average threshold
PTB patellar tendon bearing; polypyrimidine tract binding; prior to birth; proximal tubal blockage
PTb pulmonary tuberculosis
PTBA percutaneous transluminal balloon angioplasty
PTBBS peripheral type benzodiazepine binding site
PTBD percutaneous transhepatic biliary drainage; percutaneous transluminal balloon dilation
PTBE pyretic tick-borne encephalitis
PTBNA protected transbronchial needle aspirate
PTBPD posttraumatic borderline personality disorder
PTBS posttraumatic brain syndrome
PTBW peak torque to body weight
PTC papillary thyroid carcinoma; percutaneous transhepatic cholangiography; phase transfer catalyst; phenothiocarbazine; phenylthiocarbamide; phenylthiocarbamoyl; plasma thromboplastin component; plugged telescopic catheter; posttetanic count; premature termination codon; premature tricuspid closure; prior to conception; prothrombin complex; pseudotumor cerebri
PTCA percutaneous transluminal coronary angiography; percutaneous transluminal coronary angioplasty; pyrrole-2,3,5-tricarboxylic acid
PT(C)A percutaneous transluminal [coronary] angioplasty
PtcCO$_2$ transcutaneous partial pressure of carbon dioxide
PTCDA perylene-tetracarboxylic dianhydride
PTCER pulmonary transcapillary escape rate
PTCL panniculitic T-cell lymphoma; peripheral T-cell lymphoma
PtcO$_2$ transcutaneous oxygen tension
PTCR percutaneous transluminal coronary recanalization/revascularization
PTCRA percutaneous transluminal coronary rotational ablation
PTD percutaneous transluminal dilation; permanent total disability; personality trait disorder; photothermal deflection; preterm delivery; prior to delivery

PTDS posttraumatic distress syndrome

PTE parathyroid extract; posttraumatic epilepsy; pretibial edema; proximal tibial epiphysis; pulmonary thromboembolism

PTEAM particle total exposure assessment methodology

PTED pulmonary thromboembolic disease

PteGlu pteroylglutamic acid

pter end of short arm of chromosome

PTES percutaneous transcatheter ethanol sclerotherapy

PTF patient treatment file; plasma thromboplastin factor; posterior talofibular; preterm formula; proximal tubular fragment

PTFA prothrombin time fixing agent

PTFE polytetrafluoroethylene

PTFNA percutaneous transthoracic fine-needle aspiration

PTFS posttraumatic fibromyalgia syndrome

PTG parathyroid gland; prostaglandin

PTGE prostaglandin E

PTGER prostaglandin E receptor

PTH parathormone; parathyroid; parathyroid hormone; percutaneous transhepatic drainage; phenylthiohydantoin; plasma thromboplastin component; posttransfusion hepatitis

PTHC percutaneous transhepatic cholangiography

PTHL parathyroid hormone−like

PTHLP parathyroid hormone−like protein

PTH/PTHrP parathyroid hormone/parathyroid hormone−related peptide

PTHR parathyroid hormone receptor

PTHRP, PTHrP parathyroid hormone−related peptide; parathyroid hormone−related protein

PTHS parathyroid hormone secretion

PTHV Pathun Thani virus

PTI pancreatic trypsin inhibitor; penetrating trauma index; persistent tolerant infection; Pictorial Test of Intelligence; placental thrombin inhibitor; pulsatility transmission index

PTK phosphotyrosine kinase; phototherapeutic keratectomy; protein tyrosine kinase

PTL peritoneal telencephalic leukoencephalomyopathy; pharyngotracheal lumen; plasma thyroxine level; posterior tricuspid leaflet; preterm labor

pTL posterior tricuspid leaflet

PTLA pharyngeal tracheal lumen airway

PTLC precipitation thin layer chromatography

PTLD posttransplantation lymphoproliferative disorder; prescribed tumor lethal dose

PTLDS post-treatment Lyme disease syndrome

PTLV primate T-lymphotropic virus

PTLV 1, 2, 3 primate T-lymphotropic viruses 1, 2, 3

PTM posterior trabecular meshwork; posttransfusion mononucleosis; posttranslational modification; posttraumatic meningitis; prothymosin; pulse time modulation

P$_{TM}$ transmural pressure

Ptm pterygomaxillary

PTMA percutaneous transvenous mitral annuloplasty; phenyltrimethylammonium; posttransplantation thrombotic microangiopathy; prothymosin alpha

PTMDF pupils, tension, media, disc, fundus

PTMPY per thousand members per year

PTMR percutaneous transluminal myocardial revascularization

PTMS parathymosin

PTN pain transmission neuron; pleiotrophin; posterior tibial nerve; Prevention Trials Network; proximal tibial nail; public telephone network

pTNM pathologic classification of primary tumors, regional nodes, and metastases

PTO Klemperer's tuberculin [Ger. *Perlsucht Tuberculin Original*]

P$_{total}$ total pressure

PTP pancreatic thread protein; pediatric telephone protocol; percutaneous transhepatic portography; phosphotyrosine phosphatase; physical treatment planning; posterior tibial pulse; posttetanic potential; posttransfusion purpura; pretest probability; previously treated patient; protein-tyrosine phosphatase; proximal tubular pressure

Ptp transpulmonary pressure

PTPA phosphotyrosyl phosphatase activator

PTPC protein tyrosine phosphatase C

PTPG protein tyrosine phosphatase gamma

PTPI posttraumatic pulmonary insufficiency

PTPinsp inspiratory pressure-time product

PTPM posttraumatic progressive myelopathy

PTPN protein tyrosine phosphatase, non-receptor

PTPRA protein tyrosine phosphatase receptor alpha

PTPRB protein tyrosine phosphatase receptor beta

PTPRF protein tyrosine phosphatase receptor F

PTPRG protein tyrosine phosphatase receptor gamma

PTPS postthrombophlebitis syndrome; 6-pyruvoyl tetrahydropterin synthase

PTPT protein tyrosine phosphatase, T-cell

PT/PTT prothrombin time/partial thromboplastin time

PTQ parent-teacher questionnaire

PTR patellar tendon reflex; patient termination record; patient to return; peripheral total resistance; plasma transfusion reaction; prothrombin time ratio; psychotic trigger reaction

PTr porcine trypsin

Ptr intratracheal pressure

PTRA percutaneous transluminal renal angioplasty

PT Rep patient representative

PTRIA polystyrene-tube radioimmunoassay

Ptrx pelvic traction

PTS para-toluenesulfonic [acid]; patient treatment file; pediatric trauma score; postthrombotic syndrome; posttraumatic syndrome; posture training support, weighted [vest]; Pressure and Tension Scale; prior to surgery; 6-pyruvoyl tetrahydropterin synthase

Pts, pts patients

PTSD posttraumatic stress disorder

PTSM Plant, Technology, and Safety Management

PTSS posttraumatic stress syndrome

PTT partial thromboplastin time; particle transport time; posterior tibial tendon; protein truncation test; prothrombin time; pulmonary transit time; pulse transit time

ptt partial thromboplastin time

PTTI penetrating thoracic trauma index

PTU phenylthiourea; propylthiouracil

PTV patient-triggered ventilation; planning target volume; porcine teschovirus; posterior terminal vein; posterior tibial vein; Punta Toro virus

PTV$_2$ planning target volume 2

PtV pneumotropic virus

PTVT planning target volume tool

PTVV Ponteves virus

PTX palytoxin; pentoxifylline; picrotoxinin; pneumothorax

PTx parathyroidectomy; pelvic traction

Ptx pneumothorax

pTX no evidence of primary tumor

PTXT pointer to text

PTZ pentylenetetrazol

PU palindromic unit; passed urine; patient unit; pepsin unit; peptic ulcer; perfusion unit; polyurethane; pregnancy urine; 6-propyluracil; prostatic urethra

Pu plutonium; purine; purple

PUA patient unit assistant

pub public

PUBS percutaneous umbilical blood sampling; perforations, ulcers, and gastrointestinal bleeds; purple urine bag syndrome

PUC pediatric urine collector; premature uterine contractions

PUCV Puchong virus

PUD peptic ulcer disease; pudendal

PuD pulmonary disease

PUF polyurethane foam; pure ultrafiltration

PUFA polyunsaturated fatty acid

PUF-HAL polyurethane foam—hybrid artificial liver

PUH pregnancy urine hormones

PUI patient under investigation; platelet uptake index; posterior urethral injury

PUJO pelviureteric junction obstruction

PUL percutaneous ultrasonic lithotripsy

PUL, pul pulmonary

PULHEMS physique, upper extremity, lower extremity, hearing and ears, eyes and vision, mental capacity, emotional stability

pulm pulmonary

PULSES physical condition, upper limb function, lower limb function, sensory component, excretory function, and mental status/support factors

pulv. powder [L. *pulvis*]

PUM peanut-reactive urinary mucin

PUMF public use microdata file

PUMP putative metalloproteinase

PUMS patient utility measurement set; permanently unfit for military service

PUN plasma urea nitrogen

PUO pyrexia of unknown origin

PUP previously untreated patient; previously untreated product

pUPID paternal uniparental isodisomy

PUPPP pruritic urticarial papules and plaques of pregnancy

PUR polyurethrane

Pur purple

pur purulent

purg purgative

PurR purine repressor

PURSUIT Platelet Glycoprotein IIb/IIIa Underpinning the Receptor for Suppression of Unstable Ischemia Trial; Platelet Glycoprotein IIb-IIIa in Unstable Angina: Receptor Suppression Using Integrilin Therapy

PURV Purus virus

PUT provocative use test; putamen

PUU Puumala [virus]

PUUV Puumala virus

PUV posterior urethral valve

PUVA psoralen ultraviolet-A range

PV pancreatic vein; papilla of Vater; papillomavirus; paramyxovirus; parapoxvirus; paraventricular; paravertebral; partial volume; parvovirus; pemphigus vulgaris; peripheral vascular; peripheral vein; peripheral vessel; picornavirus; pityriasis versicolor; plasma viscosity; plasma volume; pneumonia virus; polio vaccine; poliovirus; polycythemia vera; polyoma virus; polyvinyl; portal vein; postvasectomy; postvoiding; poxvirus; predictive value; pressure velocity; pressure volume; process variable; progressive vaccinia; pulmonary valve; pulmonary vein

P-V pressure volume

P&V pyloroplasty and vagotomy

P$_V$ ventricular pressure

PV-1, 2, 3 human polioviruses 1, 2, 3

Pv *Proteus vulgaris*; venous pressure

PVA Paralyzed Veterans of America; peripheral venous alimentation; polyvinyl acetate; polyvinyl alcohol; pressure volume area

PV$_a$ pulmonary venous atrial

PVA-C polyvinyl alcohol cryogel

PVAc polyvinyl acetate

PVAd polyvinyladenine

PVALB parvalbumin

PVARP postventricular atrial refractory period

PVB cis-platinum, vinblastine, bleomycin; paravertebral block; pigmented villonodular bundle; premature ventricular beat

PVC peripheral venous catheterization; permanent visual circuit; persistent vaginal cornification; polyvinyl chloride; postvoiding cystogram; predicted vital capacity; premature ventricular complex; premature ventricular contraction; primary visual cortex; pulmonary venous capillaries; pulmonary venous confluence; pulmonary venous congestion

PVCM paradoxic vocal cord motion

PV$_{CO_2}$ partial pressure of carbon dioxide in mixed venous blood

PVD patient very disturbed; peripheral vascular disease; portal vein dilation; posterior vitreous detachment; postural vertical dimension; premature ventricular depolarization; pulmonary valvular dysplasia; pulmonary vascular disease

PVDF polyvinyl diisopropyl fluoride; polyvinylidene difluoride

PVE partial volume effect; perivenous encephalomyelitis; periventricular echogenicity; postvaccinial encephalopathy; premature ventricular event; premature ventricular extrasystole; prosthetic valve endocarditis

PV-ECF plasma volume/extracellular fluid [ratio]

PVEM postvaccinial encephalomyelitis

P-VEP pattern visual evoked potential

PVF peripheral visual field; portal venous flow; primary ventricular fibrillation

PVFS postviral fatigue syndrome

PVG periventricular gray matter; pulmonary valve gradient

PVH paraventricular hyperintensity; pulmonary venous hypertension

PVI patient video interview; peripheral vascular insufficiency; perivascular infiltration; positron volume imaging; protracted venous infusion

PVK penicillin V potassium

PVL perivalvular leakage; periventricular leukomalacia; permanent vision loss

PVM parallel virtual machine; pneumonia virus of mice; proteins, vitamins, and minerals; pulmonary vascular marking

PVMed preventive medicine

PVMR PRODIGY Virtual Medical Record

PVN paraventricular nucleus; predictive value negative

PVNPS post−Viet Nam psychiatric syndrome

PVNS pigmented villonodular synovitis

PVNZ parapoxvirus of red deer in New Zealand

PVO pulmonary venous obstruction

PV$_{O_2}$ partial oxygen pressure in mixed venous blood

PVOD pulmonary vascular obstructive disease; pulmonary venoocclusive disease

PVP penicillin V potassium; peripheral vein plasma; peripheral venous pressure; polyvinylpyrrolidone; portal venous phase; portal venous pressure; predictive value of positive results; pulmonary vein potential; pulmonary venous pressure

PVP-I polyvinylpyrrolidone-iodine

PVR peripheral vascular resistance; perspective volume rendering; poliovirus receptor; postvoiding residual; pulmonary valve replacement or repair; pulmonary vascular resistance; pulse volume recording

pVR perspective volume rendering

PVRI pulmonary vascular resistance index

PVS partner violence screening; percussion, vibration, suction; percutaneous vascular surgery; peritoneovenous shunt; permanent vegetative state; persistent vegetative state; persistent viral syndrome; Plummer-Vinson syndrome; poliovirus susceptibility; polyvinyl sponge; premature ventricular systole; programmed ventricular stimulation; pulmonary valvular stenosis

PV$_s$ pulmonary venous systolic

PVSA percutaneous vasal sperm aspiration

PVSG Polycythemia Vera Study Group

PVST prevertebral soft tissue

PVU Pueblo Viejo virus

PVT paroxysmal ventricular tachycardia; periventricular thalamic [nucleus]; portal vein thrombosis; pressure, volume, and temperature; private patient; psychomotor vigilance task

PVTT portal vein tumor thrombosis; portal vein tumor thrombus

PVW posterior vaginal wall

pvz pulverization

PW peristaltic wave; plantar wart; posterior wall; pressure wave; psychological warfare; pulmonary wedge; pulsed wave; pulse width

Pw progesterone withdrawal; pulsed wave; whole-cell pertussis [vaccine]

pW picowatt

PWA person with AIDS; pulse wave analysis

PWB partial weight bearing

PWBC peripheral white blood cell

PWBRT prophylactic whole-brain radiation therapy

PWBT partial weight-bearing therapy

PWC peak work capacity; physical work capacity

PWCA pure white cell aplasia

PWCR Prader-Willi chromosome region

PWCT perfusion-weighted computed tomography

PWD posterior wall in diastole; printed wiring board

pwd powder

PWDS postweaning diarrhea syndrome

PWDU pulsed wave Doppler ultrasound

PWE posterior wall excursion

PWI perfusion-weighted imaging; posterior wall infarct

PWLV posterior wall of left ventricle

PWM pulse with modulation

pw-MW prewhitening [of data] multiple window

PWP patient word processing; Prentice, Williams, and Peterson [model]; pulmonary wedge pressure

PWRQ Parental Worry of Recurrent Abdominal Pain Questionnaire

PWS port wine stain; physician workstation; Prader-Willi syndrome

PWS/AS Prader-Willi syndrome/Angelman syndrome

PWT physician waiting time; posterior wall thickness; pseudo−Winger transform

pwt pennyweight

PWTT pulsed wave transit time

PWV pulsed wave velocity

PX pancreatectomized; peroxidase; physical examination

Px past history; peroxidase; physical examination; pneumothorax; prognosis

px pancreas, pancreatic

PXA pleomorphic xanthoastrocytoma

PXE pseudoxanthoma elasticum

PXM projection x-ray microscopy; pseudoexfoliation material

PXMP peroxysomal membrane protein

PXS pseudoexfoliation syndrome

PXT piroxantrone

P$_{xy}$ propagation delay

Py phosphopyridoxal; polyoma [virus]; pyridine; pyridoxal

py pack-years

PYA psychoanalysis

PyC pyogenic culture

PYCR pyrroline-5-carboxylate reductase

PYD N-terminal pyrin domain

PYE peptone yeast extract

PYG peptone, yeast extract, glucose

PYGM peptone, yeast, glucose, maltose

PYLL potential years of life lost

PYM psychosomatic

PyNPase pyridine nucleoside phosphorylase

PYP pyrophosphate

Pyr pyridine; pyruvate

PyrP pyridoxal phosphate

PyV Polyomavirus, polyomavirus

PZ pancreozymin; phthalazinone; pregnancy zone; proliferative zone; protamine zinc

Pz 4-phenylazobenzylcarbonyl; parietal midline electrode placement [ECG]

pz pièze

PZA pyrazinamide

PZ-CCK pancreozymin cholecystokinin

PZD partial zona dissection

PZE piezoelectric

PZI protamine zinc insulin

PZP pregnancy zone protein

PZQ praziquantel

PZT lead zirconate titanate

Q

Q 1,4-glucan branching enzyme; coulomb [electric quantity]; electric charge; each, every [L. *quaque*]; flow; glutamine; heat; perfusion; qualitative; quality; quantity; quart; quartile; Queensland [fever]; query [fever]; question; quinacrine; quinidine; quinone; quotient; radiant energy; reaction energy; reactive power; temperative coefficient

Q̇ cardiac output

Q₁₀ temperature coefficient

q each, every [L. *quaque*]; electric charge; long arm of chromosome; probability of failure in a single trial; quart; quintal

q2h every two hours [L. *quaque secunda hora*]

q4h every four hours [L. *quaque quarta hora*]

QA quality assessment; quality assurance; questions and answers

QAAA quantitative amino acid analysis

QAC quaternary ammonium compound; quinacrine

QACC quality assurance coordination committee

q.a.d. every other day [L. *quaque altera die*]

QAF quality adjustment factor

QAHCS Quality of Australian Health Care Study

QA&I quality assessment and improvement

QALD quality-adjusted life-days

QALE quality-adjusted life expectancy

QALPACS quality patient care scale

QALY quality-adjusted life-year

QAM quality assurance monitoring

q.AM every day before noon [L. *quaque die ante meridiem*]

QAP quality assurance program/professional; quinine, atabrine, and pamaquine

QA/QC quality assurance and quality control

QAR quantitative autoradiography; quiet, alert, and responsive [veterinary medicine]

QARANC Queen Alexandra's Royal Army Nursing Corps

QARNNS Queen Alexandra's Royal Naval Nursing Service

QAS quality assurance standard

QAUR quality assurance and utilization review

QB whole blood

Q_B total body clearance

Q_b blood flow

QBC query by case

QBIC query by image content

QBV whole blood volume

QC quad cane; quality characteristics; quality control; quantum computing; quinine colchicine

Qc pulmonary capillary blood flow

QCA quantitative coronary arteriography or angiography

Q-CHAT quantitative checklist for autism in toddlers

QCID qualitative contingent influence diagram

QCIM Quarterly Cumulative Index Medicus

QCM quartz crystal microbalance

Q_CO₂ carbon dioxide evolution by a tissue

QCP quality care program

QCS Quebec Cardiovascular Study; Quick Confusion Scale

QCT quantitative computed tomography

QD every day [L. *quaque die*]; Qi deficiency; quantum dot

Q_d probability of detection

q.d. every day [L. *quaque die*]

QDE quantum detection efficiency

QDH/SS quick doff hood/second skin

QDPR quinoid dihydropteridine reductase

QDS, q.d.s. four times each day [L. *quater die sumendus*]

QE quantum efficiency

QEA quantitative culture of endotracheal aspirates

QED quantum electrodynamics

QEE quadriceps extension exercise

QEEG, qEEG quantitative electroencephalography

QEF quail embryo fibroblasts

QENF quantifying examination of neurologic function

QEONS Queen Elizabeth's Overseas Nursery Service

QEW quick early warning

QF quality factor; query fever; quick freeze; relative biologic effectiveness

QFCM quantitative fluorescence cytometry

QFD quality function deployment

QFES Quality Feedback Expert System

Q fever query fever

QFFV Queensland fruit fly virus

Q-FISH quantitative fluorescence in situ hybridization

QFT QuantiFERON tuberculosis test

QGS quantitative gated SPECT [single photon emission computed tomography]

QH, q.h. every hour [L. *quaque hora*]
q( )h every ( ) hours [L. *quaque hora*]
QHDS Queen's Honorary Dental Surgeon
QHFT Quinapril Heart Failure Trial
QHNS Queen's Honorary Nursing Sister
QHP Queen's Honorary Physician
QHS at every bedtime [L. *quaque hora somni*]; quantitative hepatobiliary scintigraphy; Queen's Honorary Surgeon
q.h.s. at every bedtime [L. *quaque hora somni*]
QI quality improvement; quality indicator; Quetelet Index
QID, q.i.d. four times per day [L. *quater in die*]
QIDN Queen's Institute of District Nursing
QIN quality improvement network
QIO quality improvement organization
QIP quality improvement project
QIRC quality-of-life impact of refractive correction
QISMC Quality Improvement System for Managed Care
QJ quadriceps jerk
QL as much as desired [L. *quantum libet*]; quality of life
q.l. as much as desired [L. *quantum libet*]
QLE quasi-likelihood estimation
Q-LES-Q Quality of Life Enjoyment and Satisfaction Questionnaire
QLP quality laboratory process
QLQ quality of life questionnaire
QLQ-C quality of life questionnaire-cancer
QLS Quality of Life Scale; quasielastic light-scattering spectroscopy
QLV quasi-linear viscoelastic [model]
QM every morning [L. *quaque mane*]; quality management; quantization matrix; quinacrine mustard
q.m. every morning [L. *quaque mane*]
QMAN query manager
QMB qualified Medicare beneficiary
QMC quantum Monte Carlo
QMF quadrature mirror filter
QMI Q-wave myocardial infarction
QMP Quality Management Program
QMR Quick Medical Reference
QMR-DT Quick Medical Reference-Decision Theoretic
QMR-KAT Quick Medical Reference-Knowledge Acquisition Tool
QMRP qualified mental retardation professional
QMT every month [L. *per singulos menses afferet*]; quantitative muscle test

q.m.t. every month [L. *per singulos menses afferet*]
QMWS quasi−morphine withdrawal syndrome
QN, qn quantitative
q.n. every night [L. *quaque nocte*]
QNB quinuclidinyl benzilate
QNS quantity not sufficient; Queen's Nursing Sister
qns quantity not sufficient
QO$_2$ flow of oxygen
Qo oxygen consumption
Q$_o$ flow at origin
Q$_{O_2}$ oxygen quotient; oxygen utilization
QOD, q.o.d. every other day [L. *quaque altera die*]
QOF Quality and Outcomes Framework
q.o.h. every other hour [L. *quaque altera hora*]
QOL quality of life
QOLHS Quality of Life Hypertension Study
QOLI quality-of-life index
QOLI-P quality of life index-Padilla
QOLQ quality of life questionnaire
q.o.n. every other night [L. *quaque altera nocte*]
QoR quality of recovery
QoS quality of service
QP quadrigeminal plate; quality planning; quanti-Pirquet [reaction]
Qp pulmonary blood flow
QPC quadratic phase coupling; quadrigeminal plate cistern; quality of patient care
Qpc pulmonary capillary blood flow
QPCR, qPCR quantitative polymerase chain reaction
QPD quadrature phase detector
QPEEG quantitative pharmacoelectroencephalography
Qp:Qs, Qp/Qs pulmonary-to-systemic flow ratio; pulmonic-to-systemic flow ratio
QPV quokka poxvirus
QQH, q.q.h. every four hours [L. *quaque quarta hora*]
QR quality review; quieting response; quinaldine red; quinone reductase
qr quadriradial; quarter
QRA quantitative risk assessment
QRB Quality Review Bulletin
Q$_{rbc}$ flow of red blood cells
QRFV Quaranfil virus
QRM quality and resource management
QRNG quinoline-resistant *Neisseria gonorrhoeae*
QRP quick-response program

QRS complex consisting of Q, R, and S waves, corresponding to depolarization of ventricles [ECG]; loop traced by QRS vectors, representing ventricular depolarization interval [ECG]

QRS-ST junction between the QRS complex and the ST segment [ECG]

QRS-T angle between the QRS and T vectors [vectorcardiography]

qRT-PCR quantitative reverse transcriptase polymerase chain reaction

QRZ wheal reaction time [Ger. *Quaddel Reaktion Zeit*]

QS as much as suffices [L. *quantum satis* or *quantum sufficit*]; quad set [exercise]; quality-switched; question screening; quiet sleep

Qs, Q$_s$ systemic blood flow

q.s. as much as suffices [L. *quantum satis* or *quantum sufficit*]

QSAR quantitative structure-activity relationship

QSART quantitative sudomotor axon reflex testing

QSFR quantitative structure-function relationship

QSM quality assurance and safety of medicine

QSPR quantitative structure-property relationship

QSPV quasi-static pressure volume

Q$_s$Q$_T$ shunted blood/total blood flow [ratio]

Qs/Qt shunt fraction

QSR quality system regulation

QSS quantitative sacroiliac scintigraphy

QSSR quantitative structure-stability relationship

QST quantitative sensory test

QSU Questionnaire of Smoking Urges

QT cardiac output; Quick test

Q-T time interval from the beginning of the QRS complex to the end of the T wave [ECG]

qt quantity; quart; quiet

QTc, Q-Tc Q-T interval corrected for heart rate

qter end of long arm of chromosome

QTL quantitative trait locus

Q-TWIST quality-adjusted time without symptoms of disease or subjective toxic effects of treatment

Quad quadratic

quad quadrant; quadriceps; quadriplegic

QUADS Quinapril Australian Dosing Study

QUAL qualitative attribute

qual qualitative, qualitaty

QUAL-PACS quality of patient care system

QUALYs quality-adjusted life-years

QUAN quantitative attribute

quant quantitative, quantitaty

quar quarantine

QUART quadrantectomy, axillary dissection, radiotherapy

QUASAR Quinapril Anti-Ischemia and Symptoms of Angina Reduction [trial]

QUEST Quality, Utilization, Effectiveness, Statistically Tabulated

QU.E.S.T. Quality of Life, Effectiveness, Safety, and Tolerability

QUESTAR query estimation and refinement

QUESTT question the child, use pain rating scale, evaluate behavior and physiologic changes, secure parents' involvement, take cause of pain into account, take action and evaluate results [mnemonic]

QUEXTA Quantitative Exercise Testing and Angiography [study]

QUICHA quantitative inhalation challenge apparatus

QUIET Quinapril Ischemic Event Trial

QuIC Quality Interagency Coordinating Task Force

QUIN quinolinic acid

quint fifth

QUIS Questionnaire on User Interface Satisfaction

quot quotient

quotid daily, quotidian [L. *quotidie*]

QUPV Quailpox virus

QUS quantitative ultrasound

qv which see [L. *quod vide*]

QWB quality of well-being

QWK every week

QYBV Qalyub virus

QYD Qi and Yin deficiency

R

R Behnken unit; Broadbent registration point; any chemical group [particularly an alfyl group]; a conjugative plasmid responsible for resistance to various elements; electrical resistance; in electrocardiography, far point [L. *remotum*]; first positive deflection during the QRS complex [in ECG]; gas constant; organic radical; race; racemic; radioactive; radiology; radius; ramus; Rankine [scale]; rapid accelerator; rate; rate modulation; ratio; reaction; Réaumur [scale]; receptor; rectal; rectified; red; registered trademark; regression coefficient; regular; regular insulin; regulator; rejection factor; relapse; relaxation; release; remission; remote; reperfusion; repressor; residual tumor; residue; resistance; respiration; respiratory exchange ratio; respiratory quotient; responder; response; rest; restricted; reverse; rhythm; ribose; *Rickettsia*; right; Rinne [test]; roentgen; rough; rub

® registered trademark; right

R? second positive deflection during QRS complex [ECG]

R+, +R positive Rinne test

R− negative Rinne test

°R degree of Rankine scale; degree on Reaumur scale

R0 residual tumor not assessed

R1 first repeat; longitudinal relativity; small residual tumor

R2 large residual tumor; second repeat; transverse relativity

R1, R2, R3, etc. years of resident study

r correlation coefficient; density; radius; ratio; recombinant; regional; ribose; ribosomal; ring chromosome; roentgen; sample correlation coefficient

ρ lowercase Greek letter rho; correlation coefficient; electric charge density; electrical resistivity; mass density; reactivity

r^2 coefficient of determination

RA radial artery; radioactive; radiographic absorptiometry; radiographic abstraction; radiologist's assistant; ragocyte; ragweed antigen; rapidly adapting [receptors]; reactive arthritis; reciprocal asymmetric; refractory anemia; refractory ascites; regression analysis; renal artery; renin-angiotensin; repeat action; residual air; retinoic acid; rheumatoid arthritis; right angle; right arm; right atrium;

right auricle; risk adjustment; risk assessment; rotation angiography; Roy adaptation

R$_A$ airway resistance

Ra access resistance; radial; radium; radius

rA riboadenylate

ra receptor antagonist

RAA renin-angiotensin-aldosterone; right aortic arch; right atrial appendage; ruptured abdominal aortic aneurysm

rAAA ruptured abdominal aortic aneurysm

RAADS Ritvo Autism Asperger Diagnostic Scale

RAADS-R Ritvo Autism Asperger Diagnostic Scale-Revised

RAAE robot-assisted anterior exenteration

RAAMC Royal Australian Army Medical Corps

RAAMI Randomized Angiographic Trial of Alteplase in Myocardial Infarction; Rapid Administration of Alteplase in Myocardial Infarction [trial]

RAAPI resting ankle-arm pressure index

RAAS Randomized Angiotensin II Receptor Antagonist, Angiotensin-Converting Enzyme Inhibitor Study; renin-angiotensin-aldosterone system

rAAV recombinant adeno-associated virus

RAB remote afterloading brachytherapy

Rab rabbit

RABA rabbit antibladder antibody

RAC rabeprazole, amoxicillin, clarithromycin; Recombinant Deoxyribonucleic Acid Advisory Committee; research appraisal checklist

rac racemate, racemic

RACAT rapid acquisition computed axial tomography

RACC receptor-activated calcium channel

RACE ramipril angiotensin-converting enzyme; Ramipril Cardioprotective Evaluation [trial]; rapid amplification of complementary deoxyribonucleic acid ends; rapid assessment of cardiac enzymes; rate control versus electrical cardioversion

RACGP Royal Australian College of General Practitioners

RACP Royal Australasian College of Physicians

RACS Royal Australasian College of Surgeons

RACT reasonably available control technology; research activity

RACV relative autonomic conduction velocity

RAD radial artery catheter; radiation absorbed dose; radical; radiographic, radiography; reactive airways disease; receptor affinity distribution; right atrium diameter; right axis deviation; roentgen administered dose

Rad radiology; radiotherapy; radium

rad radial; radian; radiation absorbed dose; radial; radius; root [L. *radix*]

RADA rosin amine-D-acetate

RADAI rheumatoid arthritis disease activity index

RADAR rapid assessment of disease activity in rheumatology; Research on Adverse Drug Events and Reports

RADARS Researched Abuse, Diversion, and Addiction-Related Surveillance System

RADC Royal Army Dental Corps

RADES randomly amplified differentially expressed sequence

RADES-PCR randomly amplified differentially expressed sequence polymerase chain reaction

RADIANCE Randomized Assessment of Digoxin on Inhibitors of Angiotensin-Converting Enzyme [study]

RADIO radiotherapy

radiol radiology

RADIUS Routine Antenatal Diagnostic Imaging with Ultrasound [trial]

RadLV radiation leukemia virus

RADMOS radiotherapy data management and organization system

RADP right acromiodorsoposterior

RADS reactive airways dysfunction syndrome; retrospective assessment of drug safety

rad/s rad per second; radian per second

rad/s² rad per second squared

rad ther radiation therapy

RADTS rabbit antidog thymus serum

RADTT radiation therapy technologist

RADVIS radiologic visualization

RAE right atrial enlargement

RAEB refractory anemia with excess blasts

RAEBiT, RAEB-T refractory anemia with excess blasts in transformation

RAEC rat aortic endothelial cell; rate control versus electrical cardioversion

RAEM refractory anemia with excess myeloblasts

RAF repetitive atrial firing; rheumatoid arthritis factor

RAFMS Royal Air Force Medical Services

RAFT Recurrent Atrial Fibrillation Trial; Rythmol-SR Atrial Fibrillation Trial

RAFW right atrial free wall

RAG radioautography; ragweed; recombinase activating gene; recombination activating gene; risk assessment in genetics

RAGE rapid gradient echo; receptor for advanced glycation end products

Ragg rheumatoid agglutinin

RAH radical abdominal hysterectomy; regressing atypical histiocytosis; right atrial hypertrophy

RAHM randomly amplified hybridization microsatellite

RAHO rabbit antibody to human ovary

RAHTG rabbit antihuman thymocyte globulin

RaHV ranid herpesvirus

RAI radioactive iodine; radioactive isotope; resident assessment instrument; resting ankle index; right atrial inversion; right atrial involvement

RAID radioimmunodetection; radiolabeled antibody imaging; redundant array of independent disks; redundant array of inexpensive disks

RAIS reflection-absorption infrared spectroscopy

RAITI right atrial inversion time index

RAIU radioactive iodine uptake

RALES Randomized Aldactone Evaluation Study

RALPH renal, anal, lung, polydactyly, hamartoblastoma [syndrome]

RALT routine admission laboratory tests

RAM random-access memory; rapid alternating movements; rectus abdominis muscle; rectus abdominis myocutaneous [flap]; reduced acquisition matrix; research aviation medicine; resistance-associated mutation; resource allocation methodology; right anterior measurement

RAMBA retinoic acid metabolism-blocking agent

RAMEDIS Rare Metabolic Diseases

RAMC Royal Army Medical Corps

RAM-FAST reduced acquisition matrix Fourier-acquired steady state

RaMI Ravenna Myocardial Infarction [trial]

RAMIT Ravenna Myocardial Infarction Trial

RAMM remote-access multidimensional microscopy

RAMP radioactive antigen microprecipitin; rate-modulated pacing; right atrial mean pressure

RAMPO randomly amplified microsatellite polymorphism

RAMR risk-adjusted mortality rate

RAMT rabbit antimouse thymocyte; right atrial mobile thrombi

RAN random number; remote area nurse; resident's admission notes

RANA rheumatoid arthritis nuclear antigen

RANK receptor activator of nuclear factor κB

RANKL receptor activator of nuclear factor kappa B ligand

RANO Response Assessment in Neuro-Oncology

rANP rat atrial natriuretic peptide

RANTES regulated on activation, T-cell expressed and secreted

RANTTAS Randomized Trial of Tirilazad in Acute Stroke

RAO right anterior oblique; right anterior occipital; rotational acetabular osteotomy

RaONC radiation oncology

RAP rapid atrial pacing; recurrent abdominal pain; regression-associated protein; renal artery pressure; resident assessment protocol; rheumatoid arthritis precipitin; RNA arbitrarily primed; right atrial pressure

RAPA rapamycin

RAPD randomly amplified polymorphic DNA; relative afferent pupillary defect

RAPDDIP randomly amplified polymorphic DNA for the diploid cases

RAPDHAP randomly amplified polymorphic DNA for the haploid cases

RAPID Recombinant Plasminogen Activator Angiographic Phase II International Dose Finding Study; Regional Arizona Prehospital Infarction Diagnosis [study]; Reteplase Angiographic Patency International Dose-Ranging Study

RAPK reticulate acropigmentation of Kitamura

RAPM refractory anemia with partial myeloblastosis

RAPO rabbit antibody to pig ovary

RAP-PCR ribonucleic acid [RNA arbitrarily primed polymerase chain reaction]

RAPPORT ReoPro in Acute Myocardial Infarction and Primary Percutaneous Transluminal Coronary Angioplasty Organization and Randomized Trial

RAPS Renfrew and Paisley Study; resident assessment protocols

RAPs radiologists, anesthesiologists, and pathologists

RAPT Ridogrel vs. Aspirin Potency Trial

RAR rapidly adapting receptor; rat insulin receptor; retinoic acid receptor; right arm reclining; right arm recumbent

RARA retinoic acid receptor alpha

RARB retinoic acid receptor beta

RARE rapid acquisition with relaxation enhancement; retinoic acid response element

RARG retinoic acid receptor gamma

RARLS rabbit anti-rat lymphocyte serum

RARS refractory anemia with ring sideroblasts

RARTS rabbit anti-rat thymocyte serum

RAS radiologist aid system; rapid atrial stimulation; recurrent aphthous stomatitis; reflex activating stimulus; reliability, availability, serviceability; remote access service; renal artery stenosis; renal artery stent; renin-angiotensin system; residency application service; reticular activating system; rheumatoid arthritis serum; Rokitansky-Aschoff sinus; rotational atherectomy system; routine analysis station

RA-S refractory anemia with ringed sideroblasts

ras retrovirus-associated DNA sequence

RASE rapid-acquisition spin echo

RASMC rat aortic smooth muscle dell

RASS rheumatoid arthritis and Sjögren syndrome

RAST radioallergosorbent test

RAT repeat action tablet; rheumatoid arthritis test; right anterior trigone

RATG rabbit antithymocyte globulin

RATHAS rat thymus antiserum

RATMAP Rat Genome Database

rAT-P recombinant antitrypsin Pittsburgh

RATS robotic-assisted transaxillary surgery

RATx radiation therapy

RAU radioactive uptake; remote access unit

RAV rheumatoid arthritis virus; Rous-associated virus

RAVC retrograde atrioventricular conduction; Royal Army Veterinary Corps

RAVES Reduced Anticoagulation in Saphenous Vein Graft Stent [trial]; Reduced Anticoagulation Vein Graft Study

RAVLT Rey Auditory Verbal Learning Test

RAW right atrial wall

RAW, Raw airway resistance

RAWP Resource Allocation Working Party

RAWTS RNA amplification with transcript sequencing

RAZ razoxane

RB broader semantic relationship; radial basis; radiation burn; rating board; rebreathing; reticulate body; retinoblastoma; retrobulbar; right breast; right bronchus; right bundle; rigid bronchoscopy

RB1 RB1 Gene Mutation Database

Rb retinoblastoma

RBA relative binding affinity; rescue breathing apparatus; right basilar artery; right brachial artery; rose bengal antigen

RBAC role-based access control

RBAP repetitive bursts of action potential

RbAP retinoblastoma-associated protein

RBAS rostral basilar artery syndrome

rBAT related to b$^{0,+}$ amino acid transporter

RBB right bundle branch

RBBB right bundle-branch block

RBBP retinoblastoma binding protein

RBBsB right bundle-branch system block

RBBx right breast biopsy

RBC ranitidine bismuth citrate; red blood cell; red blood count

rbc red blood cell

RBCA risk-based corrective action

RBC-ChE red blood cell cholinesterase

RBCD right border cardiac dullness

rBCG recombinant bacille Calmette-Guérin [vaccine]

RBCM red blood cell mass

RbCoV rabbit coronavirus

RBCV red blood cell volume

RBD recurrent brief depression; region binding domain; relative biologic dose; right border of dullness; RNA binding domain

RBE relative biologic effectiveness

RBF radial basis function; regional blood flow; regional bone mass; renal blood flow

RBFN radial basis function network

RBG red blue green

RBI radiographic baseline

RBI-EM rescaled block-iterative expectation maximization

Rb Imp rubber base impression

RBL rat basophilic leukemia; Reid baseline; retinoblastoma-like

RBL-ILD respiratory bronchiolitis with associated interstitial lung disease

RBM RNA binding motif

rBM reconstituted basement membrane

RBN retrobulbar neuritis

RBNA Royal British Nurses Association

RBNN recurrent backpropagation neural network

RBOW rupture of the bag of waters

RBP retinol-binding protein; riboflavin-binding protein

RBPC cellular retinol-binding protein

RBPI intestinal retinol-binding protein

rBPI recombinant bactericidal/permeability increasing [protein]

RBR risk-based response; rule-based reasoning

RB-RB right bundle to right bundle [depolarization]

RBRVS resource-based relative value scale

RBS random blood sugar; receptor binding site; remote backup service; Roberts syndrome; Rutherford backscattering

RbSA rabbit serum albumin

RBSL risk-based screening level

RBST rubber-band straightening transform

rBST recombinant bovine somatotropin

RBT resistive breathing training

RBTN rhombotin

RBTNL rhombotin-like

RBUV Rochambeau virus

RBV ribavirin; right brachial vein; Rio Bravo virus

RBW relative body weight

RBZ rubidazone

RC electronic circuit containing a resistor and capacitor in series; radiocarpal; reaction center; recrystallization; red cell; red cell casts; red corpuscle; Red Cross; referred care; regenerated cellulose; rehabilitation counseling; Renshaw cell; residential care; resistance and compliance; resistive capacity; respiration ceases; respiratory care; respiratory center; respiratory compensation; rest cure; retention catheter; retrograde cystogram; rib cage; root canal; routine cholecystography

R&C resistance and capacitance

Rc conditioned response; receptor

RCA red cell agglutination; regulator of complement activity; relative chemotactic activity; renal cell carcinoma; replication-competent adenovirus; replication-competent alphavirus; retained cortical activity; right coronary angiography; right coronary artery; rotational coronary atherectomy

RCAMC Royal Canadian Army Medical Corps

RCAVF radial-cephalic (direct wrist) arteriovenous fistula

rCBF regional cerebral blood flow

rCBV regional cerebral blood volume

RCC radiological control center; rape crisis center; ratio of cost to charges; receptor-chemoeffector complex; red cell cast; red cell concentrate; red cell count; regulator of chromosome condensation; renal cell carcinoma; reverse cumulative curve; right common carotid; right coronary cusp

RCCM Regional Committee for Community Medicine

RCCP renal cell carcinoma, papillary

RCCS remote clinical communications system

RCCT randomized controlled clinical trial

RCD relative cardiac dullness; robust change detection

RCDA recurrent chronic dissecting aneurysm

RCDP rhizomelic chondrodysplasia punctata

RCDR relative corrected death rate

RCE reasonable compensation equivalent

RCEA redo carotid endarterectomy

RCF red cell ferritin; red cell folate; refractory ceramic fiber; relative centrifugal field/force; ristocetin cofactor

RCG radioelectrocardiography

RCGP Royal College of General Practitioners

RCH rectocolic hemorrhage

RCHF right congestive heart failure

RCHMS Regional Committee for Hospital Medical Services

RCI radiation conformity index; respiratory control index; retrospective cohort incidence

RCIA red cell immune adherence

RCIRF radiologic contrast-induced renal failure

RCIS Registered Cardiovascular Invasive Specialist [examination]

RCIT red cell iron turnover

RCITR red cell iron turnover rate

RCL renal clearance; right coronary leaflet

RCLM recurrent colorectal liver metastases

RCM radial contour model; radiographic contrast medium; red cell mass; reinforced clostridial medium; remacemide; remote center of motion; replacement culture medium; retrospective cohort mortality; right costal margin; Royal College of Midwives

RCMAS Revised Children's Manifest Anxiety Scale

rCMR regional cerebral metabolism rate

rCMRGlc, rCMRglc regional cerebral metabolic rate for glucose

rCMRO$_2$ regional cerebral metabolic rate for oxygen

RCN right caudate nucleus; Royal College of Nursing

RCO right coronary ostium

RCoF ristocetin cofactor

RCOG Royal College of Obstetricians and Gynaecologists

RCoV respiratory coronavirus

RCP radiochemical purity; red cell protoporphyrin; retrocorneal pigmentation; retrograde cerebral perfusion; riboflavin carrier protein; Royal College of Physicians

rCP regional cerebral perfusion

rcp reciprocal translocation

RCPath Royal College of Pathologists

RCPCH Royal College of Paediatrics and Child Health

RCPG respiratory center pattern generator

RCPH red cell peroxide hemolysis

RCPP recurrent coronary prevention program

rCPP regional cerebral perfusion pressure

RCPSC Royal College of Physicians and Surgeons of Canada

RCPSGlas Royal College of Physicians and Surgeons, Glasgow

RCR relative consumption rate; replication-competent recombinant; replication-competent retrovirus; respiratory control ratio

RCRA Resource Conservation and Recovery Act

rCRF recombinant corticotropin-releasing factor

RCRI Revised Cardiac Risk Index

RCS rabbit aorta-contracting substance; real-time control system; red cell suspension; reference coordinate system; registered cardiovascular specialist; renal collector system; reticulum cell sarcoma; revision control system; right coronary sinus; Royal College of Science; Royal College of Surgeons

RCSE Royal College of Surgeons, Edinburgh

RCSSS resource coordination system for surgical service

RCT radiotherapy and chemotherapy; randomized clinical trial; randomized controlled trial; registered care technologist; retrograde conduction time; root canal therapy; Rorschach content test; rotator cuff tear

rct marker showing the ability of virulent strains to replicate at 40°C, while vaccine strain shows no replication

rCTB recombinant cholera toxin B

RCTE randomized clinical trial evaluator

RCU respiratory care unit

RCV rabbit calicivirus; recoverin; red cell volume

RCVS Royal College of Veterinary Surgeons

RCWI right cardiac work index

RD radial deviation; radiology department; rate difference; Raynaud disease; reaction of degeneration; registered dietitian; Reiter disease; related donor; relative dose; renal disease; resistance determinant; resistant disease; respiratory disease; resuscitation device; retinal degeneration; retinal detachment; Reye disease; rheumatoid disease; right deltoid; Riley-Day [syndrome]; Rolland-Desbuquois [syndrome]; rubber dam; ruminal drinking; ruptured disk

R&D research and development

Rd rate of disappearance

rd rutherford

RDA rapid epidemiological assessment; recommended daily allowance; recommended dietary allowance; Registered Dental Assistant; representation difference analysis; right dorsoanterior; right ductus arteriosus

RDB random double blind; relational database

RDBMS regional database management system; relational database management system

RDBP RD [gene] binding protein

RDBS relational database server

RDB-X random double-blind crossover

RDC remote data capture; research data center; research diagnostic criteria

RDCRD Rare Disease Clinical Research Database

RDD relative depth dose [radiation]

RDDA recommended daily dietary allowance

RDDB Rare Disease Database

RDDP RNA-dependent deoxynucleic acid polymerase

RDE receptor-destroying enzyme; remote data entry

RDEB recessively inherited dystrophic epidermolysis bullosa

RDE$_D$ radiation dose required

RDES remote data entry system

RDF rapid dissolution formula

RDFC recurring digital fibroma of childhood

RDG retrograde duodenogastroscopy

RDH Registered Dental Hygienist

RDHBF regional distribution of hepatic blood flow

RDHI research and development health informatics

RDI recommended daily intake; respiratory desaturation index; respiratory disturbance index; rupture-delivery interval

RDIC resuscitation device, individual chemical

RDLBBB rate-dependent left bundle-branch block

RDM readmission

RDMS registered diagnostic medical sonographer

rDNA recombinant deoxyribonucleic acid

RDOG radiology diagnostic oncology group

RDP right dorsoposterior

RDPA right descending pulmonary artery

RDQ respiratory disease questionnaire

RDR research data repository

RDRP, RdRp RNA-dependent RNA polymerase

RDRS Rapid Disability Rating Scale

RDS Raskin Depression Scale; respiratory distress syndrome; reticuloendothelial depressing substance; rhodanese; slow retinal degeneration

RDT randomized discontinuation trial; rapid diagnostic test; retinal damage threshold; routine dialysis therapy

RDW red blood cell distribution width index

RDX radixin

RE radium emanation; random error; reading epilepsy; readmission; rectal examination; reference emitter; reflux esophagitis; regional enteritis; relative effectiveness; renal and electrolyte; resistive exercise; resting energy; restriction endonuclease; reticuloendothelial; retinol equivalent; right ear; right eye

R$_E$ respiratory exchange ratio

R&E research and education

Re rhenium

R$_e$ Reynold number

REA radiation emergency area; radioenzymatic assay; regulatory effectiveness analysis; renal anastomosis; restriction endonuclease analysis; right ear advantage

rea rearrangement

REACH Research on Endothelin Antagonism in Chronic Heart Failure [study]; Resource Utilization in Congestive Heart Failure [study]

REACT Rapid Early Action in Coronary Treatment [study]

REAC/TS Radiation Emergency Assistance Center/Training Site

readm readmission

READS restriction enzyme analysis of differentially expressed sequences

REAL Revised European-American Lymphoma [classification]

REALM rapid estimate of adult literacy in medicine

REAP restriction endonuclease analysis of plasmid

REAR renal, ear, anal, and radial [syndrome]

REAS reasonably expected as safe; retained excluded antrum syndrome

REAT radiologic emergency assistance team

REB roentgen-equivalent biologic

REC receptor; recombinant, recombination

rec fresh [L. *recens*]; recessive; recombinant chromosome; record; recovery; recurrence, recurrent

RECA recombination protein A

RECAP retrosynthetic combinatorial analysis procedure

recCHO recombinant Chinese hamster ovary

R$_{ECF}$ extracellular fluid resistance

RECG radioelectrocardiography

recip recipient; reciprocal

RECIST Response Evaluation Criteria in Solid Tumors

RECIT Représentation du Contenu Informationel de Testes Médicaux

recon smallest unit of DNA capable of recombination

recond reconditioned, reconditioning

RECPAM recursive partition and amalgamation

RECREATE Rescue of Closed Arteries Treated by Stent for Threatened or Abrupt Closure [study]

recryst recrystallization

rect rectal; rectification, rectified; rectum; rectus

Rec Ther recreational therapy

recumb recumbent

recur recurrence, recurrent

RED radiation experience data; rapid erythrocyte degeneration; repeat expansion detection; rigid external distractor

red reduction

REDAP rural emergency department approved for pediatrics

RED-LIP Reduction of Lipid Metabolism [study]

redox oxidation-reduction

REDP reduced-energy diet program

REDS Retrovirus Epidemiology Donor Study

REDUCE Randomized Double-Blind Unfractionated Heparin and Placebo-Controlled Multicenter Trial; Restenosis Reduction by Cutting Balloon Evaluation [study]

REE rapid extinction effect; rare earth element; resting energy expenditure

REEDA redness, edema, ecchymosis, drainage, approximation

REEDS retention of tears, ectrodactyly, ectodermal dysplasia, and strange hair, skin and teeth [syndrome]

REEG radioelectroencephalography

R-EEG resting electroencephalography

ReEND reproductive endocrinology

REEP right end-expiratory pressure

reev reevaluate

reex reexamine

REF ejection fraction at rest; rat embryo fibroblast; referred; refused; renal erythropoietic factor; restriction endonuclease fingerprinting; right ventricular ejection fraction

ref reference; reflex

Ref-1 redox factor 1

Ref Doc referring doctor

REFI regional ejection fraction image

ref ind refractive index

refl reflex

REFLECT-1 Randomized Evaluation of Flosequinan on Exercise Tolerance—Initial Efficacy Trial

REFLECT-2 Randomized Evaluation of Flosequinan on Exercise Tolerance—Dose Response Study

REFLEX Randomized Evaluation of Flosequinan on Exercise Tolerance [study]; Restenosis Rates with Flexible GFX Stents [study]

Ref Phys referring physician

REFRAD released from active duty

REFSA Randomized European Femoral Stent vs Angioplasty Trial

RefSeq Reference Sequence [database]

REG radiation exposure guide; radioencephalogram, radioencephalography

Reg registered

reg region; regular

regen regenerated, regenerating, regeneration

ReGIS respiration-gated irradiation system

REGRESS Regression Growth Evaluation Statin Study

reg rhy regular rhythm

REGU regulation

regurg regurgitation

REGWF Ryan-Einot-Gabriel-Welsch [test]

REH renin essential hypertension

rehab rehabilitated, rehabilitation

REIN Ramipril Effect in Nephropathy [study]

REL rate of energy loss; recommended exposure limit; resource location; resting expiratory level

rel relative

RELACS Reikjavik experimental light-activated cell sorter

RELANCA relation between antineutrophil cytoplasm autoantibody [ANCA] levels and relapses of ANCA-associated glomerulonephritis and vasculitis

RELAY relayed correlation spectroscopy

RELE resistive exercise of lower extremities

RelTox Relational Toxicology [project]

REM random-effect model; rapid eye movement; recent-event memory; reticular erythematous mucinosis; return electrode monitor; roentgen equivalent—man

Rem roentgen equivalent—man

rem radiation equivalent—man; removal

REMA repetitive excess mixed anhydride

REMAB radiation equivalent—manikin absorption

REMAIN remission maintenance

REMATCH Randomized Evaluation of Mechanical Assistance in the Treatment of Congestive Heart Failure [study]

REMBRANDT Rather Exciting and Memorable Blind Randomized Assessment of a New Drug on Three Continents

REMCAL radiation equivalent-manikin calibration

remit remittent

REMO regional emergency medical organization

REMP roentgen-equivalent−man period
REMPAN radiation emergency medical preparedness
REMS rapid eye movement sleep; risk evaluation and mitigation strategy
REMT trigger-signal rapid eye movements
REN renal; renin
REn, Ren replication enhancer
RENAAL Reduction of Endpoints in Non-Insulin-Dependent Diabetes Mellitus with Angiotensin II Antagonist Losartan [trial]
rENaC rat epithelial sodium channel
RENEWAL Randomized Trial of Endoluminal Reconstruction Using the NIR Stent or Wallstent in Angioplasty of Long Segment Disease
REO respiratory enteric orphan [virus]
REOP rural elderly outreach program
REP reepithelialization; repaglinide; replication protein; rest-exercise program; restriction endonuclease profile; retrograde pyelogram; Rochester Epidemiology Project; roentgen equivalent−physical
rep replication; roentgen equivalent−physical
REPA replication protein A
REPAIR Reperfusion in Acute Infarction, Rotterdam [study]
repol repolarization
REPR reproductive
REPS reactive extensor postural synergy
reps repetitions
rept let it be repeated
req request, requested
RER renal excretion rate; replication error; respiratory exchange ratio; rough endoplasmic reticulum
RER₊ replication error positive
RERC Rehabilitation Engineering Research Center
RERF Radiation Effects Research Foundation
RES radionuclide esophageal scintigraphy; real environment sensing; Reproducibility Echocardiography Study; reticuloendothelial system; Rotterdam Elderly Study
res research; resection; resident; residue; resistance
RESAC Real-Time Expert System for Advice and Control
RESCUE Randomized Evaluation of Salvage Angioplasty with Combined Utilization of Endpoints [trial]
RESET Real Safety and Efficacy of a 3-Month Dual Antiplatelet Therapy Following Zotarolimus-Eluting Stents Implantation [trial]
Res Gen Research Genetics [database]

RESIST Restenosis After Intravascular Ultrasound-Guided Stenting [study]
RESNA Rehabilitation Engineering Society of North America
RESOLVD, RESOLVED Randomized Evaluation of Strategies for Left Ventricular Dysfunction [study]
resp respiration, respiratory; response
Resp Ther respiratory therapy
REST Raynaud phenomenon, esophageal motor dysfunction, sclerodactyly, and telangiectasia [syndrome]; regressive electroshock therapy; Restenosis Stent Trial
RESTORE Randomized Efficacy Study of Tirofiban for Outcomes and Restenosis [trial]
RESTT respiratory therapy technician
resusc resuscitation
RET retained; retention; reticular; reticulocyte; retina; right esotropia
ret rad equivalent therapeutic
RETA Registry for the Endovascular Treatment of Aneurysms
retard retardation
ret cath retention catheter
RETEST retention probability is initially estimated
retic reticulocyte
REU rectal endoscopic ultrasonography
reu radiation effect unit
REV rat encephalomyelitis virus; reticuloendotheliosis virus
ReV regulator of virion
rev reverse; review; revolution
re-x reexamination
Rex regulator x
R_ext external resistance
RF radial fiber; radiofrequency; rapid filling; readiness field; reading factor; receptive field; regurgitant fraction; Reitland-Franklin [unit]; relative flow; relative fluorescence; release factor; renal failure; replacement fluid; replication factor; replicative form; repopulation factor; resistance factor; resonant frequency; respiratory failure; respiratory frequency; reticular formation; retroperitoneal fibromatosis; rheumatic fever; rheumatoid factor; riboflavin; risk factor; root canal filling; rosette formation
R^F rate of flow
Rf ratio of distance traveled by solute to distance traveled by spot of pigment; respiratory frequency; rutherfordium
R_f distance that a spot of a substance has moved from the point of application
rf radiofrequency; rapid filling
RFA radiofrequency ablation; requirements for accreditation; resident functional atlas;

right femoral artery; right frontoanterior; risk factor of atherosclerosis

RFB retained foreign body

RFC radiofrequency coil; replication factor C; request for comments; retrograde femoral catheter; rosette-forming cell

RFCA radiofrequency catheter ablation

RFD, RfD reference dose

RFDS Royal Flying Doctors Service

RFE relative fluorescence efficiency

RfE request for erasure [subject privacy measure]

RFFIT rapid fluorescent focus inhibition test

rFGF1 recombinant fibroblast growth factor 1

rFGF2 recombinant fibroblast growth factor 2

RFH right femoral hernia

RFI radiofrequency interference; recurrence-free interval; renal failure index; request for information

RFIED round femoral inferior epiphysis dysplasia

RFK Richardson-Flory-Kops [mask]

RFL right frontolateral

RFLA rheumatoid factor−like activity

RFLP restriction fragment length polymorphism

RFLS rheumatoid factor−like substance

RFLV restriction fragment length variant

Rfm rifampin

RFNA red fuming nitric acid

RFP rapid filling period; recurrent facial paralysis; request for proposal; right fronto-posterior

RF-PMR radiofrequency percutaneous myocardial revascularization

RFPS Royal Faculty of Physicians and Surgeons

RFR rapid fluid resuscitation; refraction; relaxation-frequency relations

RFS relapse-free survival; renal function study; rotating frame spectroscopy

RFT respiratory function test; right fronto-transverse; rod-and-frame test

RFU relative fluorescence unit

RFV right femoral vein; Royal Farm virus

rFVIIa recombinant factor VIIA

rFVIII recombinant factor VIII

RFW rapid filling wave

RG right gluteal

Rg Rodgers [antigen]; roentgenium

rG regular gene

RgasD relative gas density

RGB red green blue

RGBMT renal glomerular basement membrane thickness

RGC radio gas chromatography; remnant gastric cancer; retinal ganglion cell; right giant cell

RGD range-gated Doppler; refractional geometric distortions

RGE relative gas expansion

RGEA right gastroepiploic artery

RGH rat growth hormone

RGHBV Ross' goose hepatitis B virus

RGI recovery from growth inhibition

RGL random glucose level

RGM right gluteus medius

rGM-CSF recombinant granulocyte macrophage colony-stimulating factor

RGN refinement grouper number; Registered General Nurse

RGO reciprocating gait orthosis

RGP retrograde pyelography

RGR relative growth rate

RGS regulation of G_α signaling; Rieger syndrome

RGU regional glucose utilization

RGV Rio Grande virus

RH radiant heat; radiation hybrid; radiologic health; reactive hyperemia; recurrent herpes; regulatory hormone; rehabilitation; relative humidity; releasing hormone; renal hemolysis; retinal hemorrhage; reverse hybridization; ribonuclease H; right hand, right-handed; right heart; right hemisphere; right hyperphoria; room humidifier

Rh rhesus [factor]; rhinion; rhodamine; rhodium

Rh+ rhesus positive

Rh− rhesus negative

rh recombinant human; rheumatic

r/h roentgens per hour

RHA Regional Health Authority; relative highest avidity; right hepatic artery

RhA rheumatoid arthritis

RhAG Rh-associated glycoprotein

RHB regional hospital board; right heart bypass

RHBF reactive hyperemia blood flow

rh-BMP recombinant human bone morphogenetic protein

RHBs Regional Hospital Boards

RHC rad homolog in *Cerevisiae*; resin hemoperfusion column; respiration has ceased; right heart catheterization; right hypochondrium; rural health center

RHCSA Regional Hospitals Consultants and Specialists Association

RHD radiologic health data; relative hepatic dullness; renal hypertensive disease; rheumatic heart disease

RhD rhesus factor and D antigen

RHDV rabbit hemorrhagic disease virus

RHDV-AST89 rabbit hemorrhagic disease virus AST89

RHDV-BS89 rabbit hemorrhagic disease virus BS89

RHDV-FRG rabbit hemorrhagic disease virus FRG

RHDV-V351 rabbit hemorrhagic disease virus V351

RHDV-SD rabbit hemorrhagic disease virus SD

rhDNase recombinant human deoxyribonuclease

RHE retino-hepato-endocrine [syndrome]

RHEED reflection high-energy electron diffraction

rheo rheology

rhEPO recombinant human erythropoietin

rheu, rheum rheumatic, rheumatoid

RHF restricted Hartree-Fock [level]; right heart failure

Rh F rheumatic fever

rhFSH recombinant human follicle stimulating hormone

rhFVIII recombinant human factor 8

RHG right-hand grip

rhG-CSF recombinant human granulocyte colony-stimulating factor

rhGH recombinant human growth hormone

rhGM-CSF recombinant human granulocyte—macrophage colony-stimulating factor

RHI rhesus factor immunoglobulin; Rural Health Initiative

RHIA registered health information administrator

RhIG Rh [rhesus] factor immunoglobulin

rhIGF recombinant human insulin-like growth factor [IGF]

rhIL recombinant human interleukin

RHIN regional health information network

Rhin rhinology

rhino rhinoplasty

RHIT registered health information technician

RHJSC Regional Hospital Junior Staff Committee

RHL recurrent herpes labialis; right hepatic lobe

RHLN right hilar lymph node

rhm roentgens per hour at 1 meter

RHMAP radiation hybrid mapping program

RhMK rhesus monkey kidney

RhMk rhesus monkey

RhMkK rhesus monkey kidney

RHMV right heart mixing volume

RHN Rockwell hardness number

rhnRNP recombinant heterogeneous nuclear ribonucleoprotein

Rh$_{null}$ erythrocytes that fail to express rhesus antigens

RHO rhodopsin; right heeloff

RHOA radiographic hip osteoarthritis

RHOM rhombosine

RH-PAT reactive hyperemia peripheral artery tonometry

RHR renal hypertensive rat; resting heart rate

r/hr roentgens per hour

RHRV relative heart rate variability

RHS radius head subluxation; Ramsay Hunt syndrome; Rapp-Hodgkin syndrome; reciprocal hindlimb scratching [syndrome]; Richner-Hanhart syndrome; right-hand side; right heelstrike

RHSC Royal Hospital for Sick Children

RHSIG Rehabilitation Hospitals Special Interest Group

rhSp1 recombinant human Sp1 protein

RHT renal homotransplantation

RHTC rural health training center

rH-TNF recombinant human tumor necrosis factor

rh-tPA recombinant human tissue plasminogen activator

rhTPO recombinant human thrombopoietin

RHU registered health underwriter; rheumatology

rHuEPO recombinant human erythropoietin

rHuGCF recombinant human granulocyte colony-stimulating factor

rhuMAb recombinant human monoclonal antibody

rHuTNF recombinant human tumor necrosis factor

RHV right hepatic vein

rHV recombinant hirudin variant

RI radiation intensity; radioactive isotope; radioimmunology; recession index; recombinant inbred; recurrent inhibition; refractive index; regenerative index; regional ileitis; regional information system; regular insulin; relapse incidence; relative intensity; release inhibition; remission induction; renal index; renal insufficiency; replicative intermediate; resistive index; resistance index; respiratory illness; respiratory index; response interval; reticulocyte index; retroactive inhibition; retroactive interference; ribosome; rosette index; rosette inhibition

R$_I$ intracellular resistivity

R$_i$ internal resistivity

r$_i$ intraclass correlation coefficient

RIA radioimmunoassay; reamer irrigator aspirator; reference information model; reversible ischemic attack

RIA-DA radioimmunoassay double antibody

RIAS Roter Interactional Analysis System

Rib riboflavin; ribose
RIBA recombinant immunoblot assay
ribotyping ribonucleic acid typing
RIBS Rutherford ion backscattering
RIC right internal carotid [artery]; right interventricular coronary [artery]; Royal Institute of Chemistry
RICE replicating and integrating controlled expression; rest, ice, compression, and elevation
R$_{ICF}$ intracellular fluid resistance
RICM right intercostal margin
RiCoF ristocetin cofactor
RICP recurrent intrahepatic cholestasis of pregnancy
RICS right intercostal space
RICU respiratory intensive care unit
RID radial immunodiffusion; reduced interference distribution; remission-inducing drug; ruptured intervertebral disk
RIDDOR Reporting of Injuries, Diseases, and Dangerous Occurrences Regulations
RIDL retrograde intrarenal lithotripsy
RIDT rapid influenza diagnostic test
RIE reactive ion etching
RIF radiation-induced fibrosis; radiologic interface; release-inhibiting factor; rifabutin; rifampin; right iliac fossa; rosette-inhibiting factor
RIFA radioiodinated fatty acid
RIFC rat intrinsic factor concentrate
RIFLE risk factor and life expectancy
rIFN recombinant interferon
RIFS remedial investigation/feasibility study
RIG rabies immune globulin; rat insuloma gene
RIGH rabies immune globulin, human
RIGHT Cerivastatin Gemfibrozil Hyperlipidemia Treatment [study]
RIH right inguinal hernia
RIHD radiation-induced heart disease
RIHSA radioactive iodinated human serum albumin
RIJ right internal jugular
RIKEN Institute of Physical and Clinical Research
rIL recombinant interleukin
RILT rabbit ileal loop test
RIM radioisotope medicine; recurrent induced malaria; reference information model; relative-intensity measure
RIMA reverse inhibitor of monoamino oxidase A; right internal mammary artery
riMLF rostral interstitial median longitudinal fasciculus
RIMR Rockefeller Institute for Medical Research

RIMS resonance ionization mass spectrometry
RIN radiation-induced neoplasm; radioisotope nephrography; rat insulinoma
R$_{in}$ input resistance
RINB Reitan-Indiana Neuropsychological Battery
RIND reversible ischemic neurologic deficit
RINN recommended international nonproprietary name
RIO right inferior oblique
RIOMV Rio Mamore virus
RIOSV Rio Secundo virus
RIP radioimmunoprecipitation; reflex inhibiting pattern; repeat-induced point; respiratory inductance plethysmography
RIPA radioimmunoprecipitation assay
RIPH Royal Institute of Public Health
RIPHH Royal Institute of Public Health and Hygiene
RIPP resistive-intermittent positive pressure
RIPRN Rural and Isolated Practice Registered Nurse
RIPV right inferior pulmonary vein
RIR relative incidence rates; right interior rectus
RIRB radioiodinated rose bengal
RIRL retrograde intrarenal lipotripsy
RIRS retrograde intrarenal surgery
RIS radiology information system; rapid immunofluorescence staining; relative intensity score; resonance ionization spectroscopy
R$_{is}$ resistivity of the interstitium
r$_{is}$ interstitial resistance
RISA radioactive iodinated serum albumin; radioimmunosorbent assay
RISC Radiology Information System Consortium; Research Group on Instability in Coronary Artery Disease [study]; RNA-induced silencing complex
RISK Risk Intervention Skills Study
RIS/PACS radiologic information system/ picture archiving and communication system
RIST radioimmunosorbent test
RISUG Reversible Inhibition of Sperm Under Guidance
RIT radioimmune trypsin; radioimmunotherapy; radioiodinated triolein; radioiodine treatment; rosette inhibition titer
RITA Randomised Intervention Treatment of Angina; right internal thoracic artery
RITC rhodamine isothiocyanate
RITED Italian Registry of Echo-Dobutamine
RIU radioactive iodine uptake; refractive index unit
RIV retinal image velocity

RIVC right inferior vena cava
RIVD ruptured intervertebral disk
RJA regurgitant jet area
RK rabbit kidney; radial keratotomy; reductase kinase; rhodopsin kinase; right kidney
R$_k$ restitution constant
RKG radiocardiogram
RKH Rokitansky-Küster-Hauser [syndrome]
RKIP raf-1 kinase inhibitor protein
RKM rokitamycin
RKV rabbit kidney vacuolating [virus]
RKY roentgen kymography
RL radial line; radiation laboratory; reduction level; relaxation labeling; renal dysplasia-limb defects [syndrome]; resistive load; reticular lamina; right lateral; right leg; right lung; Ringer's lactate; run length
R&L right and left
R$_L$ lung resistance
RLA Ranchos de los Amigos [Cognitive Functioning Scale]; right lung apices
RLC residual lung capacity
RLD reference-listed drug; related living donor; ruptured lumbar disc
RLE right lower extremity
RLF retrolental fibroplasia; right lateral femoral
RLG regional librarians group
RLGS restriction landmark genomic scanning
rliPCR restriction cleavage, self-ligation, inverse polymerase chain reaction
RLIU regional library and information unit
RLL right lobe of liver; right lower limb; right lower lobe; run length limited
RLLS relative laser light scattering
RLM right lower medial
rLM recombinant *Listeria monocytogenes*
RLMA reinforced laryngeal mask airway
RLN recurrent laryngeal nerve; regional lymph node; relaxin
RLNC regional lymph node cell
RLND regional lymph node dissection
RLO residual lymphatic output
RLP radiation leukemia protection; ribosome-like particle
RLPV right lower pulmonary vein
RLQ right lower quadrant
RLR right lateral rectus
RLS recursive least square; restless leg syndrome; Ringer lactate solution; Roussy-Levy syndrome; run-length statistics
RLSB right lower scapular border
R-Lsh, R-L shunt right-left shunt
RLSL recursive least square lattice
RLT ralitoline
RLU relative light unit

RLV Rauscher leukemia virus
RLWD routine laboratory work done
RLX relaxin
RLXH relaxin H
RLZ right lower zone
RM mutant reverse; radical mastectomy; radon monitor; random migration; range of movement; red marrow; reference material; rehabilitation medicine; reinforced maneuver; relative magnitude; relative mobility; resistive movement; respiratory movement; respiratory muscle; restoration maximization; Riehl melanosis; risk management; routine management; ruptured membranes
Rm relative mobility; remission
R$_m$ membrane resistance
1RM one-repetition maximum
r$_m$ membrane resistance per unit length
rm remission; room
RMA rapid membrane assay; refuses medical advice; Registered Medical Assistant; relative medullary area; right mentoanterior
RMANOVA repeated measures analysis of variance
RMAT rapid microagglutination test
Rmax maximum resistance
R$_{max}$ maximum response
Rmax,L maximum resistance, lung
Rmax,w maximum resistance, chest wall
RMB right mainstem bronchus
RMBF regional myocardial blood flow
RMC reticular magnocellular [nucleus]; right middle cerebral [artery]; Rozsos microcholecystectomy
RMCA right middle cerebral artery
RMCH rod monochromacy; rod monochromatism
RMCL recommended maximum contaminant level; right midclavicular line
RMD retromanubrial dullness
RMDP Resource Mothers Development Project
RME rapid maxillary expansion; reasonable maximum exposure; receptor-mediated endocytosis; resting metabolic expenditure; right mediolateral episiotomy
RMEC regional medical education center
RMED rural medical education
RME/FM rapid maxillary expansion and face mask
RMF recursive median filter; right middle finger
RMI recent myocardial infarction; remote method invocation; reticulocyte maturity index
R-MIM refined message information model

Rmin,L minimum resistance, lung

Rmin,rs minimum resistance, respiratory system

RMK rhesus monkey kidney

RML radiation myeloid leukemia; regional medical library; right mediolateral; right middle lobe

RMLB right middle lobe bronchus

RMLS right middle lobe syndrome

RMLV Rauscher murine leukemia virus

RMM rapid micromedia method

RMN Registered Mental Nurse

RMO regional medical officer; resident medical officer

RMP rapidly miscible pool; regional medical program; regional myocardial infarction; resting membrane potential; ribulose monophosphate pathway; rifampin; right mentoposterior; risk management planning; risk management program

RMPA Royal Medico-Psychological Association

RMR relative maximum response; repair-misrepair model; resting metabolic rate; right medial rectus

RMRS Regenstrief Medical Record System

RMS rectal morphine sulfate; red man syndrome; repetitive motion syndrome; residual mean square; resource management system; respiratory muscle strength; rhabdomyosarcoma; rheumatic mitral stenosis; rhodomyosarcoma; rigid man syndrome; root mean square

rms root mean square

RMSA regulator of mitotic spindle assembly; rhabdomyosarcoma, alveolar

RMSa rhabdomyosarcoma

RMSCR rhabdomyosarcoma chromosomal region

RMSD root mean square deviation

RMSE, rmse root mean square error

RMSF Rocky Mountain spotted fever

RMSS Ruvalcaba-Myhre-Smith syndrome

RMSSD root mean square of successive differences

RMT Registered Medical Transcriptionist; Registered Music Therapist; relative medullary thickness; retromolar trigone; right mentotransverse

RMUI relief medication unit index

RMuLV Rauscher murine leukemia virus

RMV respiratory minute volume

RMZ right midzone

RN narrower semantic relationship; radionuclide; red nucleus; reflux neuropathy; Registered Nurse; registry number; residual nitrogen; reticular nucleus

Rn radon

RNA radionuclide angiography; Registered Nurse Anesthetist; ribonucleic acid; rough, noncapsulated, avirulent

RNAA radiochemical neutron activation analysis

RNA-BP ribonucleic acid-binding protein

RNAi ribonucleic acid interference

RNAP ribonucleic acid polymerase

RNAse, RNase ribonuclease

RNase P ribonuclease P

RNasin ribonuclease inhibitor

RNC repressing nucleoprotein complex

RN-C Registered Nurse certification

RNCG relative negative charge

RNCM Registered Nurse Case Manager

RNCS Registered Nurse Certified Specialist; Registered Nurse Clinical Specialist

RND radical neck dissection; radionuclide dacryography; reactive neurotic depression; regional nodal disease; respiratory nursing diagnosis

RNFL retinal nerve fiber layer

RNFP Registered Nurse Fellowship Program

RNGF rhodamine−nerve growth factor

RNI reactive nitrogen intermediate

RNIB Royal National Institute for the Blind

RNICU regional neonatal intensive care unit

RNID Royal National Institute for the Deaf

RNINMEGLA rat integral membrane glycoprotein gene

RNL Reintegration to Normal Living [index]

RNNP Registered Nurse−Nurse Practitioner

RNP ribonucleoprotein

RNP-CS ribonucleoprotein consensus sequence

RNR ribonucleotide reductase

RNS reactive nitrogen species; reference normal serum; repetitive nerve stimulation; replacement normal saline; ribonuclease

RNSC radionuclide superior cavography

Rnt roentgenology

RNTMI transfer ribonucleic acid initiator methionine

rNTP ribonuclease-5′-triphosphate

RNV radionuclide venography; radionuclide ventriculogram/ventriculography

RNVG radionuclide ventriculogram/ventriculography

RO radiation oncology; radiation output; ratio of; reduced obesity; relative odds; renal osteodystrophy; reverse osmosis; Ritter-Oleson [technique]; routine order; rule out

R/O, r/o rule out

ro radius of orifice

ROA regurgitant orifice area; right occipitoanterior

ROAD reversible obstructive airway disease

ROAT renal organic anion transporter; repeat open application test

ROATS rabbit ovarian antitumor serum

rob robertsonian translocation

ROBCAD robotic computer-assisted diagnosis

ROBUST Recanalization of Occluded Bypass Graft with Prolonged Urokinase Infusion Site Trial

ROC receiver operating characteristic; receiver operating curve; receptor-operated channels; relative operating characteristic; resident on call; residual organic carbon; right outer canthus

ROCFT Rey-Osterrieth Complex Figure Test

ROCK Rho-associated kinase

ROCKET Regionally Organized Cardiac Key European Trial

rOCT rat organic cation transporter

ROCV Rocio virus

ROD record of decision

RODA rapid opioid detoxification under general anesthesia

RODEO rotating delivery of excitation off resonance

rOEF regional oxygen extraction fraction

roent roentgenology

ROESY rotating frame Overhauser effect spectroscopy

ROGAD radiation oncology greater area database

ROH rat ovarian hyperemia

ROI range of interest; reactive oxygen intermediate; region of interest; right occipitolateral

ROIH right oblique inguinal hernia

ROJM range of joint motion

ROLL radioguided occult lesion localization

ROM range of motion; reactive oxygen metabolite; read-only memory; reduction of movement; regional office manual; removal of metal; rupture of membranes

Rom Romberg [sign]

rom reciprocal ohm meter

ROMAS Romanian Multicenter Study

ROM CP range of motion complete and pain free

ROMI rating of medication influence; rule out myocardial infarct

ROMIO Rule Out Myocardial Infarct Observation [study]

ROMS radiation oncology management system

ROOF retro-orbital orbicular fat

ROP removal of pins or plates; removal of plaster; retinopathy of prematurity; right occipitoposterior

RO PACS radiation oncology picture archiving and communication system

ROPE respiratory-ordered phase encoding

ROPS rollover protective structure

ROR reactive oxygen radical; risk odds ratio

Ror Rorschach [test]

ROS reactive oxygen species; reflectance optical shield; relative outcome score; review of systems; rod outer segment

RoS rostral sulcus

ROSC restoration of spontaneous circulation; return of spontaneous circulation

ROSETTA Routine vs. Selective Exercise Treadmill Test After Angioplasty [trial]

ROSP rod outer segment protein

ROSS radiotherapy oncology support system; review of subjective symptoms

ROSTER Rotational Atherectomy v. Balloon Angioplasty for In-stent Restenosis [trial]

ROT real oxygen transport; remedial occupational therapy; right occipito-transverse

rot rotating, rotation

ROTA rotablator atherectomy

ROTACS rotational angioplasty catheter system

ROTASTENT Rotational Atherectomy with Adjunctive Stenting [trial]

ROU recurrent oral ulcer

R$_{out}$ outflow resistance

ROW Rendu-Osler-Weber [syndrome]; rest of the world

ROXIS Roxithromycin in Ischemic Syndromes [study]

RP radial pulse; radical prostatectomy; radiographic planimetry; radiopharmaceutical; rapid processing; rapid prototyping; Raynaud phenomenon; reactive protein; readiness potential; recessive partitioning; recreation and pastime; rectal prolapse; re-entrant pathway; refractory period; regulatory protein; relapsing polychondritis; relative power or potency; reperfusion; replication protein; resident physician; respiratory rate; responsible party; rest pain; resting position; resting potential; resting pressure; retinitis pigmentosa; retinitis proliferans; retrograde pyelogram; retroperitoneal; reverse phase; rheumatoid polyarthritis; ribonucleoprotein; ribose phosphate; ribosomal protein; Roswell Park [database]

R5P ribose-5-phosphate

R/P respiratory pulse

Rp peripheral resistance

R$_p$ pulmonary resistance

RPA radial photon absorptiometry; replication protein A; resultant physiologic acceleration; retinitis punctata albescens; retroperitoneal approach; reverse passive anaphylaxis; right pulmonary artery

r-PA reteplase

rPAF receptor for platelet activating factor

RPAHPET Royal Prince Albert Hospital Positron Emission Tomography [study]

RPase ribonucleic acid polymerase

RPC reactive perforating collagenosis; relapsing polychondritis; relative proliferative capacity; remote procedure call; restorative proctocolectomy

RPCA reverse passive cutaneous anaphylaxis

RPCF, RPCFT Reiter protein complement fixation test

RPCGN rapidly progressive crescenting glomerulonephritis

RPCH rural primary care hospital

RPD removable partial denture

R-PDQ revised prescreening developmental questionnaire

RPE rapid palatal expansion; rate of perceived exertion; recurrent pulmonary embolism; retinal pigment epithelium; ribulose 5-phosphate 3-epimerase

RPEP rabies post exposure prophylaxis

RPET rapid partial exchange transfusion

RPF relaxed pelvic floor; renal plasma flow; retroperitoneal fibrosis

rPFS radiographic progression-free survival

RPG radiation protection guide; retrograde pyelogram; rheoplethysmography; right paracolic gutter

RPGMEC Regional Postgraduate Medical Education Committee

RPGN rapidly progressive glomerulonephritis

RPGR retinitis pigmentosa guanosine triphosphatase regulator [gene]

RPh Registered Pharmacist

RPHA reversed passive hemagglutination

RPHAMCFA reversed passive hemagglutination by miniature centrifugal fast analysis

RP-HPLC, rpHPLC reverse-phase high-performance liquid chromatography

RPhT Registered Pharmacy Technician

RPI regional perfusion index; relative percentage index; reticulocyte production index; ribose 5-phosphate isomerase

RPIPP reverse-phase ion pair partition

RPK ribosephosphate kinase

RPL recurrent pregnancy loss; right precordial lead

RPLAD retroperitoneal lymphadenectomy

RPLC reverse-phase liquid chromatography

RPLD repair of potentially lethal damage

RPLES reversible posterior leukoencephalopathy syndrome

RPLND retroperitoneal lymph node dissection

RPM Rapid Pharmaceutical Management; rapid processing mode; revolutions per minute; robust point matching

rpm rapid processing mode; revolutions per minute

RPMD rheumatic pain-modulation disorder

RPMI Roswell Park Memorial Institute

RPMS relapsing-progressive multiple sclerosis; resource and patient management system

RPN Registered Practical Nurse; Registered Psychiatric Nurse

RPO right posterior oblique

RPP heart rate−systolic blood pressure product; rate-pressure product; retropubic prostatectomy

RPPA reverse-phase protein microarray

RPPI role perception picture inventory

RPPR red cell precursor production rate

RPR rapid plasmin reagin; Reiter protein reagin

RPr retinitis proliferans; rotational panoramic radiography

RPRC regional primate research center

RPRCT rapid plasma reagin cord test

RPRF rapidly progressive renal failure

Rp:Rs pulmonary/systemic vascular resistance ratio

RPS renal pressor substance; reverse pivot shift; revolutions per second; Royal Pharmaceutical Society

rps revolutions per second

RPS-BLAST reverse position-specific iterated basic local alignment search tool

RPSM residency program in social medicine

RPSP reference preparation for serum proteins

RPS4Y ribosomal protein S4, Y-linked

RPT rapid pull-through; refractory period of transmission; Registered Physical Therapist; renal parenchymal thickness; rifapentine

RPTA renal percutaneous transluminal angioplasty

RPTC regional poison treatment center

Rptd ruptured

RPTK receptor protein tyrosine kinase

RPTP receptor protein tyrosine phosphatase

RPV raccoon parvovirus; rinderpest virus; right portal vein; right pulmonary vein

RPVC resource provider of virtual center

RPVP right posterior ventricular pre-excitation

RQ recovery quotient; [Hazardous Substance] Reportable Quantities [List]; reportable quantity; respiratory quotient; risk-adjusted quantity

RQDS Revised Quantified Denver Scale of Communication

RQL rejectable quality level

RR radiation reaction; radiation response; rate ratio; rational recovery; recovery room; recurrence risk; reference reagent; regulatory region; relative resistance; relative response; relative risk; renin release; resistant relapse; respiratory rate; respiratory reserve; response rate; results reporting; retinal reflex; rheumatoid rosette; ribonucleotide reductase; risk ratio; Riva-Rocci [sphygmomanometer]; Ross River [virus]; ruthenium red

R&R rate and rhythm; rest and recuperation; rotablator and restenosis

Rr respiratory rate

RRA radioreceptor assay; registered record administrator

RRAC Research Realignment Advisory Committee

RRBAT relative rigid body accuracy test

RRC residency review committee; risk reduction component; routine respiratory care; Royal Red Cross; rural referral center

RRC-EM residency review committee for emergency medicine

RRDS radiation-resistant DNA synthesis

RRE radiation-related eosinophilia; Rev response element

RRE, RR&E round, regular, and equal

RRF ragged red fiber; residual renal function; ribosome recycling factor; rigid rectus femoris

RRFC renal reserve filtration capacity

RR-HPO rapid recompression−high-pressure oxygen

RRI recurrent respiratory infection; reflex relaxation index; relative response index

RRIS recurrent respiratory infection syndrome

RRL rabbit reticulocyte lysate; Registered Record Librarian

RRM RNA recognition motif; ribonucleotide reductase M

RRMS relapsing-remitting multiple sclerosis

RRN returning [for advanced studies] registered nurse

rRNA ribosomal ribonucleic acid

rRNP ribosomal ribonucleoprotein

RRP recurrent respiratory papillomatosis; relative refractory period

RRPCE Reduction of Recurrence and Prevention of Cerebral Emboli [study]

RRpm respiratory rate per minute

RRR regular rhythm and rate; relative risk reduction; renin release rate; renin release ratio

RR&R regular rate and rhythm

RRS result reporting repository system; retrorectal space; Richards-Rundle syndrome

R$_{RS}$ respiratory system resistance

RRT random response technique; recommended replacement time; Registered Respiratory Therapist; relative retention time; renal replacement therapy; retrieved related term

RRU respiratory resistance unit

RRV Ross River virus

RRV-TV tetravalent rhesus−human rotavirus vaccine

RS radioscaphoid; radiosurgery; random sample; rating schedule; Raynaud syndrome; reaction stimulus; recipient serum; rectal sinus; rectal suppository; rectosigmoid; reducing substance; Reed-Sternberg [cell]; reinforcing stimulus; Reiter syndrome; relative stimulus; remote sensing; remote site; renal specialist; respiratory syncytial [virus]; respiratory system; response to stimulus; resting subject; reticulated siderocyte; retinoschisis; Rett syndrome; review of symptoms; Reye syndrome; right sacrum; Reykjavik Study; right septum; right side; right stellate; Ringer solution; RNA synthetase; Roberts syndrome; Rous sarcoma

Rs *Rauwolfia serpentina*; systemic resistance

R/s roentgens per second

r$_s$ rank correlation coefficient

RSA rabbit serum albumin; regular spiking activity; relative specific activity; relative standard accuracy; respiratory sinus arrhythmia; right sacroanterior; right subclavian artery; roentgenographic stereogrammetric analysis

Rsa systemic arterial resistance

RSAC regular source of ambulatory care

RSB reticulocyte standard buffer; right sternal border

RSBA recurrent subareolar breast abscess

RSBD rapid eye movement sleep behavior disorder

RSC rat spleen cell; rested state contraction; reversible sickle cell; right subclavian

RSCA reference strand−mediated conformational analysis

RScA right scapuloanterior

RSCAAL remote-sensing chemical agent alarm

RSCN Registered Sick Children's Nurse

RScP right scapuloposterior

RSD rad surface dose; reflex sympathetic dystrophy; relative standard deviation

RSDS reflex sympathetic dystrophy syndrome

RSE rapid spin-echo; reconstruction squared error; refractory status epilepticus; relative standard error

RSEP right somatosensory evoked potential

RSES Rosenberg Self-Esteem Scale

RSF rich sequence format

RSG rosiglitazone

RSGP revised scaled gradient projection

RSH relative sitting height; Royal Society of Health

RSHT regular SNOMED (Systematized Nomenclature of Medicine) hierarchies table

RSI rapid-sequence induction; rapid sequence intubation; repetition strain injury; repetitive stress injury; Rush Sexual Inventory

RSIC Radiation Shielding Information Center

RSIL respiratory and systemic infection laboratory

R-SIRS Revised Seriousness of Illness Rating Scale

RSIVP rapid-sequence intravenous pyelography

RSK ribosomal S6 kinase

RSL radioactive seed localization; right sacrolateral; robotic suture line

RSLD repair of sublethal damage

RSLT test result

RSM risk screening model; Royal Society of Medicine

RSMR relative standard mortality rate

RSN Renal Support Network; restin; right substantia nigra

RSNA Radiological Society of North America; renal sympathetic nerve activity

RSO radiation safety officer; Resident Surgical Officer; right superior oblique

rSO$_2$ regional oxygen saturation

RSP rapid straight pacing; rat serum protein; recurrent spontaneous pneumothorax; removable silicone plug; respirable suspended particulate; ribose-5-phosphatase; right sacroposterior

RSPAC remote-sensing public access center

RSPCA Royal Society for the Prevention of Cruelty to Animals

RS-PCR RNA-specific template polymerase chain reaction

RS$_3$PE remitting seronegative symmetrical synovitis with pitting edema

RSPH Royal Society for the Promotion of Health

RSPK recurrent spontaneous psychokinesis

RSPV right superior pulmonary vein

RSR rectosphincteric reflex response/stimulus ratio; regular sinus rhythm; relative survival rate; right superior rectus

rSr an electrocardiographic complex

RSS rat stomach strip; recombination signal sequence; rectosigmoidoscopy; repetitive stress syndrome; rotary subluxation of the sphenoid; Russell-Silver syndrome; Russian spring-summer [encephalitis]

RSSE Russian spring-summer encephalitis

RSSI received signal strength indication

RSSR relative slow sinus rate

RST radiosensitivity test; rapid surfactant test; reagin screen test; repeated significance test; right sacrotransverse; rubrospinal tract

R$_{st}$ distance a spot of a substance has moved relative to a reference-standard spot

RSTD rectal−skin temperature difference

R-step restoration step

rSTERN recurrent spatiotemporal neuron

RSTI Radiological Service Training Institute

RSTL relaxed skin tension line

RSTLs relaxed skin tension lines

RSTMH Royal Society of Tropical Medicine and Hygiene

RSTS retropharyngeal soft tissue space; Rubinstein-Taybi syndrome

RSTV Rost Island virus

RSU radiologic sciences unit

RSV regurgitant stroke volume; respiratory syncytial virus; right subclavian vein; Rous sarcoma virus

RSVC right superior vena cava

RSVP rejuvenation with sparing of vascular perforators; retired senior volunteer program

RSV-Pr-C Rous sarcoma virus, Prague C

RSV-SR-D Rous sarcoma virus, Schmidt-Ruppin D

RSV-SR-B Rous sarcoma virus, Schmidt-Ruppin B

RT rabbit trachea; radiologic technologist; radiotelemetry; radiotherapy; radium therapy; random transfusion; rapid tranquilization; rational therapy; reaction time; reading test; real time; reciprocating tachycardia; recovery time; recreational therapy; rectal temperature; red tetrazolium; red top; reduction time; reference terminology; Registered Technician; related term; relaxation time; renal transplantation; repetition time; repolarization time; resistance transfer; respiratory therapist/therapy; response time; rest tremor; retention time; retransformation; retrieved term; reverse transcriptase; reverse transcription; Riedel thyroiditis; right; right thigh; robust take; room temperature; Rubinstein-Taybi [syndrome]

RT3, rT$_3$ reverse triiodothyronine

RT$_{90}$ time to 90% relaxation

Rt right; total resistance

rT recurrent tumor; ribothymidine

rt right; room temperature

RTA ray-tracing algorithm; renal tubular acidosis; reverse-transcriptase assay; road traffic accident

RTAA ruptured thoracic aortic aneurysm

RTAD renal tubular acidification defect

rTag recombinant small T antigen

rTAP recombinant tick anticoagulant peptide

RT(ARRT) Radiologic Technologist certified by the American Registry of Radiologic Technologists

RTAS radiology telephone access system

RTC rape treatment center; regional tuberculosis centre; renal tubular cell; residential treatment center; return to clinic; reverse thrust catheter

rtc return to clinic

RTCL Radiotherapy Command Language

rTCMS repetitive transcranial magnetic stimulation

RT-CT radiotherapy dedicated computed tomography

RTD real time three-dimensional; renal tubular defect; renal tubular dysgenesis; renal tubular dysplasia; resonant tunneling device; routine test dilution

RT3DE real-time three-dimensional echocardiography

RTE Registry of Toxic Effects

RTEC Regional Technology and Education Consortium

RTECS Registry of Toxic Effects of Chemical Substances

RTF resistance transfer factor; respiratory tract fluid; rich text format

RTG radioactive thermal generator; renal threshold of glucose

RTG-2 rainbow trout gonadal tissue cells

RTH resistance to thyroid hormone

RTI reproductive tract infection; respiratory tract infection; retrograde tracheal intubation; reverse transcriptase inhibition

RTK receptor tyrosine kinase; rhabdoid tumor of the kidney

rtl rectal

rt lat right lateral

RTM registered trademark

rTMS repetitive transcranial magnetic stimulation

RTN renal tubular necrosis

RTn reverse transcription intermediate

RT(N)(ARRT) Radiologic Technologist (Nuclear Medicine) certified by the American Registry of Radiologic Technologists

RTNet radiotherapy networking system

rTNF recombinant tumor necrosis factor

RTO return to office; right toe-off

RTOG radiation therapy oncology group

RTP radiation/radiotherapy treatment planning; renal transplantation patient; reverse transcriptase producing

rTPA, rtPA, rt-PA recombinant tissue plasminogen activator

RT-PACS radiotherapy picture archival and communication system

RT-PCR reverse transcriptase polymerase chain reaction

RTPV radiation therapy planning and verification; RT parvovirus

RTR Recreational Therapist, Registered; red blood cell turnover rate; retention time ratio

RT(R)(ARRT) Registered Technologist (Radiography) certified by the American Registry of Radiologic Technologists

RT-RH reverse transcriptase–ribonuclease H

RTRR return to recovery room

RTS rapid throughput screening; real-time scan; Rett syndrome; Revised Trauma Score; right toe strike; Rothmund-Thomson syndrome; Rubinstein-Taybi syndrome

RTSA reverse total shoulder arthroplasty

RTSS rest technetium-99m sestamibi scan

RTT round-trip time

RT(T)(ARRT) Radiologic Technologist (Radiation Therapy) certified by the American Registry of Radiologic Technologists

RTTP radiation therapy treatment planning

RTU real-time ultrasonography; relative time unit; renal transplantation unit

RT₃U resin triiodothyronine uptake

RTUI respiratory therapy utilization index

RTV recurrent tracheoesophageal fistula; resistance to voltage; rhinotracheitis virus; ritonavir; room temperature vulcanization

RTW return to work

RTX resiniferatoxin; robustotoxin

RU radioulnar; rat unit; reading unit; residual urine; resin uptake; resistance unit; retrograde urogram; right upper; roentgen unit

RU-1 human embryonic lung fibroblasts

RU-486 mifepristone

ru radiation unit

RUA reduced under anesthesia

RUBV rubella virus

RUC rapid update cycle

RUCAM Roussel Uclaf Causality Assessment Method

RUD recurrent ulcer of the duodenal bulb; repeating unit domain

RUE right upper extremity

RUG resource utilization group; retrograde urethrography

RUL right upper eyelid; right upper lateral; right upper limb; right upper lobe

RUMP remnants of uncertain malignant potential

RuMP ribulose monophosphate pathway

RUOQ right upper outer quadrant

RUP right upper pole
Ru1,5P ribulose-1,5-biphosphate
Ru5P ribulose-5-phosphate
rupt ruptured
RUPV right upper pulmonary vein
RUQ right upper quadrant
RUR resin uptake ratio
RURTI recurrent upper respiratory tract infection
RUS radioulnar synostosis; real-time ultrasonography
RUSB right upper sternal border
RUT rapid urease test
RUTH Raloxifene Use for the Heart [study]
RUV residual urine volume
RUX right upper extremity
RUZ right upper zone
RV ranavirus; random variable; rat virus; Rauscher virus; rectovaginal; regurgitant volume; reinforcement value; renal vein; reovirus; residual volume; respiratory volume; retroventral; retroversion; retrovesical; retrovirus; return visit; rhabdovirus; rheumatoid vasculitis; rhinovirus; right ventricle, right ventricular; rotavirus; rotavirus vaccine; rubella vaccine; rubella virus; Russell's viper
R/V, R&V record and verify
R$_V$ radius of view
Rv venous resistance
RVA rabies vaccine, adsorbed; recombinant virus assay; reentrant ventricular arrhythmia; right ventricle activation; right ventricular apex; right vertebral artery
RV-A to -G Rotaviruses A to G
RVAD right ventricular assist device
RVAW right ventricle anterior wall
RVB red venous blood
RVBF reversed vertebral blood flow
RVC reason for visit classification; rectovaginal constriction
RVD regulatory volume decrease; relative vertebral density; relative vessel diameter; relative volume decrease; right ventricular dimension; right ventricular dysplasia
RVDC right ventricular diastolic collapse
RVDO right ventricular diastolic overload
RVDV right ventricular diastolic volume
RVE right ventricular enlargement
RVECP right ventricular endocardial potential
RVED right ventricular end-diastolic
RVEDD right ventricular end-diastolic diameter
RVEDP right ventricular end-diastolic pressure
RVEDV right ventricular end-diastolic volume

RVEDVI right ventricular end-diastolic volume index
RVEF right ventricular ejection fraction; right ventricular end flow
RVESV right ventricular end-systolic volume
RVET right ventricular ejection time
RVF renal vascular failure; residual volume fraction; Rift Valley fever; right ventricular failure; right visual field
RVFP right ventricular filling pressure
RVFV Rift Valley fever virus
RVG radionuclide ventriculogram or ventriculography; right ventral gluteus; right visceral ganglion
RVH renal vascular hypertension, renovascular hypertension; right ventricular hypertrophy
RVHD rheumatic valvular heart disease
RVHR renovascular hypertensive rat
RVI relative value index; right ventricle infarction
RVID ventricular internal dimension
RVIT right ventricular inflow tract
RV-IVRT right ventricular isovolumic relaxation time
RVL right vastus lateralis
RVLG right ventrolateral gluteal
RVLM rostral ventrolateral medulla
RVM right ventricular mass; right ventricular mean
RVMM rostral ventromedial medulla
RVN radionuclide ventriculogram
RVO regional veterinary officer; relaxed vaginal outlet; right ventricular outflow
RVOT right ventricular outflow tract
RVOTO right ventricular outflow tract obstruction
RVP red veterinary petrolatum; resting venous pressure; right ventricular pressure
RVPEP right ventricular preejection period
RVPFR right ventricular peak filling rate
RVP/LVP right ventricular pressure/left ventricular pressure ratio
RVPRA renal vein plasma renin activity
RVR reduced vascular response; renal vascular resistance; repetitive ventricular response; resistance to venous return
RVRA renal vein/venous renin activity
RVRC renal vein renin concentration
RVS rectal visceral sensitivity; rectovaginal space; relative value scale; relative value study; reported visual sensation; retrovaginal space
RVSO right ventricular stroke output
RVSP right ventricular systolic pressure

RVSV right ventricular stroke volume

RVSW right ventricular stroke work

RVSWI right ventricular stroke work index

RVT radical vaginal trachelectomy; renal vein thrombosis

RVTE recurring venous thromboembolism

RV/TLC residual volume/total lung capacity

RVU relative value unit

RVV right ventricular volume; rubella vaccine−like virus; Russell's viper venom

rVV recombinant vaccinia virus

RVVO right ventricular volume overload

RVVT Russell's viper venom time

RVW right ventricular wall

RVWT right ventricle wall thickness

RW radiologic warfare; ragweed; respiratory work; Romano-Ward [syndrome]; round window

R-W Rideal-Walker [coefficient]; Romano-Ward [syndrome]

R/W return to work

RWAGE ragweed antigen E

RWC receiving water concentration; regional weaning center

RWI recreational water illness

RWIS restraint and water immersion stress

RWJF Robert Wood Johnson Foundation

RWM regional wall motion

RWMA regional wall motion abnormality

RWP ragweed pollen; R-wave progression

RWS radiology work station; ragweed sensitivity

RWT random walk theory; relative wall thickness

RWV rotating wall vessel

RX rapid exchange; reaction; residual tumor not assessed

Rx drug; medication; pharmacy; prescribe, prescription; prescription drug; take [L. *recipe*]; therapy; treatment

Rx&D Canada's Research-Based Pharmaceutical Companies

RXLI recessive X-linked ichthyosis

RXN reaction

RXR retinoid X receptor

RXRA retinoid X receptor alpha

RXRE retinoic X response element

RXRG retinoid X receptor gamma

RXT right exotropia

R-Y Roux-en-Y

RYD ryanodine

RYR, Ryr ryanodine receptor

S

S apparent power; negative deflection that follows an R wave [wave ECG]; entropy; exposure time; half [L. *semis*]; left [L. *sinister*]; mean dose per unit cumulated activity; midpoint of sella turcica; sacral; saline; *Salmonella*; saturated; scanning [pacemaker]; *Schistosoma*; schizophrenia; scleral; second; section; sedimentation coefficient; sella; semilente; senile, senility; sensation; sensitivity; septum; serine; serum; serum marker; *Shigella*; siderocyte; Siemens; sigmoid; signature; silicate; single; slope; slow accelerator; small; smooth; soft; solid; soluble; solute; sone; space; spatial; specificity; spherical; *Spirilum*; spleen; spontaneous; standard normal deviation; *Staphylococcus*; stem [cell]; stimulus; *Streptococcus*; streptomycin; subject; subjective findings; substrate; sulfur; sum of arithmetic series; supervision; supravergence; surface; surgery; suture; Svedberg; swine; Swiss [mouse]; synthesis; systole; without [L. *sine*]

Σ uppercase Greek letter sigma; syphilis; summation of series

S̄ specific heat capacity; without [L. *sine*]

S0 scleral invasion not assessed

S₁ first stimulus

s⁻¹ per second

S1 – S5 first to fifth sacral nerves

S₁ – S₄ first to fourth heart sounds

S2 supernatant, pure

s² sample variance [statistics]

4S Scandinavian Simvastatin Survival Study Group

S-100 marker protein for peripheral nervous system tumors containing α and β chains

s atomic orbital with angular momentum quantum number 0; distance; left [L. *sinister*]; length of path; sample standard deviation; satellite [chromosome]; scruple; second; section; sedimentation coefficient; sensation; series; signed; suckling

σ lowercase Greek letter sigma; conductivity; cross section; millisecond; molecular type or bond; population standard deviation; stress; surface tension; wave number

SA sacroanterior; salicylamide; salicylic acid; saline; salt added; sarcoidosis; sarcoma; scalenus anticus; secondary amenorrhea; secondary anemia; secondary arrest; self-administration; self-agglutination; self-analysis; semen analysis; sensitizing antibody;

serratus anterior; serum albumin; serum aldolase; sexual abuse; sexual addict; sexual assault; short acting; short axis; sialic acid; sialoadenectomy; signal averaged; simian adenovirus; simulated annealing; sinoatrial; sinus arrest; sinus arrhythmia; skeletal age; skin-adipose [unit]; sleep apnea; slightly active; slowly adapting; soluble in alkaline medium; Spanish American; specific activity; spectrum analysis; sperm abnormality; spiking activity; spinal abscess; spinal anesthesia; splenic artery; stable angina; standard accuracy; *Staphylococcus aureus*; status asthmaticus; stimulus artifact; Stokes-Adams [syndrome]; streptavidin; subarachnoid; substance abuse; succinylacetone; suicide alert; suicide attempt; surface antigen; surface area; surgery and anesthesia; surgical assistant; suspended animation; suspicious area; sustained action; sympathetic activity; symptom analysis; synthetic aperture; system administrator; systemic aspergillosis

S-A sinoatrial; sinoauricular

S&A sickness and accident; sugar and acetone

S/A stent/artery ratio

Sa most anterior point of the anterior contour of sella turcica; saline; *Staphylococcus aureus*

sA statampere

SAA serum amyloid A; serum amyloid – associated [protein]; severe aplastic anemia; starch ampicillin agar; synthetic amino acid

SAAG serum-ascites albumin gradient

SAAP selective aortic arch perfusion

SAAQ signal-averaged acoustic quantification

SAARD slow-acting antirheumatic drug

SAAS Substance Abuse Attitude Survey

SAAST self-administered alcohol screening test

SAB Scientific Advisory Board; serum albumin; signal above baseline; significant asymptomatic bacteriuria; sinoatrial block; Society of American Bacteriologists; spontaneous abortion; subarachnoid block

SAb spontaneous abortion

SABER Stent-Assisted Balloon Angioplasty and Its Effects on Restenosis [study]

SABOV Sabo virus

SABP spontaneous acute bacterial peritonitis; systolic arterial blood pressure

SABV Saboya virus

SAC saccharin; sacrum; screening and acute care; seasonal acute conjunctivitis; Self-Assessment of Communication; serum aminoglycoside concentration; short-arm cast; sideline assessment of concussion; small accessory chromosome; social activity [scale]; Speech-Language and Audiology Canada; splinting for acute closure; stable access cannula; stretch-activated channel; subarea advisory council; substance abuse counselor; symptomatic anomaly complex

SAC$_{cat}$ stretch-activated channel cations

sacch saccharin

SACD subacute combined degeneration

SACE serum angiotensin-converting enzyme

SACH small animal care hospital; solid ankle cushioned heel

SACK suppression of asymmetric cell kinetics

SACNAS Society for the Advancement of Chicanos and Native Americans in Science

SaCO$_2$ alveolar carbon dioxide saturation

SACS secondary anticoagulation system

SACSF subarachnoid cerebrospinal fluid

SACT sinoatrial conduction time

SAD Scale of Anxiety and Depression; seasonal affective disorder; Self-Assessment Depression [scale]; separation anxiety disorder; serially agitated solution; sinoaortic denervation; small airway disease; source-to-axis distance; standard American diet; sugar, acetone, and diacetic acid; suppressor-activating determinant

SADD Short-Alcohol Dependence Data [questionnaire]; standardized assessment of depressive disorders; Students Against Drunk Driving

SADDAN severe achondroplasia with developmental delay and acanthosis nigricans

SADIA small-angle double-incidence angiography

SADL simulated activities of daily living

SADR suspected adverse drug reaction

SADS Schedule for Affective Disorders and Schizophrenia; Sudden Adult Death Survey; sudden adult death syndrome; sudden arrhythmic death syndrome

SADS-C Schedule for Affective Disorders and Schizophrenia-Change

SADS-L Schedule for Affective Disorders and Schizophrenia-Lifetime

SADT self-accelerating decomposition temperature; Stetson Auditory Discrimination Test

SAdV simian adenovirus

SAE serious adverse event; sexual assault evaluation; short above-elbow [cast]; specific action exercise; subcortical arteriosclerotic encephalopathy; supported arm exercise

SAEB sinoatrial entrance block

SAECG, SaECG signal-averaged electrocardiogram

SAED semiautomatic external defibrillator

SAEFVSS Serious Adverse Events Following Vaccination Surveillance Scheme

SAEM Society for Academic Emergency Medicine

SAEP *Salmonella abortus equi* pyrogen

SAF scrapie-associated fibrils; self-articulating femoral; serum accelerator factor; simultaneous auditory feedback; standard analytic file

SAFA soluble antigen fluorescent antibody

SAFE Safety After Fifty Evaluation [study]; surgery, antibiotics, face washing, environmental change

SAFE-PACE Syncope and Falls in the Elderly-Role of Pacemaker [study]

SAFHS sonic-accelerated fracture-healing system

SAFIRE-D Symptomatic Atrial Fibrillation Investigation and Randomized Evaluation of Dofetilide [study]

SAFTEE Systematic Assessment for Treatment of Emergent Events

SAFTEE-GI Systematic Assessment for Treatment of Emergent Events-General Inquiry

SAFTEE-SI Systematic Assessment for Treatment of Emergent Events-Systematic Inquiry

SAFV Saint-Floris virus

SAG salicyl acyl glucuronide; sodium antimony gluconate; sonoangiography; streptavidin-gold; superantigen; Swiss agammaglobulinemia

sag sagittal

SAGE serial analysis of gene expression; Systematic Assessment of Geriatric Drug Use via Epidemiology [study]

SAGES signal-averaged electrocardiographic study

SAGM sodium chloride, adenine, glucose, mannitol

SAH S-adenosyl-L-homocysteine; subarachnoid hemorrhage

SAHA seborrhea, hypertrichosis/hirsutism, alopecia [syndrome]; suberoylanilide hydroxamic acid

SAHCS Streptokinase-Aspirin-Heparin Collaborative Study

SAHH S-adenosylhomocysteine hydrolase

SAHIGES *Staphylococcus aureus* hyperimmunoglobulinemia E syndrome

SA-HRP streptavidin-conjugated horseradish peroxidase

SAHS San Antonio Heart Study; sleep apnea-hypersomnolence [syndrome]

SAHV St. Abb's Head virus

SAI Self-Analysis Inventory; Sexual Arousability Inventory; Social Adequacy Index; suppressor of anchorage independence; systemic active immunotherapy

SAIC Science Applications International Corporation

SAICAR sylaminoimidazole carboxylase

SAID specific adaptation to imposed demand

SAIDS sexually acquired immunodeficiency syndrome; simian acquired immune deficiency syndrome

SAIF *Shigella boulardii* antiinflammatory factor

SAIMS student applicant information management system

SAKV Sakhalin virus

SAL sensorineural activity level; sterility assurance level; suction-assisted lipectomy; suction-assisted lipoplasty

Sal salicylate, salicylic; *Salmonella*

sAl serum aluminum [level]

sal salicylate, salicylic; saline; saliva

SALAD Surgery vs. Angioplasty for Proximal Left Anterior Descending Coronary Artery Stenosis [trial]

Salm *Salmonella*

SALP salpingectomy; salpingography; serum alkaline phosphatase

Salpx salpingectomy

SALT skin-associated lymphoid tissue; Swedish Aspirin in Low Dose Trial

SALTS Strategic Alternatives with Ticlopidine in Stenting [study]

SALV Salehebad virus

SAM *S*-adenosyl-L-methionine; scanning acoustic microscope; self-assembled monolayer; senescence-accelerated mouse; sex arousal mechanism; short-arc motion; smoking-attributable mortality; staphylococcal absorption method; StepWatch Activity Monitor; subject area model; substrate adhesion molecule; sulfated acid mucopolysaccharide; surface active material; system for assembling markers; systolic anterior motion

SAMA schizoaffective mania, mainly affective; South African Medical Association; Student American Medical Association

SAMBA Society of Ambulatory Anesthesiologists; Staffordshire Arthritis, Musculoskeletal, and Back Assessment

SAMD *S*-adenosyl-L-methionine decarboxylase

SaMD software as a medical device

SAM-DC *S*-adenosyl-L-methionine decarboxylase

SAMe *S*-adenosyl-L-methionine

SAMHSA Substance Abuse and Mental Health Services Administration

SAMI Streptokinase and Angioplasty in Myocardial Infarction [trial]; Streptokinase in Acute Myocardial Infarction [study]; Students for Advancement of Medical Instrumentation

SAMII Survey of Acute Myocardial Ischemia and Infarction [study]

SAMIT Streptokinase and Angioplasty Myocardial Infarction Trial

SAMMEC Smoking-Attributable Mortality, Morbidity, and Economic Costs [study]

SAMO senior administrative medical officer

SAMPLE Study on Ambulatory Monitoring of Pressure and Lisinopril Evaluation

SAMS Society for Advanced Medical Systems; substrate adhesion molecule

S-AMY salivary amylase; serum amylase

SAN sinoatrial node; sinoauricular node; slept all night; solitary autonomous nodule; storage area network

SANA sinoatrial node artery

Sanat sanatorium

SANDR sinoatrial nodal reentry

SANE sexual assault nurse examiner; Single Assessment Numerical Evaluation

SANE-A sexual assault nurse examiner-adult/adolescent

SANE-P sexual assault nurse examiner-pediatric

sang sanguineous

SANGUIS Safe and Good Use of Blood in Surgery [study]

sanit sanitary, sanitation

SANS scale for the assessment of negative symptoms

SANV Sango virus

SANWS sinoatrial node weakness syndrome

SAO small airway obstruction; splanchnic artery occlusion; subvalvular aortic obstruction

S$_{AO_2}$ oxygen saturation in alveolar gas

SaO$_2$ oxygen saturation

Sao$_2$ oxygen saturation in arterial blood

SAP sensory action potential; serum acid phosphatase; serum alkaline phosphatase; serum amyloid P; shrimp alkaline phosphatase; situs ambiguus with polysplenia; sphingolipid activator protein; stable angina pectoris; *Staphylococcus aureus* protease; subjective and physical; surfactant-associated protein; systemic arterial pressure; systolic arterial pressure

SAPA scan along polygonal approximation; spatial average, pulse average

SAPALDIA Swiss Study of Air Pollution and Lung Diseases in Adults

SAPAT Swedish Angina Pectoris Aspirin Trial

SAPD short action potential duration; signal-averaged P-wave duration; sphingolipid activator protein deficiency

SAPF simultaneous anterior and posterior fusion

saph saphenous

SAPHO synovitis, acne, pustulosis hyperostosis, osteomyelitis [syndrome]

SAPK stress-activated protein kinase

SA-PMP streptavidin-paramagnetic particle

SAPPHIRE Stanford Asian Pacific Program in Hypertension and Insulin Resistance

SAPS simplified acute physiology score; *Staphylococcus aureus* protease sensitivity

SAPV Sapphire virus

SAPX salivary peroxidase

SAQ saquinavir; self-applied questionnaire; short arc quadriceps

SAQC statistical analysis of quality control

SAR scaffold attachment region; scatter/air ratio; seasonal allergic rhinitis; sexual attitude reassessment; slowly adapting receptor; specific absorption rate; structure-activity relationship; subject access request; supplied air respirator; supraaortic ridge; supraaortic ring; synthetic aperture radar

SARA sexually acquired reactive arthritis; Superfund Amendments and Reauthorization

SARB Statistical Application and Research Branch

SARI serotonin-2 antagonist reuptake inhibitor; severe acute respiratory infection

SARS San Antonio Rotablator Study; severe acute respiratory syndrome

SARS-CoV severe acute respiratory syndrome coronavirus [emerged in 2002]

SARS-CoV-2 severe acute respiratory syndrome coronavirus-2 [the virus that causes COVID-19]

SART simultaneous algebraic reconstruction technique; Society for Assisted Reproductive Technology

SARV Santa Rosa virus

SAS sarcoma amplified sequence; Scottish Ambulance Service; sedation-agitation scale; self-rating anxiety scale; severe aortic stenosis; short arm splint; Simpson-Angus Scale; Sklar Aphasia Scale; sleep apnea syndrome; small animal surgery; small aorta syndrome; social adjustment scale; sodium amylosulfate; space adaptation syndrome; specific activity scale; statistical analysis system; sterile aqueous solution; sterile aqueous suspension; subaortic stenosis; subarachnoid space; sulfasalazine; supravalvular aortic stenosis; surface-active substance; synchronous atrial stimulation

SASA solvent-accessible surface area

SASD State Ambulatory Surgery Database

SASMAS skin-adipose superficial musculoaponeurotic system

SASP salicylazosulfapyridine

SASPP syndrome of absence of septum pellucidum with preencephaly

SASS Syngen Acute Stroke Study

SAS-SR social adjustment scale, self-report

SASSY Seniors Active Spirits Staying Young [program]

SAST selective arterial secretin injection test; Self-Administered Alcoholism Screening Test; serum aspartate aminotransferase

SAT saliva alcohol test; Saruplase Alteplase Study; satellite; satisfactibility; saturated; saturation; serum antitrypsin; shifting attention; single-agent chemotherapy; slide agglutination test; sodium ammonium thiosulfate; solitary arterial trunk; spermatogenic activity test; spontaneous activity test; subacute thrombosis; subacute thyroiditis; subcutaneous adipose tissue; sulfate adenyltransferase; symptomless autoimmune thyroiditis; systematic assertive therapy; systematic axis transform; systolic acceleration time

Sat, sat saturated, saturation

SATA spatial average, temporal average

SATB special aptitude test battery

satd saturated

SATE Safety Antiarrhythmic Trial Evaluation

SATL surgical Achilles tendon lengthening

SATP spatial average, temporal peak

SATS substance, amount ingested, time ingested, symptoms

SATSA Swedish Adoption-Twin Study of Aging

SATT Scottish Adjuvant Tamoxifen Trial

SATV Sathuperi virus

SAU statistical analysis unit

SAUDIS Sudden and Unexpected Death in Sports [study]

SAV San Angelo virus; sequential atrioventricular; Sikhote-Alyn virus

SAVD spontaneous assisted vaginal delivery

SAVE saved-young-life equivalent; sudden a ventilatory event; Survival and Ventricular Enlargement [trial]

SAVED saphenous vein de novo

SAW surface acoustic wave

SAX short axis; surface antigen, X-linked

SAx short axis

SAX-APEX short-axis plane, apical
SAX-MV short-axis plane, mitral valve
SAX-PM short-axis plane, papillary muscle
SB Bachelor of Science; Schwartz-Bartter [syndrome]; serum bilirubin; shortness of breath; sick bay; sideroblast; single blind; single breath; sinus bradycardia; small bowel; sodium balance; sodium bisulfite; Southern blotting; soybean; spike burst; spina bifida; spontaneous blastogenesis; spontaneous breathing; standard bed; Stanford-Binet [intelligence scale]; stereotyped behavior; sternal border; stillbirth; Sudan black [stain]; surface binding
S-B Sengstaken-Blakemore [tube]; suppression burst
S/β sickle cell beta-thalassemia
Sb strabismus
SBA serum bactericidal activity; serum bile acid; soybean agglutinin; spina bifida aperta; stand-by assist
SBAHC school-based adolescent health care
SBB stimulation-bound behavior
SBBT specialist in blood bank technology
SBC school-based clinic; Schwarz bayesian criterion; serum bactericidal concentration; strict bed confinement
SBCS Stockholm Breast Cancer Study
SBD selective bowel decontamination; senile brain disease
S-BD seizure−brain damage
SbDH sorbitol dehydrogenase
SBDX scanning beam digital x-ray
SBE breast self-examination; short below-elbow [cast]; shortness of breath on exertion; small bowel enema; small bowel enteroscopy; subacute bacterial endocarditis
SBEH social behavior
SBEPI sinusoidal blipped echo-planar imaging
SBET Society for Biomedical Engineering Technicians; standby emergency treatment
SBF serologic blocking factor; simulated body fluid; skin blood flow; specific blocking factor; splanchnic blood flow; systemic blood flow
SBFT small bowel follow-through
SBG selenite brilliant green
SBH Sabra hypertensive [rat]; sea-blue histiocyte; small basophilic hemocyte
SBHC school-based health center
SBI shape-based interpolation
SBIA Small Business & Industry Assistance CDER/FDA program
SBIAB secondary bacterial infection acute bronchitis
SBIS Stanford-Binet Intelligence Scale

SBL soybean lecithin
sBL sporadic Burkitt lymphoma
SBLA sarcoma, breast and brain tumors, leukemia, laryngeal and lung cancer, and adrenal cortical carcinoma
SB-LM Stanford-Binet Intelligence Test-Form L-M
SBM scientific basis of medicine; sexual intercourse between men; Solomon-Bloembergen-Morgan [equation]
SBMA spinal bulbar muscular atrophy
sBMD standardized bone mass density
SBMLC synchronous bilateral multiple lung cancers
SBN State Board of Nursing
SBN$_2$ single-breath nitrogen [test]
SBNS Society of British Neurological Surgeons
SBNT single-breath nitrogen test
SBNW single-breath nitrogen washout
SBO small bowel obstruction; spina bifida occulta
SBOM soybean oil meal
SBP schizobipolar; serotonin-binding protein; spontaneous bacterial peritonitis; steroid-binding plasma; sulfobromophthalein; symmetric biphasic; systemic blood pressure; systolic blood pressure
SBQ Smoking Behavior Questionnaire
SBQC small-base quad cane
SBR small bowel resection; small box respirator; spleen/body [weight] ratio; strict bed rest; styrene-butadiene rubber
SB-RDC sleep bruxism research diagnostic criteria
SBRN sensory branch of radial nerve
SBRS senior biomedical research service
SBRT split-beam rotation therapy
SBS secondary bilateral synchrony; shaken baby syndrome; short bowel syndrome; sick building syndrome; sinobronchial syndrome; skull base surgery; small bowel series; social breakdown syndrome; straight back syndrome; substrate-binding strand
SBSL-LTx sequential bilateral single-lung−liver transplantation
SBSP simultaneous bilateral spontaneous pneumothorax
SBSS Seligmann's buffered salt solution
SBT sequence-based typing; serum bactericidal titer; single-breath test; sulbactam
SBTI soybean trypsin inhibitor
SBTPE State Boards Test Pool Examination
SBTT small bowel transit time
SBTx small bowel transplantation
SBV singular binocular vision; soilborne virus

SB^V pentavalent antimonial
SBW standard body weight
SC conditioned stimulus; sacrococcygeal; Sanitary Corps; sarcomatous component; scalenus; scan computer; scapula; Schüller-Christian [disease]; Schwann cell; Schwarz criterion; sciatica; science; sclerosing cholangitis; secondary cleavage; secretory component; self-care; semicircular; semilunar valve closure; serum complement; serum creatinine; service connected; sex chromatin; Sézary cell; short circuit; sick call; sickle cell; sieving coefficient; sigmoid colon; silicone coated; single chemical; skin conduction; slice collimation; slow component; Snellen chart; sodium citrate; soluble complex; special care; specialty clinic; spinal canal; spinal cord; squamous carcinoma; start conversion; statistical control; stepped care; sternoclavicular; stratum corneum; subcellular; subclavian; subcorneal; subcortical; subcostal; subcutaneous; subtotal colectomy; succinylcholine; sugar coated; sulfur containing; supercoil cruciform; supercomputing; superior colliculus; supportive care; supraclavicular; surface colony; surface cooling; switching circuit; systemic candidiasis; systolic click
S/C subcutaneous; sugar coated
S-C sickle cell
S&C sclerae and conjunctivae
Sc scandium; scapula; science, scientific; screening
sC statcoulomb
sc subcutaneous
SCA self-care agency; senescent cell antigen; severe congenital anomaly; sickle cell anemia; single-camera autostereoscopy; single-channel analyzer; sperm-coating antigen; spinocerebellar ataxia; starburst calcification; steroidal-cell antibody; subclavian artery; superior cerebellar artery; suppressor cell activity; survivor of cardiac arrest
Sca-1 stem cell antigen 1
SCAA Skin Care Association of America; sporadic cerebral amyloid angiopathy
SCABG single coronary artery bypass graft
SCAD segmental colitis associated with diverticulosis [syndrome]; short-chain acyl-coenzyme A dehydrogenase; spontaneous coronary artery dissection
SCAG Sandoz Clinical Assessment-Geriatric [Rating]
SCAI Society for Cardiac Angiography and Interventions
SCAM statistical classification of activities of molecules

SCAMC Symposium on Computer Applications in Medical Care
SCAMIA Symposium on Computer Applications in Medical Care
SCAMIN Self-Concept and Motivation Inventory
SCAMP Stanford Coronary Artery Monitoring Project
SCAN Schedules for Clinical Assessment of Neuropsychiatry; suspected child abuse and neglect; systolic coronary artery narrowing
SCAP scapula
SCAR sequence characterized amplified region; severe cutaneous adverse reactions; Society for Computer Application in Radiology
SCARF skeletal abnormalities, cutis laxa, craniostenosis, psychomotor retardation, facial abnormalities [syndrome]
SCARI Spinal Cord Injury Assessment of Risk Index
SCARMD severe childhood autosomal recessive muscular dystrophy
SCAT sheep cell agglutination test; sickle cell anemia test; Simvastatin and Enalapril Coronary Atherosclerosis Trial; Sports Competition Anxiety Test
SCAV Sunday Canyon virus
SCAVF spinal cord arteriovenous fistula
SCAVM spinal cord arteriovenous malformation
SCB strictly confined to bed
SCBA self-contained breathing apparatus
SCBE single-contrast barium enema
SCBF spinal cord blood flow
SCBG symmetric calcification of the basal cerebral ganglia
SCBH systemic cutaneous basophil hypersensitivity
SCBP stratum corneum basic protein
SCC self-care center; sequential combination chemotherapy; services for crippled children; short-course chemotherapy; sickle cell disease; side-chain cleavage; small cell carcinoma; small cleaved cell; spinal cord compression; squamous cell carcinoma; standardized coding and classification; symptom cluster constraint
SC4C subcostal four-chamber [view]
SCCA single-cell cytotoxicity assay; small cell carcinoma
SCCB small cell carcinoma of the bronchus
SCCC squamous cell cervical carcinoma
SCCH sternocostoclavicular hyperostosis
SCCHN squamous cell carcinoma of the head and neck

SCCHO sternocostoclavicular hyperostosis

SCCL small cell carcinoma of the lung

SCCM Sertoli cell culture medium; Society of Critical Care Medicine

SCCOR Specialized Centers of Clinically Oriented Research

SCCT severe cerebrocranial trauma

SCD scleroderma; sequential compression device; service-connected disability; sickle cell disease; spinocerebellar degeneration; subacute combined degeneration; subacute coronary disease; sudden cardiac death; sudden coronary death; support clinical database; systemic carnitine deficiency

ScD Doctor of Science

SCDA situational control of daily activities [scale]; Special Care Dentistry Association

ScDA right scapuloanterior [L. *scapulodextra anterior*]

SCDAI simplified Crohn Disease Activity Index

SCDF skin condition data form

SCD-HeFT Sudden Cardiac Death in Heart Failure: Trial of Prophylactic Amiodarone vs. Implantable Defibrillator Therapy

SCDNT self-care deficit nursing theory

ScDP right scapuloposterior [L. *scapulodextra posterior*]

SCE secretory carcinoma of the endometrium; serious cardiac event; sister chromatid exchange; split hand, cleft lip/palate, ectodermal [dysplasia]; subcutaneous emphysema

SCe somatic cell

SCED single-case experimental design

SCEP sandwich counterelectrophoresis; spinal cord evoked potential

SCER sister chromatid exchange rate

SCES subjective computer experience scale

SCETI Stanford Computer-Based Educator Training Intervention

SceTy1V to 5V Saccharomyces cerevisiae Ty1 virus to Ty5 virus

SCF sinusoid containing blood flow; Skin Cancer Foundation; stem cell factor; subcostal frontal [view]

SCFA short-chain fatty acid

SCFE slipped capital femoral epiphysis

SCG scaled conjugate gradient; serum chemistry graft; serum chemogram; sodium cromoglycate; superior cervical ganglion

SCGE single-cell gel electrophoresis

SCH student contact hour; succinylcholine

SCh succinylchloride; succinylcholine

SChE serum cholinesterase

SCHIP State Children's Health Insurance Program

schiz schizophrenia

SCHL subcapsular hematoma of the liver

SCI Science Citation Index; Scottish Care Information; serial communication interface; sperm capacitation index; spinal cord injury; structured clinical interview

Sci science, scientific

SCID severe combined immunodeficiency; soft copy image display; Structured Clinical Interview for DSM 5

SCI/D spinal cord injury/disorder

SCIDS severe combined immunodeficiency syndrome

SCIDX severe combined immunodeficiency disease, X-linked

SCIE Social Care Institute for Excellence

SCIEH Scottish Centre for Infection and Environmental Health

SCII Strong-Campbell Interest Inventory

SCIM spinal cord injury medicine

SCINT, scint scintigraphy

SCIS spinal cord injury service

SCIU spinal cord injury unit

SCIV subcutaneous intravenous; Subcutaneous vs. Intravenous Heparin in Deep Venous Thrombosis [study]

SCIWORA spinal cord injury without radiographic abnormality

SCJ squamocolumnar junction; sternoclavicular joint; sternocostal joint

sCJD sporadic Creutzfeldt-Jakob disease

SCK serum creatine kinase

SCL scleroderma; serum copper level; sinus cycle length; skin conductance level; soft contact lens; stromal cell line; subcostal lateral [view]; symptom checklist; syndrome checklist

SCL-90 symptom checklist 90

scl sclerosed, sclerosis, sclerotic

ScLA left scapuloanterior [L. *scapulolaeva anterior*]

SCLBCL secondary cutaneous large B-cell lymphoma

SCLC small cell lung carcinoma

SCLD sickle cell chronic lung disease

SCLE subacute cutaneous lupus erythematosus

scler scleroderma, sclerosis

SCLH subcortical laminar heterotopia

ScLP left scapuloposterior [L. *scapulolaeva posterior*]

SCL-90-R symptom checklist 90, revised

SCLS systemic capillary leak syndrome

SCM scanning capacitance microscopy; Schwann cell membrane; sensation, circulation, and motion; Society of Computer Medicine; soluble cytotoxic medium; spleen cell−conditioned medium; split cord malformation; spondylitic caudal myelopathy; State Certified Midwife; sternocleidomastoid; streptococcal cell membrane; subclavius muscle; subcutaneous mastectomy; supernumerary marker chromosome; surface-connecting membrane

SCMC spontaneous cell-mediated cytotoxicity

SCMHR Society for Clinical and Medical Hair Removal

SCMO senior clerical medical officer

SCMPT sperm−cervical mucus penetration test

SCN coagulase-negative *Staphylococcus*; severe chronic neutropenia; severe congenital neutropenia; special care nursing; suprachiasmatic nucleus

SCN1A sodium channel, neuronal alpha-subunit type 1

SCN5A sodium channel gene

SCNS subcutaneous nerve stimulation

SCNT somatic cell nuclear transfer

ScNV-20S *Saccharomyces cerevisiae* narnavirus 20S

ScNV-23S *Saccharomyces cerevisiae* narnavirus 23S

SCO sclerocystic ovary; somatic crossing-over; subcommissural organ

SCOAP Surgical Care Outcomes Assessment Program

SCOFF sick, control, one stone, fat, food [questionnaire]

SCOP scopolamine; structural classification of proteins; systematic classification of proteins

SCOPE Scientific Committee on Problems of the Environment; Specialist Certification of Obesity Professionals in Europe; Study of Cognition and Prognosis in the Elderly; Surveillance and Control of Pathogens of Epidemiologic Importance [study]

SCOPEG symmetric, centrally ordered, phase-encoded group [imaging]

SCOPME Standing Committee on Postgraduate Medical and Dental Education

SCOR Specialized Center for Research

SCORE Status, Connections, Occupation, Resources, Events

SCORES Stent Comparative Restenosis [trial]; SCORES Saphenous Vein Graft Registry

SCOT social construction of technology; subcostal outflow [view]

SCP single-celled protein; smoking cessation program; sodium cellulose phosphate; soluble cytoplasmic protein; specialty care physician; standard care plan; sterol carrier protein; submucous cleft palate; superior cerebral peduncle

sCP spastic cerebral palsy

scp spherical candle power

SCPE simplified collective protective equipment

SCPK serum creatine phosphokinase

SCPL supracricoid partial laryngectomy

SCPM somatic crossover point mapping

SCPN serum carboxypeptidase N

SCPNT Southern California Postrotary Nystagmus Test

SCPR standard cardiopulmonary resuscitation

S-CPR standard postcompression remodeling

SCPS Skin Cancer Prevention Study

SCPT schizophrenic chronic paranoid type

SCQ social communication questionnaire

SCR Schick conversion rate; short consensus repeat; silicon-controlled rectifier; skin conductance response; slow-cycling rhodopsin; spondylitic caudal radiculopathy

SCr, Scr serum creatinine

sCR1 soluble complement receptor type 1

scr scruple

SCRAM speech-controlled respirometer for ambulation measurement

SCRAS Sheehan clinician-rated anxiety scale

SCRF surface coil rotating frame; Systematized Nomenclature in Medicine Cross-Reference Field

SCRIP Stanford Coronary Risk Intervention Project

SCRIPPS Scripps Coronary Radiation to Inhibit Proliferation Post Stenting [trial]

SCRIPT Smoking Cessation-Reduction in Pregnancy Trial

scRNA small cytoplasmic ribonucleic acid

SCRT stereotactic conformation radio-therapy

SCS Saethre-Chotzen syndrome; Seven Country Study; shared computer system; silicon-controlled switch; slow channel syndrome; Society of Clinical Surgery; specialized chromatin structure; spinal canal stenosis; spinal cord stimulation; splatter-control shield; splint classification system; synovial chondrosarcoma; systolic click syndrome

SCSA sperm chromatin structure assay; subcostal short axis

SCSB static charge−sensitive bed

SCSI small computer system interface

SCSIT Southern California Sensory Integration Test

SCSR standard cervical spine radiography

SCT salmon calcitonin; secretin; Sertoli cell tumor; sex chromatin test; sexual compatibility test; sickle cell trait; solid cystic tumor; sperm cytotoxicity; spinocervicothalamic; spiral computed tomography; staphylococcal clumping test; star cancellation test; stem cell transplantation; sugar-coated tablet

S-CT spiral computed tomography

S$_{CT}$ serum creatinine

SCTA spiral computed tomography angiography

SCTAT sex cord tumor with annular tubules

SCTBIFR South Carolina Traumatic Brain Injury Follow-up Registry

SCTN South Carolina Telemedicine Network

SCTR secretin receptor

SCTx spinal cervical traction

SCU self-care unit; special care unit

SCUBA self-contained underwater breathing apparatus

SCUD septicemic cutaneous ulcerative disease

SCUF slow continuous ultrafiltration

SCUP Skin Cancer Utrecht−Philadelphia [study]

SCU-PA single-chain urokinase plasminogen activator

SCUT schizophrenia, chronic undifferentiated type

SCV sensory nerve conduction velocity; smooth, capsulated, virulent; squamous cell carcinoma of the vulva; subclavian vein

ScV *Saccharomyces cerevisiae* virus

ScV-BC *Saccharomyces cerevisiae* virus L-BC

SCV-CPR simultaneous compression ventilation−cardiopulmonary resuscitation

SCVIR Society of Cardiovascular and Interventional Radiology

ScV-L-A *Saccharomyces cerevisiae* virus L-A

SCWM subcortical white matter

SCZ schizophrenia

SD Sandhoff disease; selective decontamination; semidry; senile dementia; septal defect; serologically defined; serologically detectable; serologically determined; serum defect; Shine-Dalgarno [sequence]; short dialysis; shoulder disarticulation; Shy-Draper [syndrome]; skin destruction; skin dose; solvent/detergent; somatization disorder; spatial deconvolution; spatial embedding dimension; speech delay; sphincter dilation; spontaneous delivery; sporadic depression; Sprague-Dawley [rat]; spreading depression; stable disease; standard definition; standard deviation; statistical documentation; Stensen duct; Still disease; stone disintegration; straight drainage; strength duration; streptodornase; structural deterioration; sudden death; superoxide dismutase; synchronous detector; systolic discharge

S-D sickle cell hemoglobin D; suicide-depression

S/D sharp/dull; Shine-Dalgarno [region]; systolic/diastolic

Sd standard; standard deviation of differences of sample; stimulus drive

S^d discriminative stimulus

SDA right sacroanterior [L. *sacrodextra anterior*]; Sabouraud dextrose agar; serotonin-dopamine antagonist; sialodacryoadenitis; specific dynamic action; strand displacement amplification; structural displacement amplification; succinic dehydrogenase activity

SDAI Simplified Disease Activity Index

SDAT senile dementia of Alzheimer type; surface digitalization accuracy test

SDAV sialodacryoadenitis virus

SDAVF spinal dural arteriovenous fistula

SDB shared database; sleep-disordered breathing

SDBP seated (or standing, or supine) diastolic blood pressure

SDC serum digoxin concentration; single-dispensing container; Smith delay compensator; sodium deoxycholate; sodium dichromate; subacute combined degeneration; subclavian hemodialysis catheter; succinyldicholine; symptomatic developmental complex; syndectan

SDCL symptom distress checklist

SDCN neural syndectan; N-syndectan

SDD selective decontamination of the digestive tract; Skeletal Dysplasia Diagnostician [database]; sporadic depressive disease; sterile dry dressing

SDDS 2-sulfamoyl-4,4′-diaminodiphenyl-sulfone

SDE simulation development environment; specific dynamic effect; standard-dose epinephrine; structured data entry; subdural empyema

SDEEG stereotactic depth electroencephalography

SDES symptomatic diffuse esophageal spasm

SDF slow death factor; standard data format; stress distribution factor; stromal-derived factor; structured data file

SDFV Syr-Daria Valley virus

SDG sucrose density gradient

SDGF schwannoma-derived growth factor

SDH serine dehydratase; sorbitol dehydrogenase; spinal dorsal horn; subdural hematoma; succinate dehydrogenase

SDHD sudden death heart disease

SDI selective dissemination of information; standard deviation interval; survey diagnostic instrument

SDIF standard generalized markup language document interchange format

SDIHD sudden death ischemic heart disease

SDILINE Selective Dissemination of Information Online [databank]

SDIS Stockholm Diabetes Intervention Study

SDL serum digoxin level; speech discrimination level

sdl sideline; subline

SDM semantic data model; sensory detection method; sparse distributed memory; standard deviation of the mean; system of decision making; system development method; Systematized Nomenclature in Medicine Digital Imaging and Communications in Medicine Microglossary

SDMD sulfadimethoxine

SDMS Society of Diagnostic Medical Sonography

SDN sexually dimorphic nucleus

SDNF sliding discrete Fourier transform narrow band filter

SDNV Serra do Navio virus

SDO standards development organization; sudden dosage onset

SDP right sacroposterior [L. *sacrodextra posterior*]; shared decision-making program; signal density plot

SDR shared data research; Skeletal Dysplasia Registry; spontaneously diabetic rat; standardized disease ratio; surgical dressing room

SDRI small, deep, recent infarct

SDRS social dysfunction rating scale

SDS same day surgery; school dental services; selective digestive decontamination; self-rating depression scale; sensory deprivation syndrome; sexual differentiation scale; short depression screen; Shy-Drager syndrome; single-dose suppression; sodium dodecylsulfate; specific diagnosis service; squamous [cell carcinoma] dataset; standard deviation score; sudden death syndrome; sulfadiazine silver; sustained depolarizing shift

SDSEM spinocerebellar degeneration—slow eye movements [syndrome]

SD-SK streptodornase-streptokinase

SDSL symmetric digital single line

SDS/PAGE, SDS-PGE sodium dodecylsulfate—polyacrylamide gel electrophoresis

SDT right sacrotransverse [L. *sacrodextra transversa*]; sensory detection theory; signal detection theory; single-donor transfusion; speech detection threshold

SD-T spatial deconvolution transformation

SD$_t$ standard deviation of total scores

SDU standard deviation unit; step-down unit

SDUB short double upright brace

SDV source data verification

SDW spin density weighted; system development workbench

SDYS Simpson dysmorphia syndrome

SE early systolic wave; saline enema; sanitary engineering; self-efficacy; serum; Shannon entropy; shared epitope; side effect; sleep efficiency; smoke exposure; socioeconomic; solid extract; sphenoethmoidal; spherical equivalent; spin-echo; spongiform encephalopathy; Spurway-Eddowes [syndrome]; standard error; staphylococcal endotoxin; staphylococcal enterotoxin; starch equivalent; Starr-Edwards [valve]; status epilepticus; subclinical encephalopathy; subendothelial; subependymal nodule; sulfoethyl; systematic error

S&E safety and efficiency

S-E socioeconomic; spin-echo; substantial equivalence

Se secretion; selenium

S$_e$ external skeleton

SEA sheep erythrocyte agglutination; shock-elicited aggression; soluble egg antigen; spatial envelope area; spinal epidural abscess; spontaneous electrical activity; staphylococcal enterotoxin A

SEAC Spongiform Encephalopathy Advisory Committee

SEADS Self-Efficacy and Dyspnea Strategies Scale

SEADS-C Self-Efficacy and Dyspnea Strategies-Confidence

SEAL steric and electrostatic alignment

SEAP secreted alkaline phosphatase

SEARCH Study of the Effectiveness of Additional Reductions of Cholesterol and Homocysteine

SEAT sheep erythrocyte agglutination test

SEB seborrhea; staphylococcal enterotoxin B

SE(b) standard error of regression coefficient

SEBA staphylococcal enterotoxin B antiserum

SEBI stereotactic external beam irradiation

SEBL self-emptying blind loop

SEBM Society for Experimental Biology and Medicine

SEBOV Sudan Ebola virus

SEBT Star Excursion Balance Test

SEC screening end code; secretin; *S*-ethyl-cysteine; Singapore epidemic conjunctivitis; size-exclusion chromatography; soft elastic capsule; spontaneous echo/echocardiographic contrast swollen endothelial cell

Sec Seconal; selenocysteine

sec second; secondary; section

sec-Bu sec-butyl

SeCD service for the care of drug addicts

SECG stress electrocardiography

SECON sequential continuity

SECORDS South-Eastern Consortium on Racial Differences in Stroke

SECRET stiffness of joint, elderly individuals, constitutional symptoms, arthritis, elevated erythrocyte sedimentation rate, temporal arthritis [mnemonic]

SECSY spin-echo correlated spectroscopy

sect section

SECURE Study to Evaluate Carotid Ultrasound Changes with Ramipril and Vitamin E

SED sedimentation rate; skin erythema dose; spondyloepiphyseal dysplasia; standard error of deviation; standard erythema dose; staphylococcal enterotoxin D

sed sedimentation; stool [L. *sedes*]

SEDL spondyloepiphyseal dysplasia, late

sed rt sedimentation rate

SEDT spondyloepiphyseal dysplasia tarda

SEDT-PA spondyloepiphyseal dysplasia tarda−progressive arthropathy

SEE standard error of estimate; staphylococcal enterotoxin E; substernal epicardial echocardiography

SEEG stereotactic electroencephalography

SEER Surveillance Epidemiology and End Results [program]

SEF somatosensory evoked magnetic field; spectral edge frequency; staphylococcal enterotoxin F; structured encounter form; suction effusion fluid

SEG segment; soft elastic gelatin; sonoencephalogram

SEGA subependymal giant cell astrocytoma

segm segment, segmented

SEGNE secretory granules of neural and endocrine [cells]

Se-GSH-Px selenium cofactor for glutathione peroxidase

SEH spinal epidural hemorrhage; subependymal hemorrhage

SEI Scar Elevation Index; Self-Esteem Inventory

S-EIA stick-enzyme immunoassay

SEID systemic excitation intolerance disease

SEIS slow eccentric isotonic stretch

SEISMED secure environment for information system in medicine

SE/IVH subependymal/intraventricular hemorrhage

SEL serum ethanol level

SELCA Smooth Excimer Laser Coronary Angioplasty [study]

SELDI surface-enhanced laser desorption ionization

SELDI-TOF surface-enhanced laser desorption-ionization time of flight

SELEX systemic evolution of ligands by experimental enrichment

SELF Self-Evaluation of Life Function

Sel Pt select patients

SELV Seletar virus

SEM sample evaluation method; scanning electron microphotography; scanning electron microscopy; secondary enrichment medium; standard error of measurement; standard error of the mean; stochastic expectation maximization; structural equation modeling; systolic ejection murmur

sem half [L. *semis*]; semen, seminal

SEMD spondyloepimetaphyseal dysplasia

SEMDIT spondyloepimetaphyseal dysplasia, Irapa type

SEMDJL spondyloepimetaphyseal dysplasia with joint laxity

semel in d. once a day [L. *semel in die*]

Semf seminal fluid

SEMG semenogelin; surface electromyography

sEMG surface electromyography

SEMI subendocardial myocardial infarction; subendocardial myocardial injury

SemNet semantic network

SEMSOB Stanford Self-Efficacy for Managing Shortness of Breath

SEN scalp-ear-nipple [syndrome]; State Enrolled Nurse [UK]

sen sensitive, sensitivity

SENDCAP St. Mary's Ealing, Northwick Park Diabetes Cardiovascular Prevention [study]

SENIC Study of the Efficacy of Nosocomial Infection Control

SENP sentrin-specific protease

SENS sensitivity or sensitization; Stewart evaluation of nursing scale

Sens sensitivity

sens sensation, sensorium, sensory

SENSOR Sentinel Event Notification System for Occupational Risks

SENTAC Society for Ear, Nose, Throat Advances in Children

SEOV Seoul virus

SEP self-evaluation process; sensory-evoked potential; separation; septum; somatosensory evoked potential; sperm entry point; spinal evoked potential; standard error of prediction; surface epithelium; syringe exchange program; systolic ejection period

sEP single evoked potential

separ separately, separation

SEPET extracorporeal blood purification device

SE$_{(p1-p2)}$ standard error of the difference of two proportions

SEPN selenoprotein N

SEPS subfascial endoscopic perforate ligation; Submaximal Exercise Performance Substudy

SEPT septum

SEPV Sepik virus

SEQ side effects questionnaire

seq sequence; sequel, sequela, sequelae; sequestrum

SEQOL [Bypass Angioplasty Revascularization Investigation] Substudy of Economics and Quality of Life

SER sarcoplasmic/endoplasmic reticulum; sebum excretion rate; sensitizer enhancement ratio; sensory evoked response; service; smooth endoplasmic reticulum; smooth-surface endoplasmic reticulum; somatosensory evoked response; subendocardial resection; supination, external rotation; surgical emergency room; systolic ejection rate

S/ER sero/plasmic endoplasmic reticulum

Ser serine; serology; serous; service

sER smooth endoplasmic reticulum

ser serial, series; serine

SERC State Emergency Response Commission

SERCA2 sarcoplasmic/endoplasmic reticulum Ca^{2-}

SerCl serum chloride

SER-IV supination external rotation, type 4 fracture

SERHOLD National Biomedical Serials Holding Database

SERLINE Serials Online

SERM selective estrogen receptor modulator

sero, serol serologic, serology

SERP somatosensory event−related potential

SERPIN serpine protease inhibitor

SERS Stimulus Evaluation/Response Selection [test]

SERT sustained ethanol release tube

serv keep, preserve [L. *serva*]; service

SERVHEL Service and Health Records

SES sirolimus-eluting stent; Society of Eye Surgeons; socioeconomic status; spatial emotional stimulus; sphenoethmoidal suture; subendothelial space

SESAM Study in Europe of Saruplase and Alteplase in Myocardial Infarction

SESAP Surgical Educational and Self-Assessment Program

SES-CD simple endoscopic score−Crohn disease

SESE somatosensory evoked spike epilepsy

SESIP safety engineered sharp injury protection

SET scar entry technique; secure electronic transaction; single electron transistor; single embryo transfer; surrogate embryo transfer; systolic ejection time

SET-N software evaluation tool for nursing

SETTS subjective experience of therapeutic touch survey

SEV 1 to 18, 125, 203 Simian enteroviruses 1 to 18, 125, 203

SeV Sendai virus

sev severe; severed

SEW slice excitation wave

SEWHO shoulder-elbow-wrist-hand orthosis

SE($\bar{x}$) standard error of the mean

SF Sabin-Feldman [test]; safety factor; salt free; scarlet fever; scatter factor; screen film; seminal fluid; serosal fluid; serum factor; serum ferritin; serum fibrinogen; sham feeding; shell fragment; shunt flow; sickle cell−hemoglobin F [disease]; simian foam virus; skin fibroblast; skinfold; soft feces; spinal fluid; spontaneous fibrillation; stable factor; Steel factor; sterile female; steroidogenic factor; stress formula; sugar free; superior facet; suppressor factor; suprasternal fossa; surviving fraction; Svedberg flotation [unit]; swine fever; symptom free; synovial fluid

S1F Steel factor

SF-1 steroidogenic factor 1

SF-36 short-form health survey

Sf spinal fluid; *Streptococcus faecalis*

S$_f$ Svedberg flotation unit

SFA saturated fatty acid; seminal fluid assay; serum folic acid; skinfold anthropometry; stimulated fibrinolytic activity; superficial femoral artery

SFAP single-fiber action potential

SFB Sanfilippo syndrome type B; saphenofemoral bypass; surgical foreign body

SFBL self-filling blind loop

SFC soluble fibrin complex; soluble fibrin—fibrinogen complex; spinal fluid count

SFCP Stanford Five City Project

SFD silo filler's disease; skin-film distance; small for dates; source-film distance; spectral frequency distribution

SFE slipped femoral epiphysis

SFEMG single-fiber electromyography

SFFA serum free fatty acid

SFFF sedimentation field flow fractionation

SFFV spleen focus-forming virus

SFG spotted fever group; subglottic foreign body

SFH schizophrenia family history; serum-free hemoglobin; stroma-free hemoglobin

SF/HGF scatter factor/hepatocyte growth factor

SFI Sexual Function Index; Social Function Index

SFIS structural family interaction scale

SFJ saphenofemoral junction

SFJT saphenofemoral junction thrombophlebitis

SFL scalar fuzzy logic; synovial fluid lymphocyte

SFM scanning force microscopy; Schimmelpenning-Fuerstein-Mims [syndrome]; self-fitting face mask; serum-free medium; solution-focused management; streptozocin, 5-fluorouracil, and mitomycin C

SFMC soluble fibrin monomer complex

SFMS Smith-Fineman-Myers syndrome

SFN Society for Neuroeconomics

SFNM standard finite normal mixture

SFNV Sabin virus; Sandfly fever Naples virus

SFO subfornical organ

SFP screen filtration pressure; simultaneous foveal perception; spinal fluid pressure; stopped flow pressure

SFR screen filtration resistance; stenosis flow reserve; stroke with full recovery

SFS serial foveal seizures; skin and fascia stapler; social functioning schedule; sodium formaldehyde sulfoxylate; spatial frequency spectrum; split function study

SFSV Sandfly fever Sicilian virus

SFT Sabin-Feldman test; second field tumor; sensory feedback therapy; skinfold thickness

SFTP secure file transfer protocol [telemedicine]

SFU surgical follow-up

SFV Semliki Forest virus; shipping fever virus; Shope fibroma virus; simian foamy virus; squirrel fibroma virus; swine fever virus

SFV 1, SFV 3 simian foamy viruses 1 and 3

SFW sexual function of women; shell fragment wound; slow-filling wave

SG Sachs-Georgi [test]; salivary gland; serum globulin; serum glucose; signs; skin graft; soluble gelatin; specific gravity; subgluteal; substantia gelatinosa; succinimidyl glutamate; Surgeon General; Swan-Ganz [catheter]

sg specific gravity; subgenomic

SGA second-generation antipsychotic; small for gestational age; supraglottic airway

sGAG sulfated glycosaminoglycan

SGAP superior gluteal artery perforator [flap]

SG$_{AW}$ specific airway conductance

SGB Simpson-Golabi-Behmel [syndrome]; sparsely granulated basophil

SGBI silicone gel breast implants

SGBS Simpson-Golabi-Behmel syndrome

SGC soluble guanylate cyclase; spermicide-germicide compound; Swan-Ganz catheter

SGCA subependymal giant cell astrocytoma

SGCRC German Study Group on Colo-Rectal Carcinoma

SGD *Saccharomyces* Genome Database; specific granule deficiency

SGE secondary generalized epilepsy; spoiled gradient echo

SGF sarcoma growth factor; skeletal growth factor

SGGT serum gamma-glutamyl transpeptidase

SGH subgluteal hematoma

SGHL superior glenohumeral ligament

SGL salivary gland lymphocyte; supraglottic laryngectomy

sgl sugarless

SGLD spatial gray level dependence

SGLT sodium-dependent glucose transporter

SGLT2 sodium-glucose co-transporter 2

SGM Society for General Microbiology

SGNA Society of Gastroenterology Nurses and Associates

SGNE secretory granule neuroendocrine [protein]

SGO Surgeon General's Office; surgery, gynecology, and obstetrics

SGOT serum glutamate oxaloacetate transaminase (aspartate aminotransferase)

SGP scaled gradient projection; serine glycerophosphatide; sialoglycoprotein; Society of General Physiologists; soluble glycoprotein; sulfated glycoprotein

SGPA salivary gland pleomorphic adenoma

SGPT serum glutamate pyruvate transaminase (alanine aminotransferase)

SGR Sachs-Georgi reaction; Shwartzman generalized reaction; skin galvanic reflex;

submandibular gland renin; substantia gelatinosa Rolandi; sustainable growth rate

sgRNA subgenomic ribonucleic acid

SGRQ Saint George's Respiratory Questionnaire

SGS Schinzel-Giedion syndrome

SGSG Scandinavian Glioma Study Group

S-Gt Sachs-Georgi test

SGTT standard glucose tolerance test

SGTX surugatoxin; *Scodra griseipes* toxin

SGV salivary gland virus; selective gastric vagotomy; short gastric vessel

SGVHD syngeneic graft-versus-host disease

SH Salter-Harris [fracture]; Schönlein-Henoch [purpura]; self-help; serum hepatitis; sexual harassment; sex hormone; Sherman [rat]; sick in hospital; sinus histiocytosis; social history; somatotropic hormone; spontaneously hypertensive [rat]; standard heparin; state hospital; sulfhydryl; surgical history; symptomatic hypoglycemia; syndrome of hyporeninemic hypoaldosteronism; systemic hyperthermia

S/H sample and hold

S&H speech and hearing

Sh sheep; Sherwood number; *Shigella*; shoulder

sh shoulder

SHA secure hashing algorithm; simple highest avidity; Southern hybridization analysis; staphylococcal hemagglutinating antibody; strategic hospital alliance

sHa suckling hamster

SHAA serum hepatitis associated antigen; Society of Hearing Aid Audiologists

SHAA-Ab serum hepatitis associated antigen antibody

SHAFT sad, hostile, anxious, frustrating, tenacious

SHAp stoichiometric hydroxyapatite

SHAPE Screening Health Assessment and Preventive Education [program]; Stress, Health and Physical Evaluation [program]; Study of Heparin and Actilyse Processed Electronically

SHARE source of help in airing and resolving experiences; Study of Heart Assessment and Risk in Ethnic Groups

SHARK Stroke, Hypertension and Recurrence in Kyushu [study]

SHARP school health additional referral program; Scottish Heart and Arterial Disease Risk Prevention [program]; Subcutaneous Heparin in Angioplasty Restenosis Prevention [trial]

SHAV Shamonda virus

SHAVE Steerable Housing for Atherovascular Excision

SHB sequential hemibody

S-Hb sulfhemoglobin

SHBD serum hydroxybutyric dehydrogenase

SHBG sex hormone binding globulin

SHC self-help class

SHCC state health coordinating council

SHCO sulfated hydrogenated castor oil

SHD satellite hemodialysis; sudden heart death

SHE Syrian hamster embryo; systolic hypertension of the elderly

SHEA Society for Healthcare Epidemiology of America

SHEENT skin, head, eyes, ears, nose, throat

SHEP Systolic Hypertension in the Elderly Program

SHF simian hemorrhagic fever; subfulminant hepatic failure; superhigh frequency

shf superhigh frequency

SHFD split hand/foot deformity

ShFM shear force microscopy

SHFV simian hemorrhagic fever virus

SHG sonohysterography; synthetic human gastrin

SHH sonic hedgehog [gene]; syndrome of hyporeninemic hypoaldosteronism

Shh sonic hedgehog

SHHD Scottish Home and Health Department

SHHH self-help for hard of hearing

SHHS Scottish Heart Health Study; Sleep Heart Health Study

SHHV Society for Health and Human Values

SHI severe head injury

Shig *Shigella*

SHIN skilled home health nursing

SHINE Strategic Health Informatics Network in Europe

SHIPS Shiga Pravastatin Study

SHIV Shiant Islands virus

SHL sensorineural hearing loss

SHLA soluble human lymphocyte antigen

SHLD shoulder

SHML sinus histiocytosis with massive lymphadenopathy

SHMO senior hospital medical officer

SHMO, S/HMO social health maintenance organization

SHMT serine-hydroxymethyl transferase

SHN sexual and reproductive health nurse; spontaneous hemorrhagic necrosis; subacute hepatic necrosis

SHO secondary hypertrophic osteoarthropathy; Senior House Officer [UK]; simple harmonic oscillator

SHOCK Should We Emergently Revascularize Occluded Coronaries for Cardiogenic Shock? [trial]

SHOP State Hospital Data Project

SHORT, S-H-O-R-T short stature, hyperextensibility of joints or hernia or both, ocular depression, Rieger anomaly, teething delayed

short-FRAME short stature, facial anomalies, Rieger anomaly, midline anomalies, enamel defects [syndrome]

SHOT serious hazards of transfusion; Shunt Occlusion Trial

SHOV Shokwe virus

SHP Schönlein-Henoch purpura; secondary hyperparathyroidism; Skaraborg Hypertension Project; state health plan

SHPDA state health planning and development agency

sHPT secondary hyperparathyroidism

SHR spontaneously hypertensive rat

SHRED Sedatives and Hemodynamics During Rapid-Sequence Intubation in the Emergency Department [trial]

shRNA short hairpin RNA

SHRS scanned handwritten record system

SHRSP spontaneously hypertensive rat, stroke prone

SHS Sayre head sling; sheep hemolysate supernatant; sliding hip screw; Strong Heart Study; Sutterland-Haan syndrome

SHSF split hand−split foot [malformation]

SHSP spontaneously hypertensive stroke-prone [rat]

SHSS Stanford Hypnotic Susceptibility Scale

SHT simple hypocalcemic tetany; subcutaneous histamine test

SHUA System for Hospital Uniform Accounting

SHUR System for Hospital Uniform Reporting

SHUV Shuni virus

SHV simian herpesvirus; Southampton virus

SHVRC Shiley Heart Valve Research Center

SHWI segmental hepatic warm ischemia

SI International System of Units [Fr. *Système International d'Unités*]; sacroiliac; saline infusion; saline injection; saturation index; self-inflicted; sensory integration; septic inflammation; serious illness; serum iron; severity index; sex inventory; shock index; signal intensity; Singh Index; single injection; sinus irregularities; small intestine; social interaction; soluble insulin; special

intervention; spirochetosis icterohaemorrhagica; stability index; stimulation index; stress incontinence; stroke index; structured interview; sucrase isomaltase; sulfoxidation index; superior-inferior; suppression index; syncytium inducer

S/I superior/inferior

S&I suction and irrigation

Si the most anterior point on the lower contour of the sella turcica; silicon

SIA serum inhibitory activity; small intestine atresia; stress-induced analgesia; stress-induced anesthesia; stretch-induced arrhythmia; subacute infectious arthritis; supplemental immunization activity; supplementary immunization activities

SIAD syndrome of inappropriate antidiuresis

SIADH syndrome of inappropriate secretion of antidiuretic hormone

SIAM Streptokinase in Acute Myocardial Infarction [study]

SIB self-inflating bulb; self-injurious behavior; Severe Impairment Battery [psychological assessment]; sibling [in semantic hierarchy]; Swiss Institute of Bioinformatics

sib, sibs sibling, siblings

SIBLING small integrin binding ligand N-linked glycoprotein

SIBO small intestinal bacterial overgrowth

SIB X, SIB$_X$ extended siblings in semantic hierarchy

SIC serum insulin concentration; Standard Industrial Classification

SICCO Stenting in Chronic Coronary Occlusion [study]

SICD serum isocitrate dehydrogenase

sICH symptomatic intracerebral hemorrhage

SICU spinal intensive care unit; surgical intensive care unit

SID focal spot to imaging plane distance; once per day [L. *semel in die*]; selective intestinal decontamination; single intradermal [test]; Society for Investigative Dermatology; source-image distance; source-isocenter distance; standard imaging display; state inpatient database; stress-induced depolarization; strong ion difference; sucrase-isomaltase deficiency; sudden inexplicable death; sudden infant death; suggested indication of diagnosis; systemic inflammatory disease

s.i.d. once per day [L. *semel in die*]

SIDAM Structured Interview for the Diagnosis of Dementia of the Alzheimer Type, Multi-Infarct Dementia, and Dementias of Other Etiology

SIDDT sudden infant death with dysgenesis of the testes

SIDS sudden infant death syndrome; sulfo-iduronate sulfatase

SIE sis-inducible element; stroke in evolution

SIEA superficial inferior epigastric artery

SIEB Systematized Nomenclature of Medicine International Editorial Board

SIECUS Sexuality Information and Education Council of the United States

SIESTA Snooze-Induced Excitation of Sympathetically Triggered Activity [study]

SIF sacral insufficiency fracture; serum-inhibition factor

SIFT selector ion flow tube

SIG SARS-CoV-2 Interagency Group; Self-Injury Grid; small inducible gene

SIg, sIg surface immunoglobulin

sig sigmoidoscopy; significant; write on label

SIgA, S-IgA secretory immunoglobulin A

SIGH-D Structured Interview for the Hamilton Depression Scale

SigInt signal intelligence

SIgM, S-IgM secretory immunoglobulin M

SIGMAV Sigma virus

sigmo sigmoidoscope or sigmoidoscopy

SIGN Scottish Intercollegiate Guideline Network

SIH stimulation-induced hypalgesia; stress-induced hyperthermia; suction-induced hypoxemia

SIHDSPS Stockholm Ischemic Heart Disease Secondary Prevention Study

SIHE spontaneous intramural hematoma of the esophagus

SI-HRDS structured interview Hamilton rating scale for depression

SII self-inflicted injury

SIIM Society for Imaging Informatics in Medicine

SIJ sacroiliac joint

SIL soluble interleukin; speech interference level; squamous intraepithelial lesion

SILD Sequenced Inventory of Language Development

SIM selected ion monitoring; small intestine mesentery; Society for Industrial Microbiology; Society for the Internet in Medicine; specialized intestinal metaplasia; subscriber identity module

SIMA single internal mammary artery; Stenting vs. Internal Mammary Artery for Single Left Anterior Descending Arterial Lesion [trial]

SIMD single instruction, multiple data

SIMFE severe infantile multifocal epilepsy

SIMP Schmele instrument to measure the process of nursing care; simulation of initial medical problem

SIMP-C Schmele instrument to measure the process of nursing care

SIMP-H Schmele instrument to measure the process of nursing care in home care

SIMPLE symbolic interactive modeling package and learning environment

SIMS secondary ion mass spectroscopy; situational information management system

simul simultaneously

SIMV Simbu virus; synchronized intermittent mandatory ventilation; synchronized intermittent mechanical ventilation

SIN salpingitis isthmica nodosa; self-inactivating; Sindbis [virus]

SINE short interspersed element

SIN-FM Short Indexed Nomenclature-Family Medicine

SINS Semi-Structured Intelligent Navigation System

SINV Sindbis virus

SIO sacroiliac orthosis

SIOP International Society of Pediatric Oncology [Société Internationale d'Oncologie Pédiatrique]

SIP saturation inversion projection; Short Inventory of Problems; Sickness Impact Profile; slow inhibitory potential; stroke in progression; summarized intensity projection; surface inductive plethysmography

SIPA shear-induced platelet aggregation

SIPS Strategy for Intracoronary Ultrasound-Guided Percutaneous Transluminal Coronary Angioplasty and Stenting [trial]

sIPTH serum immunoreactive parathyroid hormone

SIQ Sexual Interest Questionnaire; Symptom Interpretation Questionnaire

SIQR semiinterquartile range

SIR short intergenic region; single isomorphous replacement; sliced inverse regression; Society of Interventional Radiology; specific immune release; standardized incidence ratio; stroke index ratio; susceptible, infected, recovered; syndrome of immediate reactivities

SIRA Scientific Instrument Research Association

SIRE short interspersed repetitive element

SIREF specific immune response−enhancing factor

SIRF severely impaired renal function; significant intrarenal fragments

SIRIS sputter-initiated resonance ionization spectroscopy

siRNA small interfering ribonucleic acid

SIRS soluble immune response suppressor; Structured Interview of Reported Symptoms; systemic inflammatory response syndrome

SiRV simian rotavirus

SiRV-SA11 simian rotavirus SA11

SIS semantic indexing system; Senologic International Society [Fr. *Société International de Sénologie*]; serotonin irritation syndrome; simian sarcoma; simulator-induced syndrome; small intestinal submucosa; social information system; specialized information system; spontaneous interictal spike; sterile injectable solution; sterile injectable suspension; supplemental information seeking; Surgical Infection Society; surgical information system

SISA Stenting in Small Arteries [trial]

SISAMI Silent Ischemia in Survivors of Acute Myocardial Infarction [study]

SISCOM subtraction ictal single proton emission computed tomography coregistered to magnetic resonance imaging

SISH silver in situ hybridization; Stage I Systolic Hypertension in the Elderly [study]

SISI short increment sensitivity index

SISO single input, single output

SISRC Self-Injury and Self-Restraint Checklist

SISS Sentinel Injury Surveillance System; small inducible secreted substances

SISTEMI Southern Italian Study on Thrombolysis Early in Myocardial Infarction

SISV, SiSV simian sarcoma virus

SIT serum inhibiting titer; single inhaler therapy; sit down; Slosson Intelligence Test; specific immunotherapy; sperm immobilization test; strategic intermittent therapy; suggested immobilization test

SITA Swedish Interactive Threshold Algorithm

SITHS Swedish Secure Internet Within Healthcare

SITS supraspinatus, infraspinatus, teres minor, subscapularis

SIU International Urologic Society [Fr. *Société Internationale d'Urologie*]

SIV simian immunodeficiency virus; Sprague-Dawley-Ivanovas [rat]

SIV-agm simian immunodeficiency virus African green monkey

SIV-agm.3 simian immunodeficiency virus African green monkey 3

SIV-agm.155 simian immunodeficiency virus African green monkey 155

SIV-agm.gr simian immunodeficiency virus African green monkey gr-1

SIV-agm.sab simian immunodeficiency virus African green monkey Sab 1

SIV-agm.tan simian immunodeficiency virus African green monkey Tan 1

SIV-agm.TYO simian immunodeficiency virus African green monkey TYO

SIV-cpz simian immunodeficiency virus chimpanzee

SIVH stress-induced visceral hyperalgesia

SIV-mac simian immunodeficiency virus rhesus macaque

SIV-mnd simian immunodeficiency virus mandrill

SIV-mne simian immunodeficiency virus pig-tailed macaque

SIV-rcm simian immunodeficiency virus red-capped mangabey

SIV-sm simian immunodeficiency virus sooty mangabey

SIV-stm simian immunodeficiency virus stump-tailed macaque

SIV-syk simian immunodeficiency virus Sykes monkey

SIW self-inflicted wound

SIWI selective incomplete white matter infarction

SIWIP self-induced water intoxication and psychosis

SIWIS self-induced water intoxication and schizophrenic disorders

S$_J$ Jaccard coefficient

SJA Schwartz-Jampel-Aberfeld [syndrome]

SJAV Sandjimba virus

S$_{jb}$O$_2$ jugular bulb venous oxygen saturation

SJC swollen joint count

SjO$_2$ jugular vein oxygen saturation

SJR Shinowara-Jones-Reinhart [unit]

SJS Schwartz-Jampel syndrome; Stevens-Johnson syndrome; stiff joint syndrome; Swyer-James syndrome

SjS Sjögren syndrome

SJS/TEN Stevens-Johnson syndrome/toxic epidermal necrolysis

SJV San Juan virus

SjVO$_2$ jugular venous oxygen saturation

SK seborrheic keratosis; senile keratosis; Sloan-Kettering [Cancer Center]; spontaneous killer [cell]; squamous keratin; state of knowledge; streptokinase; swine kidney

Sk skin

SKA supracondylar knee-ankle [orthosis]

SKALP skin-derived antileukoproteinase

SKAT Sex Knowledge and Attitude Test

SKDAMI Streptokinase plus Desmopressin in Acute Myocardial Infarction [study]

skel skeleton, skeletal

SKHYDIP Skara Hypertension and Diabetes Project

SKI Sloan-Kettering Institute

SKL serum killing level

SkM skeletal muscle
SKR semantic knowledge representation
SKSD, SK-SD streptokinase-streptodornase
SKT skin temperature
sk trx skeletal traction
SKY spectral karyotyping
SL sarcolemma; scapholunar, scapholunate; sclerosing leukoencephalopathy; secondary leukemia; segment length; sensation level; sensory latency; septal leaflet; short leg [brace]; Sibley-Lehninger [unit]; signal level; Sinding-Larsen [syndrome]; Sjögren-Larsson [syndrome]; slit lamp; small lymphocyte; sodium lactate; solidified liquid; sound level; SPECIALIST Lexicon; Stein-Leventhal [syndrome]; streptolysin; sublingual; sway length
S$_L$ systolic wave, latent
S/L sublingual
Sl Steel [mouse]
sl in a broad sense [L. *sensu lato*]; stemline; sublingual
SLA left sacroanterior [L. *sacrolaeva anterior*]; single-cell liquid cytotoxic assay; slide latex agglutination; soluble liver antigen; stereo lithography; superficial linear array; surfactant-like activity
SL$_A$ segment length, anterior
SLAC scapholunate advanced collapse
SLAM scanning laser acoustic microscope; systemic lupus erythematosus activity measure
SLAP serum leucine aminopeptidase; superior labrum anterior to posterior [lesion]
SLAT simultaneous laryngoscopy and abdominal thrusts
SLB short leg brace
SLBP stem-loop binding protein
SLC short leg cast; solute carrier
SLCC short leg cylinder cast
SLD scapholunar dissociation; sublethal damage
SLD, SLDH serum lactate dehydrogenase
SLDR sublethal damage repair
SLE slit-lamp examination; St. Louis encephalitis; systemic lupus erythematosus
SLEA sheep erythrocyte antibody
SLEDAI systemic lupus erythematosus disease activity index
SLEP short latent evoked potential
SLEV St. Louis encephalitis virus
sLex sialyl Lewis x
SLF Steel factor
SL-GXT symptom-limited graded exercise test
SLH staple line height
SLHR sex-linked hypophosphatemic rickets

SLHT straight-line Hough transform
SLI selective lymphoid irradiation; somatostatin-like immunoreactivity; specific language impairment; splenic localization index
SL$_I$ segment length, inferior
SLIC scanning liquid ionization chamber; Scottish Library and Information Council; super lubricious integrated coating
SLIP serial line interface protocol; sliding linear investigative platform
SLIR somatostatin-like immunoreactivity
SLJD Sinding-Larsen-Johansson disease
SLK superior limbic keratoconjunctivitis
SLKC superior limbic keratoconjunctivitis
SLL small lymphocytic lymphoma
SL$_L$ segment length, lateral
SLM sound level meter
SLMC spontaneous lymphocyte-mediated cytotoxicity
SLN sentinel lymph node; sublentiform nucleus; superior laryngeal nerve; SYBYL line notation
SLNWBC short-leg non−weight-bearing cast
SLNWC short-leg nonwalking cast
SLO scanning laser ophthalmoscopy; Smith-Lemli-Opitz syndrome; streptolysin O
SLOS Smith-Lemli-Opitz syndrome
S-LOST sulfur mustard, for Lommel and Steinkopf
SLP left sacroposterior [L. *sacrolaeva posterior*]; segmental limb systolic pressure; sex-limited protein; single-locus probe; short luteal phase; speech language pathologist; subluxation of the patella
slp sex-limited protein
SLPI salivary leukocyte protease inhibitor; secretory leukocyte protease inhibitor
SLPP serum lipophosphoprotein
SLR Shwartzman local reaction; single-lens reflex; stentlike result; straight leg raising
SLRROM shoulder lateral rotation range of motion
SLRT straight leg-raising test
SLS Seattle Longitudinal Study; segment long spacing; short-leg splint; single-leg separation; single-limb support; Sjögren-Larsson syndrome; sodium lauryl phosphate; stagnant loop syndrome; Stein-Leventhal syndrome; synthetic lethal screening
SL$_S$ segment length, septal
SLT left sacrotransverse [L. *sacrolaeva transversa*]; selective laser trabeculoplasty; single-lumen tube; single-lung transplantation; smokeless tobacco; solid logic tech-nology
SLTEC/VTEC *Shigella*-like toxin (verotoxin) producing *Escherichia coli*

SLUD salivation, lacrimation, urination, defecation

SLUDGE salivation, lacrimation, urination, defecation, gastrointestinal upset, emesis

SLUMS St. Louis University Mental Status [examination]

SLV semilatent virus; symptomless virus

SLVDS San Luis Valley Diabetes Study

SLWC short-leg walking cast

SM Master of Science [L. *Scientiae Magister*]; sadomasochism; segmental mastectomy; self-monitoring; sensitivity matrix; serum; silicon microphysiometer; simple mastectomy; skim milk; smooth muscle; somatomedin; space medicine; sphingomyelin; splenic macrophage; splenomegaly; sports medicine; storage manager; streptomycin; Strümpell-Marie [syndrome]; submandibular; submaxillary; submucous; suckling mouse; sucrose medium; suction method; sulfomethyl; superior mesenteric; surgical microscope; surrogate mother; sustained medication; symptoms; synaptic membrane; synovial membrane; systemic mastocytosis; systolic motion; systolic murmur

S/M sadomasochism; suspicious or malignant

Sm samarium; *Serratia marcescens*; Smith [antigen]

sM small membrane [protein]; suckling mouse

sm smear

SMA sequential multichannel autoanalyzer; shape memory alloy; simultaneous multichannel autoanalyzer; smooth muscle antibody; Society for Medical Anthropology; somatomedin A; spinal muscular atrophy; spontaneous motor activity; standard method agar; superior mesenteric artery; supplementary motor area; symptomatic morphologic anomaly

SM-A somatomedin A

SMA-6 Sequential Multiple Analysis for six different serum tests

SMABF superior mesenteric artery blood flow

SMAC Sequential Multiple Analyzer Computer

SMAE superior mesenteric artery embolism

SMAF smooth muscle activating factor; specific macrophage arming factor

SMAG Special Medical Advisory Group

SM-AHNMD systemic mastocytosis with associated clonal hematologic non−mast cell lineage disease

SMAL serum methyl alcohol level

sm an small animal

SMAO superior mesenteric artery occlusion

SMAP systemic mean arterial pressure

SMART Self-Measurement for Assessment of the Response to Trandolapril [study]; semantic adaptive resonance theory; simultaneous multiple-angle reconstruction technique; small-volume multiple noncoplanar arc radiotherapy; sperm microaspiration retrieval technique; Study of Medicine vs. Angioplasty Reperfusion Trial; Study of Microstent's Ability to Limit Restenosis Trial

SMARTT Serum Markers, Acute Myocardial Infarction, and Rapid Treatment Trial

SMAS submuscular aponeurotic system; superficial musculo-aponeurotic system; superior mesenteric artery syndrome

SMASH Simultaneous Acquisition of Spatial Harmonics; Swiss Multicenter Evaluation of Early Angioplasty for Shock; Sydney Men and Sexual Health [study]

SMAST Short Michigan Alcoholism Screening Test

SMATS Seek Medical Attention in Time Study

SMB selected mucosal biopsy; standard mineral base

sMb suckling mouse brain

SMBFT small bowel follow-through

SMBG self-monitoring of blood glucose

SMC safety monitoring committee; Scientific Manpower Commission; smooth muscle cell; somatomedin C; succinylmonocholine; supernumerary marker chromosome; suture-mediated closure

SM-C, Sm-C somatomedin C

SMCA smooth muscle contracting agent; suckling mouse cataract agent

SMCC succininamidyl-4-(*N*-maleimidomethyl) cyclohexane-1-carboxylate

SMCD senile macular choroidal degeneration; systemic mast cell disease; systemic meningococcal disease

SM-C/IGF somatomedin C/insulin-like growth factor

SMCR Smith-Magenis chromosome region; 5-sulfoxymethylchrysene

SmCS smart classification

SMD senile macular degeneration; severe mental disorder; spondylometaphyseal dysplasia; standardized mean difference; submanubrial dullness

SMDA Safe Medical Devices Act; starch methylenedianiline

SMDC sodium-*N*-methyl dithiocarbamate; standards for medical device communication

SM-HDRA simulated microgravity histoculture drug response assay

SMDM Society for Medical Decision Making

SMDP semi-Markov decision process

SMDS secondary myelodysplastic syndrome; switched multimegabit data service

SME severe myoclonic epilepsy

SMEB severe myoclonic epilepsy, borderline

SMED spondylometaphyseal dysplasia

SMEDI stillbirth mummification, embryonic death, infertility [syndrome]

SMEI severe myoclonic epilepsy, of infancy

SMEM supplemented Eagle minimum essential medium

SMF selected minerals in food; streptozocin, mitomycin C, 5-fluorouracil; submembrane region containing thrombosthenin filaments; substructural molecular fragment

smf sodium motive force

SMFM shear modulation force microscopy

SMFP state medical facilities plan

SMG specialty medical group; submandibular gland

SmG supramarginal gyrus

SMH state mental hospital; strongyloidiasis with massive hyperinfection

SMHA state mental health agency

SMHC smooth muscle heavy-chain myosin

SMI Self-Motivation Inventory; senior medical investigator; serious mental illness; severe mental impairment; silent myocardial infarction; stress myocardial image; Style of Mind Inventory; supplementary medical insurance; sustained maximum inspiration

SmIg surface membrane immunoglobulin

SMILE So Much Improvement with a Little Exercise [program]; Survival of Myocardial Infarction: Long-Term Evaluation [study]

SMISS Silent Myocardial Ischemia Stress Study

SMK structured meta-knowledge

SML smouldering leukemia

SMM scintimammography; smoldering multiple myeloma

SMMD specimen mass measurement device

SMMHC smooth muscle myosin heavy chain

SMMSE Standardized Mini-Mental State Examination

SMN second malignant neoplasm; stathmin; surgical microscope navigator; survival motor neuron

SMNB submaximal neuromuscular block

SMN^T telemeric survival motor neuron

SMO second medical opinion; senior medical officer; slips made out; surveillance medical officer

SMOH senior medical officer of health; Society of Medical Officers of Health

SMON subacute myelooticoneuropathy

SMP slow-moving protease; standard medical practice; submitochondrial particle; sulfamethoxypyrazine; symmetric multiprocessor; sympathetically maintained pain

SMPC summary of product characteristics

SMPR small mannose 6-phosphate receptor

SMPV superior mesenteric portal vein

SMQ Standard MeDRA Query

SMR scatter maximum ratio; senior medical resident; sensorimotor rhythm; severe mental retardation; sexual maturity rating; significantly lower mortality rate; skeletal muscle relaxant; somnolent metabolic rate; standardized mortality rates; standardized mortality ratio; stroke with minimum residuum; submucosal resection

SMRR submucosal resection and rhinoplasty

SMRT silencing mediator of retinoid and thyroid receptors

SMRV squirrel monkey retrovirus

SMS scalable modeling system; senior medical student; serial motor seizures; Shared Medical Systems; short messaging system; Simvastatin Multicenter Study; Smith-Magenis syndrome; somatostatin; stiff-man syndrome; supplemental minimum sodium

SMSA standard metropolitan statistical area

SMSV San Miguel sea lion virus

SMT Spanish Multicentre Study; spontaneous mammary tumor; stereotactic mesencephalic tractomy; Stockholm Metoprolol Trial; surface mouth technology; Swedish massage therapy

SMTP simple mail transfer protocol

S-MUAP surface-detected motor unit action potential

SMuLV Scripps murine leukemia virus

SMV skeletal muscle ventricle; superior mesenteric vein

SMWHS Seattle Midlife Women's Health Study

SMX, SMZ sulfamethoxazole

SN school nurse; sclerema neonatorum; scrub nurse; Semantic Network; sensorineural; sensory neuron; serum neutralization; sinus node; spontaneous nystagmus; staff nurse; stromal nodule; student nurse; subnormal; substantia nigra; supernatant; suprasternal notch

S/N signal/noise ratio; supernatant

Sn subnasale

sn small nucleolar

SNA specimen not available; Student Nurses Association; sympathetic nerve activity

SNa serum sodium concentration

SNAC scaphoid nonunion advanced collapse; sertoli neuron aggregated cells; S-nitroso-*N*-acetylcysteine; sodium *N*-caprylate

SNagg serum normal agglutinator

SNAP Score for Neonatal Acute Physiology [study]; sensory nerve action potential; *S*-nitroso-*N*-acetylpenicillamine; soluble *N*-ethylmaleimide−sensitive fusion protein attachment protein; Stanford Nutrition Action Program

SNaP Study of Sodium and Blood Pressure

SNAP-25 synaptosome-associated protein of 25 kilodaltons

SNAPE Study of Nicorandil in Angina Pectoris in the Elderly

SNAP−PE Score for Neonatal Acute Physiology−Perinatal Extension

SNARE soluble *N*-ethylmaleimide−sensitive fusion protein attachment protein receptor

SNARL suggested no adverse response level

SNB scalene node biopsy

SNC spontaneous neonatal chylothorax

SNCL sinus node cycle length

SNCS sensory nerve conduction studies

SNCV sensory nerve conduction velocity

SND scatter number density; sinus node dysfunction; striatonigral degeneration; sympathetic nerve discharge; systematic nodal dissection

SNDA Student National Dental Association

SNDO Standard Nomenclature of Diseases and Operations

SNE sinus node electrogram; subacute necrotizing encephalomyelography

SNEB Sindh Nurses Examination Board; Society for Nutrition Education and Behavior

SNES suprascapular nerve entrapment syndrome

SNF sinus node formation; skilled nursing facility

SNGBF single nephron glomerular blood flow

SNGFR single nephron glomerular filtration rate

SNHL sensorineural hearing loss

SNID subnational immunization day

SNIPA seronegative inflammatory polyarthritis

SNIVT Society of Non-Invasive Vascular Technology

SNJ sebaceous nevus of Jadassohn

SNK Student-Newman-Keuls [method]

SNM Society of Nuclear Medicine; sulfanilamide

SNMA Student National Medical Association

SNMP simple network management protocol

SNMT Society of Nuclear Medical Technologists

SN-N suprasternal notch-to-nipple distance (sternal notch disease)

SNNS sentinel node navigation surgery

sno small nucleolar

SNOBOL String-Oriented Symbolic Language

SNODO Standard Nomenclature of Diseases and Operations

SNOMED Systematized Nomenclature of Medicine

SNOMED CMT Systematized Nomenclature of Medicine Convergent Medical Terminology

SNOMED CT Systematized Nomenclature of Medicine Clinical Terminology

SNOMED RT Systematized Nomenclature of Medicine Reference Terminology

SNOMED RT/CMT Systematized Nomenclature of Medicine Reference Terminology/Convergent Medical Terminology

SNOP Systematized Nomenclature of Pathology

snoRNA small nucleolar ribonucleic acid

snoRNP small nucleolar ribonucleoprotein

SNP school nurse practitioner; single nucleotide polymorphism; sinonasal papilloma; sinus node potential; sodium nitroprusside

S-NPI start nuclear polymorphism index

SNPV single nucleopolyhedrovirus

SNR selective nerve root; semantic network relationship; signal/noise ratio; substantia nigra zona reticulata; supernumerary rib

Snr substantia nigra zona reticulata

SNRB selective nerve root block

snRNA small nuclear ribonucleic acid; small nucleolar ribonucleic acid

SNRI selective serotonin-norepinephrine reuptake inhibitor

snRNP small nuclear ribonucleoprotein; small nuclear ribonucleoprotein particle

snRP small nuclear ribonucleoprotein polypeptide

snRPB small nuclear ribonucleoprotein polypeptide B

SNR$_{Pix}$ signal/noise ratio per pixel

snRPN small nuclear ribonucleoprotein polypeptide N

SNRT sinus node recovery time

SNRTd sinus node recovery time, direct measuring

SNRTi sinus node recovery time, indirect measuring

SNS Senior Nursing Sister; Society of Neurological Surgeons; supplementary nursing system; sympathetic nervous system

SNSA seronegative spondyloarthropathy

S-NSE serum neuron-specific enolase

SNST sciatic nerve stretch test

SNT sinuses, nose, and throat; spectral noise threshold

SNTB smear-negative tuberculosis

SNU skilled nursing unit

SNuPE single nucleotide primer extension

SNV Sin nombre virus; spleen necrosis virus

SNVDO Standard Nomenclature of Veterinary Diseases and Operations

SNW slow negative wave

SO salpingo-oophorectomy; Schlatter-Osgood [disease]; second opinion; sex offender; shoulder orthosis; site of origin; slow oxidative; spheno-occipital; sphincter of Oddi; standing orders; suboccipital; superior oblique; supraoccipital; supraoptic; supraorbital; sutures out; sympathetic ophthalmia

S&O salpingo-oophorectomy

SO₂ oxygen saturation

SOA serum opsonic activity; shortness of air; spinal opioid anesthesia; stimulus onset asynchrony; swelling of ankles

SoA symptoms of asthma

SOAA signed out against advice

SOAMA signed out against medical advice

SOA-MCA superficial occipital artery to middle cerebral artery

SOAP subjective, objective, assessment, and plan

SOAPIE subjective, objective, assessment, plan, implementation, and evaluation

SOAR Safety of Orbofiban in Acute Coronary Research [study]

SOB see order blank; shortness of breath; stool occult blood

SOBOE shortness of breath on exertion

SOBP spread out Bragg peak [radiotherapy]

SOC self-organized criticality; sequential oral contraceptive; Standard Occupational Classification; standards of care; state of consciousness; store-operated channel; surgical overhead canopy; synovial osteochondromatosis; syphilitic osteochondritis; system on a chip

SoC state of consciousness

SOCIAIDS Study of Cardiac Involvement in Acquired Immunodeficiency Syndrome

SoCPA stage of change for physical activity

SOCRATES Study of Coronary Revascularization and Therapeutic Evaluations

SOCS1 suppressor of cytokine signaling 1

SocSec Social Security

SocServ social services

S-OCT serum ornithine carbamyl transferase

SOD selective oropharyngeal decontamination; septo-optic dysplasia; sphincter of Oddi dysfunction; superoxide dismutase

sod sodium

SODAS spheroidal oral drug absorption system

sod bicarb sodium bicarbonate

SODF sperm outer defense fiber

SODH sorbitol dehydrogenase

SOF Study of Osteoporotic Fractures; superior orbital fissure

SOFA sequential [sepsis-related] organ failure assessment [scale]

SOFLC self-organizing fuzzy logic control

SOFM self-organization feature map

SOG supraorbital groove

SOH sympathetic orthostatic hypotension

SOHN Society of Otorhinolaryngology and Head-Neck Nurses; supraoptic hypothalamic nucleus

SOHND supraomohyoid neck dissection

SOHO self-organizing, holarchic, open

SOI severity of illness; signal of interest

SOL solution; space-occupying lesion

sol soluble, solution

SOLD Stenting After Optimal Lesion Debulking [trial]

SOLEC stand on one leg, eyes closed

Soln, sol'n solution

SOLVD Studies of Left Ventricular Dysfunction

SOM secretory otitis media; self-organizing map; sensitivity of method; serous otitis media; somatotropin; state operations manual; superior oblique muscle; suppurative otitis media; supraorbital margin; sustained outward movement

SOMA Student Osteopathic Medical Association; subjective, objective, management, and analytic

somat somatic

SOMI sternal occipital mandibular immobilization

SOMME suborbital mimetic muscle elevation

SON superior olivary nucleus; supraoptic nucleus

SONET synchronous optical network transmission

SONH spontaneous osteonecrosis of the hip

SONK spontaneous osteonecrosis of the knee

SOO structured office oral [examination]

SOOF suborbital orbicular fat

SOP service-object pair; standard operating procedure

SoP standard of performance

SOPA Survey of Pain Attitudes; syndrome of primary aldosteronism

SOPCA sporadic olivopontocerebellar ataxia

SOPED Shock Outcome Prediction in the Emergency Department [score]

SOPHE Society for Public Health Education

SOPI service object pair instance

SOPO set of possible occurrences

SOQ Suicide Opinion Questionnaire

SOR stimulus-organism response; strength of recommendation; successive over-relaxation; superoxide release

SOr supraorbitale

sOR stratified odds ratio

Sorb, sorb sorbitol

SORD sorbitol dehydrogenase

SOREM sleep-onset rapid eye movement

SORF spliceable open-reading frame

SOS self-obtained smear; son of sevenless; Southern Oxidant Study; speed of sound; supplemental oxygen system; surgery on site; Swedish Obesity Study

SoS Stent or Surgery [study]

SOSA Student Osteopathic Surgical Association

SOSF single organ system failure

SOS study Swedish Obese Subjects study

SOST sclerosteosis gene

SOT sensory organization test; solid-organ transplantation; systemic oxygen transport

SOWS subjective opiate withdrawal scale

SP sacroposterior; sacrum to pubis; salivary progesterone; schizotypal personality; secretory piece; semiprivate; senile plaque; sepiapterin; septal pore; septum pellucidum; sequence processor; sequential pulse; serine/proline; seropositive; serum protein; shunt pressure; shunt procedure; silent period; skin potential; sleep deprivation; slow pathway; small protein; smoothed periodogram; soft palate; solid phase; spastic paraplegia; specific protocol; spectrogram; speech pathology; spiramycin; spirometry; spleen; spontaneous proliferation; standard practice; standard procedure; standardized patient; standards of performance; staphylococcal protease; *Staphylococcus pneumoniae*; status post[operative]; steady potential; stimulus to P wave; stool preservative; storage phosphor; subliminal perception; substance P; sulfadoxine-pyrimethamine; sulfapyridine; sulfopropyl; summating potential; superimposed pressure; suprapatellar; suprapubic; surface polypeptide; surfactant protein; symphysis pubis; synthase phosphatase; systolic pressure

Sp most posterior point on posterior contour of sella turcica; sleep spindle; species; specific; specimen; sphenoid; spine; *Spirillum*; summation potential

S/P, s/p status post[operative]

S1P sphingosine 1-phosphate

S7P sedoheptulose-7-phosphate

S$_p$ pooled standard deviation

sP senile parkinsonism; structural protein

sp space; species; specific; spine, spinal; spirit

SPA salt-poor albumin; sheep pulmonary adenomatosis; single-photon absorptiometry; spastic ataxia; sperm penetration assay; spinal progressive amyotrophy; spondyloarth-ropathy; spontaneous platelet aggregation; staphylococcal protein A; student progress assessment; suprapubic aspiration; surface polypeptide, anonymous

SP-A surfactant protein A

SPA-Acad Acadian spastic ataxia

SPACE single potential analysis of cavernous electrical activity

sp act specific activity

SPACTO Stent vs. Percutaneous Angioplasty in Chronic Total Occlusion [trial]

SPAD stenosing peripheral arterial disease

SPAF spontaneous paroxysmal atrial fibrillation; Stroke Prevention in Atrial Fibrillation [trial]

SPAF TEE Stroke Prevention in Atrial Fibrillation-Transesophageal Echo [study]

SPAG small particle aerosol generator

SPAI steroid protein activity index

SPAM scanning photoacoustic microscopy

SPAMM spatial modulation of magnetization

sp an spinal anesthesia

sPAP systolic pulmonary artery pressure

SPAR sensitivity prediction by acoustic reflex

SPARC cysteine-rich acidic secreted protein; Stroke Prevention Assessment of Risk and Community [trial]

SPARS spatially resolved spectrometry

SPAT slow paroxysmal atrial tachycardia; spatial concept

SPB sinking pre−beta-lipoprotein

SP-B surfactant protein B

SPBI serum protein-bound iodine; sun-protector behavior index

SPBMD spinal bone mineral density

SPC safe psoriasis control; salicylamide, phenacetin, and caffeine; scaphopisocapitate; seropositive carrier; single palmar crease; single photoelectron count; soy phosphatidylcholine; spleen cell; standard plate count;

statistical process control; summary of product characteristics; synthetizing protein complex

SP-C surfactant protein C

SPCA serum prothrombin conversion accelerator; Society for Prevention of Cruelty to Animals; systemic pulmonary collateral artery

SPCC Spill Prevention, Control, and Countermeasure [plan]

SPCD syndrome of primary ciliary dyskinesia

Sp Cd, sp cd spinal cord

SPCG spectral phonocardiography

SPD schizotypal personality disorder; sociopathic personality disorder; specific paroxysmal discharge; spermidine; standard peak dilution; sterile processing department; storage pool deficiency

SPDT single pole, double throw

SPDC strio-pallido-dentate calcinosis

SpDur spike duration

SPE septic pulmonary edema; serum protein electrolytes; serum protein electrophoresis; streptococcal pyrogenic exotoxin; sucrose polyester; sustained physical exercise

SPEA strength Pareto evolutionary approach algorithm

SPEAK spectral peak [strategy]

SPEAR selective parenteral and enteral antisepsis regimen

SPE-C streptococcal pyrogenic exotoxin C

Spec specialist, specialty; specificity

spec special; specific; specificity; specimen

spec gr specific gravity

SPECT single photon emission computed tomography

SPEED Strategies for Patency Enhancement in the Emergency Department [study]

sPEEP spontaneous peak end-expiratory pressure

SPEG serum protein electrophoretogram

SPEL syndactyly, polydactyly, earlobe [syndrome]

SPEM smooth pursuit eye movement

SPEP serum protein electrophoresis; Structured Patient Education Programme

SPERM spastic paraplegia, epilepsy, mental retardation (intellectual disability) [syndrome]

SPET single-photon emission tomography; Surgical Procedure Entry Tool

SPF skin protection factor; specific pathogen free; spectrophotofluorometer; S-phase fraction; split products of fibrin; standard perfusion fluid; Stuart-Prower factor; sun protection factor; systemic pulmonary fistula

Sp Fl, sp fl spinal fluid

SPG serine phosphoglyceride; spastic paraplegia; sphenopalatine ganglion; splenoportography; sucrose, phosphate, glutamate; symmetric peripheral gangrene

SpG specific gravity

spg sponge

SPGA Bovarnik solution; sucrose, phosphate, glutamate, albumin

SPGR spoiled gradient

SpGr, sp gr specific gravity

SPGX spastic paraplegia, X-linked

SPGY spermatogenesis on Y

SPH secondary pulmonary hemosiderosis; severely and profoundly handicapped; spherocyte; spherocytosis; sphingomyelin

Sph sphenoidale; sphingomyelin

sph spherical; spherical lens; spheroid

SPHS Saskatoon Pregnancy and Health Study

sp ht specific heat

SPI selective protein index; Self-Perception Inventory; serum-precipitable iodine; serum protein index; Shipley Personal Inventory; speech processor interface; standardized patient instructor; standards for pediatric immunization; structured pain interview; Study of Perioperative Ischemia; subclinical papillomavirus infection

SPI 1, 2 *Salmonella* pathogenicity island 1, 2

SPIA solid-phase immunoabsorption; solid-phase immunoassay

SPICE Simulation Program with Integrated Circuit Emphasis; Study of Patients Intolerant to Converting Enzyme Inhibitors

SPICED TEAS Study of Pacemakers and Implantable Cardioverter Defibrillator Triggering by Electronic Article Surveillance Devices

SPICU surgical pulmonary intensive care unit

SPID summed pain intensity difference

SPIDERS Secondary Prevention of Ischemic Disease by Estrogen Replacement or Statins

SPIE International Society for Optical Engineering

SPIF solid-phase immunoassay fluorescence

SPIH superimposed pregnancy-induced hypertension

SPIHT set partitioning in hierarchical tree

SPIN signal processing in nuclear magnetic resonance; Social Phobia Inventory

spin spine, spinal

SPINAF Stroke Prevention in Nonrheumatic Atrial Fibrillation [study]

SPIO superparamagnetic iron oxide

SPIR Study of Perioperative Ischemia Research

spir spiral; spirit

SPIRIT Salvage from Perindopril in Reperfused Infarction Trial; Stroke Prevention in Reversible Ischemia Trial

SPJ saphenopopliteal junction

SPK serum pyruvate kinase; simultaneous pancreas kidney [transplantation]; superficial punctate keratitis

SPL skin potential level; sound pressure level; splanchnic; spontaneous lesion; staphylococcal phage lysate; superior parietal lobule; surfactant proteolipid

SPLATT split anterior tibial tendon

sPLM sleep-related periodic leg movement

SPLV serum parvovirus-like virus

SPlw long window spectrogram

SPM scanning probe microscopy; shocks per minute; spatiotemporal population map; spermine; statistical parametric mapping; subhuman primate model; suspended particulate matter; synaptic plasma membrane

SpM spiriformis medialis

spm spermatogonial metaphase

SPMA spinal progressive muscular atrophy

SPMD single program, multiple data

SPMR standard proportionate mortality rate; standard proportionate mortality ratio

SPMS secondary progressive multiple sclerosis

SPMSQ Short Portable Mental Status Questionnaire

SPmv medium window spectrogram

S-PMVT sustained polymorphic ventricular fibrillation

SPN senior plan network; sialophorin; Society of Pediatric Nurses; solitary pulmonary nodule; student professional nurse; supplemental parenteral nutrition; sympathetic preganglionic neuron

SpnCbT spinocerebellar tract

SpO₂ functional oxygen saturation; pulse oximetry

SPOCS Surgical Planning and Organization Computer System

SPOD spouse's perception of disease

spon, spont spontaneous

SPONASTRIME spondylar and nasal alterations with striated metaphyses; spondylar changes, nasal anomaly, associated metaphyses [dysplasia]

SPOOL simultaneous peripheral operation on-line

SPOP sequential paired opposed plaque [technique]

SPORE Specialized Programs of Research Excellence [study]

SPORT Stent Implantation Postrotational Atherectomy Trial

SPOT synthetic peptides on membrane technique

SPOV Spondweni virus

SPP Sexuality Preference Profile; skin perfusion pressure; small plaque parapsoriasis; suprapubic prostatectomy

spp plural of *species*

SPPF standard portable patient file

SPPK striate palmoplantar keratoderma

Sp Pn, Sp Pnx spontaneous pneumothorax

SPPP, sppp plural of *subspecies*

SPPS single photon planar scintigraphy; solid phase peptide synthesis; stable plasma protein solution

SPPT superprecipitation response

SPPX X-linked spastic paraplegia

SPR scanned projection radiography; selected primer; sepiapterin reductase; serial probe recognition; skin potential response; specific pathogen free; Society for Pediatric Radiology; Society for Pediatric Research; solid phase radioimmunoassay; substance P receptor; superior peroneal retinaculum

Spr scan projection radiography

spr sprain

SPRAS Sheehan patient-rated anxiety scale

SPRCA solid phase red cell adherence assay

SPRIA solid phase radioimmunoassay

SPRINT Secondary Prevention of Reinfarction Israeli Nifedipine Trial

SPRM selective progesterone receptor modulator

SPROM spontaneous premature rupture of membrane

SPRR small proline-rich protein

SPRRA small proline-rich protein A

SPRRB small proline-rich protein B

SPRRC small proline-rich protein C

SPRS Sixty Plus Reinfarction Study; Society of Pelvic Reconstructive Surgeons

SPRT sequential probability ratio test; Sixty Plus Reinfarction Trial

SPS scapuloperoneal syndrome; shoulder pain and stiffness; simple partial seizures; slow progressive schizophrenia; Society of Pelvic Surgeons; sodium polyanethol sulfonate; sodium polystyrene; sound production sample; spermidine synthase; stimulated protein synthesis; Stockholm Prospective Study; Suicide Probability Scale; systemic progressive sclerosis

SpS sphenoid sinus

sPSGL, (s)PSGL soluble P-selectin glyco-protein ligand

S-Psh, S-P shunt systemic-to-pulmonary shunt

spSHR stroke-prone spontaneously hypertensive rat

SPSS Statistical Package for the Social Sciences; Supplemental Pertussis Surveillance System

SPST Symonds Picture-Story Test

SPsw short-window spectrogram

SPT second primary tumor; secretin-pancreazymin [test]; single-patch technique; single-patient trial; skin-prick test; sleep period time; spectrin; standard psychometric test; station pull-through [technique]

SpT spinal tap

SPTA spatial peak temporal average; spectrin alpha

SPTAN spectrin alpha, nonerythroid

Sp tap spinal tap

SPTI systolic pressure time index

SPTS subjective posttraumatic syndrome

SPTx static pelvic traction

SPU short procedure unit; Society for Pediatric Urology; standardized photometric unit

SPV selective proximal vagotomy; Shope papilloma virus; sulfophosphovanillin; systolic pressure variation

SPVV sphincter pressure vector volume

SPW subxiphoid pericardial window

SPWVD smooth pseudo-Winger-Ville distribution

SPYWS Stroke Prevention in Young Women Study

SPZ sulfinpyrazone

SQ social quotient; status quo; subcutaneous; survey question; symptom questionnaire; systemizing quotient

Sq subcutaneous

sq squamous; square

SQC statistical quality control

sq cell ca squamous cell carcinoma

SQI signal quality index

SQL standard query language; structured query language

SQP sequential quadratic programming

S−QRS stimulus to QRS interval

sq rt square root

SQUID superconducting quantum interference device

SQV saquinavir

SR sample response; sarcoplasmic reticulum; saturation recovery; scanning radiometer; screen; secretion rate; sedimentation rate; seizure resistant; selection relaxation; self-recording; senior resident; sensitivity response; sensitization response; service record; sex ratio; short hair [guinea pig]; short range; side rails; sigma reaction; silicone rubber; sinus rhythm; skin resistance; sleep and rest; slow release; smooth-rough [colony]; sparse representation; spatial resolution; specific release; specific resistance; specific response; speech recognition; splenorenal; spontaneous respiration; steroid resistance; stimulus-response; stomach rumble; stress related; stress relaxation; stretch reflex; sulfonamide resistant; superior rectus; surface rendering; surface roughness; sustained release; suture removal; synchronization ratio; systemic reaction; systemic resistance; systems research; systems review

S-R smooth-rough [bacteria]; stimulus-response

Sr strontium

sr steradian

SRA segmental renal artery; serum renin activity; spleen repopulating activity

SR$_{AW}$, SR$_{aw}$ specific airway resistance

SRB sulforhodamine B

SRBC sheep red blood cells

SRBCT small round blue cell tumors

SRBD sleep-related breathing disorder

SRBSDS short-range biologic standoff detection system

SRC sedimented red cells; sheep red cells; signed reaction center; steroid receptor

src Rous sarcoma oncogene

SRCA specific red cell adherence

SRCBC serum reserve cholesterol binding capacity

SR/CP schizophrenic reaction, chronic paranoid

SRD service-related disability; Society for the Relief of Distress; Society for the Right to Die; sodium-restricted diet; specific reading disability; sustained rate duration

SRDS severe respiratory distress syndrome

SRDT single radial diffusion test

SRE Schedule of Recent Experiences; sperm recovering efficiency; standard regression effect; sterol regulatory element

SREBP sterol regulatory element binding protein

sREM stage rapid eye movement

SRF semirigid fiberglass cast; serum responsive factor; service response force; severe renal failure; skin reactive factor; somatotropin-releasing factor; split renal function; subretinal fluid

SRFA selective restriction fragment amplification

SRF-A slow-reacting−factor anaphylaxis

SRFS split renal function study

SRG specialty review group

SRH single radial hemolysis; somatotropin-releasing hormone; spontaneously responding hyperthyroidism; stigmata of recent hemorrhage

SRI serotonin reuptake inhibitor; severe renal insufficiency; sorcin; sperm recovery index; Stanford Research Institute; strain rate imaging; structured review instrument

SRID single radial immunodiffusion

SRIF somatotropin-release inhibiting factor

SRL supranational reference laboratory

SRLE schedule of recent life events

SRM spontaneous rupture of membranes; standard reference material; superior rectus muscle

SRMD stress-related mucosal damage

SRN state registered nurse

sRNA soluble ribonucleic acid

SRNG sustained-release nitroglycerin

SRNS steroid-resistant nephrotic syndrome

SRNT Society for Research on Nicotine and Tobacco

SRO sex-ratio organism; single-room occupancy; smallest region of overlap; Steele-Richardson-Olszewski [syndrome]

SROC summary receiver operating characteristic

SROF sepsis-related organ failure

SROM spontaneous rupture of membrane; self range of motion

SRP scientific review panel; short rib-polydactyly [syndrome]; signal recognition particle; Society for Radiological Protection; sponsoring residency program; state registered physiotherapist; synchronized retroperfusion

SRPG simulated respiratory pattern generator

SRPLND secondary retroperitoneal lymph node dissection

SRPR signal recognition particle receptor

SRPS short rib-polydactyly syndrome

SRQ Self-Reporting Questionnaire

SRR short R-R interval; stabilized relative response; standardized rate ratio; surgery recovery room

SRRD sleep-related respiratory disturbances

SRRS Social Readjustment Rating Scale

SR-RSV Schmidt-Ruppin Rous sarcoma virus

SRS schizophrenic residual state; sequential retrieval system; sex reassignment surgery; silencing regulatory sequence; Silver-Russell syndrome; simple repeat sequence; slow-reacting substance; Snyder-Robinson syndrome; Social and Rehabilitation Service; social relationship scale; social responsiveness scale; somatostatin receptor scintigraphy; spermidine synthase; standard rating scale; stereotactic radiosurgery; suppressor of rad six; Symptom Rating Scale

SRSA, SRS-A slow-reacting substance of anaphylaxis

SRSCB six random systematic core biopsy

SRSV small round structured virus

SRT sedimentation rate test; selective retina therapy; simple reaction time; sinus node recovery time; sitting root test; Sorbinil Retinopathy Trial; speech reception test; speech reception threshold; speech recognition technology; spontaneously resolving thyrotoxicosis; surfactant replacement therapy; sustained-release theophylline; symptom rating test

SRU sample ratio units; side rails up; solitary rectal ulcer; structural repeating unit

SRUS solitary rectal ulcer syndrome

SRV Schmidt-Ruppin virus; sheep retrovirus; simian retrovirus; small round virus; superior radicular vein

SRV 1, SRV 2 simian retroviruses 1 and 2

SRVT sustained reentrant ventricular tachyarrhythmia

SRW short ragweed [test]

SRWS super radiology workstation

SRY sex-determining region on Y chromosome

SS disulfide; sacrosciatic; saline soak; saline solution; saliva sample; saliva substitute; *Salmonella-Shigella* [agar]; salt substitute; saturated solution; Schizophrenia Subscale; Seckel syndrome; seizure sensitive; selective shunt; serum sickness; Sézary syndrome; shear stress; short sleep; short stature; siblings; sickle cell; side to side; signs and symptoms; single stranded; single strength; Sjögren syndrome; skull series; sliding scale; soapsuds; Social Security; social services; somatostatin; Spanish speaking; sparingly soluble; spatial separation; stainless steel; standard score; statistically significant; steady state; steam sterilization; sterile solution; steroid sensitivity; Stickler syndrome; stimulus separation; stromal sarcoma; structural key; subaortic stenosis; subscapular; subspinale; substernal; succinimidyl succinate; suction socket; sum of squares; supersaturated; support and stimulation; Sweet syndrome; synchronous sampling; systemic sclerosis

S/S salt substitute; signs/symptoms

S&S signs and symptoms

Ss *Shigella sonnei*; subjects

ss one half [L. *semis*]; single stranded

SSA salicylsalicylic acid; sicca syndrome A; single-stranded annealing; skin-sensitizing antibody; skin sympathetic activity; Sjögren syndrome A; smallest space analysis; Smith surface antigen; Social Security Act; Social Security Administration; social service agency; sperm-specific antiserum; stochastic simulated annealing; sulfosalicylic acid

SSAA sicca syndrome associated antigen A; Sjögren syndrome–associated antigen A; syringomyelia secondary to arachnoid adhesions

SSAV simian sarcoma–associated virus

SSB short spike burst; sicca syndrome B; single-strand break; single-stranded binding; stereospecific binding

SS-B Sjögren syndrome B

ssb single-strand break

SSBE short-segment Barrett esophagus

SSBG sex steroid–binding globulin; social services block grant

SSC salt sodium citrate; single-strand conformational [analysis]; single-stripe colitis; single-suture craniosynostosis; sister strand crossover; skin-to-skin care; somatic stem cell; somatosensory cortex; standard saline citrate; standard sodium citrate; syngeneic spleen cell

SSc systemic scleroderma; systemic sclerosis

SSCA single-strand conformational analysis; spontaneous suppressor cell activity

SSCCS slow spinal cord compression syndrome

ss(c)DNA single-stranded circular deoxyribonucleic acid

SsCEP somatosensory cortical evoked potential

SSCF sleep stage change frequency

SSCI Social Science Citation Index

SSCP single-strand conformation polymorphism, single-stranded conformational polymorphism

SSCPA single-stranded conformational polymorphism analysis

SSCr stainless steel crown

SSCT stereotactic subcaudate tractotomy

SSD shaded surface display; silver sulfadiazine; single saturating dose; Social Security disability; solid-state detector; source-skin distance; source-surface distance; speech-sound discrimination; squared sum of intensity differences; succinate semialdehyde dehydrogenase; sum of square deviations; syndrome of sudden death

SSD-BP single-stranded D-sequence binding protein

SSDBS symptom schedule for the diagnosis of borderline schizophrenia

SSDD steroid sulfatase deficiency disease

SSDI Social Security Disability Income; striatal or striatocapsular small deep infarction; Supplemental Security Disability Income

ssDNA single-stranded deoxyribonucleic acid

SSDS stepping source dosimetry system

SSE saline solution enema; skin self-examination; soap suds enema; steady state exercise; subacute spongiform encephalopathy

SSEA stage-specific embryonic antigen

SSED Summary of Safety and Effectiveness Data

SSEP somatosensory evoked potential; steady-state evoked potential

SSER somatosensory evoked response

SSES Sexual Self-Efficacy Scale

SSFP steady state free precession

SSF septic scarlet fever; solid state fermentation; soluble suppressor factor; supplemental sensory feedback

SSFSE single-shot fast spin-echo

SSG side scatter; sublabial salivary gland

SSH spinal subdural hemorrhage; suppressive subtractive hybridization

SSHM Society for the Social History of Medicine

SSHL severe sensorineural hearing

SSI segmental sequential irradiation; severity score index; shoulder subluxation inhibition; small-scale integration; Social Security increment; somatic symptom index; Somatic Symptom Inventory; strength-strain index; subshock insulin; supersonic shear-wave imaging; supplemental security income; surgical site infection; synchronous serial interface; System Sign Inventory

SSIDS sibling of sudden infant death syndrome

SSIE Smithsonian Science Information Exchange

SSISS Statewide Sentinel Immunisation Surveillance System

SSKI saturated solution of potassium iodide

SSL secure sockets layer; skin surface lipid; sufficient sleep; suppressor of stem loop

SSLI serum sickness–like illness

SSM skin-sparing mastectomy; solid-state microscopy; subsynaptic membrane; superficial spreading melanoma; system status management

SSMS saturated solution of magnesium iodide

SSN severely subnormal; Social Security Number; subacute sensory neuropathy; suprasternal notch; surgical segment navigator

SSNHL sudden sensorineural hearing loss

SSNS steroid-sensitive nephrotic syndrome

SSO sequence-specific oligonucleotide; Society of Surgical Oncology; special sense organ

ssODNs single-stranded oligodeoxynucleotides

SSOP Second Surgical Opinion Program; sequence-specific oligonucleotide probe

SSOT social services occupational therapist

SSP Sanarelli-Shwartzman phenomenon; Scottish Society of Physicians; sequence-specific primers; site-specific psoralen; slice sensitivity profile; solute-solvent property; sporozoite surface protein; stereotactic surface projection; subacute sclerosing panencephalitis; subspecies; supersensitivity perception

ssp subspecies

SSPCP service-specific practice cost percentage

SSPE salt sodium phosphate ethylenediamine tetraacetic acid; subacute sclerosing panencephalitis

SSPG steady state plasma glucose

SSPI steady state plasma insulin

SSPL saturation sound pressure level

SSPP subsynaptic plate perforation

SSPS side-to-side portacaval shunt

SS-PSE Schizophrenic Subscale of the Present State Examination

SSQ sequential scalar quantization; Social Support Questionnaire

SSQS security-related software quality standard

SSR signal sequence receptor; single sequence repeat; site-specific recombination; solar simulated radiation; somatosensory response; steady state response; sudomotor skin response; surgical supply room; sympathetic skin response

SSr single-strand region

SSrA single-strand region A

SSrB single-strand region B

SSRE shear stress response element

SSRI selective serotonin reuptake inhibitor

ssRNA single-stranded ribonucleic acid

SSRT stop signal reaction time

SSS scalded skin syndrome; secondary Sjögren syndrome; sick sinus syndrome; specific soluble substance; Stanford Sleepiness Scale; sterile saline soak; subclavian steal syndrome; subscapular skinfold; superior sagittal sinus; supplement serum substitute; systemic sicca syndrome

SSSA skin sympathetic sudomotor activity

SSSD Spanish Study on Sudden Death

SSSI Siegel Scale of Support for Innovation

SSSIII specific soluble substance III

SSSS Scandinavian Simvastatin Survival Study; staphylococcal scalded skin syndrome

SSST superior sagittal sinus thrombosis

SS-STP sum of squares simultaneous test procedure

SSSV superior sagittal sinus velocity

SST skin and soft tissue; sodium sulfite titration; somatostatin; Submacular Surgery Trials

S-STE skin—soft tissue envelope

SSTI skin and soft tissue infection

SSTL site-specific target level

SSTR somatostatin receptor

SSU Saybolt Seconds Universal; self-service unit; sterile supply unit

ssu small subunit

SSV Schoolman-Schwartz virus; simian sarcoma virus

SSVEP steady-state visual evoked potential

SSW slow spike wave; spike and sharp waves

SSWLHC Society for Social Work Leadership in Health Care

SSX sulfisoxazole

SSYM sign or symptom

SSZ sulfasalazine

ST esotropia; stable enterotoxin; scala tympani; scaphotrapezoid; sclerotherapy; sedimentation time; semantic type; semitendinosus; sensory threshold; septal thickness; serum transferrin; settling time; sharp transients; shock therapy; sickle [cell] thalassemia; sincerity test; sinus tachycardia; sinus tympani; skin temperature; skin test; skin thickness; slight trace; slow twitch; soft tissue; solid tumor; spastic torticollis; speech therapist; sphincter tone; split thickness; stable toxin; standard test; starting time; stent thrombosis; sternothyroid; stimulus; store; stress test; stretcher; stria terminalis; striation; string data; sublingual tablet; subtalar; subtotal; sulcus terminalis; sulfotransferase; supportive therapy; surface tension; surgical technologist; surgical therapy; surgical tracheostomy; surgical treatment; survival time; syndrome of the trephined; systolic time

S(T) signal-to-symbol translator

S/T spontaneous/timed

S&T science and technology

S-T portion of segment between end of the S wave and the beginning of the T wave [ECG]; sickle cell thalassemia

St, st let it stand [L. *stet*]; let them stand [L. *stent*]; stage; status; stere; sterile; stimulation;

stokes; stone; straight; stroke; stomach; stomion; subtype

sT tumor surgery classification: **sT0** surgery not done, **sT1** complete resection, **sT2** resection, 50% to 90%, **sT3** resection 5% to 50%, **sT4** biopsy, and **sT5** shunting

STA second trimester abortion; serum thrombotic accelerator; Single Tooth Anesthesia [system]; superficial temporal artery

Sta staphylion

stab stab neutrophil; stabilization

STACK Sequence Tag Alignment Consensus Knowledge-base

STAG slow-target attaching globulin; split-thickness autogenous graft; striped tag myocardial tagging [system]

STAI State Trait Anxiety Inventory

STA-MCA superficial temporal artery to middle cerebral artery

STAMI Stenting for Acute Myocardial Infarction [study]

STAMP Systemic Thrombolysis in Acute Myocardial Infarction with Prourokinase and Urokinase [trial]

STAND sutures to ambulate and discharge

STANDOUT soft thresholding and depth cueing of unspecified techniques

StanPsych standard psychiatric [nomenclature]

Staph, staph *Staphylococcus*

STAPPA State and Territorial Air Pollution Program Administration

STAR recombinant streptokinase; Specialty Training and Advanced Research; Staphylokinase Recombinant Trial; Study of Tranexamic Acid After Aneurysm Rupture

StAR steroidogenic acute regulatory [protein]

STAR*D Sequenced Treatment Alternatives to Relieve Depression [study]

STARNET South Texas Ambulatory Research Network

STARS Standard Treatment with Activase to Reverse Stroke [study]; Stent Anticoagulation Regimen Study; Stent Anticoagulation Restenosis Study; Stent Antithrombolytic Regimen Study; St. Thomas Atherosclerosis Regression Study

START Saruplase and Taprostene Acute Reocclusion Trial; selective tubal assessment to refine reproductive therapy; simple triage and rapid treatment; Stent vs. Angioplasty Restenosis Trial; Stent vs. Directional Coronary Atherectomy Randomized Trial; St. Thomas Atherosclerosis Regression Trial; Study of Thrombolytic Therapy with Additional Response Following Taprostene; Study

of Titration and Response to Tiazac; systemic arterial system

STAR TAP science, technology, and research transit access point

STARTTS Service for the Treatment and Rehabilitation of Torture and Trauma Survivors

STAS sporadic testicular agenesis syndrome

STAT immediately [L. *statim*]; Screening Tool for Autism in Toddlers; signal transducer and activator of transcription; state-trait anxiety inventory; Stent Thrombosis after Ticlopidine [study]; Stop Teenage Addiction to Tobacco; Stroke Treatment with Ancrod Trial

STaT slapped, threatened, and thrown

Stat statistical, statistics

stat immediately [L. *statim*]; radiation emanation unit

STAT-CHF Survival Trial of Antiarrhythmic Therapy in Congestive Heart Failure

STATH statherin

STATRS Stent Antithrombotic Regimen Study

STB supertropical bleach

Stb stillborn

STC sarcomatoid thymic carcinoma; serum theophylline concentration; sexually transmitted condition; soft tissue calcification; specialized treatment center; stanniocalcin; stroke treatment center; subtotal colectomy

STD selective T-cell defect; sexually transmitted disease; short-term disability; skin test dose; skin-to-tumor distance; sodium tetradecyl sulfate; source-tray distance; ST segment depression; standard test dose; standardized terminology dialog

Std standard

std saturated; standard deviation; standardized; standard walker

STDH skin test for delayed hypersensitivity

STD-MIS Sexually Transmitted Diseases Management Information System

STE Scholars for Teaching Excellence

STEAM stimulated echo acquisition mode

STEC Shiga toxin−producing *Escherichia coli*

STEEP safe, timely, effective, efficient, equitable, patient centered

STEL short-term exposure limit

STEM scanning transmission electron microscope; science, technology, engineering, and mathematics; Society of Teachers of Emergency Medicine

STEMI ST-segment elevation myocardial infarction

STEN staphylococcal toxic epidermal necrolysis

sten stenosed, stenosis

STENT-BY Stent vs. Bypass Surgery for Vessels Undergoing Abrupt Closure [trial]

STENTIM Stenting in Acute Myocardial Infarction [study]

STEP Sequential Test of Educational Progress; serial transverse enteroplasty; simultaneous transmission-emission protocol; Study of Taprostene in Elective Percutaneous Transluminal Coronary Angioplasty

STEPHY Starnberg Trial on Epidemiology of Parkinsonism and Hypertension in the Elderly

STEPP Screening Tool for Early Predictors of Posttraumatic Stress Disorder

STEPS Significance of Transesophageal Electrocardiographic Findings in Prevention of Stroke [study]

STEREO Stents and ReoPro [trial]

stereo stereogram

STESS Subjective (or Subject's) Treatment Emergent Symptom Scale

STET submaximal treadmill exercise test

STEV short-term exposure value

STF serum thymus factor; slow-twitch fiber; special tube feeding; stefin; Stoffel [buffer]; sudden transient freezing

STFeSV Snyder-Theilen feline sarcoma virus

STFM Society of Teachers of Family Medicine

STFT short-time Fourier transform; silicon thin-film transistor

STG short-term goal; split-thickness graft; superior temporal gyrus

STH soil-transmitted helminth; somatotropic hormone; subtotal hysterectomy

STh sickle cell thalassemia

ST/HR ST-segment depression with exercise divided by changes in heart rate

STHRF somatotropic hormone–releasing factor

STI Scientific and Technical Information; serum trypsin inhibitor; sexually transmitted infection; soybean trypsin inhibitor; structured therapy interruption; supervised therapy interruption; systolic time interval

STI-571 imatinib mesylate

STIC Science and Technology Information Center; serum trypsin inhibition capacity; solid-state transducer intracompartment

STILE Surgery vs. Thrombolysis for Ischemic Lower Extremity [trial]

stillb stillborn

STIM state transition information model

stim stimulated, stimulation; stimulus

STIMIS Study of Time Intervals in Myocardial Ischaemic Syndromes

STIMS Swedish Ticlodipine Multicenter Study

STIMULATE Speech, Text, Image, and Multimedia Advanced Technology Effort

STIPAS Safety Study of Tirilazad Mesylate in Patients with Acute Ischemic Stroke

STIR short tau inversion recovery

STJ subtalar joint

STK stem cell tyrosine kinase; streptokinase

STL serum theophylline level; standard template library; status thymicolymphaticus; stereolithography; swelling, tenderness, limited motion

STLI subtotal lymphoid irradiation

STLIS South Thames Library Information Service

ST-LMA stylet–laryngeal mask airway

STLOM swelling, tenderness, limitation of motion

STLS subacute thyroiditis-like syndrome

STLV simian T-lymphotropic virus

STLV 1, 2, 3 simian T-lymphotropic viruses 1, 2, 3

STM *Salmonella typhimurium*; scanning tunneling microscope; short-term memory; signature-tagged mutagenesis; specimen transport medium; streptomycin

STMS short test of mental status

sTMS single-pulse transcranial magnetic stimulation

STMV Santarem virus

STMY stromelysin

STN streptozocin; subthalamic nucleus; supratrochlear nucleus; surgical tool navigator

sTNF soluble tumor necrosis factor

sTNFr soluble tumor necrosis factor receptor

sTNM tumor-node-metastasis stage

STNR symmetric tonic neck reflex

STNV satellite tobacco necrosis virus

STO store

STO-3G Slater-type orbital comprising 3 gaussians

stom stomach

STONE Shanghai Trial of Nifedipine in the Elderly

STOP Shunt Thrombotic Occlusion Prevention by Picotamide [study]; Stenting for Total Occlusion and Restenosis Prevention [study]; Stroke Prevention in Sickle Cell Disease [study]; surgical termination of pregnancy; Swedish Trial in Older Patients

STOP 2 Swedish Trial in Older Patients with Hypertension 2

STOP-AF Systematic Trial of Pacing to Prevent Atrial Fibrillation

STOP-Hypertension Swedish Trial in Older Patients with Hypertension

STOP IT Sites Testing Osteoporosis Prevention Intervention Treatment

STOPP Selling Teens on Pregnancy Prevention [study]

STOR summary time-oriented record

STORCH syphilis, toxoplasmosis, rubella, cytomegalovirus, and herpesvirus

STP phenol-preferring sulfotransferase; scientifically treated petroleum; short-term potentiation; sodium thiopental; standard temperature and pressure; standard temperature and pulse; stiripentol; strategic technology planning

ST$_p$ settling time per patient

STPB skin transient pulse blood

STPD short-time Page distribution

STPS specific thalamic projection system

STPTUP soft tissue pinch-thickness upper pole

STQ superior temporal quadrant

STR short tandem repeat; soft tissue relaxation; statherin; stirred tank reactor; string matching

Str, str *Streptococcus*

strab strabismus

STRATIFY St. Thomas' Risk Assessment Tool in Falling Elderly Patients

STRATUS Study to Determine Rotablator and Transluminal Angioplasty Strategy

Strep *Streptococcus*; streptomycin

STRESS Stent Restenosis Study

STRETCH Symptom Tolerability Response to Exercise Trial of Candesartan Cilexetil in Patients with Heart Failure

STRICU shock, trauma, and respiratory intensive care unit

STRIP Special Turku Coronary Risk Factor Intervention Project

STROBE strengthening the reporting of observational studies in epidemiology

s-TRSV substrate of tobacco ringspot virus

STRT simultaneous thermoradiotherapy; skin temperature recovery time

struct structural, structure

STRUT stent treatment region assessed by ultrasound tomography

STS self-tensioning suture; sequence-tagged site; sequence target site; serologic test for syphilis; side to side; sodium tetradecyl sulfate; sodium thiosulfate; soft tissue sarcoma; standard test for syphilis; staphylococcal toxic syndrome; steroid sulfatase; subtrapezial space; sulcus to sulcus

STSA Southern Thoracic Surgical Association

STSD Spanish Trial on Sudden Death

STSE split-thickness skin excision

STSG split-thickness skin graft

STSS staphylococcal toxic shock syndrome

STT scaphotrapeziotrapezoid; serial thrombin time; short-term test; skin temperature test; space-time toolkit; speech task test

STTI Sigma Theta Tau International

STU skin test unit

STUMPED sclerocornea, trauma, ulcers, metabolic disorders, Peters anomaly, endothelial dystrophy, and dermoid

STUR Student Team Utilizing Research [project]

STV short-term variability; spontaneous tidal volume; superior temporal vein

STVA subtotal villous atrophy

STVS short-term visual storage

STX saxitoxin; syntaxin

Stx Shiga toxin

STY semantic type

STZ streptozocin; streptozyme

SU salicyluric acid; secretory unit; sensation unit; solar urticaria; sorbent unit; spectrophotometric unit; status uncertain; subunit; sulfonamide; sulfonylurea; supine; surface

Su sulfonamide; supine

SUA serum uric acid; single umbilical artery; single unit activity

subac subacute

subclav subclavian; subclavicular

subcut subcutaneous

subling sublingual

SubN subthalamic nucleus

SubQ, subq subcutaneous

SUBS substance

subsp subspecies

substd substandard

suc suction

Succ succinate, succinic

SUD skin unit dose; substance use disorder; sudden unexpected death

SUDAAN survey data analysis

SUDEP sudden unexpected death in epilepsy

SUDH succinyldehydrogenase

SUDI sudden unexpected death in infancy

SUDS single use diagnostic system; subjective units of distress scale

SUFE slipped upper femoral epiphysis

SuHV suid herpesvirus

SUI stress urinary incontinence; string unique identifier

SUID sudden unexplained infant death

sulf sulfate

sulfa sulfonamide

SULF-PRIM sulfamethoxazole and trimethoprim

SUMA sporadic ulcerating and mutilating acropathy

SUMAA scalable unstructured mesh algorithms and applications

SUMD Scale to Assess Unawareness in Mental Disorder

SUMIT streptokinase-urokinase myocardial infarct test

SUMMIT Stanford University Medical Media and Information Technology

SUMO small ubiquitin-related modifier

SUMSE stroke unit mental status examination

SUN serum urea nitrogen; standard unit of nomenclature

SUNA short-lasting unilateral neuralgiform headache with cranial autonomic symptoms; Society of Urologic Nurses and Associates

SUNCT short-lasting unilateral neuralgiform headache with conjunctival injection and tearing [syndrome]

SUO syncope of unknown origin

SUP schizo unipolar; supination

sup above [L. *supra*]; superficial; superior; supinator; supine

supin supination, supine

supp suppository

suppl supplement, supplementary

SUPPORT Study to Understand Prognoses and Preferences for Outcomes and Risks of Treatment

suppos suppository

SUR sulfonylurea receptor; suramin

SurDx surgical diagnosis

SURE Serial Ultrasound Analysis of Restenosis [study]

SURF surfeit

SURG, Surg surgeon; surgery, surgical

SurPROC surgical procedure

SURS solitary ulcer of rectum syndrome; Surveillance and Utilization Review System

SURVS-TB Surveillance System for Tuberculosis

SUS Saybolt Universal Seconds; solitary ulcer syndrome; stained urinary sediment; suppressor sensitive

SUSHI Stent Use Is Superior for Hospitalized Infarction Patients [study]

susp suspension, suspended

SUTAMI Saruplase and Urokinase in the Treatment of Acute Myocardial Infarction [trial]

SUTI symptomatic urinary tract infection

SUUD sudden unexpected unexplained death

SUV small unilamellar vessel; standard uptake value

SUVIMAX Supplemental Vitamins, Minerals and Anti-Oxidants [trial]

S-UVT sustained uniform ventricular tachycardia

SUX succinylcholine

SUZI subzonal insemination

SV sample volume; saphenous vein; Sapporo virus; sarcoma virus; satellite virus; scattering volume; selective vagotomy; semilunar valve; seminal vesicle; severe; sigmoid volvulus; simian virus; single ventricle; sinus venosus; snake venom; splenic vein; spontaneous ventilation; starting volume; streak virus; stroke volume; subclavian vein; subventricular; supravital; symptomless virus; synaptic vesicle; syncytial virus; systolic velocity

S/V surface/volume ratio

SV2 synaptic vesicle protein 2

SV-5, -10, -12, -40, -41 simian viruses 5, 10, 12, 40, 41

SV$_{40}$ simian vacuolating virus 40

Sv sievert

sv sievert; single vibration

SVA selective vagotomy and antrectomy; selective visceral angiography; sequential ventriculoatrial [pacing]; shell vial assay; subtotal villous atrophy

SVAS supravalvular aortic stenosis; supraventricular aortic stenosis

SVAT synaptic vesicle amine transformer

SVB saphenous vein bypass

SVBG saphenous vein bypass grafting

SVC saphenous vein cutdown; segmental venous capacitance; selective venous catheterization; slow vital capacity; spatially varying classification; subclavian vein catheterization; superior vena cava; support vector classification; supraventricular crest; supraventricular extrasystole; systemic vascular compliance

SVCCS superior vena cava compression syndrome

SVCG spatial vectorcardiogram

SVCO superior vena cava obstruction

SVCP Special Virus Cancer Program

SVCR segmental venous capacitance ratio

SVCS superior vena cava syndrome

SVD single-vessel disease; singular value decomposition; small vessel disease; spontaneous vaginal delivery; spontaneous vertex delivery; structural valve deterioration;

superficial venous thrombosis; swine vesicular disease

SVE slow volume encephalography; soluble viral extract; spontaneous ventricular event; sterile vaginal examination

SVG saphenous vein graft; scalable vector graphics; scatter and veiling glare; seminal vesiculography

SVGA super videographics array

SVH saphenous vein harvesting

SV-HUC simian virus−human uroepithelial cell

SVI seminal vesicle invasion; slow virus infection; small volume infusion; stroke volume index; systolic velocity integral

SVIN Society of Vascular and Interventional Neurology

SVL seminal HIV-1 viral load; superficial vastus lateralis

SVM seminal vesicle microsome; support vector machine; syncytiovascular membrane

SVMP snake venom metalloprotease

SVMT synaptic vesicle monoamine transformer

SVN selectively vulnerable neurons; sinuvertebral nerve; small volume nebulizer; Society for Vascular Nursing; student veterinary nurse

SvO$_2$ venous oxygen saturation

SVOC semivolatile organic compound

SVOM sequential volitional oral movement

SVP selective vagotomy and pyloroplasty; small volume parenteral [infusion]; standing venous pressure; superior vascular plexus

SVPB supraventricular premature beat

SVPC supraventricular premature complex

SVPD snake venom phosphodiesterase

SV40-PML simian vacuolating virus 40 of progressive multifocal leukoencephalopathy

SVR sequential vascular response; stroke volume ratio; support vector regression; sustained viral response, sustained virologic response; systemic vascular resistance

SVRI systemic vascular resistance index

SVS single volume spectroscopy; single voxel spectroscopy; slit ventricle syndrome; Society for Vascular Surgery

SVT sinoventricular tachycardia; subclavian vein thrombosis; supraventricular tachyarrhythmia; supraventricular tachycardia; sustained ventricular tachycardia

SVTh subvalvular thickening

SVTS Sotolol Ventricular Tachycardia Study

SVV Sal Vieja virus

SW seriously wounded; short waves; sinewave; slow wave; soap and water; social worker; spike wave; spiral wound; stab wound; sterile water; stroke work; Sturge-Weber [syndrome]; Swiss Webster [mouse]

S/W spike wave

Sw swine

SWA seriously wounded in action; slow-wave activity

SWAIDS social workers in acquired immunodeficiency syndrome

SWAP short-wavelength automated perimetry

SWASH sitting, walking, and standing hip orthosis

SWAT stationary wavelet transform; Stroke Prevention with Warfarin or Aspirin Trial

SWC submaximal working capacity

S&WC spike and wave complex

SWCM social work case manager

SWD short-wave diathermy

SWE slow-wave encephalography

SWEET Square Wave Endurance Exercise Trial

SWEHSLinC South West England Health Services Library and Information Network

SWG silkworm gut; standard wire gauge; stimulus waveform generator

SWI sterile water for injection; stroke work index; surgical wound infection; susceptibility weighted imaging

SWICE South-West Information for Clinical Effectiveness

SWIFT Should We Intervene Following Thrombolysis? [study]

SWIM sperm-washing insemination method

SWIORA spinal cord injury without radiologic abnormality

SWISH Swedish Isradipine Study in Hypertension

SWISSI Swiss Interventional Study in Silent Ischemia

SWL shock wave lithotripsy

SWM segmental wall motion

SWMA segmental wall motion analysis

SWMF Semmes-Weinstein monofilament

SWNT single-walled carbon nanotube

SWO superficial white onychomycosis

SWOG South West Oncology Group

SWOOP South Wilshire Out of Hours Project

SWORD surveillance of work-related and occupational respiratory diseases; Survival with Oral D-Sotalol [study]

SWOT strengths, weaknesses, opportunities, threats

SWPV Swinepox virus

SWR serum Wassermann reaction; slow wave ratio; surgical wound infection rate

SWRF square wave response function

SWRLIN South and West Regional Library Information Network

SWS shear wave speed; slow-wave sleep; spike-wave stupor; steroid-wasting syndrome; Sturge-Weber syndrome

SWT sine-wave threshold; systolic wall thickening

SWU septic workup

SwV swine calicivirus

SX scleral invasion cannot be assessed

Sx suction

Sx, S$_x$ signs; symptoms

S$_{\bar{x}}$ standard deviation of sampling distribution

SXA single-energy x-ray absorptiometry; single x-ray absorptiometry

SXCT spiral x-ray computed tomography

SXR skull x-ray; steroid and xenobiotic receptor

Sxr sex reversal

Sxs serologic, sex specific

SXT sulfamethoxazole-trimethoprim

SY spectroscopy; syphilis, syphilitic

SYA subacute yellow atrophy

SYB synaptobrevin

SYDS stomach yin deficiency syndrome

sym symmetric; symptom

sympath sympathetic

symph symphysis

SYMPHONY Sibrafiban vs. Aspirin to Yield Maximum Protection from Ischemic Heart Events Postacute Coronary Syndromes [trial]

sympt symptom

SYN synapse; synovitis

syn synergistic; synonym; synovial

SYNBIAPACE synchronous biatrial pacing therapy

synd syndrome

SYNDIKATE synthesis of distributed knowledge acquired from text

Synf synovial fluid

SynText symbolic text

SYP synaptophysin

syph syphilis, syphilitic

SYR Syrian [hamster]

syr syringe; syrup [L. *syrupus*]

SYREC symmetric recombinant

SYS stretching-yawning syndrome; systemic

sys system, systemic; systolic

SYS-BP systolic blood pressure

syst system; systole, systolic

SYST-CHINA Systolic Hypertension in Elderly Chinese Trial

SYST-EUR Systolic Hypertension in Europeans Study

SYT synaptotagmin

SZ schizophrenia; streptozocin

Sz schizophrenia; seizure

SZN streptozocin

T

T absolute temperature; electrocardiographic wave corresponding to the repolarization of the ventricles; large T [antigen]; life [time]; period [time]; primary tumor {**T0**, no evidence of primary tumor; **T1 to T4**, tumors in progressing sizes; **TX**, no evidence of primary tumor}; ribosylthymine; tablespoonful; *Taenia*; tamoxifen; telomere banding; temperature; temporal electrode placement [EEG]; temporary; tenderness; tension [intraocular]; tera- [trillion]; terminal banding; tesla; testosterone; tetra; tetracycline; theophylline; therapy; thoracic; thorax; threatened [animal]; threonine; thrombosis; thrombus; thymidine; thymine; thymus; thymus derived; thyroid; tidal gas; tidal volume; time; timed; tincture; tissue; tocopherol; topical; torque; total; toxicity; training [group]; transducer; transition; transmittance; transverse; treatment; *Treponema*; triangulation number; *Trichophyton*; triggered [pacemaker]; tritium; tryptamine; *Trypanosoma*; tuberculin; tuberculosis; tumor; turnkey system; type

Θ uppercase Greek letter theta; thermodynamic temperature

T- tera- [10^{12}]

T0 no evidence of primary tumor

T$_{1/2}$ half-life

T1 breast tumor smaller than 2 cm; longitudinal relaxation time

T-1, T-2, T-3 first, second, and third stages of decreased intraocular tension

T$_1$ spin-lattice or longitudinal relaxation time; time at the beginning of inspiration; tricuspid first sound; tricuspid valve closure sound

T+1, T+2, T+3 first, second, and third stages of increased intraocular tension

T1 to T4 presence of tumors progression rated by size, number, and penetration

T1 to T12 first to twelfth thoracic vertebrae

T2 breast tumor 2.0 to 5.0 cm; transverse relaxation time

T$_2$ diiodothyronine; spin-spin or transverse relaxation time

T2*, T$_2$* effective transverse relaxation time

T20 enfuvirtide

2,4,5-T 2,4,5-trichlorophenoxyacetic acid

T3 breast tumor larger than 5.0 cm

T$_3$ triiodothyronine

T4 breast tumor of any size with extension to chest wall and skin

T$_4$ thyroxine

T-7 free thyroxine factor

T$_{90}$ time required for 90% mortality in a population of microorganisms exposed to a toxic agent

t duration; small T [antigen]; student *t* test; teaspoonful; temperature; temporal; terminal; tertiary; test of significance; three times [L. *ter*]; time; tissue; tonne; transformer; translocation

t *t* value from *t* distribution

τ lowercase Greek letter tau; life [of radioisotope]; relaxation time; shear stress; spectral transmittance; transmission coefficient

θ lowercase Greek letter theta; an angular coordinate variable; customary temperature; temperature interval

t? time after infusion

t$_{1/2}$ half-life

t$_2$ time at the end of inspiration

TA alkaline tuberculin; arterial tension; axillary temperature; tactile afferent; Takayasu arteritis; technology assessment; teichoic acid; temporal abstraction; temporal arteritis; terminal antrum; therapeutic abortion; thermophilic *Actinomyces*; thymidine analogue; thymocytotoxic autoantibody; thyroarytenoid; thyroglobulin autoprecipitation; thyroid antibody; thyroid autoimmunity; tibialis anterior; tissue adhesive; titratable acid; total alkaloids; total antibody; toxic adenoma; toxin-antitoxin; traffic accident; transactional analysis; transaldolase; transaminase; transantral; transplantation antigen; transposition of aorta; trapped air; triamcinolone acetonide; tricuspid atresia; trophoblast antigen; true anomaly; truncus arteriosus; tryptamine; tryptose agar; tube agglutination; tubular atrophy; tumor associated; typical absences

T-A toxin-antitoxin; transfusion associated

T&A tonsillectomy and adenoidectomy; tonsils and adenoids

T/A time and amount

TA-4 tumor-associated antigen 4

Ta tantalum; tarsal

T1a breast tumor 0.1 to 0.5 cm

T4a breast tumor with extension to chest wall

t$_α$ *t* value corresponding to specified tail area alpha

TAA thioacetamide; thoracic aortic aneurysm; total ankle arthroplasty; transverse aortic arch; tumor-associated antigen

TAAA thoracoabdominal aortic aneurysm

TAAD type A aortic dissection

TAAF thromboplastic activity of the amniotic fluid

TA-AIDS transfusion-associated acquired immunodeficiency syndrome

TAANA The American Association of Nurse Attorneys

TAB tape-automated bonding; total autonomic blockage; typhoid, paratyphoid A, and paratyphoid B [vaccine]

TAb therapeutic abortion

tab tablet

TABC total aerobic bacteria count; typhoid, paratyphoid A, paratyphoid B, and paratyphoid C [vaccine]

TABP type A behavior pattern

Tabs tablets

T$_{abs}$ absorption time

TABT typhoid, paratyphoid A, paratyphoid B, and tetanus toxoid [vaccine]

TABTD typhoid, paratyphoid A, paratyphoid B, tetanus toxoid, and diphtheria toxoid [vaccine]

TABV Tamana bat virus

TAC tachykinin; temporary abdominal closure; terminal antrum contraction; tetracaine, adrenalin, and cocaine; time-activity curve; total abdominal colectomy; total aganglionosis coli; total allergen content; total antioxidant capacity; transient aplastic crisis; triamcinolone cream; truncus arteriosus communis

TAC-1 tachykinin-1

TAC-2 tachykinin-2

TACC thoracic aorta cross clamping

TACE chlorotrianisene; teichoic acid crude extract; transarterial chemoembolization; tumor-necrosis factor alpha—converting enzyme

tachy tachycardia

TACI total anterior circulation infarct

TACIP Triflusal vs Aspirin in Cerebral Infarction Prevention [study]

TACR tachykinin receptor

TACS Thrombolysis and Angioplasty in Cardiogenic Shock [study]

TACT thermoacoustic computed tomography; Ticlopidine Angioplasty Coronary Trial; Ticlopidine vs. Placebo for Prevention of Acute Closure After Angioplasty Trial; tuned aperture computed tomography

TACTICS Thrombolysis and Counterpulsation to Improve Cardiogenic Shock Survival [trial]

TACTICS-TIMI 18 Treat Angina with Aggrastat and Determine Cost of Therapy with an Invasive or Conservative Strategy-Thrombolysis in Myocardial Infarction [trial]

TAD test of auditory discrimination; thoracic asphyxiant dystrophy; tobacco, alcohol, and drugs; Traffic Accident Deformity [scale]; transactivation domain; transient acantholytic dermatosis

TADAC therapeutic abortion, dilation, aspiration, curettage

TAdV Turkey adenovirus

TADv 1, 2 Turkey adenoviruses 1, 2

TAE thrombotic adverse event; transcatheter arterial embolism; triacetate EDTA

TAF albumose-free tuberculin [Ger. *Tuberculin Albumose frei*]; tissue angiogenesis factor; total abdominal fat; toxin-antitoxin floccule; toxoid-antitoxin floccule; tracheobronchial aspiration fluid; transcriptional activation factor; trypsin-aldehyde-fuchsin; tumor angiogenesis factor

TAFU tumor abrasion with focused ultrasound

TAG target attaching globulin; technical advisory group; thymine, adenine, and guanine

TAg large T antigen

Tag T antigen

TAGH triiodothyronine, amino acids, glucagon, heparin

TAGV Taggert virus

TAGVHD transfusion-associated graft-versus-host disease

TAH total abdominal hysterectomy; total artificial heart

TAH BSO total abdominal hysterectomy and bilateral salpingo-oophorectomy

TAHIV transfusion-acquired human immunodeficiency virus

TAHSC Toronto Academic Health Science Council

TAHV Tahyna virus

TAI tau aggregation inhibitor; Test Anxiety Inventory

TAIAV Taiassui virus

TAIM Trial of Antihypertensive Intervention and Management

TAIS time assessment interview schedule

TAIST Tinzaparin in Acute Stroke Trial

TAIV Tai virus

TAL T-cell acute leukemia; tendon of Achilles lengthening; thick ascending limb; thymic alymphoplasia; total arm length; tumor-associated lymphocyte

talc talcum

TALH thick ascending limb of Henle's loop

TALL theoretic annual loss of life

TALL, T-ALL T-cell acute lymphoblastic leukemia

TALLA T-cell acute lymphoblastic leukemia antigen

TAM tamoxifen; technologic acceptance model; technology acceptance model; technology assessment method; teenage mother; tele-alarm management; thermoacidurans agar modified; thymidine analogue mutation; thymidine-associated mutations; time-averaged mean; total active motion; Total Atherosclerosis Management [study]; toxin-antitoxoid mixture; transient abnormal myelopoiesis

TAMC total aerobic microbial count

TAME *N*-alpha-tosyl-L-arginine methyl ester

TAMI Thrombolysis and Angioplasty in Myocardial Infarction [study]; transmural anterior myocardial infarction

TAMIS Telemetric Automated Microbial Identification System

TamMV Tamarillo mosaic virus

TAMRA tetramethylrhodamine

TAMV Tamiami virus; temporal average maximal velocity [Doppler]

TAMX time-average maximum velocity

TAN total adenine nucleotide; total ammonia nitrogen

tan tandem translocation; tangent

TANet Taiwan Network

TANF Temporary Assistance for Needy Families

TANI total axial node irradiation

TANV Tanapox virus; Tanga virus

TAO thromboangiitis obliterans; triacetyloleandomycin

TAOS total antioxidant status

TAP technology architecture project; tick anticoagulant peptide; total access plus [computer-based system]; toxicologic agent protection/protective; transesophageal atrial pacing; transluminal angioplasty; transmembrane action potential; transporter in antigen processing; trypsinogen-activating peptide

TAPA target of antiproliferative antibody

TAPE temporary atrial pacemaker electrode

TAPIRSS Triflusal vs. Aspirin in Preventing Infarction: Randomized Stroke Study

TAPS The Akita Pathology Study; Teenage Attitudes and Practices Study; trial assessment procedure scale

TAPVC total anomalous pulmonary venous connection

TAPVD total anomalous pulmonary venous drainage

TAPVR total anomalous pulmonary venous return

Taq *Thermus aquaticus*

taq DNA *Thermus aquaticus* deoxyribonucleic acid

TAQW transient abnormal Q wave

TAR thoracic aortic rupture; thrombocytopenia with absent radii [syndrome]; tissue/air ratio; total abortion rate; transactivation response; transanal resection; transaxillary resection; treatment authorization request

TARA total articular replacement arthroplasty; tumor-associated rejection antigen

TARC thymus and activation-regulated chemokine

TARGET Do Tirofiban and ReoPro Give Similar Efficacy Outcomes Trial

TARP total atrial refractory period

TAR/PD target nursing hours per patient-day

TARS threonyl transfer RNA synthetase

TART testicular adrenal rest tumor

TAS tetanus antitoxin serum; therapeutic activities specialist; thoracoabdominal syndrome; thrombolytic assessment system; transcription-based amplification system; traumatic apallic syndrome

TAS-20 20-Item Toronto Alexithymia Scale

TASA tumor-associated surface antigen

TASC tele-archive service center; time-accumulating subsurface contaminant; Trial of Angioplasty and Stents in Canada

Tase tryptophan synthetase

TASH Transcoronary Ablation of Septum Hypertrophy [study]

TASMAN Thrombolysis Anticoagulant Study: Mediterranean, Australia, New Zealand

TASO The AIDS Support Organisation

TASS thyrotoxicosis, Addison disease, Sjögren syndrome, sarcoidosis [syndrome]; Ticlopidine Aspirin Stroke Study

TASTE Ticlopidine Aspirin Stent Evaluation

TAstV Turkey astrovirus

TAT tandem autotransplantation; tetanus antitoxin; thematic apperception test; thematic aptitude test; thrombin-antithrombin complex; thromboplastin activation test; total adipose tissue; total antitryptic activity; toxin-antitoxin; transactivator; transaxial tomography; transplantation-associated thrombocytopenia; tray agglutination test; *Treponema* antibody test; tumor activity test; turnaround time; twin arginine translocation; tyrosine aminotransferase

TATA Pribnow box; tumor-associated transplantation antigen

TATD tyrosine aminotransferase deficiency

TATI tumor-associated trypsin inhibitor

TATR tyrosine aminotransferase regulator

TATRC Telemedicine and Advanced Technology Research Center

TATST tetanus antitoxin skin test

TATV Tataguine virus

TAUS transabdominal ultrasonography

TAUSA Thrombolysis and Angioplasty in Unstable Angina [trial]

TAV transcutaneous aortovelography; trapped air volume; tricuspid annular velocity

TaV *Thosea asigna* virus

TAVB total atrioventricular block

TAVR transcatheter aortic valve replacement

TAX Taxol

TB Taussig-Bing [syndrome]; terabyte; term birth; terminal bronchiole; terminal bronchus; thromboxane B; thymol blue; tissue bank; toluidine blue; total base; total bilirubin; total body; tracheobronchial; tracheal bronchiolar; tracheobronchitis; trapezoid body; triple [gene] block; tub bath; tubercle bacillus; tuberculin; tuberculosis; tumor bank; tumor bearing

T$_B$ total buffer

TB$^+$ tuberculosis positive

TB$^-$ tuberculosis negative

Tb Tbilisi [phage]; terabit [trillion bits]; terbium; tubercle bacillus; tuberculosis

T$_b$ biologic half-life; body temperature

T1b breast tumor 0.5 to 1.0 cm

T4b breast tumor with edema (including peau d'orange) or skin ulceration or satellite nodules

tb tuberculosis

TBA target [hospital] bed occupation; tertiary butylacetate; testosterone-binding affinity; tetrabutylammonium; thiobarbituric acid; to be absorbed; to be added; total bile acids; transaxillary breast augmentation; trypsin-binding activity; tubercle bacillus; tumor-bearing animal

TBAB tryptose blood agar base

TBAF tetrabutylammonium fluoride

TBAN transbronchial aspiration needle

TBARS thiobarbituric acid reactive substance

TBB transbronchial biopsy

TBBA total body bone ash

TBBM total body bone minerals

TBBx transbronchial biopsy

TBC thyroxine-binding coagulin; total body calcium; total body carbon; total body clearance; tuberculosis

Tbc tubercle bacillus; tuberculosis

TBCa total body calcium

TBCl total body chlorine

TBD to be determined; total body density

TBE tick-borne encephalitis; triborate EDTA; tris-borate EDTA; tuberculin bacillin emulsion

TBESC Tuberculosis Epidemiologic Studies Consortium

TBEV tick-borne encephalitis virus

TBF total body fat

TBFB tracheobronchial foreign body

TBFM total body fat mass

TBFVL tidal breathing flow-volume loops

TBG beta-thromboglobulin; testosterone-binding globulin; thyroglobulin; thyroid-binding globulin; thyroxine-binding globulin; tracheobronchography; tris-buffered Gey solution

TBGI thyroxine-binding globulin index

TBGP total blood granulocyte pool

TBH total body hematocrit

tBHP terbutyl hydroperoxide

TBHQ tertiary butylhydroquinone

TBHT total-body hyperthermia

TBI thyroid-binding index; thyroxine-binding index; tooth-brushing instruction; total-body irradiation; traumatic brain injury

TBII thyroid-stimulating hormone-binding inhibitory immunoglobulin

TBil, T bili, t. bili total bilirubin

TBIM thoracic bioimpedance monitoring

TBK total body potassium

tbl tablet

TBLB transbronchial lung biopsy

TBLC term birth, living child

TBLI term birth, living infant

TBLTM total-body lean tissue mass

TBM thrombomodulin; total body mass; Total Body Modification [protocol]; tracheobronchiomegaly; tracheobronchomalacia; trophoblastic basement membrane; tuberculous meningitis; tubular basement membrane

TBMC total body mineral content

TBMN thin basement membrane nephropathy

TBN bacillus emulsion; temporal belief network; total body nitrogen

Tb.N trabecular number

TBNA total-body neutron activation; transbronchial needle aspiration; treated but not admitted

TBNa total body sodium

TBNAA total-body neutron activation analysis

TBO total blood out

t-BOOH *tert*-butyl hydroperoxide

TBP bithionol; testosterone-binding protein; thyroxine-binding protein; total body protein; total bypass; tributyl phosphate; tuberculous peritonitis

TBPA thyroxine-binding prealbumin

TBPr total body protein

Tbps terabits [trillion bits] per second

TBPT total body protein turnover

TBR tumor-bearing rabbit

TB-RD tuberculosis and respiratory disease

TBS total body solids; total body solute; total body surface; total burn size; Townes-Brocks syndrome; tracheobronchial submucosa; tracheobronchoscopy; tribromosalicylanilide; triethanolamine-buffered saline; tris-buffered saline

tbs tablespoon

TBSA total body surface area

TBS-G tris-buffered saline with glycerol

Tb.Sp trabecular separation

tbsp tablespoon

TBST tris-buffered saline tween

TBT tolbutamide test; tracheobronchial toilet; tracheobronchial tree; transcervical balloon tuboplasty; tributyltin

TBTC Tuberculosis Trials Consortium

TBTO tributyltin oxide

TBTT tuberculin time test

TBTV Timboteua virus

TBV total blood volume; trabecular bone volume

TBW total body water; total body weight

TBX thromboxane; total-body irradiation

TBXA2 thromboxane A2

TBXAS thromboxane A synthase

TBZ tetrabenazine; thiabendazole

TC talocalcaneal; tandem colonoscopy; target cell; taurocholate; temperature compensation; teratocarcinoma; terminal cancer; tertiary cleavage; testicular cancer; tetanic contraction; tetracycline; theca cell; therapeutic community; thermal conductivity; thermocouple; thoracic cage; thoracic compression; thorax circumference; throat culture; thyrocalcitonin; time constant; tissue culture; to contain; total calcium; total capacity; total cholesterol; total colonoscopy; total correction; toxic concentration; transcobalamin; transcriptase complex; transcutaneous; transhepatic cholangiography; transmission control; transplant center; transverse colon; Treacher Collins [syndrome]; true channel; true conjugate; tubal catheterization; tuberculin contagiosum; tubocurarine; tumor cell; tumor of cerebrum; type and crossmatch

T&C turn and cough; type and crossmatch

T₄(C) serum thyroxine measured by column chromatography

TC₅₀ median toxic concentration; threshold concentration

Tc correlation time; Tanimoto coefficient; technetium; tetracycline; transcobalamin

Tᶜ cytotoxic T cell, cytotoxic T lymphocyte

T𝒸 critical temperature; cytotoxic T cell, cytotoxic T lymphocyte; the generation time of a cell cycle; tricuspid closure

T1c breast tumor 1.0 to 2.0 cm

t(°C) temperature on the Celsius scale

tc transcutaneous; translational control

TCA T-cell A locus; tentorium cerebelli attachment; terminal cancer; tetracyclic antidepressant; thyrocalcitonin; topological constraint algorithm; total cholic acid; total circulating albumin; total circulatory arrest; total colonic agangliosis; transcondylar axis; tricalcium aluminate; tricarboxylic acid; trichloroacetic acid; tricyclic antidepressant; tubocornual anastomosis

TCAB 3,3′,4,4′-tetrachloroazobenzene

TCABG triple coronary artery bypass graft

TCAD tricyclic antidepressant

TCADA Texas Council on Alcohol and Drug Abuse

tCAF tonic cortical activation function

TCAG triple coronary artery graft

TCAld trichloroacetaldehyde

TCAOB 3,3′,4,4′-tetrachloroazoxybenzene

TCAP trimethyl-cetyl-ammonium pentachlorophenate

TCAR T-cell antigen receptor

TCAT transmission computer-assisted tomography

TCB tetrachlorobiphenyl; total cardiopulmonary bypass; transabdominal chorionic biopsy; transcatheter biopsy; transconjunctival blepharoplasty; trusted computing base; tumor cell burden

TcB transcutaneous bilirubin

TCBF total cerebral flood flow

TCBS thiosulfate-citrate-bile salts-sucrose [agar]

TCC terminal complement complex; thromboplastic cell component; transcatheter closure; transitional cell carcinoma; transmission control computer; trauma center coordination/coordinator; trichlorocarbanilide, triclocarban

Tcc triclocarban

TCCA, TCCAV transitional cell cancer associated [virus]

TCCD transcranial color-coded Doppler

TCCDS transitional cell carcinoma dataset

TCCL T-cell chronic lymphoblastic leukemia

TCCS transcranial color-coded sonography

TCCU&C therapeutic care, understanding, and control

TCD tapetochoroidal dystrophy; T-cell depletion; thermal conductivity detector; tissue culture dose; transcranial Doppler; transverse cardiac diameter; tumoricidal dose

TCD₅₀ median tissue culture dose; tissue culture infectious dose

TCDB turn, cough, deep breathe

TcdB *Clostridium difficile* toxin B

TCDC taurochenodeoxycholate

TCDD 2,3,7,8-tetrachlorodibenzo-*p*-dioxin; threshold contrast detail detectability

TCDF 2,3,7-tetrachlorodibenzofuran

TCE T-cell enriched; tetrachlorodiphenyl ethane; total colon examination; trichloroethane; trichloroethylene

TCED$_{50}$ 50% tissue effective dose

TCES transcutaneous cranial electrical stimulation

TCESOM trichloroethylene-extracted soybean oil meal

TCET transcerebral electrotherapy

TCF T-cell factor; teleconsultation folder; tetanic contraction fatigue; tissue coding factor; total coronary flow; transcription factor; Treacher Collins–Franceschetti [syndrome]

T-CFC T-colony–forming cell

TCFU tumor colony-forming unit

TCG therapeutic care general; time-compensated gain; Thromboprophylaxis Collaborative Group

TCGF T-cell growth factor

TCH tanned-cell hemagglutination; thiophen-2-carboxylic acid hydrazide; total circulating hemoglobin; turn, cough, hyperventilate

TC/HDL total cholesterol/high density lipoprotein ratio

TChE total cholinesterase

TCI Temperament and Character Index Inventory; target-controlled infusion; Temperament and Character Index; temporal continuity index; To Come In [program]; total cerebral ischemia; transcobalamin I; transient cerebral ischemia; transitory cognitive impairment

TCi teracurie

TCID tissue culture infectious dose; tissue culture infective dose; tissue culture inoculated dose

TCID$_{50}$ median tissue culture infective dose; 50% tissue culture infective dose

TCIE transient cerebral ischemic episode

TCII transcobalamin II

TCIII transcobalamin III

TCIMC Trauma Center Information Management Center

TCI$_{pr}$ temporal continuity index for providers

TCI$_{pt}$ temporal continuity index for patients

TCIS T-cell immunodeficiency syndrome; total corrected increment score; transitional carcinoma in situ

TCKs third culture kids, trans-cultural kids

TCL tachycardia cycle length; T-cell leukemia; T-cell lymphoma; thermochemiluminescence; tibial collateral ligament; total capacity of the lung; transcallosal latency; transverse carpal ligament; triazine chlorguanide

T-CLL T-cell chronic lymphatic leukemia

TC$_{Lo}$ toxic concentration low

TCLP toxicity characteristic leachate procedure

TCM tissue culture medium; traditional Chinese medicine; transcutaneous monitor

T&CM type and crossmatch

Tc 99m technetium-99m

TCMA transcortical motor aphasia

tc-MEPS transcranial motor evoked potentials

TCMI traditional Chinese medicine informatics

Tc 99m MDP technetium-99m methylene diphosphonate

TCMP thematic content modification program

TCMS transcranial magnetic stimulation

TCMV Tacaiuma virus

TCMZ trichloromethiazide

TCN tetracycline; transcobalamin; transcultural nursing

T$_x$NM tumor with lymph node metastases

TCNS transcutaneous nerve stimulation/stimulator

TCNV terminal contingent negative variation

TCO transcutaneous oximetry

T$_{CO_2}$ total carbon dioxide

TCoV Turkey coronavirus

TCP T-complex protein; therapeutic care-psychosocial; therapeutic class profile; therapeutic continuous penicillin; thienylcyclohexylpiperidine; thrombocytopenia; tibial hole coronal positioning; tissue culture–treated plastic; tissue/tumor control probability; total cardiopulmonary; total circulating protein; toxin-coregulated pilus; transcutaneous pacemaker; transcutaneous pacing; transmission control protocol; tranylcypromine; tricalcium phosphate; trichlorophenol; tricresyl phosphate; tropical calcific pancreatitis; tumor control probability

TCPA tetrachlorophthalic anhydride

TCPC total cavopulmonary connection

tcPCO$_2$, tcpCO$_2$ transcutaneous partial pressure of carbon dioxide

TCPD$_{50}$ 50% tissue culture protective dose

TCPL tricalcium-phosphate-lysine

tcPO$_2$, tcpO$_2$ transcutaneous partial pressure of oxygen

tcP$_{O2}$, tcPO$_2$ transcutaneous oxygen pressure

2,4,5-TCPPA 2-(2,4,5-trichlorophenoxy)-propionic acid

TCPS total cavopulmonary shunt

TCR T-cell reactivity; T-cell receptor; T-cell rosette; thalamocortical relay; total cytoplasmic ribosome; transcriptional control center; transcription-coupled repair; trauma center record; true count rate; turn, cough, rebreathe

TcR T-cell receptor

TCRA T-cell receptor alpha

TCRB T-cell receptor beta

TCRBCL T-cell—rich B-cell lymphoma

TCRD T-cell receptor delta

TCRG T-cell receptor gamma

tcRNA translational control ribonucleic acid

TCRP total cellular receptor pool

TCRV Tacaribe virus; tissue culture rinderpest vaccine

TCRZ T-cell receptor Z

TCS T-cell supernatant; temporal control structure; tethered cord syndrome; total coronary score; transcranial stimulation; Treacher Collins syndrome

TCSA tetrachlorosalicylanilide

TCSEC trusted computer system evaluation criteria

TCSF T-colony—stimulating factor

TcsL *Clostridium sordelli* lethal toxin

TCSPC time-correlated single photon count

TCT thrombin clotting time; thyrocalcitonin; trachial cytotoxin; transcardial catheter therapy; transmission computed tomography

Tct tincture

tcTOFA time-constrained time-of-flight absorbance

TCU timing control unit; trauma care unit; treatment control unit

TCV thoracic cage volume; three-concept view

TCW time coincidence window

TD tabes dorsalis; tardive dyskinesia; T-cell dependent; temporal embedding dimension; temporary disability; terminal device; tetanus and diphtheria [toxoid]; tetrodotoxin; thanatophoric dwarfism; thanatophoric dysplasia; therapy discontinued; thermal dilution; thoracic duct; three times per day; threshold of detectability; threshold of discomfort; threshold dose; thymus-dependent; time delay; time dictionary; timed disintegration; tocopherol deficiency; to deliver; tone decay; topic-specific document; torsion dystonia; total disability; total discrimination; total dose; totally disabled; total dose; Tourette

disorder; toxic dose; tracheal diameter; transdermal; transverse diameter; traveler's diarrhea; treatment discontinued; tumor dose; typhoid dysentery

T-D T-cell dependent

T/D treatment discontinued

T$_D$ doubling time [time required to double the number of cells in a given population]; thermal death time

TD$_{01}$ toxic dose, 1% response

T2D type 2 diabetes

T$_4$(D) serum thyroxine measured by displacement analysis

TD$_{50}$ median toxic dose

TD$_{99}$ toxic dose, 99% response

Td doubling time; tetanus-diphtheria toxoid

T1d inflammatory breast carcinoma

TDA thyroid-stimulating hormone-displacing antibody; toluenediamine; transperitoneal direct approach

TDADF, TDAF transform domain adaptive filter

TDAP thoracodorsal artery perforator flap

Tdap tetanus toxoid, reduced diphtheria toxoid, and acellular pertussis vaccine, adsorbed

TDB terminologic database; Toxicology Data Bank; Toxicology Database

T$_{db}$ dry-bulb temperature

TDC taurodeoxycholic acid; thermal dilution catheter; time-density curve; total dietary calories

T&DC transmural and diagnostic center

Td-CIA T-cell—derived colony-inhibiting activity

TDCO thermodilution cardiac output

tDCS transcranial direct current stimulation

TDD telecommunication device for the deaf; tetradecadiene; thoracic duct drainage; total digitalizing dose; toxic doses of drugs; transverse digital deficiency

TDE tetrachlorodiphenylethane; total digestible energy; triethylene glycol diglycidyl

TDF tenofovir; testis-determining factor; thoracic duct fistula; thoracic duct flow; thoracodorsal flap; time-dose fractionation; tissue-damaging factor; tumor-dose fractionation

TdF thymidine deoxyribose

TDFA testis-determining factor, autosomal

TDFX testis-determining factor X

TDGF teratocarcinoma-derived growth factor

TDH high toxic dose; thermostable direct hemolysin; thoracic disc herniation; threonine dehydrogenase

T/DHT testosterone/dihydrotestosterone ratio

TDI temperature difference integration; three-dimensional interlocking; time-delay integration; tissue Doppler imaging; tolerable daily intake; toluene 2,4-diisocyanate; total dose infusion; total dose insulin

TDL tegmental dorsolateral [nucleus]; template definition language; thoracic duct lymph; thymus-dependent lymphocyte; toxic dose level

TDLU terminal ductal lobular unit

TDM therapeutic drug monitoring

T1DM type 1 diabetes mellitus

T2DM type 2 diabetes mellitus

TD-MCT time-domain microwave computed tomography

TDMS Trex digital mammography system

TDMV Tindholmur virus

TDN Therapeutics Development Network; total digestible nutrients

tDNA transfer deoxyribonucleic acid

TDNN time-delay neural network

TDO temporary detention order; transverse distraction osteogenesis; tricho-dento-osseous [syndrome]; tryptophan 2,3-dioxygenase

TDP thermal death point; thoracic duct pressure; thymidine diphosphate; total degradation products

TdP torsades de pointes

TDR total disk replacement; Tropical Disease Research

TDRA theory of dual radiation action

TDS temperature, depth, salinity; thiamine disulfide; total dissolved solids; transduodenal sphincteroplasty

tds three times per day

TDSD transient digestive system disorder

TDSNV Trager duck spleen necrosis virus

TDT terminal deoxynucleotidyltransferase; thermal death time; tone decay test; tumor doubling time

TdT terminal deoxynucleotidyl transferase

TdTase terminal deoxynucleotide transferase

T_DTH delayed-type hypersensitivity T lymphocyte

TDWB touch-down weight bearing

TDYV Tamdy virus

TDZ thymus-dependent zone

TE echo time; expiratory time; tennis elbow; test ear; tetanus; tetracycline; threshold energy; thromboembolism; thymus epithelium; thyrotoxic exophthalmos; tick-borne encephalitis; time estimation; tissue engineering; tissue equivalent; tonsillectomy; tooth extracted; total estrogen; toxic epidermolysis; toxic equivalent; *Toxoplasma* encephalitis; trace element; tracheoesophageal; transepithelial; transesophageal echocardiography; transposable element; treadmill exercise; trial error; trichoepithelioma; tris-ethylenediamine tetraacetic acid

T-E echo time

T&E testing and evaluation; trial and error

T_E effector T lymphocyte; exhalation time; expiratory phase time

Te effective half-life; tellurium; tetanic contraction; tetanus

TEA temporal external artery; Test of Everyday Attention; tetraethylammonium; thermal energy analyzer; thromboendarterectomy; total elbow arthroplasty; triethanolamine

TEAB tetraethylammonium bromide

TEAC tetraethylammonium chloride

TEACCH treatment and education of autistic and communication-related handicapped children

TEAE triethylammonioethyl

TEAF trimethylammonium formate

TEAHAT Thrombolysis Early in Acute Heart Attack Trial

TEAM techniques for effective alcohol management; Thrombolytic Trial of Eminase in Acute Myocardial Infarction; Total Evaluation and Acceptance Methodology; total exposure assessment method; Training in Expanded Auxiliary Management; transfemoral endovascular aneurysm management

TEAS telemetric electrode array system

teasp teaspoon

TEB thoracic electrical bioimpedance

TEBG, TeBG testosterone-estradiol−binding globulin

TEBV tissue-engineered blood vessel

TEC tissue-engineered construct; total electron count; total eosinophil count; total exchange capacity; transient erythroblastopenia of childhood; transluminal extraction catheter; trauma and emergency center

TECBEST Transluminal Extraction Catheter Before Stent [study]

TECK thymus-expressed chemokine

tecMAAP template endonuclear cleavage multiple arbitrary amplicon profiling

TECP tetrachloropropane

TECSAC tele-collaboration for signal analysis in cardiology

TECSS The European Coronary Surgery Study

TECU thermoelectric cooling unit

TECV traumatic epiphyseal coxa vara

TED Tasks of Emotional Development; threshold erythema dose; thromboembolic disease

TEDs antiembolism stockings

TEE thermic effect of exercise; total energy expenditure; transesophageal echocardiography; tyrosine ethyl ester

TEEP tetraethyl pyrophosphate

TEER transepithelial electrical resistance

TEF thermic effect of food; thoraco-epigastric flap; thyrotroph embryonic factor; toxic equivalency factor; tracheoesophageal fistula; transcriptional enhancer factor; trunk extension-flexion

T$_{eff}$ effective half-life

TEFRA Tax Equity and Fiscal Responsibility Act

TEFS transmural electrical field stimulation

TEG thromboelastogram

TEGD total esophagogastric dissociation

TEGDMA tetraethylene glycol dimethacrylate

TEHIP Toxicology and Environmental Health Program

TEIB triethyleneiminobenzoquinone

TEK total exchangeable potassium

TEL tetraethyl lead

TEL-FISH telomere fluorescent in situ hybridization

TELV Turkey entero-like virus

TEM transanal endoscopic microsurgery; transmission electron microscope/microscopy; triethylenemelamine

TEMED tetramethylethylenediamine

TEMP temporal concept

temp temperature; temple; temporal

TEMS tactical emergency medical services; Trimetazidine European Multicentre Study

TEN titanium elastic nail; total enteral nutrition; total excretory nitrogen; toxic epidermal necrolysis; transepidermal neurostimulation; Trans-European Network

TENa total exchangeable sodium

TENS toxic epidermal necrolysis syndrome; transcutaneous electrical nerve stimulation

TeNT tetanus neurotoxin

TENV Tensaw virus

TEOAE transient evoked otoacoustic emissions

TEP tetraethylpyrophosphate; totally extraperitoneal; tracheoesophageal puncture; transepithelial potential; transesophageal endoscopic plication; transesophageal pacing; triethylphosphate

TEPA triethylenephosphamide

TEPH total end-prosthetic hip implantation

TEPP tetraethyl pyrophosphate; triethylene pyrophosphate

TEPR toward an electronic patient record

TEPW temporary epicardial pacing wire

t$_{1/2eq}$ equilibration half-life

TER teratogen; terminology; total endoplasmic reticulum; transcapillary escape rate; transepithelial resistance

ter rub [L. *tere*]; terminal; terminal or end; terminus; ternary; tertiary; three times; threefold

term terminal

TERP transanal endorectal pull-through technique

TERT total end-range time

tert tertiary

TERV Termeil virus

TES thymic epithelial supernatant; toxic epidemic syndrome; *Toxocara canis* excretory/secretory [antigen]; transcutaneous electrical stimulation; transmural electrical stimulation; tutorial evaluation system

TeS terminology server

TESA testicular sperm aspiration

TESE testicular sperm extraction

TESPA thiotepa

TESS Tirilazad Efficacy Stroke Study; Toxic Exposure Surveillance System; Treatment Emergent Symptom Scale

TEST Tigecycline Evaluation Surveillance Trials; Timolol, Encainide, Sotalol Trial

TET tetracycline; total ejection time; total exchange thyroxine; transcutaneous energy transfer; treadmill exercise test

Tet tetralogy of Fallot

tet tetanus; tetracycline

TETA triethylenetetramine

TETD tetraethylthiuram disulfide

TETEV Tete virus

tet^r tetracycline resistance

TETS transcutaneous energy transmission system

tet tox tetanus toxoid

TEV tadpole edema virus; talipes equinovarus; tissue-engineered vessel

TeV temperate virus

TEVC two-electrode voltage

TEVG tissue-engineered vascular graft

TEWL transepidermal water loss

TEWM tissue-engineered wall model

TexCAPS Texas Coronary Atherosclerosis Prevention Study

TEZ transthoracic electric impedance respirogram

TF free thyroxine; tactile fremitus; tail flick; temperature factor; term formula; term frequency; testicular feminization; tetralogy of Fallot; thymol flocculation; thymus factor; time frequency; tissue-damaging factor; tissue factor; to follow; total flow; transcription factor; transfer factor; transferrin; transformation frequency; transfrontal; tube feeding; tuberculin filtrate; tubular fluid; tuning fork; typhoid fever

T/F time/frequency

Tf transferrin

T$_f$ freezing temperature

t(°F) temperature on the Fahrenheit scale

t-f time-frequency

TFA thigh-foot angle; tibiofemoral angle; total fatty acids; transfatty acid; transverse fascicular area; trifluoroacetic acid

TFIIIA transcription factor IIIA

TFAV Thiafora virus

TFB transformation buffer

TFC common form of transferrin; threadable fusion cage; triangular fibrocartilage

TFCC triangular fibrocartilage complex

TFD target-film distance; time-frequency distribution; time-frequency domain; Transcriptional Factor Database

TFd dialyzable transfer factor

TFE polytetrafluoroethylene; transcription factor for immunoglobulin heavy chain enhancer

TFF tangential flow filtration; trefoil family factor; tube-fed food

TFI Tear Function Index; thoracic fluid index; transient forebrain ischemia

TFIID transcription factor IID

TFIL transforaminal lumbar interbody fusion

TFJ tibiofemoral joint

TFJA tibiofemoral joint abduction

t-FLAS turbo-fast low-angle shot

TFM testicular feminization male; testicular feminization mutation; total fluid movement; transmission electron microscopy

TFMoV Taro feathery mottle virus

TFMPP 1-(trifluoromethylphenyl)-piperazine

TFN total fecal nitrogen; transferrin

TFO triplex-forming oligonucleotide

TFP tubular fluid plasma

TFPI tissue factor pathway inhibitor

TFPZ trifluoroperazine

TFR time-frequency representation; time to full repolarization; total fertility rate; total flavones of rhododendra; total flow resistance; traditional functional retraining; transferrin receptor

TFS testicular feminization syndrome; thyroid function study; tube-fed saline

T1FS T1 weighted fat suppressed

TFT thin-film transistor; Thought Field Therapy; thrombus formation time; thyroid function test; tight filum terminale; trifluorothymidine

TFUN tissue function

TFV Telok Forest virus; tick fever virus

TFX toxic effects

TG temperature gradient; tendon graft; testosterone glucuronide; tetraglycine; thioglucose; thioglycolate; thioguanine; thromboglobulin; thyroglobulin; tocogram; total gastrectomy; toxic goiter; transglutaminase; transmissible gastroenteritis; treated group; triacylglycerol; trigeminal ganglion; triglyceride; tumor growth

6-TG thioguanine

Tg generation time; thyroglobulin; *Toxoplasma gondii*; transglycosylation

T$_g$ glass transition temperature; globe temperature

tG$_1$ the time required to complete the G$_1$ phase of the cell cycle

tG$_2$ the time required to complete the G$_2$ phase of the cell cycle

TGA taurocholate gelatin agar; thrombin generation assay; thyroglobulin activity; total glycoalkaloids; total gonadotropin activity; transient global amnesia; transposition of great arteries; tumor glycoprotein assay

TgAb thyroglobulin antibody

TGAI technical grade active ingredient

TGAR total graft area rejected

TGase transglutaminase

TGB thromboglobulin beta; tiagabine

tGB triangular Gregory-Bézier [patches]

TGBG dimethylglyoxal bis-guanylhydrazone

TGC time gain compensation

TGD thermal-green dye

TG-DPC temperature gradient DNA probe chromatography

TGE theoretical growth evaluation; transmissible gastroenteritis; tryptone glucose extract

TGEV transmissible gastroenteritis virus

TGF T-cell growth factor; therapeutic gain factor; transforming growth factor; tubuloglomerular feedback; tumor growth factor

TG-F transforming growth factor

TGFA transforming growth factor alpha; triglyceride fatty acid

TGFb transforming growth factor beta

TGG turkey gamma globulin

TGI tracheal gas insufflation

TGL triglyceride; triglyceride lipase

TGMS telemetered glucose monitoring system

TGN thioguanine nucleotide; trans-Golgi network

TGNB transgender and gender nonbinary

TGP tobacco glycoprotein

TGPV total glucose in venous plasma

TgPVR transgenic mice that express human cellular receptor for poliovirus
TGR transgenic rat
6-TGR 6-thioguanine riboside
TGS tincture of green soap
TGs triglycerides
TGT thromboplastin generation test/time; tolbutamide-glucagon test
TGV thoracic gas volume; thoracic great vessel; transposition of great vessels
TGY tryptone glucose yeast [agar]
TGYA tryptone glucose yeast agar
TH tension headache; tetrahydrocortisol; T helper [cell]; theophylline; therapeutic hypothermia; thiohydantoin; thorax; thrill; thyrohyoid; thyroid hormone; topical hypothermia; total hysterectomy; triquetrohamate; tyrosine hydrolase; tyrosine hydroxylase
T$_H$ T helper [lymphocyte]
T&H type and hold
Th T helper [lymphocyte]; thenar; therapist; therapy; thoracic, thorax; thorium; throat
T$_h$ hypothermic temperature; T helper [lymphocyte]
th thenar; thermic; thoracic; thyroid; transhepatic
THA tacrine; tetrahydroaminoacridine; thiacetazone; total hip arthroplasty; total hydroxyapatite; *Treponema* hemagglutination
ThA thoracic aorta
THAIV Thailand virus
THAL thalassemia
THAM tris(hydroxymethyl)aminomethane
THAMES Tenormin in Hypertension and Myocardial Ischemia Epidemiological Study
THB tetrahydrobiopterin; thrombocyte B; Todd-Hewitt broth; total heart beats
THb total hemoglobin
THBD thrombomodulin
THBI thyroid hormone binding inhibitor
THBP 7,8,9,10-tetrahydrobenzo[a]-pyrene; thyroid hormone binding protein
THBS thrombospondin
THC teen health clinic; tentative human consensus; terpin hydrate and codeine; tetrahydrocannabinol; tetrahydrocortisol; thigh cuff; thiocarbanidin; thrombocytopenia; transhepatic cholangiogram; transplantable hepatocellular carcinoma
THCA alpha-trihydroxy-5-beta-cholestannic acid
THD Thomsen disease; transverse heart diameter
Thd ribothymidine
THDOC tetrahydrodeoxycorticosterone
THE tetrahydrocortisone E; tonic hind limb extension; transhepatic embolization; transhiatal esophagectomy; tropical hypereosinophilia
T-HELPER, T-Helper therapy helper
theor theoretic, theory
THER therapeutic procedure
ther therapeutic, therapy; thermometer
therap therapeutic, therapy
THERAPIS telecommunication-helped radiotherapy planning and information system
ther ex therapeutic exercise
therm thermal; thermometer
ThETT thallium stress test
THEV Tehran virus
THF tetrahydrocortisone F; tetrahydrofolate; tetrahydrofolic [acid]; tetrahydrofuran; thymic humoral factor
THFA tetrahydrofolic acid; tetrahydrofurfuryl alcohol
Thg thyroglobulin
THH telangiectasia hereditaria haemorrhagica; trichohyalin
THI transient hypogammaglobulinemia of infancy
Thi thiamine
THIP tetrahydroisoxazolopyridinol
Thio-TEPA thiotriethylenephosphamide
THIS Tissue Plasminogen Activator Heparin Interaction Study; total hospital information system
THIV Thimiri virus
THL trichohyalin
THM total heme mass
TH$_2$O titrated water
Thor thoracic
thor thoracic, thorax
THORP titanium hollow reconstruction plate
thou thousandth
THOV Thogoto virus
THP Tamm-Horsfall protein; tetrahydropapaveroline; tetrakis(hydroxymethyl) phosphonium; tissue hydrostatic pressure; total hip replacement; total hydroxyproline; transthoracic portography; trihexyphenidyl
Thp T-cell helper precursor
THPA tetrahydropteric acid
THPC tetrakis(hydroxymethyl)phosphonium chloride
THPP thiamine pyrophosphate; trihydroxy propriophenone
ThPP thiamine pyrophosphate
THPT, tHPT tertiary hyperparathyroidism
THPV transhepatic portal vein
THQ tetraquinone
THR targeted heart rate; threonine; thyroid hormone receptor; total hip replacement; transhepatic resistance

Thr thrill; threonine
thr threonine; thyroid, thyroidectomy
THRA thyroid hormone receptor alpha
THRF thyrotropic hormone—releasing factor
THRIFT Thromboembolism Risk Factors Study
THRM thrombomodulin
ThrO thrombotic occlusion
throm, thromb thrombosis, thrombus
THRV Thormódseyjarlettur virus
THS Teebe hypertelorism syndrome; tetrahydro-compound S; thrombohemorrhagic syndrome; Tolosa-Hunt syndrome; Tromsø Heart Study; Turkish Heart Study
THSC totipotent hematopoietic stem cell; totipotential stem cell
THTH thyrotropic hormone
THU tetrahydrouridine
THUG thyroid uptake gradient
THV transcatheter heart valve; Turkey hepatitis virus
ThV thebesian valve; theilovirus
THVO terminal hepatic vein obliteration; terminal hepatic vein obstruction
THVPS transhepatic portal venous sampling
Thx thromboxane
THY thymosin
Thy thymine
thy thymectomy, thymus
THYB thymosin beta
THz terahertz
TI inversion time; T-cell independent [antigen]; temporal integration; term importance; terminal ileum; thalassemia intermedia; therapeutic index; thoracic index; thymus independent; thymus irradiation; time interval; tonic immobility; topical irritation; total iron; transcallosally mediated inhibition; transient inward; transischial; translational inhibition; transverse inlet; treatment interruption; tricuspid incompetence; tricuspid insufficiency; tumor induction
T$_I$ inspiration time
T-I T-cell independent [antigen]
Ti titanium; translation imitation
TIA topical irritation arthritis; tracheoinnominate artery; transient ischemic attack; tumor-induced angiogenesis; turbidimetric immunoassay
TIA+CE transient ischemic attack plus carotid endarterectomy
TIAFO toe-inhibiting ankle-foot arthrosis
TIAH total implantation of artificial heart
TIB tibia; time in bed; tumor immunology bank
TIBA 2,3,5-triiodobenzoic acid

TIBBS Total Ischaemic Burden Bisoprolol Study
TIBC total iron-binding capacity
TIBET Total Ischemic Burden European Trial
TIBL treatment-induced bone loss
TIBS Trends in Biochemical Sciences
T-IBS T-cell immunoblastic sarcoma
TIBV Tibrogargan virus
TIC tachycardia-induced cardiomyopathy; total ion current; Toxicology Information Center; trypsin inhibitory capability; tubal intraepithelial carcinoma; tubulointerstitial cell; tumor-inducing complex
TICA traumatic intracranial aneurysm
TICC time from cessation of contraception to conception
TICO Thrombolysis in Coronary Occlusion [study]
TICU trauma intensive care unit
TID time interval difference; titrated initial dose; transient ischemic dilatation; trusted image discrimination
t.i.d. three times a day [L. *ter in die*]
TIDA tuberoinfundibular dopaminergic system
TIDAL Team Interactive Decision Analysis [software]
TIDE Technology Initiative for Disabled and Elderly People
TIDES Transdermal Intermittent Dosing Evaluation Study
TIE transient ischemic episode
TIF tumor-inducing factor; tumor infiltrating; tumor-inhibiting factor
TIFF tagged image file format
TIG Thrombosis Interest Group [study]
TIG, Tig tetanus immunoglobulin
TIGER/Line Topologically Integrated Geographic Encoding and Referencing System
TIGR The Institute for Genome Research
TIH time interval histogram
TIIAP technical information infrastructure assistance program
TIL tumor-infiltrating leukocyte; tumor-infiltrating lymphocyte
TILLV Tillamook virus
TILS temporary intraluminal shunts
TILV Tilligerry virus
TIM transthoracic intracardiac monitoring; Triflusal in Myocardial Infarction [study]; triose phosphate isomerase
Tim total imaging matrix [technology]
TIMAD Ticlodipine in Microangiography of Diabetes [study]
TIMC tumor-induced marrow cytotoxicity

TIME Teaching Immunization for Medical Education [study]; Treatment of Infarcting Myocardium Early [trials]

TIMED Trials to Investigate Morning vs. Evening Dosing [nisoldipine in hypertension]

TIMI Thrombolysis in Myocardial Infarction [score, trial]; transmural inferior myocardial infarction

TIMI-7, TIMI-9 Thrombin Inhibition in Myocardial Ischemia [trials]

TIMI IIIA, TIMI IIIB Thrombolysis in Myocardial Ischemia [trials]

TIMIKO Thrombolysis in Myocardial Infarction in Korea [study]

TIMP tissue inhibitor of metalloproteinases

TIMS Tertatolol International Multicentre Study; Tuberculosis Information Management System

TIMV Timbo virus

TIN tubulointerstitial nephropathy

tinc, tinct tincture

T$_{inf}$ infusion time

TINU tubulointerstitial nephritis-uveitis [syndrome]

TINV Tinaroo virus

TIOD total iodine organification defect

TIP telemedicine instrumentation pack; terminal interface processor; thermal inactivation point; Toxicology Information Program; translation-inhibiting protein; tumor-inhibiting principle

TIPE Thrombolysis in Peripheral Embolism [study]; Thrombolysis in Pulmonary Embolism [study]

TIPI time-insensitive predictive instrument

TIPJ terminal interphalangeal joint

TIPPS tetraiodophenylphthalein sodium

TIPS transjugular intrahepatic portacaval shunt; transjugular intrahepatic portosystemic shunt

TIPSS transjugular intrahepatic portosystemic stent shunt

TIQ tetrahydroisoquinoline

TIR terminal innervation ratio; terminal inverted repeat; totally immunoreactive

TIRES transient infrared emission spectroscopy

TIS telemedicine information service; tetracycline-induced steatosis; thoracic insufficiency syndrome; titanium interbody spacer; transdermal infusion system; triage illness scale; trypsin-insoluble segment; tumor in situ

Tis tumor in situ

TISP total immunoreactive serum pepsinogen

TISS Therapeutic Intervention Scoring System; Ticlodipine Indobufen Stroke Study

TIT *Treponema* immobilization test

TIT, TITh triiodothyronine

TIU trypsin-inhibiting unit

TIUP term intrauterine pregnancy

TIUV total intrauterine volume

TIV tomographic image visualization; total intracranial volume; trivalent inactivated influenza vaccine

TIVA total intravenous anesthesia

TIVC thoracic inferior vena cava

TIVT Thrombolysis in Deep Vein Thrombosis [study]

TIW three times a week

TIZ thermal injury zones

TJ tetrajoule; thigh junction; tight junction; triceps jerk

TJA total joint arthroplasty

TJC tender joint count; The Joint Commission

TJR total joint replacement

TK thermokeratoplasty; through knee; thymidine kinase; transketolase; triosekinase; tyrosine kinase

t(°K) absolute temperature on the Kelvin scale

tk thymidine kinase

TKA total knee arthroplasty; transketolase activity; trochanter, knee, ankle

TKase thymidine kinase

TKB tutor knowledge base

TKC torticollis, keloids, cryptorchidism [syndrome]

TKCR torticollis, keloids, cryptorchidism, renal dysplasia [syndrome]

TKD thymidine kinase deficiency; tokodynamometer

TKG tokodynagraph

TKLI tachykinin-like immunoreactivity

TKO to keep open

TKPV Turkeypox virus

TKR total knee replacement

TKT transketolase

TL temporal lobe; terminal latency; terminal lumen; thermolabile; thermoluminescence; thoracolumbar; threat to life; thymus leukemia; thymus lymphocyte; thymus lymphoma; tibia length; time lapse; time limited; tolerance limit; total laryngectomy; total lipids; total lung; true lumen; tubal ligation

T-L thoracolumbar; thymus-dependent lymphocyte

TL$_{50}$ median tolerance limit

Tl thallium

TLA thymus leukemia antigen; tissue lactase activity; tongue-to-lip adhesion; translaryngeal aspiration; translumbar aortogram; transluminal angioplasty

TLAA T-lymphocyte-associated antigen

t_lag lag time

TLam thoracic laminectomy

TLAV Tlacotalpan virus

TLC telephone-linked care; tender loving care; thin-layer chromatography; threshold limit concentration; total L-chain concentration; total library computerization; total lung capacity; total lung compliance; total lymphocyte count; transverse loop colostomy

TLCC threshold limit value ceiling

Tl_CO transfer factor for lung carbon monoxide

TLD thermoluminescent dosimeter; thermoluminescent dosimetry; thoracic lymphatic duct; tumor lethal dose

T/LD_{100} minimum dose causing 100% deaths or malformations

TLE temporal lobe epilepsy; thin-layer electrophoresis; total lipid extract

tLESRs transient lower esophageal sphincter relaxations

TLF total linear filtration; truncated Lévy flight

TLI thymidine labeling index; total lymphatic irradiation; transmitted light intensity; trypsin-like immune activity; Tucker-Lewis index

TLIF transforaminal interbody fusion

TLL T-cell leukemia or lymphoma; tissue lesion load

TLM transoral laser microsurgery

TLm median tolerance limit

TLMV TTV-like minivirus

TLOs tertiary lymphoid organs

TLPD thoracolaryngopelvic dysplasia

TLQ total living quotient

TLR tapetal-like reflex; target lesion revascularization; toll-like receptor; tonic labyrinthine reflex

TLS thoracolumbosacral; total least squares; Tourette-like syndrome; translaminar screw; tumor lysis syndrome

TLSER theoretical linear solvation energy relationship

TLSO thoracolumbosacral orthosis

TLSQL time-line standard query language

TLSS Temporary Limb Salvage Shunt

TLSSO thoracolumbosacral spinal orthosis

TLT tryptophan load test

TLTP Teaching and Learning Technology Programme

TLV threshold limit value; tidal liquid ventilation; T-lymphotropic virus; total lung volume

TLV-BLV threshold limit value-biological

TLV-C threshold limit value-ceiling

TLVM time-lapse video microscopy

TLV-STEL threshold limit value short-term exposure limit

TLV-TWA threshold limit value/threshold-weighted value

TLW total lung water

TLX trophoblast-lymphocyte cross reactivity

TM technology management; tectorial membrane; temperature by mouth; temporalis muscle; temporomandibular; tender midline; tendomyopathy; teres major; thalassemia major; Thayer-Martin [medium]; thrombomodulin; time and materials; time-motion; tobramycin; torus mandibularis; total mortality; trabecular network; trademark; traditional medicine; transatrial membranotomy; transitional mucosa; transmediastinal; transmembrane; transmetatarsal; transport mechanism; transport medium; transverse myelitis; tropical medicine; tropomyosin; tuberculous meningitis; twitch movement; tympanic membrane

T-M Thayer-Martin [medium]

T&M type and crossmatch

Tm temperature; thulium; tubular maximum excretory capacity of kidneys

T_m melting temperature; membrane immunoglobulin heavy chain polypeptide; temperature midpoint; tubular maximum excretory capacity of kidneys

tM time required to complete the M phase of the cell cycle

tm transport medium; true mean

TMA tetramethylammonium; thrombotic microangiopathy; thyroid microsomal antibody; tissue microarray; transcortical mixed aphasia; transcription-mediated amplification; transmetatarsal amputation; trimellitic anhydride; trimethoxyamphetamine; trimethoxyphenyl aminopropane; trimethylamine; true metatarsus adductus

TMACl tetramethylammonium chloride

TMAH trimethylphenylammonium (anilinium) hydroxide

TMAI trimethylphenylammonium (anilinium) iodide

TMAO trimethylamine N-oxide

TMAP transmembrane action potential

TMAS Taylor Manifest Anxiety Scale

T_max maximum threshold; time to maximum

TMB transient monocular blindness

TMB4 N,N'-trimethylenebis(pyridine-4-aldoxime bromide)

TMBA trimethoxybenzaldehyde

TMBF transmural blood flow

TMBJ thermoplastic Minerva body jacket

TMC transmyocardial mechanical channeling; triamcinolone and terramycin capsules

TMD temporomandibular disorder; transient myeloproliferative disease; transmembrane domain; transmitral Doppler [scanning]; trimethadione

t-MDS therapy-related myelodysplastic syndrome

TME total mesorectal excision; total metabolizable energy; toxic metabolic encephalopathy; transmissible mink encephalopathy; transmural enteritis; trapezium-metacarpal eburnation

TMEP telangiectasia macularis eruptiva perstans

TMES transient marrow edema syndrome

TMET treadmill exercise test

TMEV Tembe virus; Theiler's murine encephalomyelitis virus

TMF transformed mink fibroblast; transmitral flow

TM$_g$ maximum tubular reabsorption rate for glucose

TMH tetramethylammonium hydroxide

TM-HSA trimellityl–human serum albumin

TMI testing motor impairment; threatened myocardial infarction; total marrow irradiation; total medical record; transmural myocardial infarction

TMIC Toxic Materials Information Center

T1mic breast tumor microinvasion of less than 0.1 cm

TMIF tumor-cell migratory inhibition factor

TMIS Technicon Medical Information System

TMJ temporomandibular joint; trapeziometacarpal joint

TMJS temporomandibular joint syndrome

TMK thymidylate kinase

TML terminal midline; terminal motor latency; tetramethyl lead

TMLR transmyocardial laser revascularization

TMM tissue-mimicking material

TMN thin membrane nephropathy; tumor-node-metastasis

TMNST tethered median nerve stress test

TMP 2,2,4,4-tetramethylpentane; thiamine monophosphate; thymidine-5′-monophosphate; thymidine monophosphate; thymolphthalein monophosphate; transmembrane potential; transmembrane pressure; trimethaphan; trimethoprim; trimethylpsoralen

TM$_{PAH}$ maximum tubular excretory capacity for para-aminohippuric acid

TMPD tetramethyl-*p*-phenylinediamine

TMPDS temporomandibular pain and dysfunction syndrome; thiamine monophosphate disulfide

TMP-SMX trimethoprim-sulfamethoxazole

TMR the medical record; tissue maximum ratio; topical magnetic resonance; transmyocardial revascularization

TMRM tetramethylrhodamine

TMS telematic monitoring service; thallium myocardial scintigraphy; The Muscatine Study; thread mate system; thymidylate synthase; total morbidity score; transcranial magnetic stimulation; trapezoidocephaly-multiple synostosis [syndrome]; trimethylsilane

TMSE Thai Mental State Examination

TMST treadmill stem test

TMT tarsometatarsal; thiol methyltransferase; Trail-Making Test; treadmill test; trimethyllin

TMTD tetramethylthiuram disulfide

TMTJ tarsometatarsal joint

TMTX trimetrexate

TMU tetramethyl urea

TMUV Tembusu virus

TMV tobacco mosaic virus

TMX tamoxifen

TMZ transformation zone

TN talonavicular; tarsonavicular; team nursing; temperature normal; tenascin; test negative; tinea nigra; trigeminal nucleus; total negatives; toxin neutralization; trigeminal neuralgia; trochlear nucleus; true negative

T/N tar and nicotine

T$_4$N normal serum thyroxine

Tn normal intraocular tension; transposon; troponin

TNA total nutrient admixture; trinitrotoluene

TNB transnasal butorphanol

TNBP tri-n-butyl phosphate

TNBS 2,4,6-trinitrobenzene sulfonic acid

TnC troponin C

TNCC-I trauma nursing core course instructor

TNCC-P trauma nursing core course provider

TND term normal delivery

TNDM transient neonatal diabetes mellitus

t-NE total norepinephrine

TNEE titrated norepinephrine excretion

T-NEMC Tufts-New England Medical Center

TNF true negative fraction; tumor necrosis factor

TNFA tumor necrosis factor alpha

TNFAIP tumor necrosis factor, alpha-induced protein

TNFAR tumor necrosis factor alpha receptor

TNFB tumor necrosis factor beta

TNFBR tumor necrosis factor beta receptor

TNFR1 tumor necrosis factor type 1 receptor

TNFr tumor necrosis factor receptor

TNG trinitroglycerin

tng tongue

tNGF truncated nerve growth factor

TnGV *Trichoplusia ni* granulovirus

TNH teaching nursing home; transient neonatal hyperammonemia

T-NHL T-cell−derived non-Hodgkin leukemia

TNHP teaching nursing home program

TNI total nodal irradiation

TnI troponin I

TNM thyroid node metastases; tumor-node-metastasis

TNMR tritium nuclear magnetic resonance

TNP total net positive; trinitrophenyl

TNPACK truncated Newton program package

TNP-KLH trinitrophenyl keyhole limpet hemocyanin

TNP-LPS trinitrophenyl-lipopolysaccharide

TNR tonic neck reflex; true negative rate

TNS total nuclear score; Transcultural Nursing Society; transcutaneous nerve stimulation; tumor necrosis serum

TNSS total nasal symptom scores

TNT tetranitroblue tetrazolium; Transderm-Nitro Trial; Treatment to New Target [study of effectiveness of atorvastatin in coronary heart disease]; 2,4,6-trinitrotoluene

TnT troponin T

TNTC too numerous to count

TNV tobacco necrosis virus

TO old tuberculin; oral temperature; original tuberculin; target organ; telephone order; thoracic orthosis; thromboangiitis obliterans; thrombotic occlusion; tincture of opium; total obstruction; tracheoesophageal; treatment object; tubo-ovarian; turnover

T(O) oral temperature

TO₂ oxygen transport

T₀ tricuspid opening

to tincture of opium

TOA total quality assessment; tuboovarian abscess

TOAP thioguanine, Oncovin, cytosine arabinoside, and prednisone

TOAST Treatment of Acute Stroke Trial; Trial of Org 10172 in Acute Stroke Trial

TOAT The Open Artery Trial

TOB tobramycin

TOBEC total body electrical conductivity [test]

TobRV tobacco ringspot virus

TOC task-oriented coping; total organic carbon

TOCC Total Occlusion of Coronary Arteries, Chronic [study]

TOCP tri-*o*-cresyl phosphate

TOCSY total correlation spectroscopy

TOD right eye tension [L. *oculus dexter*]; target organ damage; target organ disease; time-oriented data; titanium optimized design

TOD/CCD target organ disease/clinical cardiovascular disease

TODS toxic organic dust syndrome

TOE tender on examination; tracheo-oesophageal; transesophageal echography; transferred nuclear Overhauser effect

TOEFL Test of English as a Foreign Language

TOES toxic oil epidemic syndrome

TOF tetralogy of Fallot; time of flight; tracheoesophageal fistula; train of four

ToF time-of-flight

TOFA time-of-flight absorbance; time of flight and abstinence

T of F tetralogy of Fallot

TOFHLA test of functional health literacy in adults

TOFMS, TOF-MS time-of-flight mass spectrometry

TOFS total organ failure score

TOH tower of Hanoi [test]; transient osteoporosis of hip

TOHP Trial of Hypertension Prevention

TOL trial of labor

ToL Tower of London [test]

tol tolerance, tolerated

TOLB, tolb tolbutamine

TOLC Treatment of Low-Density Lipoprotein-Bound Cholesterol [study]

TOLD top-level driver

TOM toxic oxygen metabolite

TOMA tri-octylmethylammonium chloride

TOMAS torsional ocular movement analysis system

TOMHS Treatment of Mild Hypertension Study

TOMI turkey ovomucoid inhibitor

TOMIIS Total Occlusion Postmyocardial Infarction Intervention Study

Tomo tomogram, tomography

tomos tomograms

TOMS The Oklahoma Marker Study

TON traumatic optic neuropathy

TONE tilted optimized nonsaturating excitation; Trial of Nonpharmacologic Interventions in the Elderly

tonoc tonight [to + L. *nocte*]

TOP termination of pregnancy; Thrombolysis in Older Patients [study]; topoisomerase
top topical
TOPAS Thrombolysis or Peripheral Arterial Surgery [study]
TOPCAD topical prevention or conception and disease
TOPLIT Transluminal Extraction Catheter or Percutaneous Transluminal Coronary Angioplasty in Thrombus [study]
TOPS Take Off Pounds Sensibly [program]; Thrombolysis in Old Patients Study; Treatment of Post-thrombolytic Stenosis [study]
TOPV Topografov virus; trivalent oral poliovaccine
tOPV trivalent oral poliovirus vaccine
TORCH toxoplasmosis, other [congenital syphilis and viruses], rubella, cytomegalovirus, and herpes
ToRCHeS toxoplasmosis, rubella, cytomegalovirus, herpes, syphilis
TORCHS toxoplasmosis, other diseases, rubella, cytomegalovirus, herpes, syphilis
TORDIA Treatment of Resistant Depression in Adolescents [study]
TORP total ossicular replacement prosthesis
torr mm Hg pressure
TORS transoral robotic surgery
TOS thoracic outlet syndrome; toxic oil syndrome
TOSCA Total Occlusion Study in Canada
TOSV Toscana virus
TOT The Oslo Trial; tip of the tongue; total operating time; tubal ovum transfer
TOTAL Total Occlusion Trial with Angioplasty by Using Laser Guidewire
TOTP tri-*o*-tolyl phosphate
TOV trial of voiding
TOVA test of variables of attention; trigger of ventricular arrhythmia
TOWARD Toyama Warfarin Rational Dosage [study]
Tox, tox toxicity, toxic
TOXICON Toxicology Conversational On-line Network
TOXLINE Toxicology Information On-Line
TOXLIT Toxicology Literature
TOXNET Toxicology Data Network
TP temperature and pressure; temperature probe; template; temporal peak; temporoparietal; tender point; tension pneumothorax; terminal phalanx; terminal protein; testosterone propionate; thick padding; thin plate; threshold potential; thrombocytopenic purpura; thrombophlebitis; thromboxane prostaglandin; thymic polypeptide; thymidine

phosphorylase; thymopentin; thymopoietin; thymus polypeptide; thymus protein; tissue pressure; Todd palsy; toe pressure; torsades de pointes; torus palatinus; total population; total positives; total protein; transaction processing; transforming principle; transition point; transpyloric; transverse polarization; transverse process; transverse propagation; treating physician; treatment period; treatment progress; treatment protocol; *Treponema pallidum*; triazolophthalazine; trigger point; triphosphate; true positive; tryptophan; tryptophan pyrrolase; tube precipitin; tuberculin precipitate; tumor protein
6-TP 6-thiopurine
T&P temperature and pressure; temperature and pulse
T+P temperature and pulse
Tp primary transmission; time of preparation; *Treponema pallidum*; tryptophan
T$_p$ physical half-life
TPA tannic acid, polyphosphomolybdic acid, and amino acid; 12-*O*-tetradecanoyl-phorbol-13-acetate; third-party administrator; thrombotic pulmonary artery; tissue plasminogen activator; tissue polypeptide antigen; total parenteral alimentation; *Treponema pallidum* agglutination; tumor polypeptide antigen
t-PA tissue plasminogen activator
TPAC torso phased array coil
TPAI tissue plasminogen activator inhibitor
TPase thymidine phosphorylase
TPASK Tissue Plasminogen Activator vs Streptokinase [trial]
TPAT Tissue Plasminogen Activator, Toronto Trial
TPB tetraphenyl borate; theory of planned behavior; tryptone phosphate broth
TPBF total pulmonary blood flow
TPBG trophoblast glycoprotein
TPBS three-phase bone scintigraphy; three-phase radionuclide bone scanning
TPC thromboplastic plasma component; thyroid papillary carcinoma; time to peak contrast; total patient care; total plasma catecholamines; total plasma cholesterol; total plate count; *Treponema pallidum* complement
TPCF *Treponema pallidum* complement fixation
TPCR tripartite chimeric receptor
TPCV total packed cell volume
TPD temporary partial disability; thiamine propyl disulfide; tripotassium phenolphthalein disulfate; tumor-producing dose
TP-DNA template deoxyribonucleic acid [DNA]

TPDS tropical pancreatic diabetes syndrome

TPE therapeutic plasma exchange; totally protected environment; tris-phosphate EDTA; typhoid-parathyroid enteritis

T^Pe expiratory pause time

T_peak time to peak

TPEV 1, 2 Turkey pseudoenteritis viruses 1, 2

TPEY tellurite polymyxin egg yolk [agar]

TPF thymus permeability factor; thymus to peak flow; true positive fraction

TPFR time to peak filling rate

TPG transmembrane potential gradient; transplacental gradient; transpulmonary gradient; tryptophan peptone glucose

TPGS E-alpha-tocophenyl polyethylene glycol succinate; Talairach Proportional Grid System

TPGYT trypticase-peptone-glucose-yeast extract-trypsin

TPH transplacental hemorrhage; tryptophan hydroxylase

TpH tryptophan hydroxylase

TPHA *Treponema pallidum* hemagglutination

TPHU Tropical Public Health Unit

TPI Thrombolytic Predictive Instrument; time period integrator; *Treponema pallidum* immobilization; treponemal immobilization test; triose phosphate isomerase

T^Pi inspiratory pause time

TPIA *Treponema pallidum* immune adherence

TPIIA time of postexpiratory inspiratory activity

TPK tyrosine protein kinase

TPL third-party liability; titanium proximal loading; tumor progression locus; tyrosine phenol-lyase

tpl transplantation, transplanted

TPLL T-cell prolymphocytic leukemia

TPLSM two-photon laser scanning microscopy

TPLV transient pulmonary vascular lability

TPM temporary pacemaker; thrombophlebitis migrans; topiramate; total particulate matter; total passive motion; transplant procurement management; triphenylmethane; tropomyosin; turning-point morphology

TPMT thiopurine methyltransferase

TPMV Thottapalayam virus

TPN thalamic projection neuron; total parenteral nutrition; transition protein; triphosphopyridine nucleotide

TPNH reduced triphosphopyridine nucleotide

TPO thrombopoietin; thyroid peroxidase; tryptophan peroxidase

Tpo thrombopoietin

TPP target product profile; tetraphenylporphyrin; thiamine pyrophosphate; thrust plate prosthesis; transpulmonary pressure; treadmill performance test; tripeptidyl peptidase; triphenyl phosphite

TPPase thiamine pyrophosphatase

TPPD thoracic-pelvic-phalangeal dystrophy

TPPI time-proportional phase incrementation

TPPN total peripheral parenteral nutrition

TPQ Threshold Planning Quantity

TPR temperature, pulse, and respiration; testosterone production rate; tetraricopeptide repeat; third-party reimbursement; tissue/phantom ratio; total peripheral resistance; total pulmonary resistance; true positive rate; tumor potentiating region

TPRI total peripheral resistance index

TPS thin-plate spline; time to peak shortening; topical skin protectant; treatment planning system; trypsin; tryptase; tumor polysaccharide substance

TPSE 2-(*p*-triphenyl)sulfonylethanol

TPST true positive stress test; tyrosyl protein sulfotransferase

TPT tetraphenyl tetrazolium; Thrombosis Prevention Trial; time to peak tension; topotecan; total protein tuberculin; triphalangeal thumb; typhoid-paratyphoid [vaccine]

TPTE 2-(*p*-triphenyl)thioethanol

TPTIMF soft tissue pinch-thickness at the inframammary fold

TPTX thyro-parathyroidectomized

TPTZ tripyridyltriazine

TPV tetanus-pertussis vaccine; tipranavir

TPVR total peripheral vascular resistance; total pulmonary vascular resistance

TPVS transhepatic portal venous sampling

TPW temporary pacing wire

TPX testis-specific protein

TPZ thioproperazine

TQ tocopherolquinone; tourniquet

TQD target quit date

TQE top-quality embryo

TQFCOSY triple-quantum-filtered correlated spectroscopy

TQI total quality improvement

TQM total quality management

TQS Terminology Query Service

TR recovery time; rectal temperature; repetition time; residual tuberculin; terminal repeat; tetrazolium reduction; therapeutic radiology; therapeutic ratio; therapeutic recreation; thrombin receptor; thyroid receptor; time release; time to relengthening; total resistance; total response; trachea; transfusion reaction; transmission rate; transrectal;

tricuspid regurgitation; Trinder reagent; tuberculin R; tuberculin residue; turbidity reducing; turnover ratio

T:R thickness to radius ratio

T&R treated and released

T/R transmission/[frequency] response

TR₉₀ time to 90% relengthening

t(°R) absolute temperature on the Rankine scale

Tr trace; tragion; transferrin; trypsin

T_r radiologic half-life; retention time

tr tincture; trace; traction; transaldolase; trauma, traumatic; tremor; triradial

TRA total renin activity; tumor-resistant antigen

tra transfer

TRAb thyrotoxin receptor antibody

TRAC tool for referral assessment of continuity [of health]

trac traction

TRACE Trandolapril Cardiac Evaluation [trial]

trach trachea, tracheal, tracheostomy

TRAJ timed repetitive ankle jerk

TRALI transfusion-related acute lung injury

TRALT transfusion-related acute lung trauma

TRAM transport remote-acquisition monitor; transverse rectus abdominis muscle; Treatment Rating Assessment Matrix; Treatment Response Assessment Method; trisaminomethane

TRAMAH trauma resources allocation model for ambulances and hospitals

TRANDA Trandolapril Andalusian Study

TRAPME tricho-rhino-auriculophalangeal multiple exostoses

trans transfer; transference; transverse

TRANSAX translation of axes

trans D transverse diameter

TRANSFAIR Transfatty Acids in Food in Europe [study]

transm transmission, transmitted

transpl transplantation, transplanted

TRAP carpal tunnel syndrome, Raynaud phenomenon, aching muscles, proximal muscle weakness [rheumatic disorders associated with hypothyroidism]; tartrate-resistant acid phosphatase; telomeric repeat amplification protocol; thrombin receptor-activating peptide; transport and rapid accessioning for additional procedures; triiodothyronine receptor auxiliary protein; Twin Reversed Arterial Perfusion [study]

TrAP transcriptional activator protein

trap trapezius

TRAPIST Trapidil vs Placebo to Prevent In-Stent Intimal Hyperplasia [study]

TRAS transplanted renal artery stenosis

TraSH transposition site hybridization; transposon site hybridization

TRASHES tuberculosis, radiotherapy, ankylosing spondylitis, histoplasmosis, extrinsic allergic alveolitis, silicosis [chest x-ray findings]

traum trauma, traumatic

TRB terbutalone; tropanyl benzylate

TRBF total renal blood flow

TRBV Tribec virus

TRC tanned red cell; therapeutic residential center; tissue repair cell; T-lymphocyte antigen receptor; total renin concentration; total respiratory conductance; total ridge count

TRCA tanned red cell agglutination

TRCF transcription repair coupling factor

TRCH tanned red cell hemagglutination

TRCHI tanned red cell hemagglutination inhibition

TRCV total red cell volume

TRD tongue-retaining device; traumatic rupture of diaphragm; treatment-resistant depression

TRDN transient respiratory distress of the newborn

TRE target registration error; thymic reticuloendothelial; thyroid hormone response; triplet rapid expansion; true radiation emission

TREA triethanolamine

TREAT Tranilast Restenosis Following Angioplasty Trial

treat treatment

TRECs T-cell receptor rearrangement excision circle

TREC-TCR rearrangement excision cycle

Tregs regulatory T cells

TREND Trial on Reversing Endothelial Dysfunction

Trend Trendelenburg [position]

TRENT Trial of Early Nifedipine Treatment of Acute Myocardial Infarction

Trep *Treponema*

TRF targeted RNA fingerprinting; T-cell replacing factor; thymus replacing factor; thyrotropin-releasing factor; transferrin; tubular rejection fraction

TRFC total rosette-forming cell

TRFF trough response, fine frequency

TRG T-cell rearranging gene; transfer RNA glycine

TRH tension-reducing hypothesis; thyrotropin-releasing hormone

TRHR thyrotropin-releasing hormone receptor

TRH-ST thyrotropin-releasing hormone stimulation test

TRI tetrazolium reduction inhibition; Thyroid Research Institute; total response index; Toxic Chemical Release Inventory; tubuloreticular inclusion

tri tricentric

T₃RIA, T₃(RIA) triiodothyronine radioimmunoassay

T₄RIA, T₄(RIA) thyroxine radioimmunoassay

TRIAC 3,5,3′-triiodothyroacetic acid

TRIADS time-resolved imaging by automatic data segmentation

TRIC Thrombolysis with Recombinant Tissue Plasminogen Activator During Instability in Coronary Artery Disease [trial]; trachoma inclusion conjunctivitis

TRICB trichlorobiphenyl

TRICC Transfusion Requirements in Critical Care [trial]

Trich *Trichomonas*

TRIFACTS Toxic Chemical Release Inventory Facts

trig trigger; triglycerides; trigonum

TRIM Thrombin Inhibition in Myocardial Ischemia [study]

TRIMIS Tri-Service Medical Information Systems [Department of Defense]

TRIMM Triggers and Mechanisms of Myocardial Infarction [study]

TRINS totally reversible ischemic neurological symptoms

TRIPS Trade-Related Aspects of Intellectual Property

TRIS tris-(hydroxymethyl)-aminomethane

TRISS trauma and injury severity score

TRIT triiodothyronine

trit triturate

TRITC tetrarhodamine isothiocyanate

TRK transketolase; tyrosine kinase

Trk tyrosine kinase

TrkA tyrosine kinase A

TrkB tyrosine kinase B

TRL transfer ribonucleic acid leucine

TRLP triglyceride-rich lipoprotein

TRM traditional medicines; transplant-related mortality

TRMA thiamine-responsive megaloblastic anemia

TR-MALLS time-resolved multi-angle laser light scattering

TRMC trimethylrhodamino-isothiocyanate

TRMI transfer ribonucleic acid initiator methionine

TRML, Trml terminal

TRM-SMX trimethoprim-sulfamethoxazole

TRMV Trombetas virus

TRN tegmental reticular nucleus

tRNA transfer ribonucleic acid

tRNA GLU transfer ribonucleic acid glutamic acid

tRNA-i(met) transfer ribonucleic acid initiator methionine

tRNA-SER transfer ribonucleic acid serine

TRND Therapeutics for Rare and Neglected Diseases

TRNG tetracycline-resistant *Neisseria gonorrhoeae*

TRNOE transfer nuclear Overhauser effect

TRNS transfer ribonucleic acid serine

TRO tissue reflectance oximetry

Troch trochanter

TROM torque range of motion; total range of motion

Trop tropical

TROPCAB total revascularization off pump by coronary artery bypass

TROPHY Treatment Effects of Lisinopril vs Hydrochlorothiazide in Obese Patients with Hypertension [trial]; Treatment of Obese Patients with Hypertension [trial]; Trial of Preventing Hypertension

TRP trough response phase; total refractory period; transfer ribonucleic acid proline; transient receptor potential; trichorhinophalangeal [syndrome]; tubular reabsorption of phosphate; tyrosine-related protein

TrP tricuspid valve

Trp, trp tryptophan

TRPA tryptophan-rich prealbumin

TrPl treatment plan

TRPM testosterone-repressed prostate message

TRPO tryptophan oxygenase

TRPS trichorhinophalangeal syndrome

TrPs tender trigger points; trigger points

TRPT theoretic renal phosphorus threshold

TRR temporal representation and reasoning; total respiratory resistance

TRS task routing system; testicular regression syndrome; total reducing sugars; tubuloreticular structure

TrS trauma surgery

TRST triage risk screening tool

TRSV tobacco ringspot virus

TRT targeted renal therapy; thoracic radiotherapy; transfer RNA threonine

TR/TE repetition time/echo time

T-RTS triage-revised trauma score

TRTV Turkey rhinotracheitis virus

TRU task-related unit; turbidity-reducing unit

T₃RU triiodothyronine resin uptake

TRUS transrectal ultrasonography

TRUSP transrectal ultrasonography of prostate

TRUST Trial in United Kingdom for Stroke Treatment

TRUV Trubanaman virus

TRV Tanjong Rabok virus; tobacco rattle virus

TrV Triatoma virus

TRVV total right ventricular volume

TRX thioredoxin

trx traction

Tryp tryptophan

TS Takayasu syndrome; Tay-Sachs [disease]; telemedicine system; temperature sensitivity; temperature sensor; temperature, skin; temporal stem; tensile strength; test solution; thermal stability; thoracic surgery; thymidylate synthase; time scale; tissue space; total solids; Tourette syndrome; toxic substance; toxic syndrome; tracheal sound; trachomatous scarring; transferrin saturation; transition; transitional sleep; transsexual; transverse section; transverse sinus; trauma score; treadmill score; triceps surae; tricuspid stenosis; triple strength; tropical sprue; Troyer syndrome; trypticase soy [plate]; T suppressor [cell]; tuberous sclerosis; tumor specific; Turner syndrome; type specific

T/S transverse section

T+S type and screen

Ts skin temperature; tosylate

T$_s$ secreted immunoglobulin heavy chain polypeptide; stimulus timing; T-cell suppressor; T suppressor [cell]

T$_s$1, T$_s$3 suppressor T lymphocyte subpopulations 1 and 3

tS time required to complete the S phase of the cell cycle

ts temperature sensitivity

ts, tsp teaspoon

TSA technical surgical assistance; time series analysis; toluene sulfonic acid; total shoulder arthroplasty; total solute absorption; toxic shock antigen; transcortical sensory aphasia; trypticase-soy agar; tumor-specific antigen; tumor surface antigen; type-specific antibody

T$_4$SA thyroxine-specific activity

TSAb thyroid-stimulating antibody

TSAP toxic-shock−associated protein; transport services access point

TSAS total severity assessment score

TSAT tube slide agglutination test

TSB total serum bilirubin; trypticase soy broth; tryptone soy broth

TSBA total serum bile acids

TSBB transtracheal selective bronchial brushing

TSC technetium sulfur colloid; thiazide-sensitive sodium-chloride cotransporter; thiosemicarbazide; total static compliance; total symptom complex; transient spontaneous circulation; transsodium crocetinate; transverse spinal sclerosis; tuberous sclerosis complex

TSCA Toxic Substances Control Act

TSCOHS Tri-Service Comprehensive Oral Health Survey

TSCS Tennessee Self-Concept Scale

TSD target site duplication; target-skin distance; Tay-Sachs disease; theory of signal detectability; thermionic selective detector; traditional stripchart display

TSE testicular self-examination; time since exposure; tissue-specific extinguisher; total skin electron; total skin examination; transcutaneous spinal electroanesthesia; transmissible spongiform encephalopathy; trisodium edetate; turbospin echo

TSEB total skin electron beam

T sect transverse section

TSEM transmission scanning electron microscopy

TSES Target Symptom Evaluation Scale

T-set tracheotomy set

TSF T-cell suppressor factor; testicular feminization syndrome; thrombopoiesis-stimulating factor; total systemic flow; triceps skinfold

T$_s$F T-cell suppressor factor

TSG tumor suppressor gene

TSG, TSGP tumor-specific glycoprotein

TSGE temperature sweep gel electrophoresis

TSH thyroid-stimulating hormone; transient synovitis of the hip

TSHA thyroid-stimulating hormone, alpha chain

TSHB thyroid-stimulating hormone, beta chain

TSHR thyroid-stimulating hormone receptor

TSH-RF thyroid-stimulating hormone−releasing factor

TSH-RH thyroid-stimulating hormone−releasing hormone

TSHW Thyroid Study in Healthy Women

TSI thyroid-stimulating immunoglobulin; triple-sugar iron [agar]; turbo spectroscopic imaging

TSIA total small intestine allotransplantation; triple-sugar iron agar

tSIDS totally unexplained sudden infant death syndrome

TSJ Telemedicine Society of Japan

TSL task specification language; terminal sensory latency; transport layer security

TSLP thymic stroma−derived lymphopoietin

TSM type-specific M protein

TSMDB Tuberous Sclerosis Mutation Database

TSO transient spastic occlusion; *trans*-stilbene oxide

TSOP time from symptom onset to presentation

TSP tailspin protein; testis-specific protein; thrombin-sensitive protein; thrombospondin; tibial hole sagittal positioning; total serum protein; total sleep period; total suspended particulate [matter]; tracheal sleeve pneumonectomy; trisodium phosphate; tropical spastic paraparesis

tsp teaspoon

TSPA thiotepa

TSPAP total serum prostatic acid phosphatase

TSP I thrombospondin type I

TSPL transplant

TSPP tetrasodium pyrophosphate

TSR theophylline sustained release; thyroid/serum ratio; tissue scatter ratio; tissue standard ratio; total systemic resistance

TSRI The Scripps Research Institute

TSS toxic shock syndrome; tropical splenomegaly syndrome

TSSA tumor-specific cell surface antigen

TSSE toxic shock syndrome exotoxin

TSST toxic shock syndrome toxin

TST thermoregulatory sweat test; thiosulfate sulfur-transferase; thromboplastin screening test; total sleep time; transforming sequence, thyroid; treadmill stress test; triceps skinfold thickness; tricipital skinfold thickness; tuberculin skin test; tumor skin test

TSTA toxoplasmin skin test antigen; tumor-specific tissue antigen; tumor-specific transplantation antigen

TsTX tityustoxin

TSU triple-sugar urea [agar]

TSUV Tsuruse virus

TSV total stomach volume; total stroke volume

TSVR total systemic vascular resistance

TSWT tree-structured wavelet transform

TSY trypticase soy yeast

TSYEA trypticase soy yeast enriched agar

TT tablet triturate; tactile tension; talar tilt; tandem transplant; tendon of Todaro; tendon transfer; terminal transferase; test tube; testicular torsion; tetanus toxin; tetanus toxoid; tetrathionate; tetrazol; therapeutic touch; thrombin time; thrombolytic therapy; thromboplastin time; thymol turbidity; tibial tubercle; tibial tuberosity; tick typhus; tiger top; tilt table; tiny T [antigen]; tissue tolerance; tolerance test; tonometry; total thyroidectomy; total thyroxine; total time; total transfer; trabecular thickness; transient tachypnea; transferred to; transit time; transthoracic; transtracheal; treadmill test; trend template; triple therapy; tritiated thymidine; tuberculin test; tuberculoid; tube thoracostomy; tumor thrombus; turnover time; tyrosine transaminase

T&T time and temperature; touch and tone

TT$_2$ total diiodothyronine

TT$_3$ total triiodothyronine

TT$_4$ total thyroxine

T$_t$ transition temperature

TTA tetanus toxoid antibody; timed therapeutic absence; tissue texture abnormality; total toe arthroplasty; transtracheal aspiration

tTA tetracycline-controlled transactivator

TTAP threaded titanium acetabular prosthesis

TTAT traumatic thoracic aortic transection

TTATTS Thrombolytic Therapy in Acute Thrombotic/Thromboembolic Stroke [study]

TTB third-trimester bleeding

TTC triphenyltetrazolium chloride; triple transducer connector; trying to conceive; T-tube cholangiogram

TTD temporary total disability; tetraethylthiuram disulfide; tissue tolerance dose; transfusion-transmitted disease; transient tic disorder; transverse thoracic diameter; trichothiodystrophy

TTDF time to distant failure

TTE transthoracic echocardiography

TTF thyroid transcription factor; time to failure

TTFD tetrahydrofurfuryldisulfide

TTG T-cell translocation gene; telethermography; tellurite, taurocholate, and gelatin

TTGA tellurite, taurocholate, and gelatin agar

TTH tension-type headaches; thyrotropic hormone; tritiated thymidine

TTI tension-time index; time-temperature indicator; time-tension index; time to intubation; torque-time interval; transtracheal insufflation

TTIdi tension-time index diaphragm

TTIM T-cell tumor invasion and metastasis

T-TIME tourniquet time

TTJV transtracheal jet ventilation

TTL total thymus lymphocytes; training test lung; transistor-transistor logic

TTLC true total lung capacity

TTLD terminal transverse limb defect

TTLF time to local failure; transtelephonic monitoring

TTN titin; transient tachypnea of the newborn

TT$_n$ normal trend template

TTNA transthoracic needle aspiration

TTNAB transthoracic needle aspiration biopsy

TTNB transthoracic needle biopsy

TTO time trade-off

TTO$_2$ transtracheal oxygen

TTOPP Thrombolytic Therapy in Older Patient Population [study]

TTP thiamine triphosphate; thrombotic thrombocytopenic purpura; thymidine triphosphate; time to disease progression; time to peak; time to progression; tocopherol transfer protein; transtrabecular plane; tristetraprolin; tritolyl phosphate; trusted third party

TTPA triethylene thiophosphoramide

TTR time in target range; transthoracic resistance; transthyretin; triceps tendon reflex

TTS tarsal tunnel syndrome; temporary threshold shift; The Tromsø Study; through the scope; through the skin; tilt table standing; transdermal therapeutic system; twin transfusion syndrome

TTSS type three secretion system

TTT thymol turbidity test; tolbutamide tolerance test; total twitch time; transpupillary thermotherapy; tuberculin tine test

TTTS twin-to-twin transfusion syndrome

TTTT test tube turbidity test; Tokyo Trop-T Trial

TTV tracheal transport velocity; transfusion-transmitted virus

TTVS Transfusion Transmitted Viruses Study

TTWB toe-touch weightbearing

TTX tetrodotoxin

TU texture unit; thiouracil; thyroid uptake; Todd unit; toxic unit; toxin unit; transmission unit; transurethral; tuberculin unit; turbidity unit

T$_3$U triiodothyronine uptake

TUAV Turuna virus

TUB tubulin

TUBA transumbilical breast augmentation; tubulin alpha

TUBAL tubulin alpha–like

TUBB tubulin beta

tuberc tuberculosis

TUBG tubulin gamma

TUBS traumatic unidirectional Bankart surgery

TUCC Tissue Plasminogen Activator/Urokinase Comparison in China [study]

TUCV Tucunduba virus

TUD total urethral discharge

TUG timed up and go [test]; total urinary gonadotropin

TUGMI Tsukuba University Group for Myocardial Infarction

TUGSE traumatic ulcerative granuloma with stromal eosinophilia

TuHV Tupaiid herpesvirus

TUI transurethral incision; type unique identifier

TUIP transurethral incision of prostate

TUL tumescent ultrasound liposculpture

TULIP transurethral ultrasound-guided laser-induced prostatectomy

TULV Tula virus

TUN total urinary nitrogen

TUNEL deoxyuride-5′-triphosphate biotin nick-end labeling

TUNV Tunis virus

TUP temporal utility program; transumbilical plane

TUPR transurethral prostatic resection

TUPV Tupaia virus

TUR transurethral resection

TURB, TURBT transurethral resection of bladder [tumor]

turb turbid, turbidity

turboFLASH turbo fast low-angle shot

TURBT transurethral resection of bladder tumor

TURP transurethral resection of the prostate

TURS transurethral resection syndrome

TURV transurethral resection of valves; Turlock virus

TUS trauma ultrasound

TUTase terminal uridylate transferase

TV box turtle virus; talipes varus; target volume; television; teschovirus; tetrazolium violet; thoracic vertebra; tickborne virus; tidal volume; tigré virus; Torovirus; total volume; toxic vertigo; transumbilical plane; transvaginal; transvenous; transverse; transversion; trial visit; *Trichomonas vaginalis*; tricuspid valve; trivalent; true vertebra; truncal vagotomy; tuberculin volutin; tubovesicular typhoid vaccine; tumor virus

Tv *Trichomonas vaginalis*

TVA truncal vagotomy and antrectomy

TVC timed vital capacity; total viable cells; total volume capacity; transvaginal cone; triple voiding cystogram; true vocal cords

TVCD transvaginal color Doppler sonography

TVCPD transvaginal color power Doppler

TVCV transvenous cardioversion

TVD transmissible virus dementia; triple-vessel disease

TVF tactile vocal fremitus

TVFD time-varying frequency dependence

TVG time-varied gain

TVH total vaginal hysterectomy; turkey virus hepatitis

TVHS transvaginal hysterosonography

TVI time-velocity integral; tissue velocity imaging

TVL tenth value layer; tunica vasculosa lentis

TV/L tubovesicle/lumen

TVMF time-varying magnetic field

TVOC total volatile organic compound

TVP tensor veli palatini; textured vegetable protein; transvenous pacemaker; tricuspid valve prolapse; truncal vagotomy and pyloroplasty

TVR target vessel revascularization; tonic vibratory reflex; total vascular resistance; tricuspid valve replacement; triple-valve replacement

TVRE transvaginal resection of endometrium

TVS transvaginal sonography; transvesical sonography

TVSS transient voltage surge suppressor

TVT tension-free vaginal tape; transmissible venereal tumor; tunica vaginalis testis

TVTV Trivittatus virus

TVU total volume of the urine

TVV *Trichomonas vaginalis* virus

TVX tumor virus X

TW tap water; terminal web; test weight; thyroid weight; total body water; traveling wave

Tw twist

tw twice per week

TWA time-weighted average; total wrist arthroplasty; T-wave alternans

TWAR Taiwan acute respiratory [strain]

TWB touch weight bear

T$_{wb}$ wet-bulb temperature

TWBC terminal warm blood cardioplegia; total white blood cells; total white blood count

TWD total white and differential [cell count]; traveling-wave dielectrophoresis

TWE tap water enema; tepid water enema

TWIST time without symptoms of disease and subjective toxic effects of treatment

TWISTER Trial of Within Stent Treatment of Endoluminal Restenosis

TWL transepidermal water loss

TWS tranquilizer withdrawal syndrome

TWs triphasic waves

TWT The Wellcome Trust; the whole thing; total waiting time

TWW two-week wait

TWWD tap water wet dressing

TX a derivative of contagious tuberculin; no evidence of primary tumor; tamoxifen; thromboxane; thyroidectomized; transplantation; treatment

T&X type and crossmatch

6TX 6-thioxanthine

Tx transplant or transplantation

Tx, T$_x$ therapy; traction; treatment

tx traction

TXA, TxA thromboxane A

TXA2, TXA$_2$ thromboxane A2 (A$_2$)

TXB2, TXB$_2$ thromboxane B2 (B$_2$)

TXDD transmitted data decoder

TxDD/T transmitted data decoder/timer

TXDS qualifying toxic dose

TxDE transmitted data encoder

TXN thioredoxin

Ty type; typhoid; tyrosine

TYH tyrosine hydrolase

Tymp tympanic, tympanum

TYMS thymidylate synthase

Ty-neg tyrosinase negative

Ty-pos tyrosinase positive

Tyr, tyr tyrosine

TyRIA thyroid radioisotope assay

TYRL tyrosinase-like

TYRP tyrosine-related protein

TYUV Tyuleniy virus

TZ zymoplastic tuberculin

t$_{1/2z}$ terminal half-life

TZD thiazolidinedione

U

U congenital limb absence; in electrocardiography, an undulating deflection that follows the T wave; internal energy; International Unit of enzyme activity; Mann-Whitney rank sum statistic; potential difference; ulcer; ulna; ultralente [insulin]; umbilicus; uncertain; unerupted; unit; universal application; unknown; unsharpness; upper; uracil; uranium; urea; urethra; uridine; uridylic acid; urinary concentration; urine; urology; uterus; uvula; volume velocity

Y uppercase Greek letter upsilon

U/2 upper half

U/3 upper third

u unified atomic mass unit; velocity

υ lowercase Greek letter upsilon

UA absorption unsharpness; ultraaudible; ultrasonic arteriography; umbilical artery; unauthorized absence; unicystic ameloblastoma; unit of analysis; unstable angina; upper airways; upper arm; uric acid; uridylic acid; urinalysis; urinary aldosterone; uronic acid; uterine activity; uterine aspiration

U/A uric acid; urinalysis

ua urinalysis

UAC umbilical artery catheter; unusual-appearing child; uric acid

UA/C uric acid/creatinine ratio

UAE unilateral absence of excretion; urine albumin excretion; uterine artery embolization

UAEM University Association for Emergency Medicine

UAGA Uniform Anatomical Gift Act

UAI uterine activity interval

UAI-C unprotected anal intercourse with casual partners

UAL ultrasound-assisted lipoplasty; ultrasound-assisted liposuction

U-AMY urinary amylase

UAN uric acid nitrogen

UAO upper airway obstruction

UAP unlicensed assistive personnel; unstable angina pectoris; urinary acid phosphatase; urinary alkaline phosphatase

UAPA unilateral absence of pulmonary artery

UAR upper airway resistance; uric acid riboside

UAS upper abdomen surgery; upstream activating sequence; upstream activation site

UAU uterine activity unit

UB ultimobranchial body; Unna boot; upper back; urinary bladder

UB 82 universal billing document [1982]

UBA undenatured bacterial antigen; ureidoisobutyric acid

UBB ubiquitin B

UBBC unsaturated vitamin B_{12} binding capacity

UBC ubiquitin C; University of British Columbia

UBE ubiquitin-activating enzyme

UBF uterine blood flow

UBG, Ubg urobilinogen

UBI ultraviolet blood irradiation

UBL undifferentiated B-cell lymphoma

UBM ultrasound backscatter microscopy; ultrasound biomicroscopy

UBN urobilin

UBO unidentified bright object

UBP ureteral back pressure

UBPS ultrasound bone profile score

UBS unidentified bright signal

UBT urea breath test

UBW usual body weight

UC ulcerative colitis; ultracentrifugal; umbilical cord; unchanged; unclassifiable; unconscious; undifferentiated carcinoma; undifferentiated cells; unit clerk; unsatisfactory condition; untreated cells; urea clearance; urethral catheterization; urinary catheter; urinary catheterization; urine concentrate; urine culture; usual care; uterine contractions

U&C urethral and cervical; usual and customary

UCA ultrasound contrast agent

UCAID University Corporation for Advanced Internet Development

UCARE, U-CARE Unexplained Cardiac Arrest Registry of Europe

UCB unconjugated bilirubin

UCBC umbilical cord blood culture

UCBT umbilical cord blood transplantation

UCC Uniform Code Council

UCD urine collection device; user-centered design; usual childhood diseases

UCDS uniform clinical dataset

UCE urea cycle enzymopathy

UCG ultrasonic cardiography; urinary chorionic gonadotropin

UCHD usual childhood diseases

UCI unusual childhood illness; urethral catheter in; urinary catheter in

UCL ulnar collateral ligament; upper collateral ligament; upper confidence limit; upper control limit; urea clearance

UCLP unilateral cleft of lip and palate

UCO ultrasonic cardiac output; urethral catheter out; urinary catheter out
UCOD underlying cause of death
UCP uncoupling protein; urinary coproporphyrin; urinary C-peptide
UCPT urinary coproporphyrin test
UCR unconditioned response; usual, customary, and reasonable
U$_{Cr}$ urinary creatinine
UCS ultimate compressive strength; unconditioned stimulus; unconscious; uterine compression syndrome
ucs unconscious
UCT ultrasound computed tomography; urologic care table
UCTD, uCTD undifferentiated/unclassifiable connective tissue disease
UCV uncontrolled variable; unconventional viral [disease]
UCVA uncorrected visual acuity
UD ulcerative dermatosis; ulnar deviation; underdeveloped; undetermined; unit dose; urethral dilation; urethral discharge; uridine diphosphate; uroporphyrinogen decarboxylase; use as directed; uterine delivery
UD-AHF UD-CG 115 BS in Acute Heart Failure [study]
UDB universal database
UDC University Disability Consortium; usual diseases of childhood
UDCA ursodeoxycholic acid
UDE user-defined edge
UDF user data file
UDIR underdose isodose range
UDKase uridine diphosphate kinase
UDN ulcerative dermal necrosis
UDO undetermined origin
UDP uridine diphosphate; user datagram protocol
UDPG uridine diphosphate glucose; urine diphosphoglucose
UDPGA uridine diphosphate—glucuronic acid
UDPGT uridine diphosphate glucuronosyl transferase
UDR user-defined region
UDR-BMD ultradistal radius bone mineral density
UDRP urine diribose phosphate
UDRV ulcerative disease rhabdovirus
UDS ultrasound Doppler sonography; uniform data system; unscheduled DNA synthesis
UDSTSS ultradelicate split-thickness scalp skin
UE uncertain etiology; under elbow; uninvolved epidermis; upper esophagus; upper extremity

UEA *Ulex europaeus* agglutinin
UEFFDE upper extremity fitness for duty evaluation
UEG ultrasonic encephalography; unifocal eosinophilic granuloma
UEHB uniform effective health benefits
UEL upper explosive limit
UEM universal electron microscope
UEMC unidentified endosteal marrow cell
UES upper esophageal sphincter
uE$_s$ unconjugated estriol
u/ext upper extremity
UF film unsharpness; ultrafiltrate; ultrafiltration; ultrafine; ultrasonic frequency; unaffected female; uncertainty factor; universal feeder; unknown factor; urinary formaldehyde
Uf ultrafiltration
UFA unesterified fatty acid
UFB urinary fat bodies
UFC ultrafast ceramics; urinary free cortisol
UFCT ultrafast computed tomography
UFD ultrasonic flow detector; unilateral facet dislocation
UFFI urea-formaldehyde foam insulation
UFH unfractionated heparin
UFL upper flammable limit; upper frequency limit
UFN unreamed femoral nail
UFOV useful field of view
UFP ultrafiltration pressure
UFR ultrafiltration rate; urine filtration rate; uroflowmetry
uFSH urinary follicle-stimulating hormone
UG geometric unsharpness; urogastrone; urogenital
Ug uracyl glycol
UGCR ultrasound-guided compression repair
UGD urogenital diaphragm
UGDP University Group Diabetes Project
UGDV Uasin Gishu disease virus
UGF unidentified growth factor
UGH uveitis, glaucoma, hyphema [syndrome]
UGH+ uveitis, glaucoma, hyphema plus vitreous hemorrhage [syndrome]
UGI upper gastrointestinal
UGIH upper gastrointestinal hemorrhage
UGIS upper gastrointestinal series
UGME undergraduate medical education
UGP uridyl diphosphate glucose pyrophosphorylase
UGPA undergraduate grade-point average
UGPP uridyl diphosphate glucose pyrophosphorylase
UGS urogenital sinus
UGSV Uganda S virus

UGT uridine diphosphate—glucuronosyltransferase; urogenital tract; urogenital tuberculosis

UH umbilical hernia; unaffected hemisphere; uncontrolled hemorrhage; unfavorable histology; upper half

UHC University HealthSystem Consortium

UHD universal heteroduplex generator; unstable hemoglobin disease

UHDDS uniform hospital discharge dataset

UHDRS unified Huntington disease rating scale

UHDS uniform hospital dataset

UHF ultrahigh frequency

UHID universal health care identifier

UHIS universal health care information system; university hospital information system

UHL universal hypertrichosis lanuginosa

UHMM ultrahigh-magnification mammography

UHMW ultrahigh molecular weight

UHMWPE ultrahigh molecular weight polyethylene

UHN unreamed humeral nail

UHR underlying heart rhythm

UHS uncontrolled hemorrhagic shock; university health services

UHSC university health services clinic

UHT ultrahigh temperature

UI urinary incontinence; uroporphyrin isomerase; user interface

U/I unidentified

UIBC unsaturated iron-binding capacity

UIC urinary iodine concentration

UICAO unilateral internal carotid artery occlusion

UICC International Union Against Cancer [Fr. *Union Internationale Contre le Cancer*]

UID unique identifier; unique image identifier

UIF undegraded insulin factor

UIL user interface language

UIMS user interface management system

UIP unintended pregnancy; usual interstitial pneumonia

UIQ upper inner quadrant

UIR unsolicited information retrieval

UIS utilization information service

UJT unijunction transistor

UK unknown; uridine kinase; urinary kallikrein; urokinase

UKA unicompartmental knee arthroplasty

UKα urinary kallikrein

UKAEA United Kingdom Atomic Energy Authority

UKase uridine kinase

UKCCSG United Kingdom Children's Cancer Study Group

UK-COMA United Kingdom Committee on Medical Aspects [of food and nutrition]

UKCSG United Kingdom Collaborative Study Group

UKEGNS United Kingdom Epidemiology Group for the Nutrition Society

UKHAS United Kingdom Heart Attack Study

UKHEART United Kingdom Heart Failure Evaluation and Assessment of Risk Trial

UK in USA Urokinase in Unstable Angina [study]

UKM urea kinetic modeling

ukn unknown

UKNCSPAIVS United Kingdom National Collaborative Study of Pulmonary Atresia with Intact Ventricular Septum

UKPACE United Kingdom Pacing and Cardiovascular Events [study]; United Kingdom Pacing and Clinical Events [study]

UKPDS United Kingdom Prospective Diabetes Study

UKR unicompartmental knee replacement

UKSAT United Kingdom Small Aneurysm Trial

UK-TIA United Kingdom Transient Ischemic Attack [trial]

UKTSSA United Kingdom Transplant Support Service Authority

UL ultrasonic; Underwriters Laboratories; undifferentiated lymphoma; upper limb; upper limit; upper lobe

U&L upper and lower

U/Li units per liter

ULAM United Network for Organ Sharing Liver Allocation Model

ULBW ultralow birth weight

ULD Unverricht-Lundborg disease

ULDH urinary lactate dehydrogenase

ULDR ultralow dose rate

ULF ultralow frequency

ULL ultra-lipo-lift

ULLE upper lid of left eye

ULM unprotected left main

ULN upper limit of normal

uln ulna, ulnar

ULP ultralow profile; User Liaison Program

ULPA ultralow-penetration air filter

ULPE upper lobe pulmonary edema

ULQ upper left quadrant

ULR universal leukoreduction

ULRE upper lid of right eye

ULSB upper left sternal border

ULT ultrahigh temperature

ult ultimate

ULTC urban level trauma center

ULTIMA Unprotected Left Main Trunk Intervention Multicenter Assessment

ULTRA utilizing GFX 2.5 stent in small diameter arteries

UltraSTAR ultrasound structured attribute reporting

ULV ultralow volume

ULvWF unusually large von Willebrand factor

UM movement unsharpness; ultrarapid metabolizer; unaffected male; upper motor [neuron]; uracil mustard; utilization management

uM, μM micromole, micromolar

UMA ulcerative mutilating acropathy; upright membrane assay; urinary muramidase activity

UMAV Umatilla virus

Umax maximum urinary osmolality

umb umbilicus, umbilical

UMBV Umbre virus

UMC unidimensional chromatography; university medical center

UM-CIDI University of Michigan Composite International Diagnostic Interview

UMCV-TO ulnar motor conduction velocity across thoracic outlet

UMD unmodified domain

UMDNS Universal Medical Device Nomenclature System

UME undergraduate medical education

UMHDS uniform minimum health dataset

UMI unrecognized myocardial infarction; urinary meconium index

UMIN university medical information network

UMKase uridine monophosphate kinase

UML unified modeling language

UMLS Unified Medical Language System

UMN upper motor neuron

UMNL upper motor neuron lesion

UMNS upper motor neuron syndrome

UMP uridine monophosphate

UMPH uridine 5′-monophosphate phosphohydrolase

UMPK uridine monophosphate kinase

UMPS uridine monophosphate synthase

UMS urethral manipulation syndrome

UMT units of medical time

UN ulnar nerve; undernourished; unilateral neglect; updraft nebulizer; urea nitrogen; urinary nitrogen

UNa, U_Na urinary sodium

UNAI Uniform Needs Assessment Instrument

UNAIDS United Nations Acquired Immunodeficiency Syndrome [program]

UNASEM Unstable Angina Study Using Eminase

UNAV Una virus

uncomp uncompensated

uncond unconditioned

UNCV ulnar nerve conduction velocity

undet undetermined

UNDP United Nations Development Program

UNDRO United Nations Disaster Relief Organization

UNE urinary norepinephrine

UNEP United Nations Environmental Program

UNEX Unexplained Deaths Project

UNFPA United Nations Population Fund

UNG uracil deoxyribonucleic acid glycosylase

UNGASS United Nations General Assembly Special Session [on HIV/AIDS]

UNHCR United Nations High Commission on Refugees

UniGene Unique Human Gene Sequence Collection

unilat unilateral

UNIS Urological Nursing Information Systems

univ universal

unk, unkn unknown

UNL upper normal limit

UNLS Unified Nursing Language System

UNODC United Nations Office on Drugs and Crime

UNOS United Network for Organ Sharing

UNRPCA Use of Nicardipine to Retard the Progression of Coronary Atherosclerosis [trial]

UNSA Unstable Angina Study

unsat unsatisfactory; unsaturated

UNSCEAR United Nations Scientific Committee on the Effects of Atomic Radiation

UNT untreated

UNTS unilateral nevoid telangiectasia syndrome

UNX uninephrectomy

UO under observation; undetermined origin; urethral orifice; urinary output

U/O urinary output

u/o under observation

UOP urinary output

UOQ upper outer quadrant

UOsm urinary osmolality

UOV units of variance

UOX urate oxidase

UP parallax unsharpness; ulcerative proctitis; ultrahigh purity; unipolar; upright posture; ureteropelvic; uridine phosphorylase; uroporphyrin; urticaria pigmentosa

U/P urine/plasma ratio

uPA, u-PA urokinase plasminogen acti-vator

uPAR urokinase-type plasminogen activator receptor

UPase uridine phosphorylase

UPC usual provider continuity

UPD ulcerative periodontal disease; uniparental disomy; urinary production

UPDIC Uppsala Prospective Diabetes Control [study]

UPDRS Unified Parkinson's Disease Rating Scale

UPEC uropathogenic *Escherichia coli* signature-tagged mutagenesis A

UPEP urinary protein electrophoresis; urine protein electrophoresis

UPET Urokinase Pulmonary Embolism Trial

UPF universal proximal femur [prosthesis]

UPG uroporphyrinogen

UPGMA unweighted pair group method with averages

UPI unique patient identifier; uteroplacental insufficiency; uteroplacental ischemia

UPID uniparental isodisomy

UPIF uniform provider [electronic] interchange format

UPIN universal physician identifier number

UPJ ureteropelvic junction

UPJO ureteropelvic junction obstruction

UPL unusual position of limbs

UPLN upper limit of normal

UPOV Upolu virus

UPP urethral pressure profile

UPPP uvulopalatopharyngoplasty

UPPRA upright peripheral plasma renin activity

UPS ultraviolet photoelectron spectroscopy; uninterruptible power supply; uroporphyrinogen synthetase; uterine progesterone system

UPSC uterine papillary serous carcinoma

UPSIT University of Pennsylvania Smell Identification Test

UPSIZE Ultrasound-Controlled Percutaneous Transluminal Coronary Angioplasty with Optional Balloon Size [study]

UpU uridyl (3′-5′) uridine

UQ ubiquinone; upper quadrant

UQAC unit quality assurance committee

UQCRC ubiquinol-cytochrome Creductase core

UQL unacceptable quality level

UQS upper quadrant syndrome

UR unconditioned reflex; upper respiratory; uridine; urinal; urology; utilization review

Ur urea; urinary, urine

URA unilateral renal agenesis

URA, Ura uracil

URAC American Accreditation Health Care Commission; Utilization Review Accreditation Commission

URALMI Urokinase and Alteplase in Myocardial Infarction [study]

URC upper rib cage; utilization review committee

URD unrelated donor; unspecified respiratory disease; upper respiratory disease

Urd uridine

ureth urethra

URF unidentified reading frame; unique recombinant form; uterine relaxing factor

URG urogastrone

URI uniform resource identifier; upper respiratory illness; upper respiratory infection

URISA Urban and Regional Information Systems Association

URK urokinase

URL uniform resource locator; upper rate limit [pacemaker]; upper reference level

URN uniform resource name

U-RNA uridylic acid–ribonucleic acid

URO urology; uroporphyrin; uroporphyrinogen; utilization review organization

UROD ultrarapid opioid detoxification; uroporphyrinogen decarboxylase

URO-GEN urogenital

Urol urologist, urology

UROS uroporphyrinogen synthase

URQ upper right quadrant

URR upstream regulatory region

URS ultrasonic renal scanning; upstream repressing sequence

URSB upper right sternal border

UR2SV UR2 sarcoma virus

URT upper respiratory tract

URTI upper respiratory tract infection

URUV Urucuri virus

URVD unilateral renovascular disease

US screen unsharpness; ultrasonic, ultrasonography, ultrasound; unconditioned stimulus; unique sequence; unit separator; upper segment; upper strength; urinary sugar; Usher syndrome

US1 Usher syndrome type I

US1A Usher syndrome type IA

US1B Usher syndrome type IB

US1C Usher syndrome type IC

US2 Usher syndrome type II

US2A Usher syndrome type IIA

US2B Usher syndrome type IIB

US3 Usher syndrome type III
US4 Usher syndrome type IV
u/s ultrasonic; ultrasound
USAID United States Agency for International Development
USAN United States Adopted Name
USAR urban search and rescue
USASI United States of America Standards Institute
USAT ultrasmall aperture terminal
USB upper sternal border
USBS United States Bureau of Standards
USCA ultrasound contrast agent
USCG ultrasonic cardiography
USCR universal self-care requisites
USCT ultrasound computed tomography
USD United States Dispensary
USDA United States Department of Agriculture
USDHEW United States Department of Health, Education, and Welfare
USDHHS United States Department of Health and Human Services
USE ultrasonic echography
USEIR United States Eye Injury Registry
USF upstream stimulatory factor
USFA United States Fire Administration
USFAE ultrasonic superficial femoral artery endarterectomy
USFMG United States foreign medical graduate
USFMS United States foreign medical student
USG ultrasonography; user semantic group
USH Usher syndrome
USH1 Usher syndrome type 1
USH1A Usher syndrome type 1A
USH1B Usher syndrome type 1B
USH1C Usher syndrome type 1C
USH2 Usher syndrome type 2
USH2A Usher syndrome type 2A
USH2B Usher syndrome type 2B
USH3 Usher syndrome type 3
USH4 Usher syndrome type 4
US+HC ultrasound-driven hydrocortisone
USHL United States Hygienic Laboratory
USI universal serial interface; urinary stress incontinence
USIMG United States [citizen] international medical school graduate
USL ultrasound lithotripsy
US/LS upper strength/lower strength ratio
USMG United States or Canada medical school graduate
USMLE United States Medical Licensing Examination
USN ultrasonic nebulizer; unilateral spatial neglect

USNCHS United States National Center for Health Statistics
USNRP United States National Reference Preparation
USO unilateral salpingo-oophorectomy
USP ultrasound-guided puncture; United States Pharmacopeia
US+P ultrasound and placebo
USPC United States Pharmacopeia Convention
USPDI United States Pharmacopeia Drug Information
USPET Urokinase Streptokinase Pulmonary Embolism Trial
USPHS United States Public Health Service; United States Physicians' Health Study
USPIO ultrasmall particle superparamagnetic iron oxide
USPSTF United States Preventive Services Task Force
USPTA United States Physical Therapy Association
USR unheated serum reagin
USRDS United States Renal Data System
USS ultrasound scanning; universal spine system; user support system
USUV Usutu virus
USVMD urine specimen volume measuring device
USW ultrashort waves
UT total unsharpness; Ullrich-Turner [syndrome]; Unna-Thost [syndrome]; untested; untreated; urinary tract; urticaria
uT unbound testosterone
UTBG unbound thyroxine-binding globulin
UTC ultrasonic tissue characterization; upper thoracic compression
UTD up to date
UT-ETT ultrathin endotracheal tube
UTI urinary tract infection; urinary trypsin inhibitor
util rev utilization review
UTIV Utinga virus
UTO upper tibial osteotomy; urinary tract obstruction
UTOPIA Utilization of Platelet Inhibition in Angina [trial]
UTP unilateral tension pneumothorax; unshielded twisted pair; uridine triphosphate
UTR untranslated region
UTS Ullrich-Turner syndrome; ulnar tunnel syndrome; ultimate tensile strength
UTTS-ETT two-stage ultrathin-walled endotracheal tube
UTZ ultrasound
UU urinary urea; urine urobilinogen
UUID universal unique identifier
UUKV Uukuniemi virus

UUN urinary urea nitrogen
UUO unilateral urethral obstruction
UUP urinary uroporphyrin
uUTI uncomplicated urinary tract infection
UV ultraviolet; umbilical vein; Uppsala virus; ureterovesical; urinary volume
UVA ultraviolet A; ultraviolet germicidal irradiation; ureterovesical angle
UV-A ultraviolet A
UVAL-MED universal visual associative language for medicine
UVB, UV-B ultraviolet B
UVC Ullucus virus C; ultraviolet C; umbilical venous catheter
UV-C ultraviolet C
UVEB unifocal ventricular ectopic beat

UVER ultraviolet-enhanced reactivation
UVGI ultraviolet germicidal irradiation
UVI ultraviolet irradiation
UVJ ureterovesical junction
UVL ultraviolet light
UVO uvomorulin
UVP ultraviolet photometry
UVR ultraviolet radiation
UVV Utive virus
UW unilateral weakness
UWB unit of whole blood
UWD Urbach-Wiethe disease
UWSC unstimulated whole saliva collection
UWW underwater weight
UX uranium X, proactinium
UYP upper yield point

V

V coefficient of variation; electrical potential [volts]; a logical binary relation that is true if any argument is true and false otherwise; luminous efficiency; potential; potential energy; unipolar chest lead [ECG]; vaccinated, vaccine; vagina; valine; valve; vanadium; variable, variation; varnish; vector; vegetarian; vein; velocity; venom, venomous; venous; venous tumor invasion; ventilation; ventricle; ventricular; verbal comprehension; vertebra; vertex; vertex sharp transient [EEG]; vestibular; Vibrio; vincristine; violet; viral; virion; virulence; virus; vision; visual acuity; volt; voltage; volume; vomiting
V0 no evidence of venous [tumor] invasion
V$_{0.5}$ midpoint voltage
V1 primary visual area; venous [tumor] invasion assessed
V$_1$ mean flow velocity
V1 to V6 ventral 1 to ventral 6 [chest leads in ECG]
v rate of reaction catalyzed by an enzyme; specific volume; valve; vein; velocity; venous; ventricular; versus; very; virus; vision; volt; volume
VA alveolar ventilation; vacuum aspiration; valproic acid; vasodilator agent; ventricular aneurysm; ventricular arrhythmia; ventriculoatrial; ventroanterior; Veterans Administration; Veterans Affairs; vincristine, Adriamycin; viral antigen; visual acuity; visual aid; visual axis; volt-ampere; volume average
V$_A$ alveolar ventilation
V/A volt/ampere
V-A venoarterial
Va activated factor V
V$_a$ alveolar ventilation
va volt-ampere
VAAE vaccine-associated adverse events
VAB vincristine, actinomycin D, and bleomycin; violent antisocial behavior
VAB-6 vincristine, actinomycin, bleomycin, cisplatin, Cytoxan
VABP venoarterial bypass pumping; ventilator-associated bacterial pneumonia
VABS Vineland Adaptive Behavior Scales
VAC vacuum-assisted closure; ventriculoatrial conduction; vincristine, doxorubicin, and cyclophosphamide; virus capsid antigen
vac vacuum

VACA Valvuloplasty and Angioplasty of Congenital Anomalies [registry]
VAcc visual acuity with correction
vacc vaccination
VACO Veterans Affairs Central Office
VACS Veterans Administration Cooperative Study
VACSDM Veterans Affairs Cooperative Study on Glycemic Control and Complications in Non-Insulin Dependent Diabetes Mellitus
VACT Veterans Administration Cooperative Trial
VACTERL vertebral abnormalities, anal atresia, cardiac abnormalities, tracheoesophageal fistula and/or esophageal atresia, renal agenesis and dysplasia, and limb defects [association]
VACV vaccinia virus
VAD venous access device; ventricular assist device; vinblastine and dexamethasone; virus-adjusting diluent; vitamin A deficiency
VaD vascular dementia
VADD vitamin A deficiency disorder
VAE venous air emboli; vertical attachment energy
VA-ECMO venoarterial extracorporeal membrane oxygenation
VAEG visual and auditory environment generator
VAERS Vaccine Adverse Events Reporting System
VAEV Vearoy virus
VAF viral-free antigen
VAFC vacuum-assisted fascial closure
VAG vibroarthrography
vag vagina, vaginal, vaginitis
VAG HYST vaginal hysterectomy
VAH vertebral ankylosing hyperostosis; Veterans Affairs Hospital; virilizing adrenal hyperplasia
VA-HIT Veterans Affairs High-Density Lipoprotein Intervention Trial
VAHS virus-associated hemophagocytic syndrome
VAIN vaginal intraepithelial neoplasm
V$_{ak}$ atrial volume constant
VAL valproate
Val valine
val valine; valve
VALE visual acuity, left eye
Val-HeFT Valsartan-Heart Failure Trial
VALIANT Valsartan in Acute Myocardial Infarction [study]
VALID Velocity Assessment for Lesions of Intermediate Severity [trial]

VALID II Velocity Assessment for Lesions of Indeterminate Severity [trial]

ValRS valyl ribonucleic acid synthetase

VALUE Valsartan Antihypertensive Long-Term Use Evaluation

VAM ventricular arrhythmia monitor; virtual archive manager

VAMC Veterans Affairs Medical Center

VAMCS Veterans Affairs Medical Center Score

VAMP venous arterial blood management protection [system]; vincristine, amethopterine, 6-mercaptopurine, and prednisone

VAN value-added network; vein, artery, nerve

VANQWISH Veterans Affairs Non-Q-Wave Infarction Strategies In-Hospital [study]

VAP vaginal acid phosphatase; variant angina pectoris; venous access port; ventilator-associated pneumonia; virulence-attenuated pool

vap vapor

VAPP vaccine-associated paralytic poliomyelitis

VAPS visual analog pain score

VAPSE variation affecting protein structure or expression

VAPSHCS Veterans Affairs Puget Sound Health Care System

V$_a$/Q alveolar ventilation/perfusion ratio

VA/Q$_c$ ventilation/perfusion ratio

VAR vector autoregressive [model algorithm]; venoarteriolar reflex; visual-auditory range

Var variable; variant, variation, variety; varicella

var variable; variant, variation, variety; varicose

VARE visual acuity, right eye

VARETA variable-resolution electromagnetic tomography

VA RNA virus-associated ribonucleic acid

VARPRO variable projection

VARS valyl-transfer ribonucleic acid synthetase

VARV variola virus

VAS vagal afferents; vascular; vascular access service; ventricular assist system; ventriculoatrial shunt; Verapamil Angioplasty Study; vesicle attachment site; vestibular aqueduct syndrome; Veterans Adjustment Scale; vibroacoustic stimulation; video-assisted surgery; viral arthritis syndrome; visual analog scale

VASC vascular; Verbal Auditory Screening for Children; visual-auditory screening

VAsc visual acuity without correction

vasc vascular

VASD Vascular Access Service Database

VASER Vibration Amplification of Sound Energy at Resonance [study]

VASP vasodilator-stimulated phosphoprotein

VASPNAF Veterans Administration Stroke Prevention in Nonrheumatic Atrial Fibrillation [study]

VAS RAD vascular radiology

VAST visual analysis systems technology

VAST/STT visual analysis systems technology/space-time toolkit

VAT variable antigen type; vasoocclusive angiotherapy; ventricular accommodation test; ventricular activation time; vesicular amine transformer; video-assisted thoracoscopy; visceral adipose tissue; visual action therapy; visual action time; visual apperception test; vocational apperception test

VATER vertebral defects, imperforate anus, tracheoesophageal fistula, and radial and renal dysplasia [association]

v-ATPase vascular adenosine triphosphatase

VATS Veterans Administration medical center transference syndrome; video-assisted thoracic surgery

VATs surface variable antigen

VATT vascular anatomy teaching tool

VAV variable air volume

VAWC vacuum-assisted wound closure

VB vaginal bulb; valence bond; venous blood; ventrobasal; veronal buffer; vertebrobasilar; viable birth; vinblastine; virus buffer; voided bladder

Vb vinblastine

VBAC vaginal birth after cesarean section

VBAIN vertebrobasilar artery insufficiency nystagmus

VBAS ViewSite Brain Access System

VBC vincristine, bleomycin, and cisplatin; visualization in biomedical computing; volumetric-based capnometry

VBD vanishing bile duct; veronal-buffered diluent

VBE visualized bronchus endoscope

VBF variable bandwidth filter

VBG vagotomy and Billroth gastroenterostomy; venous blood gases; venous bypass graft; vertical-banded gastroplasty

VBI ventral blood island; vertebrobasilar insufficiency; vertebrobasilar ischemia

VBL vinblastine

VBM voxel-based morphometry

VbMF vinblastine, methotrexate, 5-fluorouracil

VBNC viable but nonculturable [microorganism]

vBNS very-high-bandwidth network service; very-high-performance backbone network service

VBOS veronal-buffered oxalated saline

VBP vagal body paraganglia; venous blood pressure; ventricular premature beat

VBR ventricular brain ratio; vertebral body replacement; vertebral body repositioning; voxel-based relaxometry

VBS veronal-buffered saline; vertebrobasilar system

VBS:FBS veronal-buffered saline–fetal bovine serum

VBT vascular brachytherapy

VBWG Vascular Biology Working Group

VBX visual basic controls

VC color vision; variance cardiography; variation coefficient; vascular changes; vasoconstriction; vena cava; venereal case; venous capacitance; ventilatory capacity; ventral column; ventricular contraction; vertebral canal; Veterinary Corps; videocassette; video conference; vincristine; vinyl chloride; virtual coloscopy; virus C; visual capacity; visual cortex; vital capacity; vocal cord

V/C ventilation/circulation ratio

Vc vital capacity

V$_c$ volume of [central] compartment

vc verbal cues

VCA vancomycin, colistin, and anisomycin; viral capsid antigen

VCAM vascular cell adhesion molecule

VCAP vincristine, cyclophosphamide, Adriamycin, and prednisone

VCB ventricular capture beat

vCBF venous cerebral blood flow

VCC vasoconstrictor center; ventral cell column

VC-CFMV volume-controlled constant-flow mechanical ventilation

VCD Van Capelle–Durrer [model]; vibrational circular dichroism

VCE vagina, ectocervix, and endocervix; videocapsule endoscopy

VCF velocardiofacial [syndrome]; velocity of circumferential fiber [lengthening]; ventricular contractility function

VCFG volume-cycled flow generator

VCF$_{min}$ minimum velocity of circumferential fiber [lengthening]

VCFS velocardiofacial syndrome

VCG vectorcardiogram, vectorcardiography; voiding cystourethrography; volumetric cardiogram

VCHS Virginia Center for Health Statistics

VCL vinculin; visual concept library; Voxtool Command Language

VCM vinyl chloride monomer

V$_{cM}$ volume of [central] compartment for metabolite

VCMP vincristine, cyclophosphamide, melphalan, and prednisone

VCN vancomycin, colistomethane, and nystatin; *Vibrio cholerae* neuraminidase

VCO endogenous production of carbon monoxide; voltage-controlled oscillator

V$_{CO}$ endogenous production of carbon monoxide

VCO$_2$ carbon dioxide elimination rate; carbon dioxide output

V$_{CO_2}$ carbon dioxide output

VCP vincristine, cyclophosphamide, and prednisone

VCR vasoconstriction rate; vincristine; volume clearance rate

VCRS virtual center for renal support; voluntary cardiorespiratory synchronization

VCS vasoconstrictor substance; vesicocervical space; virtual chart system

VCSA viral cell surface antigen

VCSF ventricular cerebrospinal fluid

VCT venous clotting time; volume computed tomography; voluntary counseling and testing

VCU video conference unit; videocystourethrography; voiding cystourethrogram, voiding cystourethrography

VCUG vesicoureterogram; voiding cystourethrogram

VCV vein chlorosis virus; vein clearing virus

VD vapor density; vascular disease; vasodilation, vasodilator; venereal disease; venous dilation; ventricular dilator; ventrodorsal; verbal dysphasia; vertical deviation; vertical divergence; video disk; viral diarrhea; voided; volume of dead space; volume of distribution

V&D vomiting and diarrhea

V$_D$ dead space; volume of distribution

Vd value of [drug] distribution; viroid; voided, voiding; volume of dead space; volume of distribution

V$_d$ apparent volume of distribution

V$_D$ dead space

V/D vomiting and diarrhea [veterinary medicine]

VDA vascular disrupting agent; virtual DNA analysis; visual discriminatory acuity

VDAC voltage-dependent anion channel

VDB virtual database

VdB van der Bergh [test]

VDBR volume of distribution of bilirubin

VDC vasodilator center

VDCC voltage-dependent calcium channel

VDD atrial synchronous ventricular inhibited [pacemaker]; vitamin D dependent

VDDR vitamin D–dependent rickets

VDE vertical detachment energy

VDEL Venereal Disease Experimental Laboratory

VDEM vasodepressor material

VDF ventricular diastolic fragmentation

VDG, VD-G venereal disease–gonorrhea

vdg voiding

VDH valvular disease of the heart

VDI venous distensibility index; virtual desktop infrastructure; virus defective interfering [particle]

V$_{dia}$ diastolic potential

VDL vasodepressor lipid; visual detection level

VDM vasodepressor material

vDOC virtual distributed online clinic

VDP ventricular premature depolarization

VDPV vaccine-derived poliovirus

VDR venous diameter ratio; vitamin D receptor

VDRG vitamin D receptor gene

VDRL Venereal Disease Research Laboratory [syphilis test]

VDRR vitamin D–resistant rickets

VDRT venereal disease reference test

VDS vasodilator substance; vindesine

VDS, VD-S venereal disease–syphilis

VDT vector distance transform; vibration disappearance threshold; visual display terminal; visual distortion test

VDU video display unit

VDV ventricular end-diastolic volume

V$_D$/V$_T$ dead space/tidal volume ratio

Vd/Vt dead space ventilation/total ventilation ratio

VDWS Van der Woude syndrome

VE vaccine effectiveness; vaginal examination; valve equivalent [mechanical]; vascular endothelial; Venezuelan encephalitis; venous emptying; venous extension; ventilation; ventilatory equivalent; ventricular elasticity; ventricular extrasystole; vertex; vesicular exanthema; viral encephalitis; virtual endoscopy; virtual environment; visual efficiency; vitamin E; volume ejection; voluntary effort

V&E vinyl and ether (Vinethene)

V$_E$ environmental variance; respiratory minute volume

V$_E$ minute ventilation

Ve ventilation

V$_e$ volume of effect compartment

VEA ventricular ectopic activity; ventricular ectopic arrhythmia; viral envelope antigen

VEB ventricular ectopic beat

VEC velocity encoding cine; virtual environment control

VEcad vascular endothelial cadherin

VECG vector electrocardiogram

VEC-MR velocity encoded cine–magnetic resonance

VECP visually evoked cortical potential

VED vacuum erection device; ventricular ectopic depolarization; virtual environment display [system]; vital exhaustion and depression

VEE vagina, ectocervix, and endocervix; Venezuelan equine encephalomyelitis

VEEV Venezuelan equine encephalitis virus

VEF ventricular ejection fraction; visually evoked field

VEG vegetation; von Egner gland

VEGAS Vein Graft Angiojet Study; ventricular enlargement with gait apraxia syndrome

VEGF vascular endothelial growth factor

VEGF-A vascular endothelial growth factor type A

VEGP von Ebner gland protein

vehic vehicle

VEI volume [lung] at the end of inspiration

VEID Vein Entry Indicator Device

VEINES Venous Insufficiency Epidemiologic and Economic Study

vel, veloc velocity

VELV Vellore virus

VEM vasoexcitor material

VEMR virtual electronic medical record

VENC velocity encoding

vent ventilation; ventral; ventricle, ventricular

vent fib ventricular fibrillation

ventric ventricle

VENUS Very Early Nimodipine Use in Stroke [trial]

VEP visual evoked potential

VEPID video-based electronic portal imaging device

VEPT volume of electrically participating thoracic tissue

VEPTR vertical expandable prosthetic titanium rib

VER ventricular evoked response; visual evoked response

Verc vervet kidney cells

VERDI Verapamil vs. Diuretics [trial]

VERDICT Verapamil Digoxin Cardioversion Trial; Veterans Evidence-Based Research, Dissemination, and Implementation Center

VERP visual event-related potential

vert vertebra, vertebral

VES virtual endoscope system; viscoelastic substance

ves bladder [L. *vesica*]; vesicular; vessel

VESA virtual endoscopy software application

vesic blister [L. *vesicula*]

VEST Vesnarinone Trial

vest vestibular

ves ur urinary bladder [L. *vesica urinaria*]

VET ventricular ejection time; vestigial testis

Vet veteran; veterinarian; veterinary

VETF vaccinia early transcription factor

VetMB Bachelor of Veterinary Medicine

Vet Med veterinary medicine

VETS Veterinary Expert Technology System

Vet Sci veterinary science

VEUD virtual emergency and urgency department

VF left leg [electrode]; ventricular fibrillation; ventricular fluid; ventricular flutter; ventricular function; videofluorography; virologic failure; visual field; vitreous fluorophotometry; vocal fremitus

Vf visual frequency

V$_f$ final voltage; variant frequency

vf visual field

VFA volatile fatty acid

VFC vaccine for children; ventricular function curve

VFD vacuum fluorescent display; visual feedback display; visual field defect

VFDP variant familial developmental pattern

VFI vascularization flow index; venous filling index; visual field intact

V fib ventricular fibrillation

VFID virtual focus isocenter distance

VFL ventricular flutter

VFOS vector fast orthogonal search

VFP ventricular filling pressure; ventricular fluid pressure; vocal fold pathology

VFR visiting friends and relatives; voiding flow rate

VFS vascular fragility syndrome; very fast sedimentation; visual file system

VFT venous filling time; ventricular fibrillation threshold

VF/VT ventricular fibrillation/ventricular tachycardia

VG van Gieson [stain]; ventricular gallop; volume of gas

V$_G$ genetic variance

VGA video graphics array

VGAS visual grading analysis score

VGAT vesicular gamma-aminobutyric acid transporter

VGB vigabatrin

VGCC voltage-gated calcium channels

VGH very good health

vGI ventral giant interneuron

VGKC voltage-gated potassium channels

VGLUT vesicular glutamate transporter

VGM venous graft myringoplasty

VGP viral glycoprotein

VGPO volume-guaranteed pressure options [ventilation]

VGS video game–induced seizures

VH vaginal hysterectomy; venous hematocrit; ventral hippocampus; ventricular hypertrophy; veterans hospital; viral hepatitis; virtual hospital; Visible Human [project]

V$_H$ variable domain of heavy chain; variable heavy chain

Vh volt-hours

VHA Veterans Health Administration; Voluntary Hospital Association

V/Hallu visual hallucinations

VHAS Verapamil in Hypertension Atherosclerosis Study

VHCD virtual health care databank

VHD valvular heart disease; viral hematodepressive disease; Visible Human Dataset

VHDL very-high-density lipoprotein

V-HeFT Vasodilator Heart Failure Trial; Veterans Administration Heart Failure Trial

VHEV Vilyuisk human encephalomyelitis virus

VHF very high frequency; viral hemorrhagic fever; visual half-field

VH-IVUS virtual histology intravascular ultrasound

VHL Virtual Health Library; von Hippel–Lindau [disease]

VHN Vickers hardness number

VHP vaporized hydrogen peroxide; Visible Human Project

VHR ventricular heart rate

VHS Veterans Health Study

VHS&RA Veterans Health Service and Research Administration

VHSV viral hemorrhagic septicemia virus

VI vaginal irrigation; variable interval; vascularization index; vastus intermedius; ventilation index; virgo intacta; virtual document; virulence, virulent; viscosity index; visual impairment; visual inspection; vitality index; volume index

V$_I$ initial voltage

Vi virulence, virulent

VIA virus inactivating agent; virus infection-associated antigen; visual inspection with acetic acid

VIB viral inclusion body

vib vibration

VIBE volumetric interpolated breath-hold examination

vib & perc vibration and percussion

VIC valvular interstitial cell; variable impedance characterization; vasoinhibitory center; virtual information center; visual communication therapy; voice intensity control

VICP Vaccine Injury Compensation Program

VICTOR Vioxx in Colorectal Cancer Therapy: Definition of Optimal Regime [trial]

VI-CTS vibration-induced carpal tunnel syndrome

VID visible iris diameter

VIDA viability identification with dipyridamole-dobutamine administration

VIDE Virus Identification Data Exchange

VIDERO virtual delivery room

VIDRL Victorian Infectious Diseases Reference Laboratory

VIF variance inflation factor; virus-induced interferon

VIG, VIg vaccinia immune globulin; vaccinia immunoglobulin

VIGIM intravascular vaccinia immunoglobulin

VIGIV intravenous vaccinia immunoglobulin

VIGOUR Virtual Coordinating Center for Global Collaborative Cardiovascular Research

VIGRE velocity imaging with gradient-recalled echos

VIIag factor VII antigen

VIIIAGN factor VIII antigen

VIIIc factor VIII clotting activity

VIII$_{vwf}$ factor VIII von Willebrand factor

VIL villin

VILI ventilator-induced lung injury

VIM video-intensification microscopy; vimentin

VIN vulvar intraepithelial neoplasm

vin vinyl

VINDICATE vascular, inflammatory/infectious, neoplastic/neurologic/psychiatric, degenerative/dietary, intoxication/idiopathic/iatrogenic, congenital, allergic/autoimmune, trauma, endocrine/metabolic [mnemonic]

VINV Vinces virus

VIP vaccine information pamphlet; vasoactive intestinal peptide; vasoinhibitory peptide; venous impedance plethysmography; ventricular inotropic parameter; Viability Impact on Prognosis [study]; video interface processor; voluntary interruption of pregnancy

vip vegetative insecticidal enterotoxin

VIPERS virtual intelligent patient electronic record system

VIPoma vasoactive intestinal polypeptide−secreting tumor

VIPOR Vermont Integrated Problem Oriented Record

VIQ Verbal Intelligence Quotient

vIQ virtual inhibitory quotient

VIR virology

Vir virus, viral

vir virulent

Virahep-C Viral Resistance to Antiviral Therapy of Chronic Hepatitis C [study]

VIRTUOS virtual radiotherapy simulation and verification

VIS vaccine information statement; vaginal irrigation smear; value-intensity-strength; venous insufficiency syndrome; vertebral irritation syndrome; visible; visual information storage

vis vision, visual

VISA vancomycin-intermediate *Staphylococcus aureus*

VISC vitreous infusion suction cutter

visc viscera, visceral; viscosity

VISI volar intercalated segment instability

VISIR Verification and Information System in Radiology

VISN veterans Integrated Service Network

VISNA visna-maedi virus

VISP Vitamin Intervention for Stroke Prevention [trial]

Vit vitamin

vit vital

VITA Vicenza Thrombophilia and Atherosclerosis Project

VITALS vital indicators of teaching and learning success

vit cap vital capacity

VIVAS Vaccination Information Vaccination Administration System

VIVIAN virtual intracranial visualization and navigation

VJ ventriculojugular

VJC ventriculojugular cardiac

VK vervet kidney [cells]

VKC vernal keratoconjunctivitis

VKG videokymography

VKH, VKHS Vogt-Koyanagi-Harada [syndrome]

VL left arm [electrode]; vastus lateralis; ventralis lateralis; ventrolateral; viral load; visceral leishmaniasis; vision, left [eye]

V$_L$ lung volume; variable domain of the light chain; variable light chain

VLA very late activation; viruslike agent

VLAB, VLA-β very late activation protein beta

V LACT venous lactate

VLAN virtual online area network

VLAS vector least squares

VLB vinblastine; vincaleukoblastine
VLBR very low birth rate
VLBW very low birth weight
VLC variable length coding
VLCAD very long chain acyl-coenzyme A dehydrogenase
VLCD very low calorie diet
VLCFA very long chain fatty acid
VLD very low density; volume limiter disk
VLDL, VLDLP very-low-density lipoprotein
VLDLR very-low-density lipoprotein receptor
VLDL-TG very-low-density lipoprotein–triglyceride complex
V$_{LES}$ volume of lesion
VLF very low frequency
VLG ventral nucleus of the lateral geniculate body
VLH ventrolateral nucleus of the hypothalamus
VLIA viruslike infectious agent
VLIS Virtual Laboratory Information System
VLM ventrolateral medulla; visceral larva migrans
VLO vastus lateralis obliquus
VLP vincristine, L-asparaginase, and prednisone; viruslike particle
VLp viruslike particle
VLPA ventrolateral pressure area
VLR vinleurosine
VLS vascular leak syndrome; visible light spectroscopy
VLSI very-large-scale integration
VLTF vaccinia late transcription factor
VM Valsalva maneuver; vasomotor; ventilator management; ventralis medialus; ventricular mass; ventriculomegaly; ventriculometry; ventromedial; vestibular membrane; video microscopy; viomycin; viral myocarditis; voltmeter
V/m volts per meter
V$_m$ membrane potential; maximum velocity; muscle volume
VMA vanillylmandelic acid; vastus medialis advancement; ventilator management advisor; vitreomacular adhesion
VMAC Vasodilatation in the Management of Acute Congestive Heart Failure [trial]
VMAP, Vmap velocity mapping
VMAT vesicular monoamine transformer
Vmax maximum velocity
V$_{max}$ maximum volume
VMC vasomotor center
VMCG vector magnetocardiogram
VMCHN Victorian Maternal and Child Health Nurses

VMD Doctor of Veterinary Medicine; virtual medical device; vitelliform macular dystrophy
VMDS virtual medical device system
vMDV virulent Marek disease virus
VME Volunteers for Medical Engineering
VMF vasomotor flushing
VMGT Visual Motor Gestalt Test
VMH ventromedial hypothalamus
VMI, VMIT visual-motor integration test
VML vector markup language; ventriculomegaly
VMLS virtual medical library system
VMN ventromedial nucleus
VMO vastus medialis obliquus; visiting medical officer
VMP virtual machine platform
VMR vasomotor rhinitis
VMRS Vermont Medical Record System
VMS virtual medical school; virtual memory system; visual memory span
VMST visual motor sequencing test
VMT vasomotor tonus; ventilatory muscle training; ventromedial tegmentum
V$_m$(t) time-averaged membrane potential
V$_m$(x,t) absolute transmembrane potential
VN vesical neck; vestibular nucleus; virus neutralization; visceral nucleus; visiting nurse; vitronectin; vocational nurse; vomeronasal
VNA Visiting Nurse Association
VNAA Visiting Nurse Associations of America
VNDPT visual numerical discrimination pretest
VNO vomeronasal organ
VNQ variable N-Quoit filter [imaging]
VNR vitronectin receptor
VNRA vitronectin receptor alpha
VNS vagal nerve stimulation; virtual notebook system; visiting nursing service
VNTR variable number of tandem repeats; variable copy number tandem repeats
VO verbal order; volume overload; voluntary opening
Vo standard volume; vascular volume
V$_O$ rest volume
VO$_2$, V$_{O2}$ volume of oxygen utilization
VOC vasoocclusive crisis; volatile organic compound
VOCC voltage-operated calcium channel
VOD venoocclusive disease; video on demand
VOI value of information; volume of interest
VO$_2$I volume of oxygen utilization index
VoIP voice over Internet protocol

vol volar; volatile; volume; voluntary, volunteer
VOM volt-ohm-milliammeter
VO₂ Max, V̇O₂max maximum volume of oxygen utilization
VON Victorian Order of Nurses
v-onc viral oncogene
VOO ventricular asynchronous [pacemaker]
vOOMM visual object-oriented matrix model
VOP vasoocclusive pain; venous occlusion plethysmography
VOPS vector optimal parameter search [algorithm]
VOR vestibuloocular reflex; volume of regret
VORd vestibuloocular reflex in darkness
VORe vestibuloocular reflex enhancement
VORs vestibuloocular reflex suppression
VOS videothoracoscopic operator staging; vision, left eye [L. *visio, oculus sinister*]
VOT voice onset time
VOTE Value of Transesophageal Echocardiography [study]
VP physiologic volume; vapor pressure; Varadi-Papp [orofaciodigital syndrome]; variegate porphyria; vascular permeability; vasopressin; velopharyngeal; venipuncture; venous pressure; ventricular pacing; ventricular pericardium; ventricular premature [beat]; ventroposterior; VePesid; verbal paraphrasia; vertex potential; vestibular papillae; vincristine and prednisone; virion protein; visual presentation; Voges-Proskauer [medium, test]; voiding pressure; volume-pressure; vulnerable period
V/P ventilation/perfusion ratio
V&P vagotomy and pyloroplasty
Vp paced ventricular output; peak velocity; peak voltage; phenotype variance; plasma volume; ventricular premature [beat]
vp vapor pressure
VPA valproic acid
VPAP variable positive airway pressure
VPB ventricular premature beat
VPC vapor-phase chromatography; ventricular premature complex; ventricular premature contraction; volume-packed cells; volume percent
VPCT ventricular premature contraction threshold
VPD vaccine-preventable disease; ventricular premature depolarization
VPF vascular permeability factor
VPFRU vapor-protective, flame-resistant undergarment
VPG velopharyngeal gap

VPg genome-linked protein
VPGSS venous pressure gradient support stockings
VPI vapor phase inhibitor; velopharyngeal insufficiency
VPL ventroposterolateral; vertical partial laryngectomy
VPM ventilator pressure manometer; ventroposteromedial
vpm vibrations per minute
VPN ventral pontine nucleus; virtual private network
VPO velopharyngeal opening; vertical pendular oscillation
VPP Vaccine Provision Project; vacuolar proton pump; viral porcine pneumonia
VPR vascular permeability reaction; ventricular paced rhythm; virtual patient record; Voges-Proskauer reaction; volume/pressure ratio
VPRBC volume of packed red blood cells
VPRC volume of packed red cells
VPRS variable precision rough set [model]
VPS Vasovagal Pacemaker Study; ventriculoperitoneal shunt; verbal pain scale; virtual point source; visual pleural space; volume performance standard
vps vibrations per second
VPT vibratory perception threshold
VQ vector quantization
V̇/Q̇ ventilation/perfusion ratio
VQE visa qualifying examination
VQI ventilation-perfusion index
V-QRS QRS ventricular potential
2VR double valve replacement
VR right arm [electrode]; Valsalva ratio; valve replacement; valvular regurgitation; vanilloid receptor; variable rate; variable ratio; variable region; vascular resistance; vasopressin receptor; venous flow reversal; venous reflux; venous resistance; venous return; ventilation rate; ventilation ratio; ventral root; ventricular rale; ventricular response; ventricular rhythm; vesicular rosette; virtual reality; vision, right [eye]; vital records; vocal resonance; vocational rehabilitation; volume ratio; volume regulation; volume rendering
Vr relaxation volume
V2R vasopressin 2 receptor [*AVPR* gene]
VRA visual reinforcement audiometry
VRBC red blood cell volume
VRC Vaccine Research Center; venous renin concentration
VRCP vitreoretinochoroidopathy
VRD vascular reconstruction device; ventricular radial dysplasia; viral reference division

VRE vancomycin-resistant *Enterococcus*
VR&E vocational rehabilitation and education
VREF vancomycin-resistant *Enterococcus faecium*
V$_{rest}$ resting potential
VRI viral respiratory infection; virtual reality imaging
VRL lumbar ventral root; vanilloid receptor-like [protein]; Virus Reference Laboratory
VRML Virtual Reality Modeling Language
VRNA viral ribonucleic acid
VRNI neovascular inflammatory vitreoretinopathy
VROM voluntary range of motion
VRP ventral root potential; ventricular refractory period
VRPV vaccine-related poliovirus
VRR ventral root reflex
VRS verbal rating scale; Virchow-Robin space
VRSA vancomycin-resistant *Staphylococcus aureus*
VRT vehicle rescue technician; virtual reality therapy; volume ray tracing; volume-rendering technique
VRV ventricular residual volume; viper retrovirus; Virgin River virus
VRX variable resolution x-ray
VS vaccination scar; vaccine serotype; vagal stimulation; vascular surgeon; vasospasm; venesection; ventricular septum; verapamil shock; verification/recording system; vesicular stomatitis; veterinary surgeon; vibration syndrome; virtual simulator; visual storage; vital sign; Vogt-Spielmeyer [disease]; volatile solid; volume support; volumetric solution; voluntary sterilization
Vs stressed volume; venesection
V·s vibration second; volt-second
V$_s$ system tissue volume
V × s volts by seconds
vs see above [L. *vide supra*]; single vibration; versus; vibration seconds; vital signs
VSA variant-specific surface antigen
VSAT very small aperture terminal
VSAV vesicular stomatitis Alagoas virus
VSBE very short, below elbow [cast]
VSC visual sequence comparison; voluntary surgical contraception
VSCC volume-sensitive chloride channel
VSCT ventral spinocerebellar cell tract
VSD ventricular septal defect; vesicular stomatitis virus; virtually safe dose
VSFP venous stop flow pressure
VSG variant surface glycoprotein; Vesnarinone Study Group

VSHD ventricular septal heart defect
VSIE volume surface integral equation
VSINC Virus Subcommittee of the International Nomenclature Committee
VSIV vesicular stomatitis Indiana virus
VSM vascular smooth muscle
VSMC vascular smooth muscle cell
VSMS Vineland Social Maturity Scale
vsn vision
VSNJV vesicular stomatitis New Jersey virus
VSO vertical supranuclear ophthalmoplegia
VSOK vital signs normal
VSP variable spine plating; very short patch [DNA repair]
VSR venous stasis retinopathy; visceral/subcutaneous [adipose tissue] ratio
VSRA variable speech rate audiometry
VSS vital signs stable
V$_{ss}$ volume at steady state
VST ventral spinothalamic tract; video see-through; volume-selective excitation
VSTA Virus-Serum-Toxin Act
v-STM vaginal specimen transport medium
VSV vesicular stomatitis virus
VSV-G G protein of gibbon ape leukemia virus
VSW ventricular stroke work
VT tetrazolium violet; tidal volume; total ventilation; vacuum tube; vacuum tuberculin; vasotonin; velocity of tension; venous thrombosis; ventricular tachyarrhythmia; ventricular tachycardia; verocytotoxin; verotoxin; vibration threshold; vitronectin
V$_T$ tidal volume; T-lymphocyte antigen receptor variable region; total ventilation
+VT maximum velocity of tension
−VT decline in velocity of tension
V&T volume and tension
V̇$_T$ tidal volume
Vt total vascular volume; volume of tissue
VTA ventral tegmental area
VTach, Vtach, V tach ventricular tachycardia
VTB virtual tracheobronchoscopy
VTE venous thromboembolism; ventricular tachycardia event
VTEC verotoxin-producing *Escherichia coli*
VTEU Vaccine and Treatment Evaluation Unit
VTG volume thoracic gas
VTI velocity-time integral; volume thickness index
VTK visualization tool kit
VTL ventricular tracking limit
VTM mechanical tidal volume; viral transport media; virus transport medium

VT-MASS Metoprolol and Sotalol for Sustained Ventricular Tachycardia [study]
VTN Vaccine Trials Network; vitronectin
VTNPA Vermont Nurse Practitioners Association
VTOP vaginal termination of pregnancy
VTR variable tandem repeats; vesicular transport system; videotape recording; vitronectin receptor
VTSRS Verdun Target Symptom Rating Scale
V$_{T\ T}$ tidal volume
VT/VF ventricular tachycardia/ventricular fibrillation
VTVM vacuum tube voltmeter
VTX verocytotoxin; vertex
vtx vertex
VU varicose ulcer; volume unit
vu volume unit
VUC voided urinary cytology
VUD voluntary unrelated donor
VUJ vesicoureteral junction
VUO vesicoureteral orifice
VUR vesicoureteral reflux
V-US volumetric ultrasonography
VUSE variable angle uniform signal excitation
VUV vacuum ultraviolet
2VV double valve replacement
VV vaccinia virus; variable volume; varicose veins; venous volume; venovenous; vertical vein; viper venom; vulva and vagina
V&V verification and validation
V-V venovenous [bypass]
vv varicose veins; veins
v/v percent volume in volume
VVAS vertical visual analog scale
VVC vulvovaginal candidiasis
VVD vaginal vertex delivery
VVDL venovenous double-lumen [catheter]
VVFR vesicovaginal fistula repair

VVGF vaccinia virus growth factor
VVI ventricular inhibited [pacemaker]; vocal velocity index
VVI/R ventricular demand, rate-responsive [pacemaker]
v$_{vk}$ ventricular volume constant
VVLBW very very low birth weight
vvMDV very virulent Marek disease virus
VVol venous volume
VVS vesicovaginal space; vestibulo-vegetative syndrome; vulvar vestibulitis syndrome
VVT ventricular triggered [pacemaker]
VW Van der Woude [syndrome]; vascular wall; vessel wall; Volterra-Wiener [approach]; von Willebrand [disease, factor]
v/w volume per weight
vWAg von Willebrand antigen
VWD ventral wall defect
vWD von Willebrand disease
VWDFAg, vWDFAg von Willebrand disease factor antigen
VWF velocity waveform; vibration-induced white finger; von Willebrand factor; von Willebrand Factor Database
vWF, vWf von Willebrand factor
VWM ventricular wall motion; verbal working memory
VWS Van der Woude syndrome
vWS viewing work station; von Willebrand syndrome
VX no evidence of venous [tumor] invasion; virus X
Vx vertex
VYS visceral yolk sac
VZ varicella-zoster
V$_z$ volume of distribution in the terminal phase
VZIG, VZIg varicella zoster immunoglobulin
VZV varicella-zoster virus

W dominant spotting [mouse]; energy; section modulus; series of small triangular incisions in plastic surgery [w-plasty]; tryptophan; tungsten [Ger. *Wolfram*]; wakefulness; ward; water; watt; Weber [test]; week; wehnelt; weight; white; widowed; width; wife; Wilcoxon rank sum statistic; Wistar [rat]; with; word fluency; work; wound

W3 World Wide Web

W+ weakly positive

w velocity (m/s); water; watt; while; with

WA when awake; white adult; Wiskott-Aldrich [syndrome]

W/A watt/ampere

W&A weakness and atrophy

WAAT Warfarin Plus Aspirin vs. Aspirin Trial

WAB Western Aphasia Battery

WACS Women's Atherosclerosis Cardiovascular Study

WAF weakness, atrophy, and fasciculation; white adult female

WAFUS Warfarin Anticoagulation Follow-up Study

WAGR Wilms tumor, aniridia, genitourinary abnormalities, and mental retardation (intellectual disability)

WAI Web Accessibility Initiative

WAIS Wechsler Adult Intelligence Scale; Western Angiographic and Interventional Society; wide area information server; Workplace Advocacy Information System

WAIS-R revised Wechsler Adult Intelligence Scale

WAK wearable artificial kidney

WALK Walking with Angina-Learning Is the Key [program]

WALV Wallal virus

WAM white adult male; work area model; worksheet for ambulatory medicine

WAN wide area network

WANV Wanowrie virus

WAP wandering atrial pacemaker; whey acid protein

WAR Wasserman antigen reaction; without additional reagents

WARCRY Wegener and Related Diseases Compassionate Regimen Yield [study]

WARF warfarin; Wisconsin Alumni Research Foundation

WARIS Warfarin Reinfarction Study

WARIS II Warfarin-Aspirin Reinfarction Study—Norwegian

WARSS Warfarin-Aspirin Recurrent Stroke Study

WARV Warrego virus

WAS weekly activities summary; Wiskott-Aldrich syndrome

WASH Warfarin-Aspirin Study of Heart Failure

WASID Warfarin-Aspirin Symptomatic Intracranial Disease [study]

WASP Weber Advanced Spatial Perception [test]; Wiskott-Aldrich syndrome protein

Wass Wasserman [reaction]

WAST Woman Abuse Screening Tool

WAT word association test

WATCH Warfarin Antiplatelet Trial in Chronic Heart Failure; Worcester-area Trial for Counseling in Hyperlipidemia

WATSMART Waterloo Spatial Motion Analysis and Recording Technique

WAVE Women's Angiographic Vitamin and Estrogen [trial]

WAXS wide-angle x-ray scattering

WB waist belt; washable base; washed bladder; water bottle; Wechsler-Bellevue [scale]; weight-bearing; well baby; Western blot; wet bulb; whole blood; whole body; Willowbrook [virus]; Wilson-Blair [agar]

Wb weber; well-being

WBA wax bean agglutinin; Western blot assay; whole-body activity

Wb/A webers/ampere

WBAPTT whole-blood activated partial thromboplastin time

WBAT weight bearing as tolerated

WBC well-baby care; well-baby clinic; white blood cell; white blood cell count; whole blood cell count

WBCT whole-blood clotting time

WBDC whole-body digital scanner

WBE whole-body extract

WBF whole-blood folate

WBGT wet bulb global temperature

WBH whole-blood hematocrit; whole-body hyperthermia

WBI Web-based instruction; whole bowel irrigation

WBLT Watson-Barker Listening Test

Wb/m² weber per square meter

WBMP wireless bitmap

WBN whole-blood nitrogen

WBPTT whole-blood partial thromboplastin time

WBR whole-body radiation

WBRT whole-blood recalcification time; whole-breast radiation therapy

WBS Wechsler-Bellevue Scale; whole-blood serum; whole-body scan; whole-body scintiscan; Wiedemann-Beckwith syndrome; Williams-Beuren syndrome; withdrawal body shakes

WBT wet bulb temperature

WBUS whole-breast ultrasound

WBV waterborne virus; whole-blood volume; whole-body vibration; whole-brain volume

WC waist circumference; ward clerk; warty carcinoma; water closet; Weber-Christian [syndrome]; wheelchair; white cell; white cell casts; white cell count; white child; whooping cough; wild caught; work capacity; workers' compensation; writer's cramp

WC? whole complement

W/C watch carefully; wheelchair

W3C World Wide Web Consortium

wc wheelchair

WCB working cell bank

WCC Walker carcinosarcoma cells; white cell count; windowed cross correlation; wound-care certified

WCD Weber-Christian disease

WCE white coat effect; whole-cell extract; wireless capsule endoscopy; work capacity evaluation

WCGS Western Collaborative Group Study

WCL Wenckebach cycle length; whole-cell lysate

w/cm² watts per square centimeter

WCP well-characterized product

WCPs whole-chromosome paints

WCS white clot syndrome; Wisconsin Card Sort [test]; worst-case scenario

WCST Wisconsin Card-Sorting Test

WCT wide complex tachycardia; word categorization test

WCTU Women's Christian Temperance Union

WCUS Wiktor Stent and Cutting Balloon Angioplasty Study

WD wallerian degeneration; well developed; well differentiated; wet dressing; Whitney Damon [dextrose]; Wilson disease; Winger distribution; with disease; withdraw, withdrawn; without dyskinesia; Wolman disease; wrist disarticulation

W/D warm and dry

Wd ward

wd well developed; wound, wounded

WDCC well-developed collateral circulation

WDG water-dispersible granule

WDHA watery diarrhea, hypokalemia, achlorhydria [syndrome]

WDHH watery diarrhea, hypokalemia, and hypochlorhydria [syndrome]

WDI warfarin dose index; World Drug Index

WDL well-differentiated lymphocytic

WDLL well-differentiated lymphatic lymphoma

WDMF wall-defective microbial forms

WDR wide dynamic range

WDS watery diarrhea syndrome; wet dog shakes [veterinary medicine]

WDSCC well-differentiated squamous cell carcinoma

WDTC well-differentiated thyroid cancer

WDWN, wdwn well developed and well nourished

WE wax ester; Wernicke encephalopathy; western encephalitis; western encephalomyelitis; wound of entry

We weber

WEB Women's Experience with Battering [scale]

WEDI Workgroup for Electronic Data Interchange

WEE western equine encephalitis/encephalomyelitis

WEEV western equine encephalitis virus

WEL wave equivalent length

WELL-HART Women's Estrogen/Progestin and Lipid-Lowering Hormone Atherosclerosis Regression Trial

WELV Weldona virus

W3-EMRS World Wide Web Electronic Medical Records System

WENR Workgroup of European Nurse Researchers

WEP wired equivalent privacy

WER wheal erythema reaction

WES wall echo shadow; wall echo sign; work environment scale; wound evaluation scale

WESDR Wisconsin Epidemiologic Study of Diabetic Retinopathy

WESH West European Study of Health

WESSV Wesselsbron virus

WEST Western European Stent Trial; Women's Estrogen for Stroke Trial

WEXV Wexford virus

WF Weil-Felix reaction; white female; Wistar-Furth [rat]; workflow

W/F, wf white female

WFA weight for age

WFC workflow cycle

WFD word-finding difficulty

WFDB waveform database

WFE Williams flexion exercise

WFG wavefront-guided

WFI water for injection

WFL within function limits

WFLC weighted-frequency Fourier linear combiner [algorithm]

WfMS workflow management system

WFOT World Federation of Occupational Therapists

WFPHA World Federation of Public Health Associations

WFR Weil-Felix reaction; wheal-and-flare reaction

WFRT wide-field radiation therapy

WFS Waterhouse-Friderichsen syndrome; World Fertility Survey

WFSL workflow specification language

WFT windowed Fourier transform

WG water gauge; Wegener granulomatosis; Wright-Giemsa [stain]

WGA wheat germ agglutinin

WGE wheat germ extract

WGO World Gastroenterology Organization

WG-RH whole-genome radiation hybrid task

WGRV Wongorr virus

WGS whole-genome shotgun

wgt weight

WH well hydrated; Werdnig-Hoffmann [syndrome]; whole homogenate; wound healing

Wh watt/hours; white

wh wheeled walker; white

w·h watt-hour

WHA warm and humid air; World Health Assembly

WHAP Women's Health Australia Project

WHAS Women's Health and Aging Study; Women's Heart Attack Study

WHAT Worcester Heart Attack Trial

WHAV Whataroa virus

wh ch wheelchair; white child

WHCOA White House Conference on Aging

WHCR Wolf-Hirschhorn chromosome region

WHD Werdnig-Hoffmann disease

WHEASE What Happens Eventually to Asthmatics Sociologically and Epidemiologically? [study]

WHHHIMP Wernicke encephalopathy/withdrawal, hypertensive encephalopathy, hypoglycemia, hypoxemia, intracranial bleeding/infection, meningitis/encephalitis, poison/medication

WHHL Watanabe heritable hyperlipidemia; Watanabe heritable hyperlipidemic [rabbit]

WHI Women's Health Initiative

WHIMS Women's Health Initiative Memory Study

WHML Wellcome Historical Medical Library

WHNP Women's Health Nurse Practitioner

WHO World Health Organization; wrist-hand orthosis

WHO/ISH World Health Organization/International Society of Hypertension

whp whirlpool

WHR waist/hip ratio

whr watt-hour

WHS Werdnig-Hoffmann syndrome; Wolf-Hirschhorn syndrome; Women's Health Study

WHT Walsh-Hadamard transform; Warm Heart Trial

WHTVS Women's Health Trial Vanguard Study

WHV woodchuck hepatic virus

WHVP wedge hepatic venous pressure

WHYMPI West Haven−Yale Multidimensional Pain Inventory

WI human embryonic lung cell line; walk in; water ingestion; weaning index; Wistar [rat]

WIA wounded in action

WIBC Wiggins Interpersonal Behavior Circle

WIC walk-in clinic; women, infants, and children; Women, Infants, and Children [program]

WICHEN Western Interstate Commission for Higher Education in Nursing

WIHS Women's Interagency HIV Study

WIL workflow intermediate language

WIMP windows, icons, menus, pointing

WIN Wallstent in Native Vessel [study]; Weight Control Information Network; Western Institute of Nursing

WINS Wallstent in Saphenous Vein Grafts [study]

WIPI Word Intelligibility by Picture Identification

WIS Wechsler Intelligence Scale

WISC Wechsler Intelligence Scale for Children

WISCR Wisconsin clinical record

WISC-R Wechsler Intelligence Scale for Children-Revised

WISE Women's Ischemic Syndrome Evaluation [study]

WISER Wireless Information System for Emergency Responders

WISH wearable information system for human health care

WISHIN Wisconsin Statewide Health Information Network

WISP-2 Wnt-1−induced signaling protein 2

WIST Whitaker Index of Schizophrenic Thinking

WIT warm ischemia time

WITS Women and Infants Transmission Study

WITT Wittenborn [Psychiatric Rating Scale]

WITV Witwatersrand virus

W-J Woodcock-Johnson [Psycho-Educational Battery]

WJG Wilders-Jongsma-van Ginneken [model]

WK week; Wernicke-Korsakoff [syndrome]; Wilson-Kimmelstiel [syndrome]; Windkessel [model]

wk weak; week; work

WKD Wilson-Kimmelstiel disease

W/kg watts per kilogram

WKS Wernicke-Korsakoff syndrome

WKY Wistar-Kyoto [rat]

WL waiting list; warning letter; waterload; wavelength; weighted least squares; weight loss; window level [imaging]; withdrawal; wire localization; Wood's lamp; working level [exposure]; workload

wl wavelength

WLAN wireless local area network

WLE white-light endoscopy; wide local excision

WLF whole lymphocytic fraction

WLI weight-length index

WLM white-light microscopy; working level month [exposure]

WLS weighted least square; wet lung syndrome

WLT whole lung tomography

WM Waldenström macroglobulinemia; wall motion; ward manager; warm and moist; Wernicke-Mann [hemiplegia]; wet mount; white male; white matter; whole milk; Wilson-Mikity [syndrome]; working memory

W-M Weill-Marchesani [syndrome]

W/M white male

wm white male; whole milk; whole mount

w/m² watts per square meter

WMA wall motion abnormality; wall motion analysis; World Medical Association

WMBT weighted moving beam therapy

WMC weight-matched control

WMD weapon of mass destruction; weighted mean difference

WME Williams' medium E

WMF wavelet multiresolution filter

WMH white matter hyperintensities

WML white matter lesion; wireless markup language

WMO ward medical officer

WMP weight-management program

WMR work metabolic rate; World Medical Relief

WMS wall motion scoring; Wechsler Memory Scale; Weill-Marchesani syndrome; Williams syndrome; workflow management system

WMS-R Wechsler Memory Scale−Revised

WMV Wad Medani virus

WMX whirlpool, massage, exercise

WN, wn well nourished

WNE West Nile encephalitis

WNF well-nourished female

WNL within normal limits

WNM well-nourished male

WNN wavelet neural network

WNPW wide, notched P wave

WNSA weighted negative surface area

WNV West Nile virus

WO wash out; will order; written order

W/O water in oil [emulsion]

wo weeks old

w/o without

WOB work of breathing

WOB$_I$ imposed work of breathing

WOB$_P$ physiologic work of breathing

WOB$_T$ total work of breathing

WOB$_V$ work of breathing performed by ventilator

WOCN wound, ostomy, continence nurse

WOCNS Wound, Ostomy and Continence Nurses Society

WOE wound of entry

WOLF Work, Lipids, Fibrinogen [study]

WOMAC Western Ontario and McMaster University Osteoarthritis Index

WONCA World Organization of Family Doctors

WONV Wongal virus

WOOFS Warfarin Optimized Outpatient Follow-up Study

WooV Woot virus

WOP without pain; whole-organ pancreas [transplantation]

WOPN walled-off pancreatic necrosis

WORC Western Ontario Rotator Cuff Index

WORM write once read many times

WOSCOPS West of Scotland Coronary Prevention Study

WOSI Western Ontario Shoulder Instability Score

WOU women's outpatient unit

WOWS weak opiate withdrawal scale

WOX wound of exit

WP wavelet packet; weakly positive; weak-plate; wedge pressure; wet pack; wettable powder; whirlpool; white phosphorus; white pulp; word processor; working point

W/P water/powder ratio

wp wettable powder

WPAI Work Productivity and Activity Impairment [Questionnaire]

WP-ANAT weak plate with anatomic information

WPB whirlpool bath

WPCU weighted patient care unit

WPDL workflow process definition language

Wpf wave at a pilot frequency

WPFM Wright peak flowmeter

WPk Ward's pack; wet pack

WPPSI Wechsler Preschool and Primary Scale of Intelligence

WPR written progress report

WPRS Wittenborn Psychiatric Rating Scale

WPS wasting pig syndrome

WPV wild poliovirus

WPW Wolff-Parkinson-White [syndrome]

WQAC ward quality assurance committee

W-QLI Wisconsin quality-of-life index

WR Wassermann reaction; water retention; weakly reactive; weak response; whole response; Wiedemann-Rautenstrauch [syndrome]; wiping reaction; work rate

W$_R$ radiation weighting factor

Wr wrist; writhe

WRA weight-related amenorrhea

WRAC wide-ranging aerosol classifier

WRAML Wide Range Assessment of Memory and Learning

WRAT Wide Range Achievement Test

WRBC washed red blood cell

WRC washed red cell; water retention coefficient

WRE wahole ragweed extract

WR HA-NP Western Reserve hemagglutinin and nucleoprotein [replication-competent vaccinia virus]

WRISS Weapons Related Injury Surveillance System

WRIST Washington Radiation for In-Stent Restenosis Trial

WRK Woodward reagent K

WRMD work-related musculoskeletal disorder

WRMT Woodcock Reading Mastery Tests

WRN Werner [syndrome]

WRS Ward-Romano syndrome; war research service; Wiedemann-Rautenstrauch syndrome

WRSI Work-related Strain Inventory

WRSS weighted residual sum of squares

WRVP wedge renal vein pressure

WS Waardenburg syndrome; Wallenberg syndrome; ward secretary; Warkany syndrome; warning stimulus; Warthin-Starry [stain]; water soluble; water swallow; watt-second; Wellens syndrome; Werner syndrome; West syndrome; Whickham striae;

Wiener spectrum [x-ray]; Wilder silver [stain]; Williams syndrome; Wolfram syndrome; word sense; work station

W&S wound and skin

W·s watt-second

ws water-soluble

WSA water-soluble antibiotic

WSACS World Society of the Abdominal Compartment Syndrome

WSB wheat-soy blend

WSC water-soluble contrast [medium]

WSD word sense disambiguation

WSDRN Western Satellite Data Relay System

w-sec watt-second

WSI Waardenburg syndrome type I; whole-slide imaging

WSL Wesselsbron [virus]

WSM women who have sex with men

WSP withdrawal seizure prone

WSPHU Western Sector Public Health Unit [Australia]

WSQ wavelet scalar quantization

WSR Westergren sedimentation rate; withdrawal seizure resistant

W/sr watts per steradian

WSS Weaver-Smith syndrome; wrinkly skin syndrome

WSW women who have sex with women

WT wall thickness; water temperature; wavelet transform; wild type; Wilms tumor; wisdom teeth; work therapy

wt weight; white; wild type

WT1 Wilms tumor gene 1

WTA Wound Treatment Associate

wtAAV wild-type adeno-associated virus

wtAd wild-type adenovirus

WTCC wavelet transform cross correlation

WTE whole time equivalent

WTF weight transferral frequency

WTH Women Take Heart [project]

WTO World Trade Organization

WTP willingness to pay

wtPSGL wild type P selectin glycoprotein ligand

WTR waist/thigh [circumference] ratio

WTS Wilson-Turner syndrome

WTV wound tumor virus

WTW white-to-white [diameter]

W/U workup

WUT wake-up test

WV walking ventilation; weighting vector; Wrath virus

W/V, w/v percent weight in volume, weight/volume

W^v variable dominant spotting [mouse]

WVD wavelet-vaguelette decomposition; Winger-Ville distribution

WVTR water vapor transmission rate

WW Weight Watchers; wet weight; whisker weaving; window width [imaging]

W/W, w/w percent weight; weight-to-weight ratio

WWAV Whitewater Arroyo virus

WWBV Weddel waterborne virus

WWICT Western Washington Intracoronary Streptokinase Trial

WWIST Western Washington Intravenous Streptokinase Trial

WWM world wide microscope

W/wo with or without

WWS Walker-Warburg syndrome; Wieacker-Wolff syndrome; Working Well Study

WWSIMIT Western Washington Streptokinase in Myocardial Infarction Trials

WWU weighted working unit

WWW World Wide Web

WX wound of exit

WxB wax bite

WxP wax pattern

WY women-years

WYOV Wyeomyia virus

WYSIWYG what you see is what you get

WZα wide-zone alpha

WZS Weissenbacher-Zweymuller syndrome

X androgenic; cross; crossbite; exophoria distance; exposure; extra; female sex chromosome; ionization exposure; ionization exposure rate; Kienböck's unit of x-ray exposure; magnification; multiplication symbol; reactance; removal of; respirations; Roman numeral ten; start of anesthesia; "times"; translocation between two X chromosomes; transverse; unknown quantity; xanthosine; X unit; xylene

Ξ uppercase Greek letter xi

ξ lowercase Greek letter xi

X̄ sample mean

X², χ² chi-square

X3 orientation as to time, place, and person

x except; extremity; horizontal axis of a rectangular coordinate system; mole fraction; multiplication symbol; position; roentgen [rays]; sample mean; "times"; unknown factor; xanthine

XA xanthurenic acid; x-ray analysis

X-A xylene and alcohol

Xa activated factor X; chiasma

Xaa unknown amino acid

XAD External Atrial Defibrillation [trial]

Xam examination

Xan xanthine

Xanth xanthomatosis

Xao xanthosine

XBP xanthophyll-binding protein; X-box binding protein

XBSN X-linked bulbospinal neuropathy

XC, Xc excretory cystogram

XCCL exaggerated craniocaudal lateral [view]

XCE X-chromosome controlling element

X-CGD X-linked chronic granulomatous disease

Xcv *Xanthomonas campestris vesicatoria*

XD x-ray diffraction

XDH xanthine dehydrogenase

XDP xanthine diphosphate; xeroderma pigmentosum

XDR extensively drug-resistant; transducer

XDR-TB extensively drug-resistant tuberculosis

Xe electric susceptibility; xenon

XECT, XeCT xenon-enhanced computed tomography

XEF excess ejection fraction

XES x-ray energy spectrometry

Xfb cross-linked Gibrin

XFD x-ray flat detector

XGP xanthogranulomatous pyelonephritis

XGPT xylosylprotein-4-beta-galactosyltransferase

Xi inactive X chromosome

XIAP X-linked inhibitor of apoptosis

XIBV Xiburema virus

XIC X chromosome inactivation center; X-inactivation center

X-IEP crossed immunoelectrophoresis

XINV Xingu virus

XIP exchanger inhibitory peptide; x-ray-induced polypeptide; x-ray in plaster

XISHF Xamoterol in Severe Heart Failure [study]

XIST inactive X-chromosome specific transcript; X-inactivation specific transcript

XL excess lactate; X-linked; xylose-lysine

XLA, X-LA X-linked agammaglobulinemia

XLAS X-linked aqueductal stenosis

XLCM X-linked dilated cardiomyopathy

XLD X-linked dominant; xylose-lysine-deoxycholate

XLH X-linked hydrocephalus; X-linked hypophosphatemia

XLHED X-linked hypohidrotic ectodermal dysplasia

XLI X-linked ichthyosis

XLIF extreme lateral interbody fusion

XLMR X-linked mental retardation (intellectual disability)

XLMTM, XLMTm X-linked myotubular myopathy

XLOS X-linked Opitz syndrome

XLP X-linked lymphoproliferative [syndrome]

XLPD X-linked lymphoproliferative disease

XLR X-linked recessive

XLRP X-linked retinitis pigmentosa

XLS X-linked recessive lymphoproliferative syndrome

XLSP X-linked spastic paraplegia

XM crossmatch

XM, Xm maternal chromosome X

xma chiasma

X-mas Christmas [factor]

x-mat crossmatch

X-match crossmatch

XME xenobiotic-metabolizing enzyme

XML extensible markup language

XMMR *Xenopus* molecular marker resource

XMP xanthine monophosphate

XMR X-linked mental retardation (intellectual disability)

XMRV xenotropic murine leukemia virus—related virus

XN night blindness
XO presence of only one sex chromosome; xanthine oxidase
XOAD X-linked ocular albinism with deafness
XOM extraocular movements
XOP x-ray out of plaster
XOR exclusive operating room
XP xanthogranulomatous pyelonephritis; xeroderma pigmentosum
XP, Xp paternal chromosome X; short arm of chromosome X
XPA xeroderma pigmentosum group A
XPC xeroderma pigmentosum group C
XPN xanthogranulomatous pyelonephritis
XPS x-ray photoelectron spectroscopy; x-ray photoemission spectroscopy
XPTB extrapulmonary tuberculosis
Xq long arm of chromosome X
XR extended release; xeroradiography; X-linked recessive; x-ray
x-rays roentgen rays
XRD x-ray diffraction
XRE xenobiotic response element
XRF x-ray fluorescence
XRFDC x-ray film digitization console
XRII x-ray image intensifier
XRMR X-linked recessive mental retardation (intellectual disability)
XRN X-linked recessive nephrolithiasis
XRS x-ray sensitivity
XRT x-ray therapy
XS cross-section; excessive; xiphisternum
X/S cross-section
xs excess
XSA cross-section area

XSCID X-linked severe combined immunodeficiency [syndrome]
XSCLH X-linked subcortical laminar heterotopia
X-sect cross-section
XSP xanthoma striatum palmare
XT exotropia
Xt extra toe
Xta chiasmata
Xtab cross-tabulating
XTE xeroderma, talipes, and enamel defect [syndrome]
XTM xanthoma tuberosum multiplex
XTP xanthosine triphosphate
X-TUL external tumescent ultrasound liposculpture
XU excretory urogram; X unit
Xu X-unit
X$_u$ cumulative amount of urine
Xu5P, Xu5p xylulose-5-phosphate
XUC extended use case [format]
XuMP xylulose monophosphate
XX chromosome X disomy; double strength; female chromosome type
46,XX 46 chromosomes, 2 X chromosomes (normal female)
XXL xylocaine
XXX chromosome X trisomy
XXXX chromosome X tetrasomy
XXXXX chromosome X pentasomy
XX/XY sex karyotypes
XY male chromosome type
46,XY 46 chromosomes, one X and one Y chromosome (normal male)
Xyl xylose

Y coordinate axis in a plane; electrical admittance; male sex chromosome; mean of y values; tyrosine; year; yellow; *Yersinia;* yield; yttrium

Y- yotta- [10^{24}]

Y see *upsilon*

υ see *upsilon*

y vertical axis of a rectangular coordinate system

y- yocto- [10^{-24}]

YA *Yersinia* arthritis

Y/A years of age

YAC yeast artificial chromosome

YACP young adult chronic patient

YACV Yacaaba virus

YADH yeast alcohol dehydrogenase

YAG yttrium-aluminum-garnet [laser]

YAOV Yaounde virus

YATAV Yata virus

Yb ytterbium

YBOCS Yale-Brown Obsessive Compulsive Scale

YBV Yug Bogdanovac virus

YCB yeast carbon base

YCMI Yale Center for Medical Informatics

YCT YMCA Cardiac Therapy

YCVDS Yugoslavia Cardiovascular Disease Study

yd yard

YDV yeast-derived hepatitis B vaccine

YDYES yin deficiency yang excess syndrome

YE yeast extract; yellow enzyme

YEH$_2$ reduced yellow enzyme

YEI *Yersinia enterocolitica* infection

Yel yellow

YEL-AND yellow fever vaccine—associated neurotropic disease

YEL-AVD yellow fever vaccine—associated viscerotrophic disease

YF yellow fever

YFI yellow fever immunization

YFMD yellow fever membrane disease

YFV yellow fever virus

YHV Yaquina Head virus

YKV yokapoxvirus

YLC youngest living child

YLD years lived with disability

YLF yttrium lithium fluoride

YLL years of life lost

YLS years of life saved

YM yeast and mannitol; yeast and mold; Young's modulus

Y$_{max}$ maximum yield

YMB yeast malt broth

YMRS Young Mania Rating Scale

YMS Young Men's Survey

YMTV Yaba monkey tumor virus

YNB yeast nitrogen base

YNS yellow nail syndrome

YO years old

y/o years old

YOB year of birth

Y$_{obs}$ observed value

YOGV Yogue virus

YOKV Yokose virus

Yops *Yersinia* outer membrane proteins

YOS Yale Observation Scale

YP yeast phase; yield pressure

YPA yeast, peptone, and adenine sulfate

YPAS Yale Preoperative Anxiety Score

YpkA *Yersinia* protein kinase A

YPLL years of potential life lost

yr year

YRBS Youth Risk Behavior Survey

YRD Yangtze River disease

YRRM Y ribonucleic acid recognition motif

YS yellow spot; yield strength; yolk sac

ys yellow spot; yolk sac

YSHR younger spontaneously hypertensive rat

YST yolk sac tumor

Y73SV Y73 sarcoma virus

YT, yt yttrium

YTs yoga therapists

Y-TZP yttria-stabilized tetragonal zirconia polycrystalline

Y1V Yaba-1 virus

Y7V Yaba-7 virus

yWACC younger woman with aggressive cervical cancer

YWKY younger Wistar-Kyoto rat

Z

Z acoustic impedance; atomic number; complex impedance; contraction [Ger. *Zuckung*]; glutamine; impedance; ionic charge number; no effect; point formed by a line perpendicular to the nasion-menton line through the anterior nasal spine; proton number; section modulus; standardized deviate; standard normal score; standard score; zero; zone; a Z-shaped incision in plastic surgery

Z uppercase Greek letter zeta

ζ lowercase Greek letter zeta

Z- zetta- [10^{21}]

Z?, Z?? increasing degrees of contraction

z algebraic unknown or space coordinate; axis of a three-dimensional rectangular coordinate system; catalytic amount; standard normal deviate; zero

z- zepto- [10^{-21}]

ZAG, ZA2G zinc-alpha-2-glycoprotein

ZAM Zhao-Atlas-Marks [distribution]

ZAMSTAR Zambia, South Africa Tuberculosis and AIDS Reduction [program]

ZAP zeta-associated protein [rabbit]; zymosan-activated plasma

ZAPF zinc adequate pair-fed

ZAPS zonal air pollution system

ZAS zymosan-activated autologous serum

ZB zebra body

ZBG zinc-binding group

ZCA zone of cortical abnormality

ZCAP zinc-calcium−phosphorous oxide

ZCP zinc chloride poisoning

ZD zero defects; zero discharge; zinc deficiency

Z-D Zamorano-Duchovny [digitizer]

ZDDP zinc dialkyldithiophosphate

Z-DNA zig-zag (left-handed helical) deoxyribonucleic acid

ZDO zero differential overlap

ZDS zinc depletion syndrome

ZDV zidovudine

ZE Zollinger-Ellison [syndrome]

ZEBOV Zaire Ebola virus

ZEBRA zero balanced reimbursement account

ZEC Zinsser-Engman-Cole [syndrome]

ZEEP zero end-expiratory pressure

ZEGV Zegla virus

ZEPI zonal echo planar imaging

Z-ERS zeta erythrocyte sedimentation rate

ZES Zollinger-Ellison syndrome; Zutphen Elderly Study

ZEST Zocor Early Start Trial

ZF zero frequency; zinc finger [protein]; zona fasciculata

ZFA *N*-benzyloxcarbonyl Phe-Ala omefluoromethylketone

ZFF zinc fume fever

ZFP zinc finger protein

ZFX X-linked zinc finger protein

Zfy zinc finger [protein]

ZG zona glomerulosa

ZGM zinc glycinate marker

ZIAR zona-induced acrosome reaction

ZIFT zygote intrafallopian tube transfer

ZIG, ZIg zoster immunoglobulin

ZIKV Zika virus

ZIP zoster immune plasma

ZIRV Zirqa virus

zJ zeptojoule

ZK Zuelzer-Kaplan [syndrome]

ZLS Zimmerman-Laband syndrome

Zm zygomaxillare

ZMA zinc meta-arsenite

ZMC zygomaticomaxillary complex

ZN Ziehl-Neelsen [staining]

ZNF zinc finger [protein]

ZnOE zinc oxide and eugenol

ZnPP/H zinc protoporphyrin/heme ratio

ZNS zonisamide

ZO Zichen-Oppenheim [syndrome]; *Zonula occludens*; Zuelzer-Ogden [syndrome]

Zo impedance; thoracic fluid

ZOA zinc orthoarsenate

ZOE zinc oxide−eugenol

ZOL zoladex

ZOMC zygomatico-orbito-maxillary complex

Zool zoology

ZOT *Zonula occludens* toxin

ZP zona pellucida

ZPA zone of polarizing activity

ZPC zero point of change

ZPG zero population growth

ZPO zinc peroxide

ZPP zinc protoporphyrin

ZPS, Zps zwitterionic polysaccharides

ZPT zinc pyridinethione

ZR zona reticularis

Zr zirconium

ZRK zona receptor kinase

ZS Zellweger syndrome; Zutphen Study

ZSC zone of slow conduction

ZSR zeta sedimentation ratio

ZSV signature-tagged mutagenesis; zonate spot virus

ZT Zwolle Trial

ZTS zymosan-treated serum

Z-TSP zephiran-trisodium phosphate
ZTT zinc turbidity test
ZTV Zaliv Terpeniya virus
ZVAD *N*-benzyloxcarbonyl Val-Ala-Asp omefluoromethylketone
ZVD zidovudine
ZVT cell-binding test [Ger. *Zehlenverbindungstest*]
ZW Zellweger [syndrome]
ZWCHRS Zellweger cerebrohepatorenal syndrome

ZWOLLE Primary Coronary Angioplasty Compared with Intravenous Streptokinase [trial]
ZWS Zellweger syndrome
ZXF zero crossing frequency
Zy zygion
ZyC zymosan complement
zyg zygotene
Zz ginger [L. *zingibar*]